Clinician's Guide to Laboratory Medicine

A Practical Approach

3rd Edition

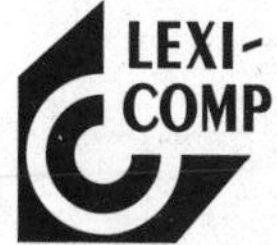

TABLE OF CONTENTS

PART III: ENDOCRINOLOGY

PART IV: PULMONARY

PART V: NEUROLOGY

PART VI: NEPHROLOGY

PART VII: GASTROENTEROLOGY

PART VIII: RHEUMATOLOGY

PART IX: INFECTIOUS DISEASE

PART X: CARDIOLOGY

PART XI: OBSTETRICS & GYNECOLOGY

ALGORITHMS

PART I: HEMATOLOGY

PART II: FLUIDS, ELECTROLYTES, AND ACID-BASE

PART III: ENDOCRINOLOGY

PART IV: PULMONARY

PART VI: NEPHROLOGY

PART VII: GASTROENTEROLOGY

PART X: CARDIOLOGY

ABOUT THE AUTHOR

Samir P. Desai, MD

Dr. Samir Desai serves on the faculty of the Baylor College of Medicine in the Department of Medicine. Dr. Desai has educated and mentored both medical students and residents, work for which he has received teaching awards.

Dr. Desai is the author of the popular *101 Biggest Mistakes 3rd Year Medical Students Make And How to Avoid Them,* a book that has helped students reach their full potential during the third year of medical school. In the book, *The Residency Match: 101 Biggest Mistakes And How To Avoid Them,* Dr. Desai shows applicants how to avoid commonly made mistakes during the residency application process. In the *Internal Medicine Clerkship: 150 Biggest Mistakes And How To Avoid Them,* students can not only learn about the errors their predecessors made but also avoid these pitfalls, which is crucial for success during this very important rotation.

Dr. Desai conceived and authored the "Clinician's Guide Series," a series of books dedicated to providing clinicians with practical approaches to commonly encountered problems. *The Clinician's Guide to Laboratory Medicine* and *Clinician's Guide to Diagnosis* have become popular books for healthcare professionals, providing a step-by-step approach to laboratory test interpretation and symptom evaluation, respectively. The *Clinician's Guide to Internal Medicine* offers quick access to key information that is needed in the care of patients with a wide variety of medical problems.

Dr. Desai is also the founder of www.md2b.net, a website committed to helping today's medical student become tomorrow's doctor. Founded in 2002, www.md2b.net is dedicated to providing medical students with the tools needed to tackle the challenges of the clinical years of medical school.

After completing his residency training in Internal Medicine at Northwestern University in Chicago, Illinois, Dr. Desai had the opportunity of serving as chief medical resident. He received his MD degree from the Wayne State University School of Medicine in Detroit, Michigan, graduating first in his class.

PREFACE

In 2000, Lexi-Comp, Inc published the first edition of the Clinician's Guide to Laboratory Medicine: A Practical Approach. The goal of the book was to provide healthcare professionals with a practical guide to laboratory test interpretation. In the four years that have passed, we have appreciated the feedback you have shared with us regarding our efforts. In hearing and reading your thoughts, it has become clear to us that the book's goals have been realized. Many of you have praised the step-by-step approach to laboratory test interpretation. In particular, you have valued the emphasis that we have placed on the interpretation of lab tests in the context of the patient's clinical presentation.

There are many laboratory test books that offer clinicians a long list of causes for an abnormal lab test. Some stop right there, offering no guidance on how to determine the etiology of the abnormality. Others focus exclusively on the lab test, without any consideration of the patient's clinical presentation. Our goal is to provide you with so much more than just a differential diagnosis for an abnormal lab test. Our goal is to walk you from abnormal lab test to diagnosis through a series of logical steps, without ever losing track of the patient's clinical situation. It is precisely this exercise that the accomplished clinician performs when confirming or excluding a possible diagnosis.

In this third edition, we have updated the entire text without altering the practical approaches that readers feel is one of the major strengths of this book. Nearly 40 new chapters have been added, including a new section on obstetrics/gynecology and expanded sections covering laboratory testing in infectious disease, neurology, and nephrology. Because so many of you have found the boxes, tables, and algorithms useful, we have added many more, again to help you utilize the information that is presented quickly.

In the nearly 4 years that have passed since the publication of the first edition, the book has been warmly received by medical students and residents, many of whom have informed us that the book has provided them with the tools necessary to tackle even the most challenging laboratory data. Other healthcare professionals, including established physicians, nurse practitioners, nurses, and physician assistants have also found the book very useful. It is our hope that the third edition of this book will continue to offer you, the clinician, the practical approaches that are not readily available in standard textbooks, guidance to help make informed diagnoses, and readily accessible information at the point of care.

Samir Desai, MD

ACKNOWLEDGMENTS

The development of this book required the concerted efforts of so many people. Robert D. Kerscher, president of Lexi-Comp, Inc, has always given this book his full support. This effort would not have been possible without the time, energy, attention to detail, and drive of Lynn Coppinger, managing editor. Matt Kerscher, product manager, deserves special thanks for his efforts to raise awareness of this book's existence among health care professionals. Many thanks are also extended to Tracey Reinecke for her assistance with the cover design, Jeanne Wilson for her work and design of the web page product, and David C. Marcus for his expertise in indexing. I also appreciate the efforts of so many other individuals at Lexi-Comp, both in production and marketing.

I would also like to thank the faculty at the Northwestern University School of Medicine. It was while I was a resident there in the Department of Medicine that the idea for this book came to mind. Without the guidance and encouragement of so many people, it is unlikely that this book would have ever come to fruition. I am particularly grateful to Drs. Lewis Landsberg, Dale Gerding, Robert Rosa, Warren Wallace, David Neely, Robert Hirschtick, and Vinky Chadha for creating an atmosphere of intellectual curiosity that allowed me to grow professionally.

As a faculty member at the Baylor College of Medicine, I am blessed with the opportunity to work with some outstanding colleagues including Drs. Jeffrey Bates, Richard Hamill, Daniel Musher, Biykem Bozkurt, and Douglas Mann. Although not directly involved in the development of this book, it has been a pleasure to work with all of them on a regular basis. I have appreciated their encouragement and advice.

It would be remiss of me not to express my appreciation to the students, interns, and residents at the Baylor College of Medicine. This is an outstanding group of future and young doctors, who continue to be an inspiration for me. It is a pleasure for me to have the opportunity to work with them.

Samir Desai, MD

HOW TO USE THIS HANDBOOK

The *Clinician's Guide to Laboratory Medicine: A Practical Approach* is divided into 11 parts, each of which addresses an organ system. Within each part are a number of chapters, each dealing with a different laboratory test abnormality or suspected clinical disorder. When appropriate, the chapter is written in a step-by-step approach that guides the reader from the laboratory test abnormality to a diagnosis.

Each step begins with a question. The reader is encouraged to answer the question based upon the information gathered from the patient's clinical presentation. An example from the chapter entitled "Hematuria" follows.

STEP 1 – What Is Hematuria?

Hematuria is defined as the presence of blood in the urine. It may either be gross or microscopic. When it is gross, it understandably causes considerable anxiety in both patients and clinicians alike. In particular, there is concern that the hematuria may be caused by a serious condition (ie, malignancy). It is important to realize, however, that the causes of gross and microscopic hematuria are the same. Therefore, a thorough evaluation is necessary regardless of whether the patient presents with gross or microscopic hematuria.

If the patient complains of gross hematuria, **proceed to Step 2**.

If the patient has microscopic hematuria, **proceed to Step 3**.

As shown in the example above, the body of the step contains the information that is necessary to answer the question as it relates to the patient at hand. At the end of each step is a decision point. The next step in the evaluation will differ depending upon which decision point is chosen. In the example given above, the reader who has a patient with gross hematuria will travel to Step 2. The reader who has a patient with microscopic hematuria, however, will skip Step 2 (thus bypassing information that is relevant to patients with gross hematuria) and travel to Step 3.

The steps in these chapters are designed to guide the reader from laboratory test abnormality to diagnosis. By proceeding through these steps, the long list of causes of a particular laboratory test abnormality will be quickly narrowed until the correct diagnosis is ultimately established. As laboratory test abnormalities must always be interpreted with the patient's clinical presentation in mind, this information is integrated into the decision-making process at each step.

In some of the chapters not written in a step-by-step format, the Socratic question and answer format is used. In other chapters, information is separated by headings. Both formats allow the information to be separated into blocks that the reader can actively process.

This book contains over 50 algorithms. The algorithms serve to help the reader quickly organize a strategy for approaching the particular laboratory test abnormality. Each algorithm closely parallels the information in its respective chapter. Also at the end of each chapter is a list of references that can be referred to for further information.

PART I:

HEMATOLOGY

Mean Corpuscular Hemoglobin (MCH)

The MCH refers to the weight of hemoglobin in the average red blood cell. The reference range for MCH is 26-34 pg. In general, increases or decreases in the MCH parallel changes in the MCV.

Mean Corpuscular Hemoglobin Concentration (MCHC)

The MCHC is a measure of the amount of hemoglobin present in the average red blood cell when compared to its size. In men, the reference range for MCHC is 31-37 g/dL. In women, the reference range is 30-36 g/dL. Fifty percent of patients with hereditary spherocytosis have a MCHC >36 g/dL.

Red Cell Distribution Width (RDW)

Normally, most red blood cells are about equal in size. In many types of anemia, however, there is variability in red blood cell size, also known as anisocytosis. The red blood cell distribution width or RDW is a measure of this variability. This difference in size between cells is reflected in the RDW. Any process that leads to a wide variation in cell size will manifest with an increased RDW. It is important to note that an increased RDW may precede an abnormality in hemoglobin or MCV. Anemia may be classified based on red blood cell size and distribution width, as shown in the following table.

Classification of Anemia Based on Red Blood Cell Size and Distribution Width

Cell Size	Normal RDW	High RDW
Microcytosis	Thalassemia minor Anemia of chronic disease Some hemoglobinopathy traits	Iron deficiency Hemoglobin H disease Some anemia of chronic disease Some thalassemia minor Fragmentation hemolysis
Normocytosis	Anemia of chronic disease Hereditary spherocytosis Some hemoglobinopathy traits Acute bleeding	Early or partially treated iron or vitamin deficiency Sickle cell anemia
Macrocytosis	Aplastic anemia Some myelodysplasias	Vitamin B_{12} deficiency Folate deficiency Autoimmune hemolytic anemia Cold agglutinin disease Some myelodysplasias Liver disease Thyroid disease Alcohol

Adapted from Kjeldsberg C, *Practical Diagnosis of Hematologic Disorders*, 3rd ed, Chicago, IL: ASCP Press, 2001, 10.

Peripheral Blood Smear

The peripheral blood smear should be examined when the CBC reveals abnormal blood counts. In these cases, the smear will often reveal morphologic abnormalities that are not detectable by automated cell counters. This information is often the key to elucidating the etiology of the abnormal CBC.

No evaluation of anemia is complete without inspection of the peripheral blood smear, which may reveal clues to the etiology of the anemia. The quality of the information gleaned from the peripheral blood smear is dependent upon how well prepared the peripheral blood smear is. In addition, systematic examination of the smear is necessary so important findings are not missed.

It is important to search for the best area on the peripheral blood smear. The best area is usually the thinner part of the smear, where red blood cells are not overlapping one another. Examination of this area will provide the clinician with the opportunity to describe abnormalities in red cell size, shape, or number. Anisocytosis refers to variations in cell size, whereas poikilocytosis indicates variation in cell shape. Many laboratories grade anisocytosis and poikilocytosis on a 0-4+ scale, but it is important to realize that no standardization of this scoring method exists. It is not sufficient to merely take note of anisocytosis or poikilocytosis on the peripheral blood smear; rather, the clinician should strive to describe the abnormalities present.

MORE DEFINITIONS...

Anisocytosis: Variation of cell size
Poikilocytosis: Variation of cell shape

The following table lists some important abnormalities of cell shape and conditions associated with these changes.

Abnormalities of RBC Shape

Cell Shape	Synonym	Features	Associated Conditions
Spherocyte	—	Smaller than normal RBC, no central pallor	Autoimmune hemolysis Hereditary spherocytosis Hemoglobinopathies Artifact
Tear drop cells	Dacrocyte	Single spicule with blunt end	Myeloid metaplasia with myelofibrosis Myelophthisic process Thalassemia Pernicious anemia
Target cell	Codocyte	Target-like	Chronic liver disease Thalassemia Hemoglobin C, S, or D disease Iron deficiency Splenectomy
Macroovalocyte	—	Large oval-shaped cell	Megaloblastic anemia
Stomatocyte	—	Slit-like central pallor	Hereditary stomatocytosis Alcoholic cirrhosis
Schistocyte	—	Fragmented cell with two or more points	MAHA* (DIC, TTP) Heart valve hemolysis Severe burns
Echinocyte	Burr cell	Short evenly-spaced spicules	Kidney disease Heart disease Untreated hypothyroidism Artifact Bleeding ulcers Gastric carcinoma
Acanthocyte	Spur cell	Irregularly spaced spicules of varying lengths	Liver disease Abetalipoproteinemia Hypothyroidism Vitamin E deficiency Splenectomy
Sickle cell	Drepanocyte	Sickle shape, pointed at both ends	Sickle cell anemia Other hemoglobinopathies
Rouleau formation†	—	Stack of coins appearance	Multiple myeloma Chronic liver disease Hypergammaglobulinemia Artifact

*MAHA = microangiopathic hemolytic anemia.

†True Rouleau formation is characterized by this appearance along with the presence of free red blood cells. The presence of Rouleau formation suggests that an abnormal serum protein may be present (eg, multiple myeloma). It is important not to examine the thick part of the smear as stacking can be appreciated here even in the normal patient. This, however, is not true Rouleau formation but an artifact of preparation.

Besides anisocytosis and poikilocytosis, the clinician should look for immature red blood cells. Normally, the peripheral blood smear is free of immature red blood cells except for reticulocytes and the occasional nucleated red blood cell. Larger numbers of nucleated red blood cells may be seen in conditions associated with extreme demand on the bone marrow, extramedullary hematopoiesis, or marrow replacement.

MORE DEFINITIONS...
Reticulocytes: Red blood cells that are slightly larger than normal red blood cells and appear polychromatic **Polychromasia**: Grayish-blue color of the cytoplasm in reticulocytes (secondary to ribosomes)

Erythrocytic inclusions may also be appreciated on review of the peripheral blood smear. Some erythrocytic inclusions and their associated conditions are listed in the following table.

Erythrocytic Inclusions

Erythrocytic Inclusion	Associated Conditions
Howell-Jolly body	Splenectomy Hemolytic anemia Megaloblastic anemia
Basophilic stippling	Lead poisoning Thalassemia Hemolytic anemias Megaloblastic anemia Alcoholism Arsenic intoxication
Cabot's ring	Megaloblastic anemia Thalassemia Splenectomy Hemolytic anemias
Pappenheimer body	Sickle cell anemia Thalassemia Splenectomy Megaloblastic anemias Sideroblastic anemia
Heinz body	Splenectomy Hemoglobinopathies Hemolytic anemia (G6PD deficiency)

Examination of the peripheral blood smear also provides information about white blood cells and platelets. Peripheral blood smear findings pertaining to white blood cells and platelets will be discussed in the other chapters of this book.

Reticulocyte Count

It is essential to determine the reticulocyte count in the evaluation of the anemic patient. Recall that the mature red blood cell is not nucleated, because it is extruded during the maturation of red blood cells at the normoblast phase. Reticulocytes are produced with extrusion of the nucleus. Reticulocytes are young red blood cells that contain residual RNA, explaining their tendency to stain with certain dyes, such as methylene blue. They are reported as a percent of circulating red blood cells. The reticulocyte count reflects the ability of the bone marrow to produce mature red blood cells. In the absence of anemia, a normal reticulocyte count varies from 1% to 2%. In an anemic patient, an increase in the reticulocyte count provides evidence that the bone marrow is adequately responding to the anemia. When the bone marrow is significantly stimulated, nucleated red blood cells may be seen as well on the peripheral blood smear. It is important to note that if nucleated red blood cells are observed, they are usually few in number and are often further along in maturation. This is in contrast to disease states, characterized by the invasion of bone marrow, in which nucleated red blood cells may be found in increased numbers and with less maturity.

When anemia develops, the bone marrow should respond with an increase in the reticulocyte count in an effort to maintain the hemoglobin level. The absence of an increase in the reticulocyte count reflects an inability of the bone marrow to compensate for the anemia. The laboratory will report the reticulocyte count as a percentage of the total RBC count. To interpret the reticulocyte count, several corrections must be made. The first correction involves adjusting the reticulocyte count for the degree of anemia as shown below:

$$\textbf{Reticulocyte } \%_{\textbf{corrected}} = \text{reticulocyte } \%_{\text{reported}} \times (\text{patient's Hct}) / 45$$

Another factor the clinician should be aware of is that an anemic patient may release reticulocytes prematurely into the blood. Under normal circumstances, reticulocytes circulate in the blood for only 1 day before becoming mature RBCs. If, however, reticulocytes are released early from the bone marrow, they may circulate in the blood for 2-3 days. This is usually seen in the setting of severe anemia that results in marked bone marrow stimulation. As reticulocytes should only be present in the peripheral blood for one day, in cases where they are circulating for more than one day, a correction factor accounting for this needs to be used. Using the correction factor and the corrected reticulocyte percentage (see equation above), the reticulocyte production index (RPI) can be calculated as follows:

$$\textbf{RPI} = \text{reticulocyte } \%_{\text{corrected}} / \text{ correction factor}$$

Appropriate hematocrit correction factors are listed in the following table.

Patient's Hct (%)	Correction Factor
40-45	1.0
35-39	1.5
25-34	2.0
15-24	2.5
<15	3.0

An RPI value <2 indicates inadequate bone marrow response, whereas an RPI >2 suggests that bone marrow response is appropriate for the degree of anemia.

Because reticulocytes are slightly larger than normal red blood cells, it is not uncommon for the MCV to be elevated with a reticulocytosis.

Another important point to recognize is that reticulocytosis may take between 48-96 hours to manifest, following conditions that cause bone marrow stimulation. There are really only three situations where reticulocytosis is appreciated and these are listed in the following box.

RETICULOCYTOSIS DIFFERENTIAL DIAGNOSIS
ACUTE BLOOD LOSS
HEMOLYTIC ANEMIA
RESPONSE TO IRON, FOLATE, OR B_{12} REPLACEMENT

References

Bessman JD, Gilmer PR Jr, and Gardener FH, "Improved Classification of Anemias by MCV and RDW," *Am J Clin Pathol*, 1983, 80(3):322-6.

Flynn MM, Reppun TS, and Bhagavan NV, "Limitations of Red Cell Distribution Width (RDW) in Evaluation of Microcytosis," *Am J Clin Pathol*, 1986, 85(4):445-9.

Gulati GL and Hyun BH, "The Automated CBC: A Current Perspective," *Hematol Oncol Clin North Am*, 1994, 8(4):593-603.

Kaye FJ and Alter BP, "Red-Cell Size Distribution Analysis: An Evaluation of Microcytic Anemia in Chronically Ill Patients," *Mt Sinai J Med*, 1985, 52(5):319-23.

Snower DP and Weil SC, "Changing Etiology of Macrocytosis: Zidovudine as a Frequent Causative Factor,"*Am J Clin Pathol*, 1993, 99(1):57-60.

APPROACH TO THE PATIENT WITH ANEMIA

STEP 1 – *Does the Patient Have Anemia?*

Anemia is defined as a hemoglobin or hematocrit below the lower limit of normal. The reference range for hemoglobin and hematocrit includes 95% of the normal population. Five percent of the normal population falls outside the reference range, with 2.5% having hemoglobin and hematocrit levels below the lower limit of normal. This means that 2.5% of normal, healthy individuals will be considered to be anemic when, in fact, they are not. These individuals should be considered, however, to have anemia until proven otherwise and deserve a careful evaluation. Anemia should always be considered a symptom or sign of an underlying disease. As such, it is never appropriate to ignore this important finding. When the presence of anemia is discovered, it is incumbent upon the clinician to determine the etiology.

Proceed to Step 2.

STEP 2 – *What Is the Reticulocyte Production Index (RPI)?*

Although there are many ways to approach the patient with anemia, most clinicians begin with a measurement of the reticulocyte count. When anemia develops, the bone marrow should respond with an increase in the reticulocyte count in an effort to maintain the hemoglobin level. The absence of an increase in the reticulocyte count reflects an inability of the bone marrow to compensate for the anemia. In these cases, the anemia is caused by a bone marrow underproduction process.

The laboratory will report the reticulocyte count as a percentage of the circulating red blood cells (typically 0.5% to 1.5%). To interpret the reticulocyte count appropriately, several corrections must be made to the reticulocyte count reported by the laboratory. The first correction involves adjusting the reticulocyte count for the degree of anemia, as shown in the following box.

Reticulocyte $\%_{corrected}$ = reticulocyte $\%_{reported}$ x (patient's Hct) / 45

This calculation will yield the corrected reticulocyte count. To calculate the reticulocyte production index (RPI) from the corrected reticulocyte count, another correction must be made, as shown in the following box.

RPI = reticulocyte $\%_{corrected}$ / correction factor

Patient's Hct (%)	Correction Factor
40-45	1.0
35-39	1.5
25-34	2.0
15-24	2.5
<15	3.0

An RPI value <2 is indicative of inadequate bone marrow response while a level >2 suggests that the bone marrow is responding appropriately for the degree of anemia. By calculating the RPI, the clinician can narrow the differential diagnosis of anemia.

If the RPI is >2, ***proceed to Step 17*** *on page 51.*

If the RPI is <2, ***proceed to Step 3***.

STEP 3 – *What Is the MCV?*

When the RPI is <2, the differential diagnosis can be narrowed even further by consideration of the mean corpuscular volume (MCV). The MCV can be used to categorize patients into one of the following groups.

- Microcytic anemia (MCV <80 fL)
- Normocytic anemia (MCV between 80 and 96 fL)
- Macrocytic anemia (MCV >96 fL)

If the patient has microcytic anemia, ***proceed to Step 4***.

If the patient has normocytic anemia, ***proceed to Step 9*** *on page 32.*

If the patient has macrocytic anemia, ***proceed to Step 10*** *on page 41.*

STEP 4 – *What Is the Approach to the Patient With Microcytic Anemia and RPI <2?*

The causes of microcytic anemia and RPI <2 are listed in the following box.

CAUSES OF MICROCYTIC ANEMIA AND RPI <2	
IRON DEFICIENCY ANEMIA	HEMOGLOBINOPATHIES (Hgb Lepore trait, E trait, etc)
ANEMIA OF CHRONIC DISEASE	SIDEROBLASTIC ANEMIA
α-THALASSEMIA	
β-THALASSEMIA	

The evaluation of microcytic anemia begins with a thorough history and physical examination along with appropriate laboratory testing. Laboratory testing plays a key role in elucidating the etiology of the microcytic anemia. Laboratory tests that should be considered in the evaluation of microcytic anemia are listed in the following box.

RECOMMENDED LABORATORY TESTING TO ELUCIDATE ETIOLOGY OF MICROCYTIC ANEMIA

ESSENTIAL

DEGREE OF MICROCYTOSIS
IRON STUDIES
- Serum iron
- Total iron binding capacity (TIBC)
- Serum ferritin

RED CELL DISTRIBUTION WIDTH (RDW)
PERIPHERAL BLOOD SMEAR

MAY BE INDICATED

HEMOGLOBIN ELECTROPHORESIS
FREE ERYTHROCYTE PROTOPORPHYRIN
BONE MARROW BIOPSY
SERUM SOLUBLE TRANSFERRIN RECEPTOR
DNA TESTING FOR GLOBIN CHAIN SYNTHESIS

The essential tests listed above are described in further detail in the remainder of this step.

Degree of Microcytosis

Even before other laboratory studies are obtained, the degree of microcytosis may provide clues to the etiology. An MCV <70 fL is unlikely to be due to the anemia of chronic disease. This degree of microcytosis should prompt the clinician to consider other etiologies of microcytic anemia such as iron deficiency anemia and thalassemia minor. It is important to realize, however, that an MCV between 70 and 80 fL may be due to any of the causes of microcytic anemia.

Iron Studies

It is essential to obtain iron studies (serum iron, TIBC, ferritin) in every patient with microcytic anemia. The results of the iron studies are often useful in elucidating the etiology, as shown in the following table.

Using Iron Studies to Elucidate the Etiology of Microcytic, Hypochromic Anemia

	Serum Iron*	TIBC†	TS‡	Ferritin#	Serum Soluble Transferrin Receptor
Iron deficiency anemia	Decreased	Increased	Decreased	Decreased	High
Anemia of chronic disease	Decreased	Decreased	Decreased	Normal or increased	Normal
Thalassemia	Normal	Normal	Normal	Normal	Variable, may be high
Sideroblastic anemia	Increased	Normal	Increased	Increased	Variable, may be high

TS = transferrin saturation; TIBC = total iron binding capacity

*Serum iron levels should be obtained in the morning since there is diurnal variability in iron levels, with the highest values occurring in the morning. It is preferable to obtain the level before a meal since even one meal containing a large amount of iron can normalize the serum iron level. Levels may be normal or high in iron deficiency anemia patients if the blood specimen is obtained after the patient has received iron therapy. It is best to hold oral iron therapy for at least 24 hours prior to testing. Low serum iron levels are also a hallmark of the anemia of chronic disease, which is why this test alone cannot be used to make the distinction between these two causes of microcytic anemia.

†The total iron binding capacity is usually increased in iron deficiency anemia. In contrast, anemia of chronic disease is associated with decreased total iron binding capacity. If both iron deficiency anemia and anemia of chronic disease are present together, however, the total iron binding capacity may not be elevated. The clinician should realize that pregnancy and oral contraceptive use can also increase the TIBC.

‡Transferrin saturation is calculated by dividing the serum iron by the serum TIBC. The quantity obtained should then be multiplied by 100. Normal transferrin saturation ranges between 25% and 45%. While both anemia of chronic disease and iron deficiency anemia are associated with decreased transferrin saturation, levels <16% are more suggestive of iron deficiency anemia. Even when 16% is used as a cutoff, however, there remain some patients with anemia of chronic disease who present with transferrin saturation less than 16%.

#Serum ferritin levels <10 ng/mL are virtually diagnostic for iron deficiency anemia (sensitivity = 59%, specificity = 99%). Levels between 10 and 20 ng/mL are very suggestive of the diagnosis. It is important to realize, however, that ferritin is an acute phase reactant. Therefore, if inflammation and iron deficiency are present together, the ferritin level may be in the normal range. Levels >150-200 ng/mL argue against the diagnosis of iron deficiency anemia. In pregnant women, the serum ferritin is the best test to assess for iron deficiency. Using 30 ng/mL as the cutoff, the sensitivity and specificity are 90% and 85%, respectively. The transferrin saturation is not as useful because pregnancy is associated with an increase in the TIBC.

Red Cell Distribution Width (RDW)

The red cell distribution width, which is a measure of variability in red blood cell size, is also helpful in determining the etiology of the microcytic anemia, as shown in the following table.

Using the RDW to Elucidate the Etiology of Microcytic Anemia

Red Cell Distribution Width (RDW)	Etiology of Microcytic Anemia Suggested
Normal	Thalassemia minor; anemia of chronic disease
High	Iron deficiency anemia; anemia of chronic disease (some cases); thalassemia minor (some cases)

Peripheral Blood Smear

A review of the peripheral blood smear may provide clues to the etiology, as shown in the following table.

Using the Peripheral Blood Smear to Elucidate the Etiology of Microcytic Anemia

Cause of Microcytic Anemia	Peripheral Blood Smear Findings
Iron deficiency anemia	Anisocytosis Poikilocytosis Microcytic, hypochromic red blood cells Elliptocytes Pencil cells Platelet count normal, increased, or decreased
Anemia of chronic disease	Microcytic, hypochromic red blood cells
Thalassemia minor	Microcytic, hypochromic red blood cells Target cells Basophilic stippling
Sideroblastic anemia	Anisocytosis Poikilocytosis Microcytic, hypochromic red blood cells Dimorphic population ± dysplastic features in WBCs

Bone Marrow Biopsy

Even with the use of iron studies, red cell distribution width, and peripheral blood smear, the clinician may encounter difficult cases, in which the etiology of the microcytic anemia is not clear. In these cases, bone marrow biopsy may be very revealing. In iron deficiency anemia, Prussian blue staining of the bone marrow specimen will reveal the absence of iron stores. In other causes of microcytic anemia, bone marrow iron is present. Bone marrow biopsy is also needed to establish the diagnosis of sideroblastic anemia. In this condition, the hallmark finding is the presence of increased numbers of ringed sideroblasts. Although bone marrow evaluation is useful for establishing the diagnosis, the clinician should realize that results may be misleading in certain situations (after blood transfusion or treatment with parenteral iron).

If the patient has iron deficiency anemia, ***proceed to Step 5.***

If the patient has thalassemia minor, ***proceed to Step 7.***

If the patient has sideroblastic anemia, ***proceed to Step 8.***

If the patient has anemia of chronic disease, ***proceed to discussion*** *on page 26.*

STEP 5 – *Does the Patient Have Iron Deficiency Anemia?*

Iron deficiency anemia is the major cause of microcytic anemia. Because some of the causes of iron deficiency anemia are serious conditions (ie, malignancy), it behooves the clinician to be comfortable differentiating iron deficiency anemia from other causes of microcytic anemia.

History

In some cases, the history may be quite revealing. Although not always present, risk factors for iron deficiency anemia, such as frank or occult gastrointestinal bleeding, may be elicited. A minority of patients may present with food cravings for dirt, starch, ice, or clay (pica).

Physical Examination

Although the physical examination may be normal, in some cases, characteristic skin and nail changes may be appreciated. Skin atrophy and koilonychia (spoon-shaped nails) are findings that should prompt consideration of iron deficiency anemia. Other examination findings include angular stomatitis (painful cracks at angle of mouth) and glossitis.

Laboratory Testing

In most cases, the diagnosis rests upon the results of the iron studies. These as well as other laboratory test abnormalities seen in iron deficiency anemia are listed in the following box.

LABORATORY TEST FINDINGS IN IRON DEFICIENCY ANEMIA

- LOW SERUM IRON
- LOW SERUM FERRITIN*
- HIGH TOTAL IRON BINDING CAPACITY
- LOW TRANSFERRIN SATURATION (<15%)†
- HIGH SERUM SOLUBLE TRANSFERRIN RECEPTOR
- HIGH FREE ERYTHROCYTE PROTOPORPHYRIN LEVELS
- ELEVATED RDW (earliest finding)
- DECREASED RETICULOCYTE COUNT / RPI
- PERIPHERAL BLOOD SMEAR
  - Microcytic, hypochromic red blood cells‡
  - Anisocytosis (earliest recognizable morphologic change)
  - Poikilocytosis
  - Elliptocytes
  - Pencil cells
- THROMBOCYTOPENIA / THROMBOCYTOSIS (platelet count can be normal)
- BONE MARROW WITH ABSENT IRON STORES

*Because serum ferritin is an acute phase reactant, ferritin levels may rise to normal levels in iron deficient patients who have concomitant inflammation. In general, serum ferritin levels <10 ng/mL are indicative of iron deficiency anemia while levels between 10 and 20 ng/mL are strongly suggestive of the diagnosis. Levels >150-200 ng/mL strongly argue against the diagnosis. Levels between 20 and 150-200 ng/mL may be seen in iron deficiency anemia as well as other causes of microcytic anemia.

†Transferrin saturation is calculated by dividing the serum iron by the total iron binding capacity. The quantity obtained should then be multiplied by 100. This percentage is known as the transferrin saturation.

‡Early iron deficiency anemia is characterized by normocytic, normochromic red blood cells.

D...erentiating Iron Deficiency Anemia From Anemia of Chronic Disease

The two most common causes of microcytic anemia are iron deficiency anemia and anemia of chronic disease. Therefore, the clinician must be familiar with the laboratory test features used to differentiate between these two conditions.

Iron Deficiency Anemia vs Anemia of Chronic Disease

	Iron Deficiency Anemia	Anemia of Chronic Disease
RDW	High	Normal
Serum iron	Decreased	Decreased
TIBC	Increased	Decreased
Ferritin	Normal / decreased	Normal / increased
Transferrin saturation	Decreased but usually <16%	Decreased but usually >16%
Serum soluble transferrin receptor	High	Normal
Bone marrow (Prussian blue stain)	(-)	(+)

Some advocate a therapeutic trial of iron recognizing that in patients with anemia of chronic disease, iron replacement is not likely to be helpful. It must be recognized, however, that the two disorders can coexist and concomitant treatment of both, or the spontaneous resolution of chronic disease while on iron replacement therapy may lead to a confusing picture. Although there are some who are not advocates of the therapeutic trial of iron, many others favor it, maintaining that it is a cost-effective and definitive way of establishing the diagnosis, particularly in cases where iron studies are inconclusive. When administering a therapeutic trail, oral iron therapy should result in reticulocytosis, with the peak response occurring after 1-2 weeks. With continued therapy, hemoglobin levels should normalize within 2-4 months.

If reticulocytosis is not noted, other causes of microcytic anemia should be considered. Before considering other causes of microcytic anemia, it is worthwhile to exclude noncompliance with iron supplementation, administration of an ineffective iron preparation, concomitant antacid use (increased gastric pH may interfere with iron absorption), presence of a malabsorption syndrome, or ongoing blood loss that prevents the body from responding to the iron replacement.

Differentiating Iron Deficiency Anemia From Thalassemia Minor

At times, it can be quite challenging to differentiate iron deficiency anemia from thalassemia minor. The following table highlights the differences between these two causes of microcytic anemia.

Iron Deficiency Anemia vs Thalassemia Minor

	Iron Deficiency Anemia	Thalassemia Minor
Ethnicity	No ethnic predilection	African American / Asian / Mediterranean descent
MCV*	↓	↓↓
RBC count	<5 x 10^6/mm^3	>5 x 10^6/mm^3
Mentzer index†	>13	<13
Serum iron	Decreased	Normal
Serum ferritin	Decreased / normal	Normal
TIBC	Increased	Normal
RDW	Increased	Normal (usually)
Free erythrocyte protoporphyrin	High	Normal
Hemoglobin electrophoresis‡	Normal	Increased A_2/F

*A decrease in MCV is disproportionate to the hemoglobin level in patients with thalassemia minor. There is often microcytosis in the presence of normal or mildly decreased hemoglobin levels in these patients. In patients with iron deficiency anemia, the decrease in MCV is not usually as impressive and is only appreciated if the anemia is particularly severe.

†Mentzer index = MCV / RBC.

‡Hemoglobin electrophoresis revealing an elevated hemoglobin A_2 is consistent with β-thalassemia minor, but it is not seen with iron deficiency or anemia of chronic disease. The quantification of hemoglobin A_2 is very helpful in distinguishing β-thalassemia minor from iron deficiency anemia. However, it is not uncommon for thalassemia minor and iron deficiency anemia to coexist. When they do occur together, hemoglobin A_2 elevation is no longer appreciated. In these cases, the patient may seem only to have iron deficiency anemia. With adequate treatment of iron deficiency anemia, however, the anemia may not correct completely and elevated hemoglobin A_2 will be seen on a subsequent hemoglobin electrophoresis. It is important to realize that α-thalassemia minor is also associated with normal hemoglobin A_2 levels. The definitive diagnosis of α-thalassemia can only be established by DNA analysis.

If the patient has iron deficiency anemia, ***proceed to Step 6***.

If the patient has anemia of chronic disease, ***proceed to the discussion*** *on page 33.*

If the patient has thalassemia minor, ***proceed to Step 7***.

STEP 6 – *What Are the Causes of Iron Deficiency Anemia?*

Once the presence of iron deficiency anemia has been established, the clinician should make every effort to identify the cause of the iron deficiency anemia. Causes of iron deficiency anemia are listed in the following box.

CAUSES OF IRON DEFICIENCY ANEMIA

BLOOD LOSS
- Gastrointestinal
- Genitourinary
- Intrapulmonary / respiratory tract hemorrhage
- Hemolysis (hemoglobinuria)
- Self-inflicted blood loss
- Phlebotomy
- Blood donation
- Therapeutic (eg, PCV)

DECREASED DIETARY INTAKE

IMPAIRED ABSORPTION
- Gastrectomy
- Malabsorption (gluten-induced enteropathy)

INCREASED REQUIREMENTS
- Pregnancy
- Growth

For further information regarding workup to elucidate the cause of iron deficiency anemia, ***proceed to Iron Deficiency Anemia*** *on page 733.*

STEP 7 – *Does the Patient Have Thalassemia Minor?*

Thalassemia syndromes are another cause of microcytic anemia. An insufficient synthesis of either the alpha or beta chain of hemoglobin is the hallmark of thalassemia. Based on the globin chain that is affected, thalassemia syndromes may be divided into α-thalassemia and β-thalassemia.

β-*Thalassemia*

Commonly encountered among individuals of Mediterranean descent, the severity of the β-thalassemia depends on the number of abnormal genes inherited. If the patient has only inherited one abnormal gene, the patient is said to have β-thalassemia minor. This disease is characterized by a mild microcytic anemia, with an MCV often between 60 and 70 fL. The hemoglobin is typically normal but can be mildly depressed (10-13 g/dL).

If two abnormal genes have been inherited, the affected patient will present with β-thalassemia major. This illness manifests in infancy and childhood. Clinical manifestations include hepatosplenomegaly, bony deformities from marked erythroid hyperplasia, and failure to grow. A severe hemolytic anemia is typically present, with hemoglobin levels between 2 and 6 g/dL.

α-*Thalassemia*

As with β-thalassemia, the severity of α-thalassemia depends on the number of abnormal genes present. Because there are normally four alpha chain genes, four forms of the disease with varying severity are recognized.

The deletion of all four genes is not compatible with life. In fact, this form of α-thalassemia, also known as hydrops fetalis, is a common cause of stillbirth in Southeast Asia.

When only one alpha chain gene is functioning, the patient is said to have Hb H disease. This disease manifests as a moderately severe hemolytic anemia that usually becomes apparent during childhood.

α-thalassemia minor or α-thalassemia trait is said to be present if two functioning alpha chain genes are present. Although these patients do have microcytic, hypochromic anemia, the anemia is characteristically mild.

Patients who have three normally functioning alpha chain genes are known as silent carriers. These patients do not manifest with anemia.

Establishing the Diagnosis

The severe forms of α-thalassemia and β-thalassemia will not escape detection during infancy and childhood. It can be particularly difficult, however, to distinguish the milder forms of α- and β-thalassemia (ie, β-thalassemia minor and α-thalassemia minor) from other causes of microcytic anemia, especially iron deficiency anemia. For these reasons, it is important for the clinician to become familiar with the laboratory features of α- and β-thalassemia minor, as shown in the following box.

LABORATORY FEATURES OF α- AND β-THALASSEMIA MINOR
IRON STUDIES Normal serum iron Normal serum ferritin Normal total iron binding capacity Normal transferrin saturation NORMAL FREE ERYTHROCYTE PROTOPORPHYRIN LEVELS* NORMAL TO SLIGHTLY INCREASED RED BLOOD CELL COUNT MILD MICROCYTIC, HYPOCHROMIC ANEMIA MICROCYTOSIS OUT OF PROPORTION TO THE ANEMIA PERIPHERAL BLOOD SMEAR Microcytosis Target cells Basophilic stippling HEMOGLOBIN ELECTROPHORESIS REVEALING ELEVATED HEMOGLOBIN A_2 (only β-thalassemia minor)

*Free erythrocyte protoporphyrin (FEP) levels are elevated in patients with iron deficiency anemia, anemia of chronic disease, and sideroblastic anemia. In thalassemia minor, FEP levels are normal. FEP levels are therefore useful in differentiating iron deficiency anemia from thalassemia minor.

Particularly useful in establishing the diagnosis of β-thalassemia minor is measurement of hemoglobin A_2 (Hb A_2), which may be performed by hemoglobin electrophoresis or chromatography. Healthy adults have three forms of hemoglobin, as shown in the following table.

Types of Hemoglobin Found in Healthy Adults

Hemoglobin Type	% Total Hemoglobin
Hb A (α_2 β_2)	>95
Hb A_2 (α_2 δ_2)	≤3.5
Hb F (α_2 γ_2)	1

In β-thalassemia minor, Hb A_2 is elevated, usually ranging between 3.5% to 8%. Levels of Hb F may be mildly elevated in up to 30% of β-thalassemia minor patients.

α-thalassemia minor is usually a diagnosis of exclusion in patients with microcytic anemia. This is because laboratory testing for α-thalassemia minor is not readily available. Elevations in Hb A_2 and Hb F seen in β-thalassemia minor are not observed in patients with α-thalassemia minor. When thalassemia minor is the suspected diagnosis (iron deficiency, anemia of chronic disease, and sideroblastic anemia have been ruled out), a normal hemoglobin electrophoresis (ruling out β-thalassemia minor) should prompt consideration of α-thalassemia minor. If necessary, the definitive diagnosis can be established by DNA testing, which is available in specialized laboratories. Determination of globin chain synthetic ratios may be the only way to make the diagnosis of milder forms of α-thalassemia. In most cases, the diagnosis can be securely made without DNA testing once other causes of microcytic anemia have been excluded.

Differentiating Thalassemia Minor From Iron Deficiency Anemia

At times, it can be quite challenging to differentiate thalassemia minor from iron deficiency anemia. The following table highlights the differences between these two causes of microcytic anemia.

Iron Deficiency Anemia vs Thalassemia Minor

	Iron Deficiency Anemia	**Thalassemia Minor**
Ethnicity	No ethnic predilection	African American / Asian / Mediterranean descent
MCV*	↓	↓↓
RBC count	$<5 \times 10^6/mm^3$	$>5 \times 10^6/mm^3$
Mentzer index†	>13	<13
Serum iron	Decreased	Normal
Serum ferritin	Decreased / normal	Normal
TIBC	Increased	Normal
RDW	Increased	Normal (usually)
Free erythrocyte protoporphyrin	High	Normal
Hemoglobin electrophoresis‡	Normal	Increased A_2/F

*The decrease in MCV is disproportionate to the hemoglobin level in patients with thalassemia minor. There is often microcytosis in the presence of normal or mildly decreased hemoglobin levels in patients with thalassemia minor. In patients with iron deficiency anemia, the decrease in MCV is not usually as impressive and is only appreciated when the anemia is particularly severe. In general, thalassemia minor patients have hematocrit levels >30% with MCV <75. In iron deficiency anemia, however, the MCV will not become microcytic until the hematocrit has fallen below 30%.

†Mentzer index = MCV / RBC.

‡Hemoglobin electrophoresis revealing an elevated hemoglobin A_2 is consistent with β-thalassemia minor, but it is not seen with iron deficiency or anemia of chronic disease. The quantification of hemoglobin A_2 is very helpful in distinguishing β-thalassemia minor from iron deficiency anemia. However, it is not uncommon for thalassemia minor and iron deficiency anemia to coexist. When they do occur together, hemoglobin A_2 elevation is no longer appreciated. In these cases, the patient may seem only to have iron deficiency anemia. With adequate treatment of iron deficiency anemia, however, the anemia may not correct completely and elevated hemoglobin A_2 will be seen on a subsequent hemoglobin electrophoresis. It is important to realize that α-thalassemia minor is also associated with normal hemoglobin A_2 levels. The definitive diagnosis of α-thalassemia can only be established by DNA analysis.

If the patient has α- or β-thalassemia minor, ***stop here***.

If the patient has iron deficiency anemia, ***proceed to Step 5*** *on page 25.*

STEP 8 – *Does the Patient Have Sideroblastic Anemia?*

Sideroblastic anemia is an uncommon cause of microcytic anemia. Sideroblastic anemias are characterized by a defect in heme synthesis. Iron is not able to be incorporated into heme and as a result, accumulates within mitochondria. This gives rise to accumulation of iron in the perinuclear region of the developing red blood cell. These cells are called ringed sideroblasts.

Laboratory test features consistent with sideroblastic anemia are listed in the following box.

LABORATORY TEST FINDINGS IN SIDEROBLASTIC ANEMIA
INCREASED SERUM IRON
INCREASED TRANSFERRIN SATURATION
DECREASED OR NORMAL TOTAL IRON BINDING CAPACITY
INCREASED SERUM FERRITIN
PERIPHERAL BLOOD SMEAR: Dimorphic population, dysplastic cells
LOW, NORMAL, OR HIGH MCV
RDW VARIABLE
± Leukopenia
± Thrombocytopenia

The clinician should realize that sideroblastic anemia and iron deficiency anemia can coexist. This can occur, for example, in some patients with sideroblastic anemia who have thrombocytopenia. The low platelet count may lead to gastrointestinal loss of blood. In these cases, establishing the diagnosis can be difficult.

Although laboratory testing can be suggestive of sideroblastic anemia, the definitive diagnosis can only be established at the time of bone marrow biopsy. Bone marrow biopsy revealing increased numbers of ringed sideroblasts establishes the diagnosis of sideroblastic anemia.

Once the presence of sideroblastic anemia has been established, the clinician should determine the etiology of the sideroblastic anemia. Causes of sideroblastic anemia are listed in the following box.

CAUSES OF SIDEROBLASTIC ANEMIA

- HEREDITARY
  - X-linked
  - Autosomal
- ACQUIRED
  - Idiopathic (myelodysplastic syndrome)
  - Secondary
    - Drug-induced: Isoniazid, cycloserine, pyrazinamide, chlorambucil, chloramphenicol
    - Alcohol
    - Lead poisoning
    - Other: Copper deficiency (of all causes including that due to overdose of chelators such as penicillamine or triethylene tetramine dihydrochloride), zinc overload, rheumatoid arthritis, lymphoma, multiple myeloma, hypothermia

Acquired sideroblastic anemia is much more common than the hereditary type. Among the various causes of acquired sideroblastic anemia, drugs and toxins are the most common etiology. If no secondary causes of sideroblastic anemia are identified, it is likely the patient has acquired idiopathic sideroblastic anemia. In fact, acquired idiopathic sideroblastic anemia is more common than secondary causes of sideroblastic anemia and is generally considered to be a type of myelodysplastic syndrome (refractory anemia with ringed sideroblasts).

Hemoglobin levels can vary considerably in sideroblastic anemia patients but typically range between 4-10 mg/dL. If the condition is suspected, a thorough history focusing on toxin or drug exposure is essential. A complete family history should also be obtained to exclude hereditary sideroblastic anemia. Although most cases of the hereditary type will be detected in childhood, milder cases may not come to clinical attention until adulthood.

End of Section.

STEP 9 – *What Is the Approach to the Patient With Normocytic Anemia and RPI <2?*

The causes of normocytic anemia and RPI <2 are listed in the following box.

CAUSES OF NORMOCYTIC ANEMIA AND RPI <2
IRON DEFICIENCY ANEMIA (early or mild)
ANEMIA OF CHRONIC DISEASE
ANEMIA SECONDARY TO ACUTE BLOOD LOSS
APLASTIC ANEMIA
PURE RED BLOOD CELL APLASIA
MYELODYSPLASTIC SYNDROME
MYELOPHTHISIS
ANEMIA OF RENAL INSUFFICIENCY
ANEMIA OF LIVER DISEASE
ANEMIA OF ENDOCRINE DISEASE
SIDEROBLASTIC ANEMIA
MEGALOBLASTIC ANEMIA
MIXED ANEMIA
ANEMIA ASSOCIATED WITH AIDS

The evaluation of the patient presenting with normocytic anemia and RPI <2 can be quite challenging. This is because many of the anemias traditionally considered to be microcytic or macrocytic may present with normocytosis, especially in the early stages of the anemia. For example, iron deficiency anemia and megaloblastic anemia (folic acid or vitamin B_{12} deficiency) which are classically categorized as microcytic and macrocytic, respectively, are frequently normocytic. In addition, mixed anemias (ie, combined folic acid and iron deficiency anemia) often present with MCV in the normal range.

As with all types of anemia, the peripheral blood smear is essential in the evaluation of normocytic anemia and RPI <2. It is particularly important in identifying a mixed anemia. In these cases, two populations of red blood cells, one microcytic and the other macrocytic, may be noted on examination of the smear. Because of the presence of both microcytic and macrocytic red blood cells, the MCV, which is a measure of average red blood cell size, may be reported as normal.

The peripheral blood smear may also reveal findings suggestive of certain causes of normocytic anemia and RPI <2, as shown in the following box.

Using the Peripheral Blood Smear to Elucidate the Etiology of Normocytic Anemia and RPI <2

Peripheral Blood Smear Finding	Peripheral Blood Smear Findings
Decrease in white blood cells and/or platelets	Aplastic anemia Myelophthisis Myelodysplastic syndrome Megaloblastic anemia Anemia of liver disease (due to hypersplenism)
Leukoerythroblastosis	Myelophthisis
Abnormal white blood cells	Leukemia Lymphoma Myelodysplastic syndrome
Rouleaux formation	Multiple myeloma
Hypersegmented PMNs	Megaloblastic anemia
Target cell	Anemia of liver disease
Dimorphic population	Sideroblastic anemia
Burr cell	Uremia (anemia of renal insufficiency)

The red blood cell distribution width may also provide clues to the etiology of the normocytic anemia and RPI <2, as shown in the following table.

Classification of Normocytic Anemia and RPI <2 Based on RDW

RDW	Causes of Normocytic Anemia and RPI <2
Normal	Anemia of chronic disease Anemia of acute blood loss Myelodysplastic syndrome
Elevated	Early iron deficiency anemia Partially treated iron deficiency anemia Megaloblastic anemia Myelodysplastic syndrome Anemia of liver disease

Although there are many causes of normocytic anemia, the two major causes are iron deficiency anemia and anemia of chronic disease. Therefore, iron studies (serum iron, TIBC, ferritin) are indicated in the evaluation of normocytic anemia. Vitamin B_{12} and folate levels should be obtained as well. Even with consideration of the iron studies, peripheral blood smear, RDW and other noninvasive laboratory tests, many patients will require bone marrow biopsy to establish the definitive diagnosis.

The causes of normocytic anemia and RPI <2 will be discussed in the remainder of this step.

Iron Deficiency Anemia

Early or mild iron deficiency anemia may present with a normocytic, normochromic anemia. As a general rule, the MCV does not fall into the microcytic range until the hematocrit drops below 30. For this reason, iron studies are recommended in all patients with normocytic anemia and RPI <2. For further information regarding the diagnosis of iron deficiency anemia, please refer to Step 5 *on page 25*

Anemia of Chronic Disease

In terms of incidence, anemia of chronic disease trails only iron deficiency anemia. Anemia of chronic disease is characterized by an impairment in the delivery of iron to the developing red blood cells. Although most patients present with normocytic anemia, approximately 30% to 40% are found to have a microcytic anemia, with MCV usually between 70 and 80 fL. Other characteristics of the anemia of chronic disease are listed in the following box.

CHARACTERISTICS OF THE ANEMIA OF CHRONIC DISEASE
CLINICAL
Development of anemia 1-2 months after onset of chronic disease
BLOOD
Usually normocytic, normochromic anemia with normal MCV, MCHC, and RDW
Anemia of variable severity (20% present with hemoglobin levels <8 g/dL)
Inappropriately low reticulocyte count
IRON STUDIES
Decreased serum iron
Decreased total iron binding capacity
Decreased transferrin saturation, but typically near-normal (20%, however, with transferrin saturation as low as 10%)
Normal to increased serum ferritin
ACUTE PHASE REACTANTS
Increased ESR, CRP, and other acute phase reactants
BONE MARROW*
Normal numbers of erythroid precursors
Decreased sideroblasts (iron-containing precursors)
Increased storage iron

*Bone marrow biopsy is not indicated in all cases of anemia of chronic disease. It should be considered, however, in cases in which the diagnosis of anemia of chronic disease is not secure.

Adapted from Kjeldsberg CR, *Practical Diagnosis of Hematologic Disorders*, 3rd ed, Chicago, IL: ASCP Press, 2001, 40.

There are a number of chronic diseases associated with the anemia of chronic disease, as shown in the following box.

DISEASES COMMONLY ASSOCIATED WITH ANEMIA OF CHRONIC DISEASE	
CONNECTIVE TISSUE DISEASES	MALIGNANCY
Rheumatoid arthritis	Carcinomas
Systemic lupus erythematosus	Lymphomas
INFECTION	Leukemias
HIV	LIVER DISEASE
Tuberculosis	ENDOCRINOLOGIC DISORDERS
Osteomyelitis	Adrenal insufficiency
Chronic fungal infections	Diabetes mellitus
Subacute bacterial endocarditis	Hyperparathyroidism
	Hypothyroidism
	Hyperthyroidism
	Hypopituitarism

When the presence of anemia of chronic disease is established, every effort should be made to identify the chronic disease. In most cases, the underlying disease is readily apparent. At times, however, the finding of anemia of chronic disease precedes diagnosis of the underlying disease. It is in these patients that a thorough search should be undertaken to identify the underlying disease.

It is also important to note that there are certain chronic conditions that are not characterized by the anemia of chronic disease. These include chronic obstructive pulmonary disease, congestive heart failure, and hypertension. If an anemia is present in patients with one of these conditions, the clinician should search for another etiology.

Several of the diseases associated with the anemia of chronic disease, including liver disease, HIV, and malignancy, will be discussed as separate entities because the pathogenesis of the anemia, in these conditions, is often multifactorial or even due to another etiology rather than the anemia of chronic disease.

Differentiating Anemia of Chronic Disease From Iron Deficiency Anemia

Test	Anemia of Chronic Disease	Iron Deficiency Anemia
Serum iron	↓	↓
Serum TIBC	↓	↑
Serum ferritin	↑	↓
Free erythrocyte protoporphyrin	↑	↑
Soluble transferrin receptor	Normal or ↓	Normal or ↑
Bone marrow iron	Present	Absent

Megaloblastic Anemia

Megaloblastic anemia due to either folic acid or vitamin B_{12} deficiency should be a consideration in every patient with normocytic anemia. In one study of 86 patients with vitamin B_{12} deficiency, 36% had an MCV ≤100. Normocytic anemia is more likely in early megaloblastic anemia. Another explanation for normocytosis includes the presence of a mixed anemia (ie, combined folic acid and iron deficiency anemia). For more information regarding the diagnosis of megaloblastic anemia, the reader is referred to Step 10 *on page 41.*

Anemia of Malignancy

Malignancy that has been present for more than several weeks can lead to the development of anemia of chronic disease. The clinician should realize, however, that there are other reasons why patients with cancer may develop anemia. Bone marrow infiltration (myelophthisis) is one cause, characterized by a leukoerythroblastic peripheral blood smear (presence of immature red and white blood cells). Leukopenia and/or thrombocytopenia may accompany the anemia of myelophthisis.

Patients with gastrointestinal cancers are predisposed to blood loss, which may present with anemia of acute blood loss or iron deficiency anemia. Malnutrition is quite common among cancer patients, raising concern for the possibility of nutritional anemia (ie, folate deficiency).

Disseminated carcinoma is one cause of microangiopathic hemolytic anemia characterized by the presence of schistocytes and helmet cells in the peripheral blood smear. In patients with lymphoproliferative malignancy, hemolytic anemia may be immune-mediated. Finally, chemotherapy and radiotherapy are well known causes of anemia in cancer patients.

The causes of anemia in patients with malignancy are listed in the following box.

CAUSES OF ANEMIA IN THE PATIENT WITH MALIGNANCY
ANEMIA OF CHRONIC DISEASE
GASTROINTESTINAL BLOOD LOSS
HYPERSPLENISM
IATROGENIC
Chemotherapy
Radiotherapy
IMMUNE HEMOLYSIS (usually B-cell neoplasms)
MICROANGIOPATHIC HEMOLYTIC ANEMIA
Disseminated carcinoma
Drug-induced (ie, mitomycin C)
MYELOPHTHISIS (bone marrow replacement)
NUTRITIONAL DEFICIENCY (iron, folate)
MYELODYSPLASTIC SYNDROME (from chemotherapy)

Anemia of Liver Disease

While patients with chronic liver disease do develop the anemia of chronic disease, it is important to realize that there may be other reasons causing or contributing to anemia in this patient population. Because these patients are prone to gastrointestinal blood loss, they may develop iron deficiency anemia or the anemia of acute blood loss. The portal hypertension that often accompanies liver disease can lead to hypersplenism, which results in decreased red blood cell survival. These as well as other factors involved in the pathogenesis of the anemia of liver disease are listed in the following box.

FACTORS CONTRIBUTING TO THE ANEMIA OF LIVER DISEASE
ANEMIA OF CHRONIC DISEASE
FOLIC ACID DEFICIENCY
IRON DEFICIENCY ANEMIA
DECREASED RED BLOOD CELL SURVIVAL
TOXIC EFFECTS OF ALCOHOL
HEMODILUTION
HYPERSPLENISM

Anemia Associated With AIDS

Anemia is common in HIV/AIDS patients, with the incidence depending upon the status of the disease. In HIV patients who are asymptomatic, anemia is found in about 15% to 20%. The incidence rises to about 80% in advanced AIDS.

There are many causes of anemia in patients with AIDS. There is evidence to suggest that HIV may suppress hematopoiesis by invading bone marrow precursor cells. Other causes of anemia in the AIDS patient are listed in the following box.

CAUSES OF ANEMIA IN AIDS
ANEMIA OF CHRONIC DISEASE
SUPPRESSION OF BONE MARROW BY HIV
MEDICATION-INDUCED SUPPRESSION OF BONE MARROW
MYELOPHTHISIS SECONDARY TO INFECTION OR MALIGNANCY
IMMUNE-MEDIATED
PARVOVIRUS INFECTION CAUSING PRCA
GI BLOOD LOSS (due to opportunistic infection and malignancy)
NUTRITIONAL DEFICIENCY (ie, iron)

Anemia of Acute Blood Loss

The hemoglobin after an acute bleed is often normal. This is because sufficient time has not passed for hemodilution to occur. After about 24 hours or so, there will be a shift of volume from the extravascular space to the intravascular space to replenish the volume deficit. This will lead to a fall in the hemoglobin level.

In most cases, the bleeding event is quite apparent but on occasion, bleeding may occur into soft tissues or into a body cavity.

The reticulocyte count may be normal for the first several days after the acute event but will increase shortly thereafter. A brisk reticulocytosis may result in a mildly macrocytic anemia. Prior to the decrease in the hemoglobin level, laboratory studies may reveal leukocytosis and thrombocytosis. Immature red and white blood cells, including metamyelocytes, myelocytes, and nucleated red blood cells may be seen with severe hemorrhage.

Anemia of Chronic Renal Insufficiency

Anemia is quite commonly encountered in patients with chronic renal insufficiency. Playing a major role in the pathogenesis of the anemia of chronic renal insufficiency is decreased erythropoietin production. As with the anemia of malignancy and the anemia of liver disease, the pathogenesis of the anemia of renal disease may be more complex. Causes of anemia in patients with chronic renal insufficiency are listed in the following box.

MAJOR CAUSES OF ANEMIA IN PATIENTS WITH CHRONIC RENAL INSUFFICIENCY
DECREASED ERYTHROPOIETIN PRODUCTION
IRON DEFICIENCY
FOLIC ACID DEFICIENCY
GASTROINTESTINAL BLOOD LOSS
DECREASED RED BLOOD CELL SURVIVAL

In general, anemia of renal disease is normocytic and normochromic. Its severity usually correlates with the severity of the renal insufficiency.

Aplastic Anemia

Aplastic anemia should be a consideration in every patient who presents with pancytopenia. The red blood cells may be normocytic or macrocytic. Examination of the peripheral blood smear usually reveals decreased numbers of red blood cells, white blood cells, and platelets. The presence of immature myeloid forms, large or abnormal platelets, and nucleated red blood cells are not features of aplastic anemia and their presence should prompt consideration of other causes of pancytopenia.

The definitive diagnosis of aplastic anemia is based on bone marrow biopsy findings. Bone marrow aspiration usually leads to a "dry tap". Very characteristic of aplastic anemia is a hypocellular marrow. It is important to realize, however, that patchy areas of normocellularity and hypercellularity may be present. The bone marrow biopsy helps to exclude other causes of pancytopenia that may present with infiltrative or fibrotic marrow.

Once the presence of aplastic anemia has been established, every effort should be made to identify the etiology. The causes of aplastic anemia are listed in the following box.

CAUSES OF APLASTIC ANEMIA

- HEREDITARY
- ACQUIRED
  - Idiopathic
  - Infection
    - Epstein-Barr virus
    - Hepatitis
    - HIV
    - Influenza
    - Parvovirus B19
    - Others
  - Medications
    - Anticonvulsants
    - Chloramphenicol
    - Felbamate
    - Gold
    - Chemotherapy
    - Nifedipine
    - Sulfonamides
    - Others
  - Pregnancy
  - Radiation
  - Toxins / chemicals
    - Benzene
    - Insecticides
    - Solvents
  - Paroxysmal nocturnal hemoglobinuria
  - Malignancy (CLL, thymoma, thymic cancer)
  - Immune disorders

Workup to evaluate for causes of aplastic anemia may include viral serology (EBV, HIV) and liver function tests (increased levels suggest hepatitis). Ham's test or flow microfluorometry of granulocytes may be needed to exclude paroxymal nocturnal hemoglobinuria. In younger patients or in those who have a positive family history, cytogenetic studies are recommended.

Pure Red Cell Aplasia (PRCA)

Pure red cell aplasia, as its name suggests, affects only the red blood cell line. Most cases are characterized by normocytic red blood cells but macrocytosis has been described. The red blood cell distribution width is typically normal. When parvovirus infection occurs in the patient with hemolytic anemia, however, PRCA may present with an elevated RDW. Otherwise, the peripheral blood smear is unremarkable in patients with PRCA.

The definitive diagnosis can only be established by bone marrow biopsy. Bone marrow biopsy will reveal a significant decline in erythroid precursors but normal numbers of megakaryocytic and granulocytic precursors. The presence of giant proerythroblasts is considered to be characteristic of PRCA that is due to parvoviral infection. The serum can also be assayed for anti-parvovirus B19 IgM antibodies.

Other causes of PRCA should also be considered. These causes are listed in the following box. In a Mayo clinic review of 47 cases of PRCA, the most common cause was found to be T-cell large granular lymphocyte leukemia. Immunophenotypic analysis can be performed to help establish the diagnosis of large granular lymphocyte leukemia. Depending on the patient's clinical presentation, other tests that can be obtained include serologic testing for other viruses (besides parvovirus) and autoantibodies (to assess for connective tissue disease). Because of the association between pure red cell aplasia and thymoma, a chest CT should be obtained in patients thought to have idiopathic PRCA.

CAUSES OF PRCA

IDIOPATHIC (50% of cases)
THYMOMA
VIRAL INFECTION
- Parvovirus B19
- Hepatitis
- Adult T-cell leukemia virus
- Epstein-Barr virus

MALIGNANCY
- Lymphoma
- Solid tumors

CONNECTIVE TISSUE DISEASE
- Systemic lupus erythematosus
- Juvenile rheumatoid arthritis
- Rheumatoid arthritis

PREGNANCY
MEDICATIONS
- Dilantin
- Azathioprine
- Chlorambucil
- Procainamide
- Antibiotics
- Antithyroid
- Tacrolimus
- Allopurinol
- Recombinant human erythropoietin therapy
- Isoniazid

Myelophthisis

Myelophthisis, which refers to infiltrated bone marrow, may be due to a variety of conditions. The severity of the anemia of myelophthisis varies. Not uncommonly, thrombocytopenia and/or leukopenia accompanies the anemia. Anisopoikilocytosis is quite common with the presence of the teardrop cell being a particularly helpful feature supporting the diagnosis. Very characteristic of myelophthisis is a leukoerythroblastic peripheral blood smear. Leukoerythroblastosis is said to be present if the peripheral blood smear reveals immature red (nucleated red blood cells, teardrop-shaped red blood cells) and white blood cells cells (promyelocytes, metamyelocytes). The presence of leukoerythroblastic findings is not synonymous with myelophthisis. Causes of leukoerythroblastosis are listed in the following box.

CAUSES OF LEUKOERYTHROBLASTOSIS

In addition to causes of myelophthisis (see box below), other causes include:
- Acute hemolysis
- Hemorrhage
- Severe infection
- Sickle cell anemia (crises)
- Severe megaloblastic anemia
- Rebound following bone marrow failure/suppression

If the myelophthisis is due to leukemia or lymphoma, malignant cells may actually be present in the peripheral blood smear.

The causes of myelophthisis are listed in the following box.

CAUSES OF MYELOPHTHISIS
HEMATOLOGIC MALIGNANCY / DISORDERS
Acute lymphocytic leukemia
Acute myelogenous leukemia
Chronic lymphocytic leukemia
Chronic myelogenous leukemia
Hairy cell leukemia
Hodgkin's lymphoma
Non-Hodgkin's lymphoma
Malignant histiocytosis
Multiple myeloma
Myeloid metaplasia with myelofibrosis
Polycythemia vera
SOLID MALIGNANCY
Breast
Lung
Gastrointestinal
Prostate
Renal
INFECTION
Fungal diseases
Tuberculosis
SARCOIDOSIS
LIPID STORAGE DISEASES

Myelodysplastic Syndrome

Myelodysplastic syndromes refer to a group of disorders that are also known as preleukemic states. This is an inaccurate term since only 25% develop into acute leukemia. This disorder is characterized not only by ineffective erythropoiesis, but also by the ineffective production of white blood cells and platelets. Patients may present with anemia, bicytopenia, or pancytopenia. There is considerable anisocytosis. Although red blood cells are usually normocytic, they may be mildly macrocytic in some cases. The peripheral blood smear may reveal Howell-Jolly bodies and basophilic stippling. It is not uncommon to appreciate nucleated red blood cells and immature white blood cells. Very characteristic is the presence of mature neutrophils with hypolobulated nuclei. This is the pseudo-Pelger-Huet anomaly. One form of myelodysplastic syndrome, called chronic myelomonocytic leukemia (CMML), is characterized by a striking monocytosis. Platelet abnormalities that may be noted include the presence of large platelets, megakaryocyte fragments, and hypogranulation. Definitive diagnosis requires an evaluation of the bone marrow. Myelodysplastic syndromes are divided into subtypes based on cellularity, the number of blasts and ringed sideroblasts, and the presence of dysplastic changes. Myelodysplastic syndromes have been subdivided based on the FAB classification, as shown in the following table.

MYELODYSPLASTIC SYNDROMES FAB CLASSIFICATION
CHRONIC MYELOMONOCYTIC LEUKEMIA REFRACTORY ANEMIA REFRACTORY ANEMIA WITH EXCESS BLASTS REFRACTORY ANEMIA WITH EXCESS BLASTS IN TRANSFORMATION REFRACTORY ANEMIA WITH RINGED SIDEROBLASTS

The different types of myelodysplastic syndromes listed in the above box can be distinguished from one another by examining the peripheral blood and bone marrow, as shown in the following table.

Differentiating Among the Different Types of Myelodysplastic Syndrome (Based on FAB Criteria)

Type	Bone marrow blasts, %	Peripheral blood blasts, %	Monocytes >1000/ microliter	Ringed sideroblasts, >15% of nucleated erythroid cells
RA	<5	≤1	No	No
RARS	<5	≤1	No	Yes
RAEB	5-20	<5	No	±
RAEB-T	21-30 OR	≥5	±	±
CMML	≤20	<5	Yes	±

RA = refractory anemia

RARS = refractory anemia with ringed sideroblasts

RAEB = refractory anemia with excess blasts

RAEB-T = refractory anemia with excess blasts in transformation

CMML = chronic myelomonocytic leukemia

Modified from Up-to-Date article "Clinical Manifestations and Diagnosis of the Myelodysplastic Syndromes," by Donald C Doll and Stephen A Landlaw

The above disorders are different from the myeloproliferative disorders which include polycythemia vera, chronic myelogenous leukemia, essential thrombocytosis, and agnogenic myeloid metaplasia.

Recently, new classification systems for the myelodysplastic syndrome have been proposed, which may gain wider acceptance.

Sideroblastic Anemia

For more information regarding sideroblastic anemia, please refer to Step 8 *on page 30.*

End of Section.

STEP 10 – *What Is the Approach to the Patient With Macrocytic Anemia and RPI <2?*

The causes of macrocytic anemia and RPI <2 are listed in the following box.

CAUSES OF MACROCYTIC ANEMIA AND RPI <2	
MEGALOBLASTIC ANEMIA	ALCOHOLISM
Vitamin B_{12} deficiency	LIVER DISEASE
Folic acid deficiency	DRUG-INDUCED
Others	APLASTIC ANEMIA
Inborn errors	MYELODYSPLASTIC SYNDROME
Drug-induced	PREGNANCY
Myelodysplastic syndrome	MYELOMA
Acute myelogenous leukemia	HYPOTHYROIDISM

The causes of macrocytic anemia may be categorized as megaloblastic or nonmegaloblastic. In most cases, the findings of the peripheral blood smear allow the clinician to make the distinction. The presence of oval macrocytes and hypersegmented neutrophils is consistent with megaloblastic anemia. The absence of neutrophil hypersegmentation along with the presence of round macrocytes should prompt consideration of nonmegaloblastic anemia.

The clinician should realize, however, that the use of the peripheral blood smear alone may not always allow separation of megaloblastic from nonmegaloblastic anemia. This is because the neutrophil hypersegmentation characteristic of megaloblastic anemia may be subtle or absent. In one study of 86 patients with vitamin B_{12} deficiency (major cause of megaloblastic anemia), 33% of these patients had an unremarkable peripheral blood smear. In addition, many clinicians do not feel comfortable examining the peripheral blood smear.

For these reasons, most clinicians will obtain serum vitamin B_{12} and folate levels to exclude vitamin B_{12} and folic acid deficiency, the two major causes of megaloblastic anemia, irrespective of the peripheral blood smear findings. The interpretation of serum vitamin B_{12} and folate levels are discussed in further detail in Step 11.

If the patient has megaloblastic anemia, ***proceed to Step 11***.

If the patient has nonmegaloblastic anemia, ***proceed to Step 16*** *on page 49.*

STEP 11 – *Does the Patient Have Megaloblastic Anemia?*

Megaloblastic anemia is an important cause of macrocytic anemia. Megaloblastic refers to an abnormality in DNA synthesis leading to impaired maturation of the nucleus relative to the cytoplasm. Megaloblastic and macrocytic are not interchangeable terms. Not all macrocytic anemias are megaloblastic and conversely not all megaloblastic anemias are macrocytic. The most common causes of megaloblastic anemia are vitamin B_{12} and folic acid deficiency. Other causes include administration of medications which interfere with DNA synthesis, myelodysplastic syndrome, and erythroleukemia.

Because neurological damage can be seen with B_{12} deficiency, it is important to make this diagnosis. Folic acid deficiency, however, is not characterized by neurologic abnormalities. Mistakenly diagnosing a patient with folate deficiency when in reality a B_{12} deficiency exists can have serious consequences for the patient. The neurologic abnormalities of B_{12} deficiency can worsen with folic acid supplementation. For these reasons, it is important to not only establish the diagnosis of megaloblastic anemia but also differentiate vitamin B_{12} from folic acid deficiency.

CBC and peripheral blood smear findings of megaloblastic anemia may be the first clue to the diagnosis. These findings are described in the following box.

CBC AND PERIPHERAL BLOOD SMEAR FINDINGS IN MEGALOBLASTIC ANEMIA

CBC
- Normocytic (early) or macrocytic anemia*
- Variable severity of anemia
- ± Leukopenia†
- ± Thrombocytopenia†
- Elevated RDW

PERIPHERAL BLOOD SMEAR
- Normocytic (early) or macrocytic anemia
- ± Leukopenia
- ± Thrombocytopenia
- Hypersegmented PMNs‡
- Macroovalocytes
- Anisopoikilocytosis
- Nucleated red blood cells#
- Target cells
- Schistocytes
- Spherocytes
- Erythrocytic inclusions
  - Howell-Jolly bodies
  - Cabot's rings
  - Basophilic stippling

LAB TEST ABNORMALITIES OF INEFFECTIVE ERYTHROPOIESIS
- Elevated LDH¶
- Elevated serum bilirubin

*Very high MCV values (>110 fL) are very suggestive of the presence of megaloblastic anemia. Other types of macrocytic anemia are not associated with this degree of MCV elevation. Macrocytic anemia with MCV <110 fL may be seen in megaloblastic as well as nonmegaloblastic causes of macrocytic anemia.

†Anemia is much more common than leukopenia and thrombocytopenia. Megaloblastic anemia should always be considered, however, in the differential diagnosis of pancytopenia.

‡One of the hallmark peripheral blood smear findings of megaloblastic anemia is the presence of hypersegmented PMNs. PMN hypersegmentation is said to be present if one or more of the following criteria are met: Presence of at least one PMN containing ≥6 lobes; 5-lobe PMNs account for ≥5% of the total neutrophil count; neutrophil lobe average ≥3.4.

#Nucleated red blood cells are more commonly encountered in severe megaloblastic anemia.

¶Serum LDH is often elevated in megaloblastic anemia. This elevation results from the increased destruction of red blood cell precursors in bone marrow (ineffective erythropoiesis). This, then, may be a clue to the diagnosis. However, it must be kept in mind that elevations in LDH are nonspecific. If increased LDH is secondary to megaloblastic anemia, the degree of elevation tends to be proportional to the severity of the anemia. Therefore, it is easy to understand that LDH may be normal in mild cases.

Of note, bone marrow biopsy is not necessary for the diagnosis of vitamin B_{12} or folic acid deficiency. If performed, bone marrow examination reveals nuclear-cytoplasmic dissociation. In megaloblastic states, maturation of the nucleus falls behind cytoplasmic maturation of all hematopoietic precursors. The bone marrow is hypercellular with a reversal in the myeloid to erythroid ratio. The normal ratio is 3:1 but in megaloblastic anemia it can approach 1:3. Very characteristic is the presence of megaloblastic erythroblasts and giant metamyelocytes.

In summary, the presence of the above CBC and peripheral blood smear findings supports the diagnosis of megaloblastic anemia. On occasion, the peripheral blood smear may fail to show the characteristic red blood cell and neutrophil abnormalities. Therefore, every patient with macrocytic anemia should be tested for vitamin B_{12} and folic acid deficiency, the two major causes of megaloblastic anemia. Testing begins with the measurement of serum vitamin B_{12} (cobalamin) and folate levels.

Serum Folate

Despite adequate body stores of folate, serum folate levels may decline within several days after folate intake has been curtailed. Conversely, serum folate levels often increase after the ingestion of food. In fact, serum folate levels can normalize after just one hospital meal in patients with folate deficiency. As a result, fasting determinations are recommended in the patient suspected of having folate deficiency. Every effort must be made to avoid hemolysis during venipuncture because even the slightest degree of hemolysis can falsely elevate serum folate levels. Serum folate levels may decrease after recent alcohol intake. It is not uncommon for serum folate levels to increase in patients with vitamin B_{12} deficiency. Falsely normal serum folate levels may be encountered in patients with combined folic acid and iron deficiency, particularly when the iron deficiency anemia is severe.

Because of the limitations of the serum folate level in the diagnosis of folate deficiency, the use of the red blood cell folate level was advocated with its arrival in the 1960s. Since folate levels in red blood cells are not affected by recent changes in dietary intake, many favored red blood cell folate determinations in lieu of the serum folate level. Recent studies have revealed, however, that a significant number of pregnant women and alcoholics with folic acid deficiency had either normal or low normal RBC folate levels. In addition, a major limitation of the red blood cell folate is that a falsely low value may be obtained in patients with vitamin B_{12} deficiency. In fact, 60% of patients with pernicious anemia have low red blood cell folate levels.

The initial enthusiasm which greeted the arrival of the red blood cell folate level has been tempered by the limitations discussed above. Furthermore, the methodology used to assay the red blood cell folate has changed. In recent years, the early microbiologic assays have been replaced by radioassays. These assays have not been validated clinically. Because both the serum and RBC folate tests have some limitations, it is reasonable to obtain both in patients suspected of having folate deficiency. If need be, the clinician can measure serum homocysteine levels for the diagnosis of folic acid deficiency. In folate deficiency, serum homocysteine levels increase because folate is required for the conversion of homocysteine to methionine.

Serum Cobalamin (Vitamin B_{12})

While a low serum cobalamin level should raise concern about the presence of vitamin B_{12} deficiency, the clinician should realize that there are other causes of a low serum cobalamin level.

These include those listed in the following box.

CAUSES OF DECREASED VITAMIN B_{12} LEVEL
VITAMIN B_{12} DEFICIENCY
FOLIC ACID DEFICIENCY (33% of patients)
PREGNANCY
ORAL CONTRACEPTIVES
ELDERLY
LEUKOPENIA
MULTIPLE MYELOMA
MEGADOSE VITAMIN C THERAPY
TRANSCOBALAMIN I DEFICIENCY
HYPOCHLORHYDRIA
HIV

Conversely, serum cobalamin levels may be falsely normal or elevated in patients having true vitamin B_{12} deficiency. The causes of false elevation of the serum cobalamin levels in the setting of vitamin B_{12} deficiency include those listed in the following box.

CAUSES OF FALSELY NORMAL OR ELEVATED VITAMIN B_{12} LEVEL
MYELOPROLIFERATIVE DISORDERS
HEPATOMAS
FIBROLAMELLAR HEPATIC TUMORS
AUTOIMMUNE DISEASES
MONOBLASTIC LEUKEMIAS
LYMPHOMAS
LIVER DISEASE
IRON DEFICIENCY
HEMOGLOBINOPATHY

Approach to the Diagnosis of Vitamin B_{12} and Folate Deficiency

In the patient with megaloblastic anemia or the patient with neurologic findings consistent with vitamin B_{12} deficiency, the initial evaluation begins with the measurement of serum folate and cobalamin levels.

Studies have been performed to assess the distribution of serum cobalamin levels in patients with clinically substantiated cobalamin deficiency. These studies have shown about 10% of patients with clinically confirmed cobalamin deficiency will have cobalamin levels exceeding the lower limit of normal (usually 200-300 pg/mL). Similar studies have been performed in patients with clinically confirmed folic acid deficiency. These studies have revealed that 25% of patients have serum folate levels above the lower limit of normal (usually 2.5-5.0 ng/mL). These studies highlight the fact that serum cobalamin and folate levels in the low normal range do not exclude the diagnosis of megaloblastic anemia.

In these patients, metabolite testing (serum homocysteine and methylmalonic acid) is useful in establishing or excluding the diagnosis of megaloblastic anemia. The basis behind the usefulness of these two tests has to do with the fact that folic acid and vitamin B_{12} are essential in a number of intracellular biochemical reactions. Deficiency of either can lead to an impairment in the function of certain enzymes. This impairment can lead to a buildup in the substrates of these reactions. Two such substrates include methylmalonic acid (MMA) and homocysteine.

Measurement of serum homocysteine and methylmalonic acid cannot only establish the diagnosis of megaloblastic anemia in patients with low normal cobalamin or folate levels but can also help to differentiate folate from B_{12} deficiency. Homocysteine and methylmalonic acid levels will be increased in vitamin B_{12} deficiency. In folic acid deficiency, however, only the homocysteine level is increased. The clinician should realize that there are other causes of increased methylmalonic (renal insufficiency, congenital disorders of cobalamin metabolism, hypovolemic states) and homocysteine levels (renal failure, homocystinuria, inborn errors of metabolism). The patient's clinical presentation often allows these other conditions to be differentiated from vitamin B_{12} or folic acid deficiency.

The following results obtained after measurement of the vitamin B_{12} and folate levels will guide the clinician in determining whether further metabolite testing is necessary.

Cobalamin (pg/mL)	Folate (ng/mL)	Provisional Diagnosis	Need for Metabolite Testing
>300	>4	Cobalamin or folate deficiency unlikely	No
>300	<2	Folate deficiency	No
<200	>4	Cobalamin deficiency	No
200-300*	>4	Possible cobalamin deficiency	Yes
<200†	<2	Isolated folate deficiency vs combined deficiency	Yes
>300‡	2-4	Isolated folate deficiency vs another cause of anemia	Yes

*10% of patients with vitamin B_{12} deficiency will have serum cobalamin levels in the low normal range (200 and 300 pg/mL). Measurement of serum methylmalonic acid and homocysteine levels will establish the diagnosis.

†It is difficult to distinguish isolated folate deficiency from combined deficiency in the patient found to have low serum levels of both folate and cobalamin. This is because folic acid deficiency is associated with depression of the serum cobalamin levels in up to 33% of patients in the absence of true vitamin B_{12} deficiency. Measurement of the serum homocysteine and methylmalonic acid levels will help in distinguishing between these two possibilities.

‡The patient with normal serum cobalamin level but a low normal serum folate level (2-4 ng/mL) may have either isolated folate deficiency or an anemia secondary to another process. To differentiate between the two, metabolite testing is necessary.

If metabolite testing is deemed necessary, the results outlined below will help in the diagnosis of vitamin B_{12} or folate deficiency.

Methylmalonic Acid	Homocysteine	Diagnosis
Normal	↑	Folate deficiency likely; <5% have cobalamin deficiency
↑	↑	Cobalamin deficiency; cannot exclude folate deficiency
Normal	Normal	B_{12} or folate deficiency unlikely

Adapted from Snow CF, "Laboratory Diagnosis of Vitamin B_{12} and Folate Deficiency," *Arch Intern Med*, 1999, 159:1289-98.

Once the diagnosis of vitamin B_{12} or folate deficiency is established, it is then important to determine the underlying cause of the vitamin B_{12} or folate deficiency.

If the patient has folic acid deficiency ***proceed to Step 12***.

If the patient has vitamin B_{12} deficiency, ***proceed to Step 13***.

If the patient does not have vitamin B_{12} or folic acid deficiency, ***proceed to Step 16*** *on page 49.*

STEP 12 – *What Are the Causes of Folate Deficiency?*

The causes of folate deficiency are listed in the following box.

FOLATE DEFICIENCY DIFFERENTIAL DIAGNOSIS	
DECREASED INTAKE	INCREASED NEEDS
Alcoholics	Pregnancy
Old age	Lactation
Poverty	Hyperthyroidism
	Skin diseases (psoriasis)
MALABSORPTION	Dialysis
Tropical sprue	Rapid cell turnover
Nontropical sprue	Phenytoin
Infiltrative diseases	Phenobarbital
Gastrectomy	Primidone
	Hemolytic anemia
IMPAIRED METABOLISM	Multiple myeloma
Alcohol	Metastatic cancer
Methotrexate	Acute leukemia
Triamterene	
Pyrimethamine	
Trimethoprim	

Establishing the etiology of the folate deficiency begins with a thorough history and physical examination.

End of Section.

STEP 13 – *What Are the Causes of Vitamin B_{12} Deficiency?*

The causes of vitamin B_{12} deficiency are listed in the following box.

B_{12} DEFICIENCY DIFFERENTIAL DIAGNOSIS	
POOR ORAL INTAKE	MALABSORPTION
Strict vegetarians	Chronic pancreatic insufficiency
Alcoholics	Sprue (tropical, nontropical)
INCREASED NEEDS	Ileal resection
Pregnancy	Regional ileitis
Lactation	Zollinger-Ellison syndrome
Cancer	FISH TAPEWORM
Hyperthyroidism	*Diphyllobothrium latum*
POSTGASTRECTOMY	TRANSPORT PROTEIN DEFECTS
PERNICIOUS ANEMIA	MEDICATIONS
BACTERIAL OVERGROWTH	Colchicine
Fistula	PAS
Diverticulosis	NITROUS OXIDE ADMINISTRATION
Blind loops	
Strictures	
CONGENITAL INTRINSIC FACTOR DEFICIENCY	

Proceed to Step 14.

STEP 14 – *Does the Patient Have Pernicious Anemia?*

The initial step in determining the etiology of vitamin B_{12} deficiency is to assay for antiparietal and anti-intrinsic factor antibodies to evaluate for the presence of pernicious anemia, the most common cause of vitamin B_{12} deficiency.

Pernicious anemia is characterized by the presence of a variety of autoantibodies. Antiparietal cell antibodies are present in approximately 85% of patients with pernicious anemia. While these autoantibodies are present in many patients with pernicious anemia, they may also be demonstrated in patients with autoimmune endocrinopathies. In addition, up to 10% of normal individuals may have detectable antiparietal cell antibodies.

In contrast, anti-intrinsic factor antibodies are highly specific for pernicious anemia. These antibodies have been found in a minority of Graves' disease patients and in up to 20% of patients with the Lambert-Easton myasthenic syndrome. Sensitivity of the anti-intrinsic factor antibody, however, is only 50%. Therefore, negative results do not exclude the diagnosis of pernicious anemia and demand further workup for this disorder. Of note, falsely-negative test results have been reported if the test is performed within a few days after the parenteral administration of vitamin B_{12}.

If the antibody testing is positive and suspicion for pernicious anemia is high, no further testing is necessary.

If the antibody testing is negative, ***proceed to Step 15.***

STEP 15 – *What Are the Results of the Schilling Test?*

Although negative results of antibody testing do not definitively exclude the diagnosis of pernicious anemia, it certainly becomes less likely. In these patients, the clinician should consider other causes of vitamin B_{12} deficiency. The key to elucidating the etiology is a thorough history and physical examination in combination with the Schilling test. To interpret the results of the Schilling test, the clinician must be familiar with vitamin B_{12} absorption.

Foods of animal origin are rich in vitamin B_{12}. Ingested B_{12} binds to gastric R binder. Upon entry into the duodenum, this complex separates and B_{12} binds to intrinsic factor (secreted by parietal cells). This complex travels to the distal ileum where it binds to receptors and is subsequently absorbed. Any condition that affects this process can lead to vitamin B_{12} deficiency.

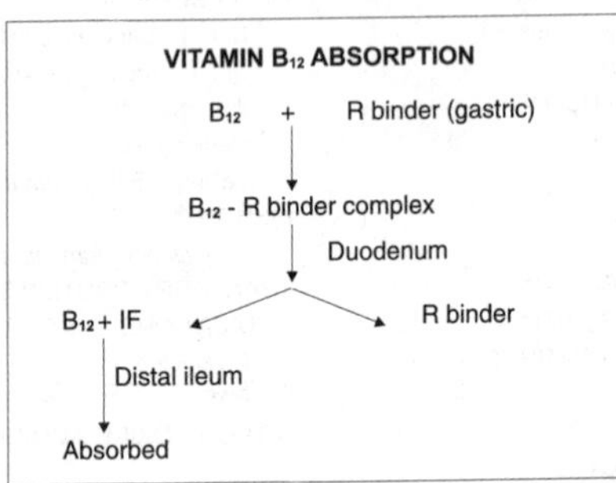

The Schilling test involves the simultaneous administration of unlabeled vitamin B_{12} (intramuscular) and radiolabeled vitamin B_{12} (oral). Intramuscular B_{12} serves to saturate tissue binding sites so some of the radiolabeled B_{12} will be excreted in the urine. Normally, >7% of the radiolabeled B_{12} is excreted in the urine over a 24-hour period. An abnormal result should be followed by a repeat test using intrinsic factor as well. If excretion normalizes, a diagnosis of pernicious anemia can be made. If the test remains abnormal, a repeat test adding an antibiotic may be administered. Correction with an antibiotic suggests that bacterial overgrowth is the cause of the B_{12} deficiency. If the test still remains abnormal after the antibiotic, then the underlying etiology is malabsorption. Accuracy of the Schilling test requires normal renal function and a 24-hour urine collection that is complete.

SCHILLING TEST

Schilling test is performed in 2 stages. However, stage 2 is performed only if stage 1 results are abnormal.

In stage 1, patient receives, simultaneously, 1 mg of unlabeled vitamin B_{12} (intramuscular injection) to saturate vitamin B_{12}-binding proteins and 1 microgram of radiolabeled crystalline vitamin B_{12} (oral). A 24-hour urinary collection follows immediately; if detected radioactivity in the urine is >7% of ingested load, result is normal, and patient has no problem absorbing "crystalline" vitamin B_{12}.

- Normal stage 1 results rule out pernicious anemia but not malabsorption from gastric atrophy. (Elderly patients may have difficulty absorbing food-bound vitamin B_{12}, which requires gastric acid and pepsin to release vitamin B_{12}.)
- Abnormal stage 1 results suggest either pernicious anemia or a primary intestinal malabsorption disorder. Rare instances of intestinal bacterial overgrowth and pancreatic insufficiency also may cause abnormal stage 1 results.

Correction of abnormal stage 1 results by adding intrinsic factor (60 mg) to oral vitamin B_{12} dose (stage 2) establishes the diagnosis of pernicious anemia. However, abnormal stage 2 results do not rule out the possibility of pernicious anemia because the disease may secondarily affect intestinal epithelium and mimic a primary malabsorptive syndrome. Therefore, the best time to do the Schilling test is after 2 weeks of treatment with vitamin B_{12}, which allows healing of absorptive surface.

From Tefferi A, "Anemia in Adults: A Contemporary Approach to Diagnosis," *Mayo Clin Proc*, 2003, 78:1274-1280 (this box from page 1279).

There are several limitations of the Schilling's test that the clinician should be aware of, including the following.

- 24-hour urine collection is cumbersome (can lead to incomplete collection)
- Test validity depends upon the presence of normal renal function
- Test validity depends upon the presence of normal intestinal mucosa

An incomplete urine collection is a common cause of invalid Schilling's test results, which is why it is important to measure the urine creatinine in the sample to ensure the adequacy of the collection. The clinician should keep these factors in mind when interpreting the results of the Schilling's test.

End of Section.

STEP 16 – *What Are the Causes of Nonmegaloblastic Anemia?*

Once vitamin B_{12} and folic acid deficiency have been excluded, the clinician should focus on the other causes of macrocytic anemia. The other causes of macrocytic anemia include the following.

- Alcoholism

  Alcoholism is a common cause of macrocytosis. In many patients who drink excessive amounts of alcohol, macrocytosis may be present in the absence of anemia. With the development of alcoholic liver disease, the hemoglobin may fall, resulting in macrocytic anemia.

- Liver disease

  Excessive lipid deposition on red blood cell membranes occurs in patients with liver disease. This may lead to the development of macrocytic anemia. Although any type of liver disease may be associated with macrocytic anemia, the rise in MCV seems to be more pronounced in alcoholic liver disease.

- Myelodysplastic syndrome

  Myelodysplastic syndrome may present with anemia alone or anemia in combination with leukopenia and/or thrombocytopenia. In addition to decreased numbers of red blood cells, platelets, and white blood cells, qualitative changes in the cells may also be present (dysplastic changes). The definitive diagnosis requires bone marrow biopsy. See Myelodysplastic Syndrome *on page 40* for more information.

- Aplastic anemia

  Aplastic anemia needs to be considered in every anemic patient with macrocytosis who has a pancytopenia. This is not specific for aplastic anemia as pancytopenia may also be appreciated in other causes of macrocytic anemia (ie, myelodysplastic syndrome, megaloblastic anemia). The definitive diagnosis requires bone marrow biopsy. See Aplastic Anemia *on page 37* for more information.

- Pure red cell aplasia

  Pure red cell aplasia, as its name suggests, affects only the red blood cell line. See Pure Red Cell Aplasia *on page 38* for more information.

- Hypothyroidism

  The diagnosis of hypothyroidism can be established by obtaining thyroid function tests.

- Multiple myeloma

  MCV may be elevated in the presence of a paraproteinemia such as multiple myeloma.

- Drug-induced

  Many drugs including antiretroviral agents and chemotherapeutic agents can interrupt DNA synthesis, manifesting with macrocytosis.

In these patients, the workup should include liver and thyroid function tests to exclude liver disease and hypothyroidism, respectively. Aplastic anemia should be a consideration if all three cell lines are depressed. Depression of other cell lines should also prompt consideration of myelodysplastic syndrome although, in some cases, only anemia is present. One clue to the presence of a primary bone marrow abnormality (ie., aplastic anemia, myelodysplastic syndrome, pure red cell aplasia) is the presence of marked macrocytosis. In general, the most common causes of impressive macrocytosis are vitamin B_{12} deficiency, folic acid deficiency, and medications but if these are excluded, the most likely explanation is primary bone marrow disease. The clinician should realize, however, that primary bone marrow disorders may also present with mild macrocytosis. The definitive diagnosis of aplastic anemia, pure red cell aplasia, and myelodysplastic syndrome requires bone marrow biopsy.

End of Section.

STEP 17 – *What Is the Approach to the Patient With Anemia and RPI >2?*

There are only three causes of anemia associated with a RPI >2, as shown in the following box.

CAUSES OF ANEMIA AND RPI >2
ANEMIA OF ACUTE BLOOD LOSS HEMOLYSIS RESPONSE TO THERAPY

Response to therapy (iron, B_{12}, or folate repletion in deficiency states) should be readily apparent. Most patients with anemia and RPI >2 will have the anemia of acute blood loss or hemolysis. It is important to realize, however, that hemolysis and acute blood loss can be associated with a low RPI if the patient has a condition that is impairing red blood cell production (eg, iron or folate deficiency). Both conditions may also present with a low RPI if the reticulocyte count is determined early in the disease process. Another cause of a low RPI in the patient with hemolysis include antibody-mediated destruction of red blood cell precursors.

In usual clinical practice, it is not difficult to differentiate between these two causes of anemia. In the anemia of acute blood loss, the source of blood loss is usually quite clear. The gastrointestinal tract is most often implicated. Other sources of bleeding need to be considered as well, including genitourinary, retroperitoneal, intrapulmonary, and intra-articular blood loss.

The hemoglobin after an acute bleed is often normal. This is because sufficient time has not passed for hemodilution to occur. After about 24 hours or so, there will be a shift of volume from the extravascular space to the intravascular space to replenish volume deficit. This will lead to a fall in the hemoglobin level.

The reticulocyte count may be normal for the first several days after the acute event but will increase shortly thereafter. A brisk reticulocytosis may result in a mildly macrocytic anemia. Prior to the decrease in the hemoglobin level, laboratory studies may reveal leukocytosis and thrombocytosis. Immature red and white blood cells, including metamyelocytes, myelocytes, and nucleated red blood cells may be seen with severe hemorrhage.

If the patient has the anemia of acute blood loss, ***stop here.***

If the patient does not have the anemia of acute blood loss, ***proceed to Step 18.***

STEP 18 – *Does the Patient Have Hemolysis?*

Once the anemia of acute blood loss has been excluded, the clinician should consider hemolysis as the etiology of the anemia. Laboratory testing plays a key role in establishing whether or not the patient has a hemolytic anemia. The laboratory test findings supportive of hemolysis are listed in the following box.

LABORATORY TEST FINDINGS INDICATIVE OF HEMOLYSIS
DECREASED HAPTOGLOBIN*
ELEVATED BILIRUBIN (unconjugated)†
ELEVATED LDH
POSITIVE URINE HEMOGLOBIN‡
POSITIVE URINE HEMOSIDERIN§
INCREASED PLASMA HEMOGLOBIN (hemoglobinemia)¶

*Released hemoglobin from damaged red blood cells complexes with haptoglobin. This complex is cleared by the liver. In states of hemolysis, then, haptoglobin is often low. Haptoglobin may also be low in patients with hepatic disease secondary to decreased production. Haptoglobin deficiency has also been reported in some African-Americans (genetic). One important point is that haptoglobin, like ferritin, is an acute phase reactant. If there is accompanying inflammation, the haptoglobin may be misleadingly normal or even high. In general, low haptoglobin levels are usually noted in patients with intravascular hemolysis. Low levels may not always be seen, however, in extravascular hemolysis.

†Unconjugated hyperbilirubinemia results from hemolysis. Rarely does the bilirubin exceed 5 mg/dL in uncomplicated hemolysis.

‡When the hemoglobin that is released overwhelms the binding ability of haptoglobin, hemoglobin is freely filtered at the glomerulus. In this setting, renal tubular cells absorb the hemoglobin. However, if the absorptive ability is exceeded, free hemoglobin may be detected on the urinalysis. The presence of free hemoglobin should be suspected when the urinalysis reveals positive blood but few red blood cells (ie, disparity between the dipstick test for blood and microscopic analysis of the urine for red blood cells).

§Hemosiderin is produced from hemoglobin in renal tubular cells. Several days after the hemolytic episode, renal tubular cells may be shed in the urine leading to a positive test for urine hemosiderin. Therefore, a negative result for urine hemosiderin does not exclude hemolysis in cases in which hemolysis has been recent. This test is most useful in patients with intravascular hemolysis.

¶Normal plasma hemoglobin levels are <10 mg/dL. Levels >50 mg/dL are consistent with hemolysis. Plasma becomes cherry-red at levels >150-200 mg/dL. This test is most useful in patients with intravascular hemolysis.

It is important to note that any of the above tests may be normal in the presence of hemolysis. For this reason, it is necessary to obtain several of these tests, as at least one of them will be abnormal in the setting of hemolytic disease. After hemolysis has been established, the cause needs to be identified.

Once the presence of hemolysis has been established, it is often useful to determine if the patient is having intravascular or extravascular hemolysis. Intravascular hemolysis refers to hemolysis occurring within blood vessels. Hemolysis that takes place in the spleen and liver is known as extravascular hemolysis. The distinction can be made by carefully considering the patient's clinical presentation, as shown in the following table.

Differentiating Intravascular From Extravascular Hemolysis

Type	All Types of Hemolytic Anemia	Intravascular Hemolytic Anemia	Extravascular Hemolytic Anemia
Reticulocyte count	↑	↑	↑
LDH	↑	↑	↑
Indirect bilirubin	↑ or normal	↑	↑ or normal
Haptoglobin	↓	↓	↓
Urinary hemosiderin	±	+	–

From Tefferi A, "Anemia in Adults: A Contemporary Approach to Diagnosis," *Mayo Clin Proc*, 2003, 78:1274-80 (this box from page 1276).

Proceed to Step 19.

STEP 19 – *What Are the Results of the Direct Coombs' Test (Direct Antiglobulin Test)?*

Once the presence of hemolysis has been established, a direct Coombs' test, also known as the direct antiglobulin test, should be obtained to differentiate between immune and nonimmune hemolytic anemia.

This test was first described in 1945 when Coombs injected human serum into rabbits. As a result, antibodies were produced against the antibodies present in human serum. These antibodies that are produced can be referred to as antihuman antibodies. When the red blood cells of a patient are coated with immunoglobulin or complement, the addition of these antihuman antibodies will cause agglutination to occur. This is referred to as a positive Coombs' or direct antiglobulin test. In the setting of anemia, a positive direct Coombs' test is consistent with the possibility of immune hemolysis.

It is important to realize, however, that a positive direct Coombs' test is not synonymous with the presence of autoimmune hemolytic anemia. Causes of positive direct Coombs' test in the absence of hemolysis include advancing age, systemic lupus erythematosus, HIV/AIDS, multiple myeloma, sickle cell disease, renal disease, transplantation, and medications (hydralazine, procainamide, IVIG, antilymphocyte globulin, antithymocyte globulin, Rh immune globulin, others). Of note, up to 0.1% and 8% of healthy blood donors and hospitalized patients, respectively, have a positive direct Coombs' test without having any evidence of autoimmune hemolytic anemia. Therefore, a positive direct Coombs' test merely suggests that if hemolysis is present, an immune mechanism is very possible.

A negative direct Coombs' test does not exclude the possibility of immune hemolytic anemia. For example, transfusion with incompatible blood may result in massive and complete hemolysis. In this case, the direct Coombs' test may be negative. The clinician should understand the limitations of using the direct Coombs' test to classify hemolytic anemia as immune or nonimmune.

If the direct Coombs' test is negative, ***proceed to Step 20.***

If the direct Coombs' test is positive, ***proceed to Step 21.***

STEP 20 – *What Is the Approach to the Patient With Nonimmune Hemolytic Anemia?*

A negative direct Coombs' test provides evidence against an immune etiology for the hemolysis. The clinician should consider causes of nonimmune hemolytic anemia, which are listed in the following box.

NONIMMUNE HEMOLYTIC ANEMIA
DIFFERENTIAL DIAGNOSIS

ABNORMALITIES OF THE RED CELL MEMBRANE
- Hereditary spherocytosis
- Hereditary elliptocytosis
- Hereditary stomatocytosis
- Paroxysmal nocturnal hemoglobinuria (PNH)
- Spur cell anemia

ARSINE GAS

COPPER
- Intoxication during suicide attempts
- Wilson's disease

DISORDERS WITHIN THE RBC
- Enzyme deficiency (G6PD, pyruvate kinase)
- Hemoglobinopathies

(continued)

NONIMMUNE HEMOLYTIC ANEMIA DIFFERENTIAL DIAGNOSIS
HYPERSPLENISM INFECTION Babesiosis Bartonellosis Clostridia Malaria MICROANGIOPATHIC HEMOLYTIC ANEMIA Allograft rejection Disseminated intravascular coagulation Disseminated cancer Eclampsia Hemangioma Hemolytic-uremic syndrome Malignant hypertension Thrombotic thrombocytopenic purpura PROSTHETIC HEART VALVE SEVERE BURNS SNAKE / SPIDER BITES

The peripheral blood smear can provide clues to the etiology of the nonimmune hemolytic anemia, as shown in the following table.

Using the Peripheral Blood Smear to Elucidate the Etiology of Nonimmune Hemolytic Anemia

Peripheral Blood Smear Finding	Etiology of Nonimmune Hemolytic Anemia Suggested
Spherocytes	Burns Hereditary spherocytosis
Target cells	Hemoglobinopathies
Schistocytes	Microangiopathic hemolytic anemia
Helmet cells	Prosthetic heart valves Microangiopathic hemolytic anemia
Other cell fragments	Severe burns
Bite or blister cell	G6PD deficiency
Elliptocytes	Hereditary elliptocytosis
Stomatocytes	Hereditary stomatocytosis
Sickle cells	Sickle cell anemia
Intraerythrocytic inclusions	Malaria Babesiosis Bartonellosis
Heinz bodies	G6PD deficiency

Some of the major causes of nonimmune hemolytic anemia will be discussed in the remainder of this step.

Hereditary Spherocytosis (HS)

Although hereditary spherocytosis is more common among those of Northern European descent, it is seen in all races. This autosomal dominant condition manifests considerable variability in its severity, ranging from a relatively well compensated to a fairly severe hemolytic anemia. The variability in severity explains the broad age range at which it may be initially diagnosed. The more severe forms of the disease are usually diagnosed in children. However, it is not unusual for milder forms of the disease to escape detection until adulthood.

HS should be considered in the patient with chronic hemolysis found to have spherocytes on examination of the peripheral blood smear. When such a patient is encountered, evaluation of family members may reveal asymptomatic individuals with spherocytes as well. The hemoglobin level typically ranges between 9 and 12 g/dL (can be normal as well). Very characteristic of this disease is an increase in MCHC (may also be at the upper end of normal range). An osmotic fragility test is often performed to help establish the presence of osmotically fragile red blood cells. A positive osmotic fragility test only establishes the presence of spherocytes. It does not, however, differentiate HS from other disorders characterized by spherocytes, such as autoimmune hemolytic anemia. The Coombs' test is helpful in this regard, being negative in HS. The diagnosis of HS can be established by flow cytometry or quantification of spectrin and other red blood cell membrane proteins.

Paroxysmal Nocturnal Hemoglobinuria (PNH)

PNH, a rare disorder, often presents with pancytopenia. In this condition, the red blood cell membrane has a defect which makes the cell abnormally sensitive to complement-mediated lysis. The anemia may vary from mild to severe and is usually normocytic and normochromic. Patients with PNH may also become iron deficient, resulting in the appearance of microcytic hypochromic cells in the peripheral blood smear. A leukocyte alkaline phosphatase (LAP) score can help distinguish PNH from aplastic anemia. PNH is characterized by a low LAP score, whereas aplastic anemia usually has a normal or elevated level. Urine hemosiderin is usually detectable. Bone marrow examination usually reveals erythroid hyperplasia, but, in some patients, cellularity may be decreased. Prussian blue staining for iron usually reveals the absence of iron stores. Tests that are commonly performed to establish the diagnosis include the sucrose hemolysis and Ham's tests.

PNH LABORATORY VALUES
NORMOCYTIC NORMOCHROMIC ANEMIA*
WBC AND PLATELETS OFTEN DECREASED
DECREASED LAP SCORE
POSITIVE HAM'S TEST
POSITIVE SUCROSE HEMOLYSIS TEST
POSITIVE URINE HEMOSIDERIN

*Can also be microcytic.

Recently, a flow cytometric test has been developed and found to have a high sensitivity and specificity for the diagnosis.

G6PD Deficiency

Glucose-6-phosphate dehydrogenase (G6PD) is the initial enzyme of the pentose phosphate pathway. It is integral in the production of NADPH which helps red blood cells resist oxidant stress. The normal G6PD variant is referred to as the B variant. The A variant is found in 16% of African-American males and is not associated with disease. A defective A variant exists and is known as the A- variant. It is the A- variant that predisposes to the development of hemolytic anemia when oxidant stress occurs. Under normal conditions, anemia is absent in most patients. These variants can be demonstrated by electrophoresis.

The G6PD gene is carried on the X chromosome and is therefore inherited in a sex-linked pattern. As a result, the disease is fully expressed in affected males. In women who are heterozygous for the abnormal G6PD gene, the blood will contain both normal and G6PD RBCs. Some of these women are fully affected while others are completely healthy.

G6PD deficiency manifests as hemolysis when susceptible patients are infected or exposed to certain medications. Offending medications include primaquine, nitrofurantoin, sulfa drugs, and quinine. These as well as other precipitants of hemolysis in G6PD deficient patients are listed in the following box.

PRECIPITANTS OF HEMOLYSIS IN G6PD DEFICIENCY

- INFECTION
- EXPOSURE TO FAVA BEANS
- MEDICATIONS
  - Antimalarial drugs
    - Primaquine
    - Quinacrine
  - Antibacterial agents
    - Sulfonamides
    - Nitrofurantoin
    - Nitrofurazone
    - Nalidixic acid
    - Para-aminosalicylic acid
  - Acetanilid
  - Sulfones
    - Diaminodiphenyl sulfone
    - Thiazolsulfone
  - Dimercaprol
  - Methylene blue
  - Naphthalene
  - Trinitrotoluene

Oxidant stress leads to intravascular hemolysis, which is characterized by hemoglobinemia, hemoglobinuria, and decreasing hemoglobin. When precipitated by an offending medication, the manifestations of the acute hemolysis become evident within 1-3 days after drug administration. In most cases, the hemolysis is self-limited because younger red blood cells with enough G6PD remain to combat the stress.

The peripheral blood smear reveals fragmented red blood cells as well as blister cells. The blister cell results from the oxidative denaturation of hemoglobin which appears to separate from the membrane of the red blood cell (looking like a blister). Heinz bodies are characteristic red blood cell inclusions that develop in this disorder as well. Supravital staining is required to appreciate these inclusions.

Screening tests that are available for the diagnosis of G6PD deficiency include the fluorescein spot and the methemoglobin reduction tests. These tests are not so useful in the patient with active hemolysis, because the remaining cells (those that have not hemolyzed) as well as the newly produced RBCs, are not deficient in G6PD. In these cases, it is best to repeat the test in several weeks to months.

Hemoglobinopathy (ie, Sickle Cell Anemia)

Sickle cell anemia (Hb SS disease) is characterized by severe anemia. Patients with sickle cell anemia lack normal hemoglobin A since they are homozygous for hemoglobin S. Individuals have a moderate to severe hemolytic anemia complicated, at times, by episodes of increased hemolysis known as hemolytic crisis, as well as aplastic crisis. Aplastic crisis usually involves the acquisition of a virus, most commonly parvovirus, which results in bone marrow aplasia. Cessation of erythropoiesis leads to an impressive decrease in hemoglobin, often to life-threatening levels. Aplastic crisis can also occur in patients not receiving folic acid supplementation.

The hemoglobin level is typically between 6 and 10 g/dL. The peripheral blood smear reveals considerable target cells, fragmented red blood cells, nucleated red blood cells, polychromasia, and sickle cells. Sickle cells may comprise 6% to 18% of all red blood cells. It is not uncommon to have an accompanying leukocytosis or thrombocytosis. During painful crises, leukocytosis is quite common, with white blood cell counts sometimes rising to very high levels (40-50 X 10^9/L). The reticulocyte count is typically elevated except when sickle cell anemia is complicated by an aplastic crisis. Bone marrow examination is not necessary but will reveal erythroid hyperplasia except when complicated by aplasia.

Screening solubility tests are available that detect the presence of sickle hemoglobin. One such test is the sodium metabisulfite test, a reducing agent which induces sickling. False-negative test results may occur if outdated metabisulfite reagent is used.

The gold standard, however, is hemoglobin electrophoresis. Since the patient with sickle cell anemia does not produce any normal chains, electrophoresis will not show the presence of any hemoglobin A (Hb A). However, Hb A may be appreciated if hemoglobin electrophoresis is done on a blood specimen after transfusion. Usually, >80% of the hemoglobin is represented by hemoglobin S.

Many other hemoglobinopathies besides sickle cell anemia are recognized. It is important to realize that these disorders can only be definitively diagnosed by laboratory tests that establish the presence of an abnormal hemoglobin. In this regard, hemoglobin electrophoresis is essential. In normal individuals, approximately 97% of the hemoglobin found in red blood cells is hemoglobin A. The remainder consists of hemoglobin A_2 and F. In the hemoglobinopathies, electrophoretic analysis will often establish the presence of an abnormal hemoglobin and the hemoglobin that is separated can be quantitated. Using all this information, most hemoglobinopathies can be detected. However, it is important to realize that some of the more uncommon hemoglobinopathies may be silent electrophoretically.

Microangiopathic Hemolytic Anemia

A microangiopathic hemolytic anemia occurs when capillaries are partially occluded by fibrin. This leads to the fragmentation of red cells. The peripheral blood smear characteristically shows schistocytes and helmet cells as well as a decrease in the number of platelets. The causes of microangiopathic hemolytic anemia have been considered earlier in this step.

End of Section.

STEP 21 – *What Is the Approach to the Patient With Autoimmune Hemolytic Anemia?*

A positive direct Coombs' test is consistent with the presence of an autoimmune hemolytic anemia. It is important to understand that a positive direct Coombs' test result does not definitively establish the presence of immune hemolysis. A positive result connotes that an immune mechanism may be involved if hemolysis is present.

In autoimmune hemolytic anemia, red blood cells are destroyed by antibodies directed against red blood cell antigens. The three major types of autoimmune hemolytic anemia include the following:

- Warm autoimmune hemolytic anemia
- Drug-induced hemolytic anemia
- Cold autoimmune hemolytic anemia

The terms "warm" and "cold" refer to the temperature at which the autoantibody is most active. Warm-type antibodies are most active at 37°C while cold-type autoantibodies are most active at 0-4°C. Occasionally, patients have a combination of warm and cold autoantibodies.

Warm Autoimmune Hemolytic Anemia

Warm autoimmune hemolytic anemia is much more common than cold autoimmune hemolytic anemia. In fact, warm autoimmune hemolytic anemia accounts for about 70% of cases. Most cases involve IgG autoantibodies. When the red blood cell is significantly coated by IgG, however, complement may also bind to the membrane of the red blood cell.

Warm autoimmune hemolytic anemia can vary from a mildly compensated disorder to a particularly severe anemia. Hemoglobinemia and hemoglobinuria are uncommon. The peripheral blood smear shows polychromasia and spherocytes. Nucleated red blood cells and granulocytic precursors may be appreciated in more severe cases. The smear may also reveal findings consistent with an underlying disease such as chronic lymphocytic leukemia, large granular lymphocytic leukemia, or non-Hodgkin's lymphoma. It is not uncommon for leukocytosis and thrombocytosis to accompany the autoimmune hemolytic anemia. Some patients, however, may have an associated immune thrombocytopenia, which is termed the Evans' syndrome.

As discussed above, the direct Coombs' test will be positive using a polyspecific or "broad spectrum" antiglobulin reagent. A polyspecific antiglobulin reagent is one that contains antibodies directed against immunoglobulin and complement. If agglutination with polyspecific sera is appreciated, further evaluation includes the direct Coombs' test using a monospecific antiglobulin reagent. Monospecific sera refers to the use of first antisera directed against immunoglobulin, and then against complement, to determine the specific pattern of red blood cell sensitization. This test will be positive for both IgG and C3 in 24% to 63% of cases. In the remaining cases, IgG (20% to 66% of cases) or C3 (7% to 14% of cases) will be positive alone. Rarely, the direct Coombs' test may be negative in the setting of a warm autoimmune hemolytic anemia.

Warm autoimmune hemolytic anemia may be idiopathic or secondary to an underlying disease. Although it varies depending upon the type of population studied, a secondary cause can be identified in 20% to 80% of cases. Among the secondary causes, lymphoproliferative disorders account for about 50% of cases with autoimmune disorders representing the second most common cause.

WARM AIHA DIFFERENTIAL DIAGNOSIS	
CONNECTIVE TISSUE DISEASES	MALIGNANCY
Rheumatoid arthritis	Chronic lymphocytic leukemia
Scleroderma	Lymphoma (Hodgkin's, non-Hodgkin's)
Systemic lupus erythematosus	Multiple myeloma
Ulcerative colitis	Waldenström's macroglobulinemia
IDIOPATHIC	Solid tumors (rare)
IMMUNODEFICIENCY STATES	Ovarian dermoid cysts
Dysglobulinemia	Teratomas
AIDS	Kaposi's sarcoma
Hypogammaglobulinemia	Carcinomas
INFECTION	Thymoma

In some cases of warm autoimmune hemolytic anemia, the etiology is readily apparent. For example, there may be little diagnostic difficulty in the systemic lupus erythematosus patient who develops an immune hemolytic anemia. In other cases, the etiology is not so clear. In these cases, antinuclear antibody testing (ANA) should be performed, particularly in women. A positive test result should prompt consideration of systemic lupus erythematosus or another connective tissue disease. The clinician should realize that warm autoimmune hemolytic anemia may precede other manifestations of connective tissue disease by months or even years.

Another major cause of warm autoimmune hemolytic anemia is lymphoma. In some cases, the immune hemolytic anemia precedes the diagnosis of lymphoma by years. In other cases, the diagnosis of warm autoimmune hemolytic anemia prompts an examination that results in the discovery of lymphoma. In all patients with warm autoimmune hemolytic anemia, a thorough physical examination of lymph node areas, liver, and spleen is warranted. If lymphadenopathy, hepatomegaly, or splenomegaly are detected, a biopsy should be performed.

Drug-Induced Hemolytic Anemia

Drug-induced hemolytic anemia must also be considered in the differential diagnosis of a Coombs' positive hemolytic anemia. The three major mechanisms of drug-induced hemolytic anemia include the following:

- Hapten type
- Immune complex type
- Warm-type autoantibodies

Features of drug-induced hemolytic anemia are described in the following table.

Features of Drug-Induced Hemolytic Anemia

Parameter	Drug Absorption, Hapten Formation	Toxic Immune Complex	Warm-Type Autoantibodies
Associated drugs	Penicillin and penicillin-type drugs	Quinine Quinidine NSAIDs	Alpha-methyldopa Procainamide Mefenamic acid
Role of drug	Binds to RBC membrane	Forms antigen-antibody complex that binds to RBC	Unknown
Antibody formed	To drug	To drug	To RBC
Antibody class	IgG	IgM or IgG	IgG
Proteins detected with direct antiglobulin test	IgG, rarely complement	Complement	IgG, rarely complement

Adapted from Kjeldsberg CR, *Practical Diagnosis of Hematologic Disorders*, 3rd ed, Chicago, IL: ASCP Press, 2001, 210.

Cold Autoimmune Hemolytic Anemia

Cold autoimmune hemolytic anemia is less common than warm autoimmune hemolytic anemia. Nevertheless, it remains a consideration in all patients with a Coombs' positive hemolytic anemia. A positive direct Coombs' test using polyspecific sera should be followed by a direct Coombs' test using monospecific sera. In cold autoimmune hemolytic anemia, a direct Coombs' test using monospecific sera will only reveal complement.

The pathogenesis of cold autoimmune hemolytic anemia involves IgM autoantibodies. These autoantibodies have been termed "cold agglutinins" because they have a predilection to cause red blood cell agglutination at low temperatures (<16°C).

Many healthy individuals have low titers of cold agglutinins (≤1:32). Although these antibodies (cold agglutinins) are present in low titers in normal serum, they are not pathologic. In certain conditions, however, there may be increased production of IgM. At times, these higher titers of cold agglutinins may be clinically significant, manifesting as cold autoimmune hemolytic anemia.

When increased cold agglutinins (high titer) are present or the agglutinins are associated with a large thermal amplitude, the patient is said to have cold autoimmune hemolytic anemia. A titer ≤1:32 is considered to be physiologic. A titer ≥1:64 is considered to be pathologic.

Quite often, it is laboratory testing that first brings patients with cold agglutinin syndrome to clinical attention. After determination of the CBC and inspection of the peripheral blood smear, the lab may report that clumping is present. The MCV may be artifactually elevated due to the red blood cell clumping. In addition to agglutination, the peripheral blood smear may also reveal anisocytosis, poikilocytosis, and polychromasia.

Once the presence of cold autoimmune hemolytic anemia has been established, the clinician should then try to ascertain the cause of the immune hemolytic anemia. The causes of cold autoimmune hemolytic anemia are listed in the following box.

CAUSES OF COLD AUTOIMMUNE HEMOLYTIC ANEMIA

IDIOPATHIC

INFECTION
- *M. pneumoniae*
- Epstein-Barr virus
- CMV
- Adenovirus
- Influenza
- Varicella-zoster virus
- HIV
- *L. monocytogenes*
- *E. coli*

MALIGNANCY
- Lymphoma
- Leukemia
- Carcinoma
  - Squamous cell (lung)
  - Colon
  - Adrenal
  - Basal cell
- Myeloma

Depending on the patient population studied, a secondary cause of cold autoimmune hemolytic anemia can be found in 20% to 80% of cases. Lymphoproliferative disorders are responsible for approximately 50% of secondary cases while infection is the second most common cause. The disease tends to be transient in cases associated with infection while idiopathic or secondary cold autoimmune hemolytic anemia due to lymphoproliferative disorder runs a chronic course.

In some cases of cold autoimmune hemolytic anemia, the cause may be readily apparent. For example, the cold autoimmune hemolytic anemia secondary to mycoplasmal pneumonia or infectious mononucleosis typically develops during or following the illness. In other cases, however, the etiology may not be so clear. In these cases, further evaluation to determine the etiology of cold autoimmune hemolytic anemia may include antibody testing for viral causes (EBV, CMV) or radiologic evaluation for an occult lymphoproliferative disorder.

The clinical and laboratory features of warm and cold autoimmune hemolytic anemia are listed in the following table.

Clinical Laboratory Characteristics of Autoimmune Hemolytic Anemia

Clinical or Laboratory Finding	WAHA	CAHA
Onset	Abrupt	Insidious
Jaundice	Usually present	Often absent
Splenomegaly	Yes	Absent
Age	All ages	All ages
Sex	Slightly more women	Women predominate
Autoantibody origin		
idiopathic	50% to 60%	30% to 40%
drug-induced	25% to 30%	1% to 5%
LPD	10% to 15%	15% to 20%
viral or *Mycoplasma*	0%	25% to 35%
Other (inflammatory diseases, other malignancy)	5% to 10%	5% to 10%
Usual immunoglobulin type	IgG	IgM

Clinical Laboratory Characteristics of Autoimmune Hemolytic Anemia *(continued)*

Clinical or Laboratory Finding	WAHA	CAHA
Direct antibody test		
Monospecific sera		
anti-IgG only	1+	0
anti-IgG + anti-CI	1+	0
anti-CI only	Rare	1+
Complement activation	Little or none	Yes
Serum complement levels	Normal or decreased	Decreased
Peripheral blood findings	Spherocytes Nucleated RBCs	RBC agglutination

WAHA = warm autoimmune hemolytic anemia.

CAHA = cold autoimmune hemolytic anemia.

LPD = lymphoproliferative disorder.

Adapted from Kjeldsberg CR, *Practical Diagnosis of Hematologic Disorders*, 3rd ed, Chicago, IL: ASCP Press, 2001, 220-1.

Paroxysmal Cold Hemoglobinuria (PCH)

PCH also deserves mention as a cause of autoimmune hemolytic anemia. It is the least common type of autoimmune hemolytic anemia. It was originally described in patients with syphilis but is now rarely seen in this setting. Most cases seen today are transient and due to infection, primarily in children. Infectious agents that have been identified in PCH patients include EBV, CMV, adenovirus, *M. pneumoniae, E. coli, H. influenzae*, VZV, influenza, measles, and mumps. Hemolysis in this disease is secondary to a cold autoantibody, known as an autohemolysin. This autohemolysin reacts with the patient's red cells at a low temperature leading to complement activation, which is more prominent at higher temperatures (37°C). Interestingly, this autoantibody is IgG in nature and is termed the Donath-Landsteiner antibody. The Donath-Landsteiner test allows paroxysmal cold hemoglobinuria to be distinguished from cold autoimmune hemolytic anemia.

References

Balaban EP, Sheehan RG, Demian SE, et al, "Evaluation of Bone Marrow Iron Stores in Anemia Associated With Chronic Disease: A Comparative Study of Serum and Red Cell Ferritin," *Am J Hematol*, 1993, 42(2):177-81.

Bessman JD, Gilmer PR, and Gardener FH, "Improved Classification of Anemias by MCV and RDW," *Am J Clin Pathol*, 1983, 80(3):322-6.

Carmel R, "A Focused Approach to Anemia," *Hosp Pract*, 1999, 34(2):71-8, 81-5, 89-90.

Eldibany MM, Totonchi KF, Joseph NJ, et al, "Usefulness of Certain Red Blood Cell Indices in Diagnosing and Differentiating Thalassemia Trait From Iron-Deficiency Anemia," *Am J Clin Pathol*, 1999, 111(5):676-82.

Erslev AJ and Soltan A, "Pure Red-Cell Aplasia: A Review," *Blood Rev*, 1996, 10(1):20-8 (review).

Green R, "Metabolite Assays in Cobalamin and Folate Deficiency," *Baillieres Clin Haematol*, 1995, 8(3):533-66 (review).

Guinan EC, "Clinical Aspects of Aplastic Anemia," *Hematol Oncol Clin North Am*, 1997, 11(6):1025-44 (review).

Guyatt GH, Oxman AD, Ali M, et al, "Laboratory Diagnosis of Iron Deficiency Anemia: An Overview," *J Gen Intern Med*, 1992, 7(2):145-53 (review).

Hashimoto C, "Autoimmune Hemolytic Anemia," *Clin Rev Allergy Immunol*, 1998, 16(3):285-95 (review).

Hocking WG, "Hematologic Abnormalities in Patients With Renal Diseases," *Hematol Oncol Clin North Am*, 1987, 1(2):229-60 (review).

Mason PJ, "New Insights Into G6PD Deficiency," *Br J Haematol*, 1996, 94(4):585-91.

Mast AE, Blinder MA, Gronowski AM, et al, "Clinical Utility of the Soluble Transferrin Receptor and Comparison With Serum Ferritin in Several Populations," *Clin Chem*, 1998, 44(1):45-51.

Moliterno AR and Spivak JL, "Anemia of Cancer," *Hematol Oncol Clin North Am*, 1996, 10(2):345-63 (review).

North M, Dallalio G, Donath AS, et al, "Serum Transferrin Receptor Levels in Patients Undergoing Evaluation of Iron Stores: Correlation With Other Parameters, and Observed Versus Predicted Results," *Clin Lab Haematol*, 1997, 19(2):93-7.

Packman CH, "Pathogenesis and Management of Paroxysmal Nocturnal Hemoglobinuria," *Blood Rev*, 1998, 12(1):1-11 (review).

Petz LD, "Drug-Induced Autoimmune Hemolytic Anemia," *Transfus Med Rev*, 1993, 7(4):242-54 (review).

Toh BH, van Driel IR, and Gleeson PA, "Pernicious Anemia," *N Engl J Med*, 1997, 337(2):1441-8 (review).

Wickramasinghe SN, "The Wide Spectrum and Unresolved Issues of Megaloblastic Anemia," *Semin Hematol*, 1999, 36(1):3-18 (review).

Worwood M, "The Laboratory Assessment of Iron Status: An Update," *Clin Chim Acta*, 1997, 259(1-2):3-23 (review).

Zittoun J and Zittoun R, "Modern Clinical Testing Strategies in Cobalamin and Folate Deficiency," *Semin Hematol*, 1999, 36(1):35-46 (review).

ANEMIA

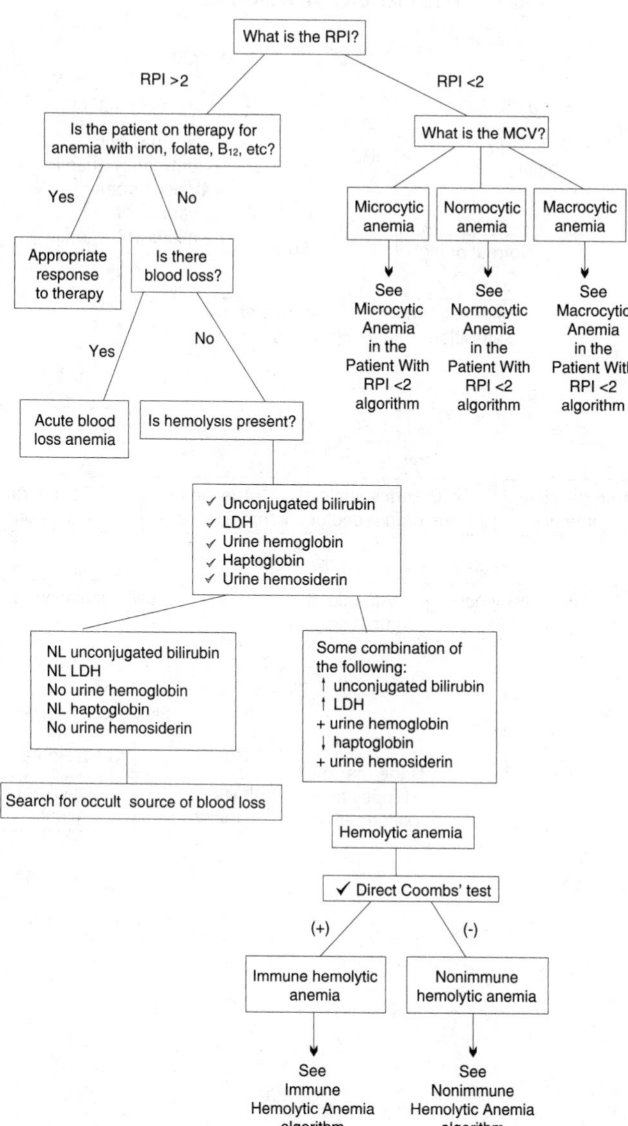
What is the RPI?
RPI >2
RPI <2
Is the patient on therapy for anemia with iron, folate, B12, etc?
What is the MCV?
Yes
No
Microcytic anemia
Normocytic anemia
Macrocytic anemia
Appropriate response to therapy
Is there blood loss?
See Microcytic Anemia in the Patient With RPI <2 algorithm
See Normocytic Anemia in the Patient With RPI <2 algorithm
See Macrocytic Anemia in the Patient With RPI <2 algorithm
Yes
No
Acute blood loss anemia
Is hemolysis present?
✓ Unconjugated bilirubin
✓ LDH
✓ Urine hemoglobin
✓ Haptoglobin
✓ Urine hemosiderin
NL unconjugated bilirubin
NL LDH
No urine hemoglobin
NL haptoglobin
No urine hemosiderin
Some combination of the following:
↑ unconjugated bilirubin
↑ LDH
+ urine hemoglobin
↓ haptoglobin
+ urine hemosiderin
Search for occult source of blood loss
Hemolytic anemia
✓ Direct Coombs' test
(+)
(-)
Immune hemolytic anemia
Nonimmune hemolytic anemia
See Immune Hemolytic Anemia algorithm
See Nonimmune Hemolytic Anemia algorithm

MICROCYTIC ANEMIA IN THE PATIENT WITH RPI <2

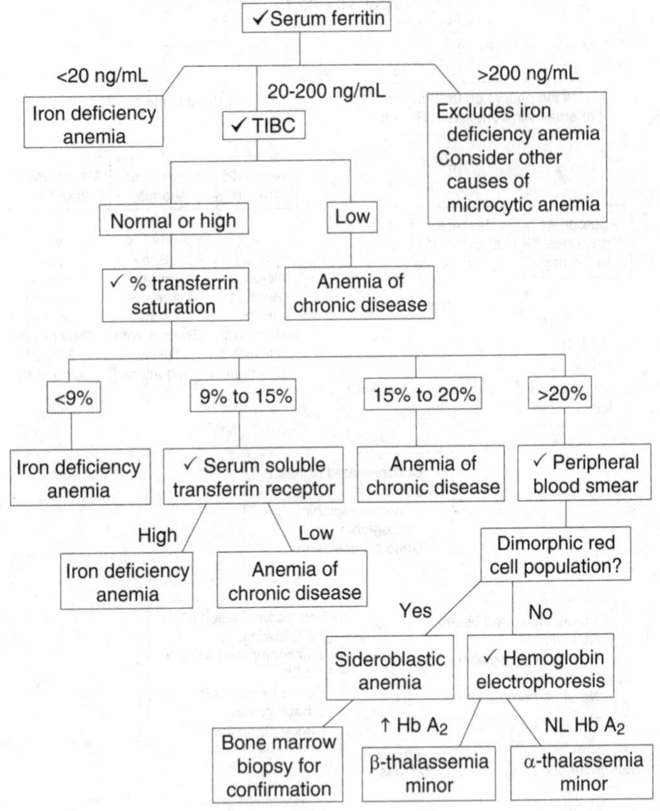

NORMOCYTIC ANEMIA IN THE PATIENT WITH RPI <2

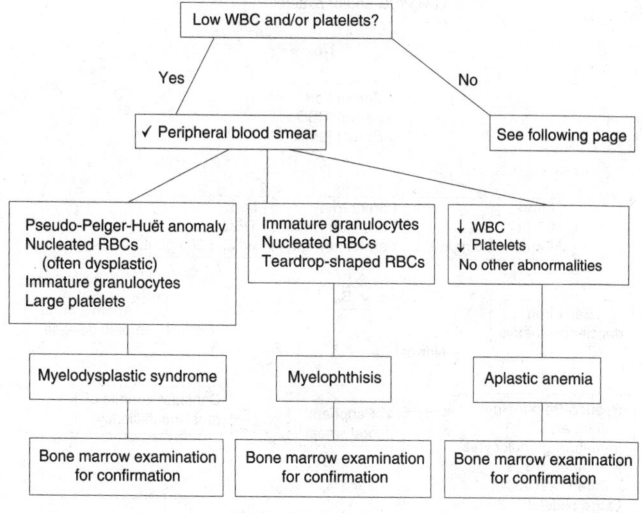
Low WBC and/or platelets?
Yes
No
✓ Peripheral blood smear
See following page
Pseudo-Pelger-Huët anomaly
Nucleated RBCs
(often dysplastic)
Immature granulocytes
Large platelets
Immature granulocytes
Nucleated RBCs
Teardrop-shaped RBCs
↓ WBC
↓ Platelets
No other abnormalities
Myelodysplastic syndrome
Myelophthisis
Aplastic anemia
Bone marrow examination for confirmation
Bone marrow examination for confirmation
Bone marrow examination for confirmation

NORMOCYTIC ANEMIA IN THE PATIENT WITH RPI <2 (*continued*)

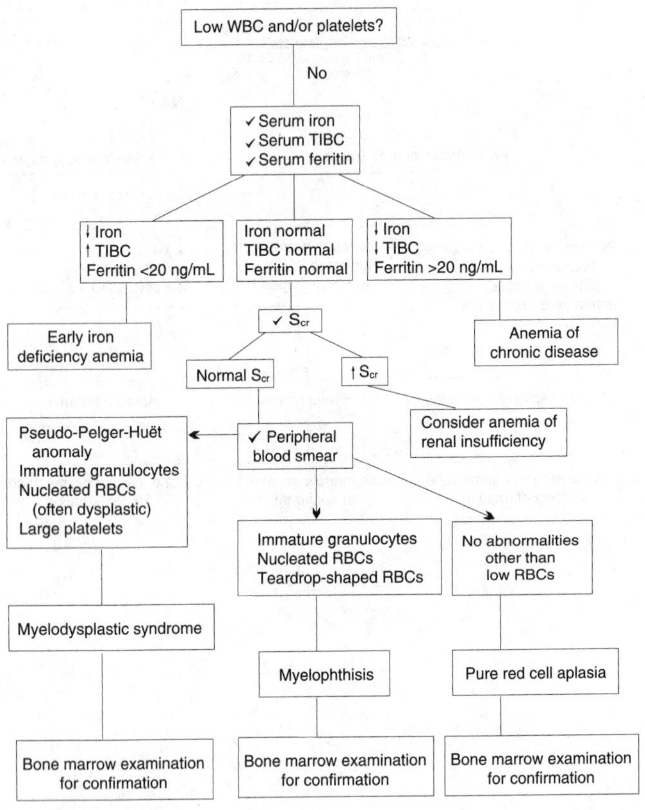

S_{cr} = serum creatinine

MACROCYTIC ANEMIA IN THE PATIENT WITH RPI <2

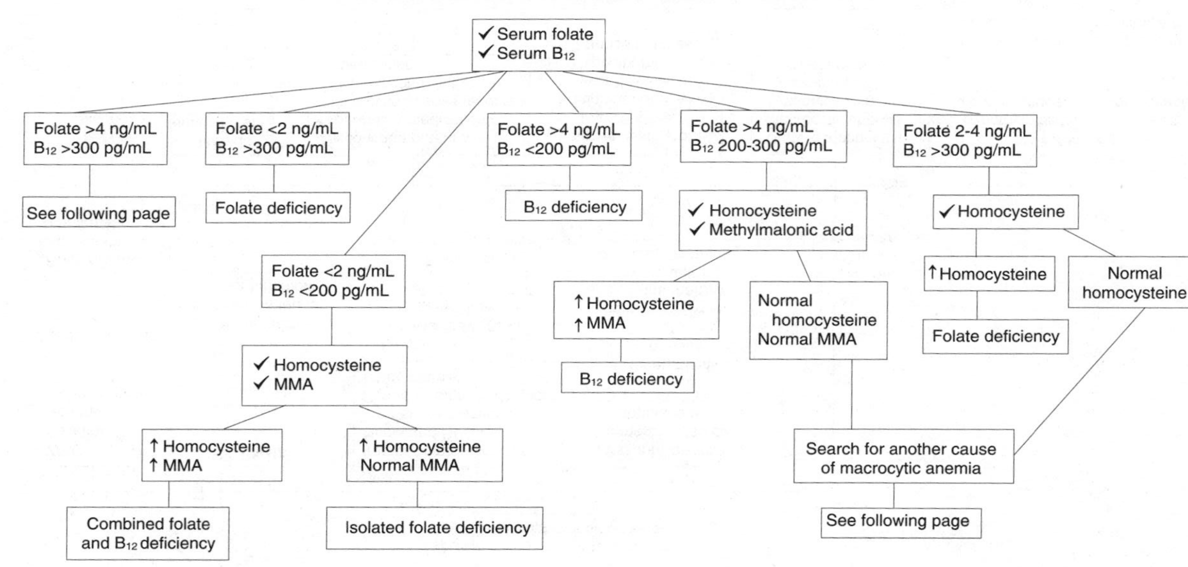

MMA = methylmalonic acid

MACROCYTIC ANEMIA IN THE PATIENT WITH RPI <2 *(continued)*

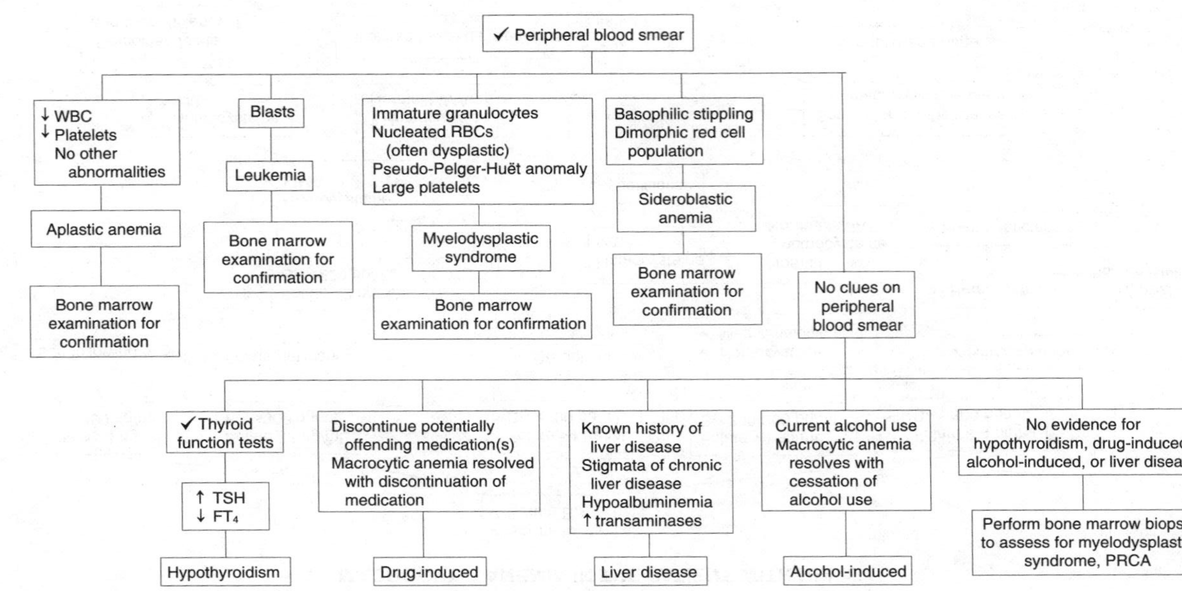

NONIMMUNE HEMOLYTIC ANEMIA

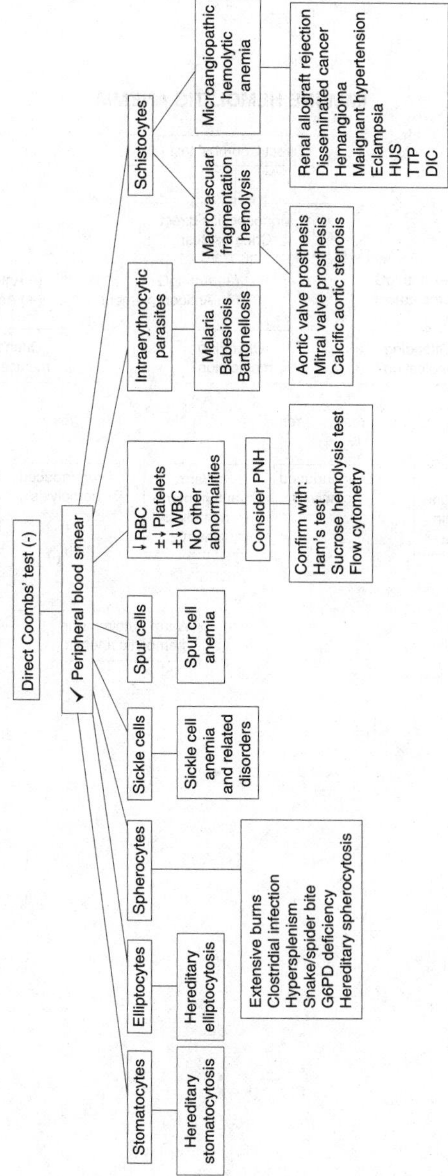
Direct Coombs' test (-)
✓ Peripheral blood smear
Stomatocytes
Hereditary stomatocytosis
Elliptocytes
Hereditary elliptocytosis
Spherocytes
Extensive burns
Clostridial infection
Hypersplenism
Snake/spider bite
G6PD deficiency
Hereditary spherocytosis
Sickle cells
Sickle cell anemia and related disorders
Spur cells
Spur cell anemia
↓RBC
±↓ Platelets
±↓ WBC
No other abnormalities
Consider PNH
Confirm with:
Ham's test
Sucrose hemolysis test
Flow cytometry
Intraerythrocytic parasites
Malaria
Babesiosis
Bartonellosis
Schistocytes
Macrovascular fragmentation hemolysis
Aortic valve prosthesis
Mitral valve prosthesis
Calcific aortic stenosis
Microangiopathic hemolytic anemia
Renal allograft rejection
Disseminated cancer
Hemangioma
Malignant hypertension
Eclampsia
HUS
TTP
DIC

IMMUNE HEMOLYTIC ANEMIA

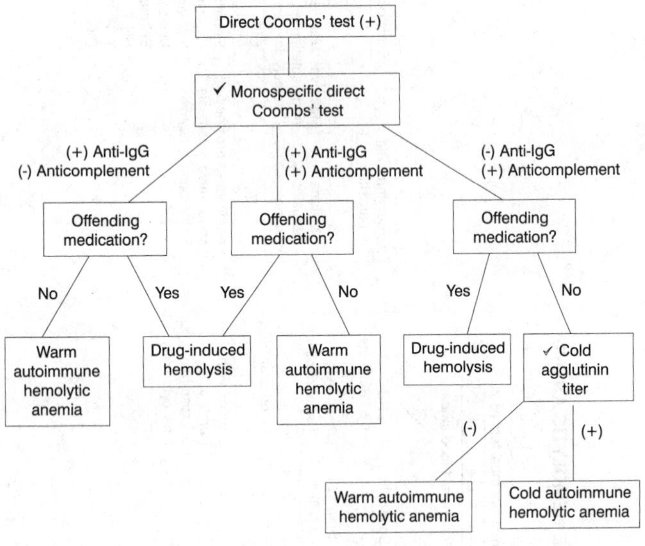

POLYCYTHEMIA

STEP 1 – *What Are the Different Types of Polycythemia?*

Polycythemia can be categorized into absolute and relative types.

DEFINITIONS...

Absolute polycythemia: An increase in total red cell mass which includes both polycythemia vera and secondary polycythemia

Relative polycythemia: An elevated hematocrit which results from a decrease in blood volume

Proceed to Step 2.

STEP 2 – *What Is the RBC Mass?*

The determination of a red blood cell mass using chromium-51 labeled erythrocytes is the first step in elucidating the etiology of polycythemia. This measurement will help separate patients with relative polycythemia from patients with absolute polycythemia.

If the red blood cell mass is increased, ***proceed to Step 3.***

If the red blood cell mass is not increased, the patient has relative polycythemia. It is important to make the distinction because patients with relative polycythemia do not need further evaluation.

CAUSES OF RELATIVE POLYCYTHEMIA
HEMOCONCENTRATION GAISBOCK'S SYNDROME*

*Gaisbock's syndrome, or stress erythrocytosis, is characterized by a normal red blood cell mass, but a decrease in plasma volume, resulting in an elevated hematocrit. The typical patient is an obese, middle-aged white male who suffers from anxiety and hypertension.

End of Section.

STEP 3 – *What Is the Arterial Oxygen Saturation?*

Once relative polycythemia has been excluded, attention should focus on distinguishing the causes of secondary polycythemia from polycythemia vera.

CAUSES OF SECONDARY POLYCYTHEMIA
PHYSIOLOGIC INCREASE IN EPO* PRODUCTION SECONDARY TO TISSUE HYPOXIA
High altitude
Carbon monoxide intoxication
Pulmonary disease (ie, COPD)
Sleep-apnea syndrome
High O_2-affinity hemoglobin
NONPHYSIOLOGIC INCREASE IN EPO PRODUCTION
RENAL DISEASE
Renal cyst
Renal artery stenosis
Renal transplant
Hydronephrosis
MALIGNANCY
Renal
Hepatic
Cerebellar hemangioblastoma
Adrenal adenoma
Pheochromocytoma
Uterine fibromyoma
Meningioma

*EPO refers to erythropoietin.

Tissue hypoxia is a major cause of secondary polycythemia. To determine whether tissue hypoxia is the cause of the polycythemia, an arterial oxygen saturation should be obtained. A saturation that is <92% argues for hypoxia as the cause of polycythemia. It is important to note that a single saturation >92% does not exclude hypoxia as a cause of polycythemia. Low arterial oxygenation should prompt the clinician to pursue one of the causes listed above.

If arterial oxygen saturation is <92%, the patient has tissue hypoxia as the secondary cause of polycythemia. ***Stop here.***

If arterial oxygen saturation is >92%, ***proceed to Step 4***.

STEP 4 – *What Is the Carboxyhemoglobin Level?*

Carboxyhemoglobin decreases the oxygen carrying capacity of the blood. Increases in the carboxyhemoglobin level may lead to polycythemia. This is known as smoker's polycythemia. Measurement of the carboxyhemoglobin level will detect the presence of this disorder.

If the patient has smoker's polycythemia, ***stop here***.

If the patient does not have smoker's polycythemia, ***proceed to Step 5***.

STEP 5 – *What Is the $P_{50}O_2$ of the Blood?*

Normal arterial oxygen saturation does not exclude all causes of tissue hypoxia. It is merely a measure of the amount of oxygen delivered to the tissues. It does not provide any information about the amount of oxygen released at the tissue level.

High oxygen affinity hemoglobin is an example of a condition that is characterized by a normal arterial oxygen saturation, yet results in tissue hypoxia because of an impairment in its ability to release oxygen to the tissues. Another example is a rare deficiency of red blood cell 2,3-DPG.

An excellent screening test for high oxygen affinity hemoglobin is the determination of the $P_{50}O_2$ of the blood.

DEFINITIONS...

$P_{50}O_2$ = Partial pressure of oxygen in the blood at which the hemoglobin is 50% saturated

Normal $P_{50}O_2$ = 26 mm Hg

High oxygen affinity hemoglobin is characterized by a lower $P_{50}O_2$. This will result in less oxygen released at the tissue level.

If the $P_{50}O_2$ is normal, ***proceed to Step 6.***

If the $P_{50}O_2$ is low, the patient likely has high oxygen affinity hemoglobin. ***Stop here.***

STEP 6 – *What Is the Erythropoietin (EPO) Level?*

A normal oxygen saturation and $P_{50}O_2$ in the patient with polycythemia should prompt the clinician to obtain an erythropoietin level. Unfortunately, there is considerable overlap in levels that may be obtained in patients who have either secondary polycythemia or polycythemia vera. For this reason, multiple specimens are recommended.

DEFINITIONS...

Erythropoietin (EPO): Growth factor produced by the juxtaglomerular cells of the kidney in response to a reduction in the amount of oxygen reaching the tissues

EPO level:

Normal: 18-35 mU/mL

Secondary polycythemia: 18 to >200 mU/mL

PCV: <22 mU/mL

If the erythropoietin level is high, the patient has secondary polycythemia. ***Proceed to Step 7.***

If the erythropoietin level is low, the patient has polycythemia vera. ***Proceed to Step 8.***

STEP 7 – *What Is the Result of the Abdominal CT?*

The remaining causes of secondary polycythemia include various malignancies and renal disorders. Because hepatic and renal cell carcinoma are the two most common malignancies that give rise to polycythemia, an abdominal CT is recommended. An abdominal CT is also helpful in the detection of a pheochromocytoma or an adrenal adenoma.

If needed, a head CT or MRI can also be obtained to exclude a hemangioblastoma or a meningioma.

The multiple causes of malignancy-associated polycythemia are listed in the following box.

MALIGNANCY-ASSOCIATED POLYCYTHEMIA
HEPATIC CARCINOMA
RENAL CELL CARCINOMA
CEREBELLAR HEMANGIOBLASTOMA
PHEOCHROMOCYTOMA
ADRENAL ADENOMA
UTERINE FIBROMYOMA
MENINGIOMA

If malignancy is not present, then the patient may have one of several renal disorders. A renal cyst or hydronephrosis may be detected by abdominal CT scan. Renal artery stenosis or transplantation should be suspected, in the appropriate clinical setting.

End of Section.

STEP 8 – *Does the Patient Have Polycythemia Vera (PCV)?*

DEFINITION...

PCV: Myeloproliferative disorder characterized by the autonomous production of red blood cells leading to polycythemia. Elevations in white blood cell and/or platelet counts may be appreciated because the pluripotent stem cell is often involved.

The other myeloproliferative disorders are essential thrombocytosis, chronic myelogenous leukemia, and agnogenic myeloid metaplasia.

The diagnosis of polycythemia vera is established when the other causes of polycythemia, both relative and secondary, are excluded.

Laboratory Features

The laboratory features of polycythemia vera are listed in the following box.

POLYCYTHEMIA VERA LABORATORY FEATURES
INCREASED HEMOGLOBIN
INCREASED WBC (<20 x 10^9 cells/L in 66%)
INCREASED PLATELETS (>400 x 10^9 cells/L in 50%)*
INCREASED URIC ACID
INCREASED SERUM COBALAMIN
INCREASED SERUM COBALAMIN - BINDING CAPACITY
INCREASED LAP SCORE
DECREASED / NORMAL SERUM IRON

*Occasionally the platelet count may climb above 1000 x 10^9 cells/L.

Peripheral Blood Smear Findings

The peripheral blood smear findings in PCV include the following.

1. Erythrocytes

   In the absence of phlebotomy treatment, most patients with polycythemia have normocytic, normochromic red blood cells. With repeated phlebotomy, however, iron deficient erythropoiesis leads to the appearance of microcytic, hypochromic red blood cells. Rarely, polycythemia vera patients may present with iron deficiency in the absence of treatment due to occult blood loss. This may lead to microcytosis in the setting of a normal to high hemoglobin, resembling thalassemia. Nucleated red blood cells may also be appreciated in polycythemia vera.

2. Leukocytes

   A left shift of the granulocytic series may be appreciated, with myelocytes and metamyelocytes. The presence of promyelocytes and blast cells is unusual. An increased number of eosinophils and basophils may also be noted. Some patients with polycythemia vera develop myelofibrosis as the disease progresses. In these cases, examination of the peripheral blood smear may reveal immature red and white blood cells.

3. Platelets

   In some patients, giant platelet forms may be noted.

Bone Marrow Examination Findings

There are no pathognomonic features of polycythemia vera that may be appreciated on bone marrow examination. Rather, a number of features should prompt the clinician to consider this disease. These include:

1. Hypercellularity

   Bone marrow examination typically reveals hypercellularity. There is an increase in myeloid, erythroid, and megakaryocytic precursors (in contrast, patients with secondary polycythemia only have erythroid hyperplasia). As a result, the myeloid to erythroid ratio often remains normal.

2. Positive reticulin staining

   Reticulin is a type of collagen fiber. It can be stained by various silver stains. When bone marrow specimens in patients with polycythemia vera are stained for the presence of reticulin, 30% to 40% have a slight to marked increase in reticulin at the time of their presentation. As these patients are followed, reticulin staining often becomes more impressive. In fact, marked reticulin staining is appreciated in polycythemia vera patients in the so-called "spent phase" of the disease. The spent phase is really the progression of polycythemia vera to myelofibrosis.

Criteria for the Diagnosis

The diagnostic criteria are listed in the following box.

POLYCYTHEMIA VERA DIAGNOSTIC CRITERIA

MAJOR CRITERIA

ELEVATED RBC MASS
NORMAL ARTERIAL OXYGEN SATURATION (≥92%)
SPLENOMEGALY

MINOR CRITERIA

PLATELET COUNT >400 x 10^9 cells/L
WBC COUNT >12 x 10^9 cells/L
INCREASED LAP SCORE
INCREASED B_{12} LEVEL OR BINDING CAPACITY

Using the above criteria, the diagnosis of PCV can be established if:

1. All three major criteria are fulfilled **or**
2. The first two major, plus any two minor, criteria are fulfilled.

PCV vs Secondary Polycythemia vs Relative Polycythemia

	PCV	Secondary Polycythemia	Relative Polycythemia
RBC mass	↑	↑	Normal
Erythropoietin	Usually ↓	Normal or ↑	Usually normal
PaO_2	Usually normal	↓ (some cases)	Normal
LAP score	↑	Usually normal	Usually normal
B_{12} level	↑	Normal	Normal
B_{12} binding capacity	↑	Normal	Normal
Uric acid	↑	Normal	Normal
Iron	↓	Normal	Normal
Bone marrow iron	↓	Normal	Normal
Platelet aggregation	Abnormal	Normal	Normal
Marrow chromosome abnormality	Present in some	Absent	Absent

References

Berlin NI, "Diagnosis and Classification of the Polycythemias," *Semin Hematol*, 1975, 12:339-51.

Messinezy M and Pearson TC, "The Classification and Diagnostic Criteria of the Erythrocytoses (Polycythaemias)," *Clin Lab Haematol*, 1999, 21(5):309-16.

Pearson TC, "Diagnosis and Classification of Erythrocytoses and Thrombocytoses," *Baillieres Clin Haematol*, 1998, 11(4):695-720.

Pearson TC, "Evaluation of Diagnostic Criteria in Polycythemia Vera," *Semin Hematol*, 2001, 38(1 Suppl 2):21-4.

Tefferi A, "Diagnosing Polycythemia Vera: A Paradigm Shift," *Mayo Clin Proc*, 1999, 74(2):159-62.

Tefferi A, Solberg LA, and Silverstein MN, "A Clinical Update in Polycythemia Vera and Essential Thrombocythemia," *Am J Med*, 2000, 109(2):141-9.

POLYCYTHEMIA

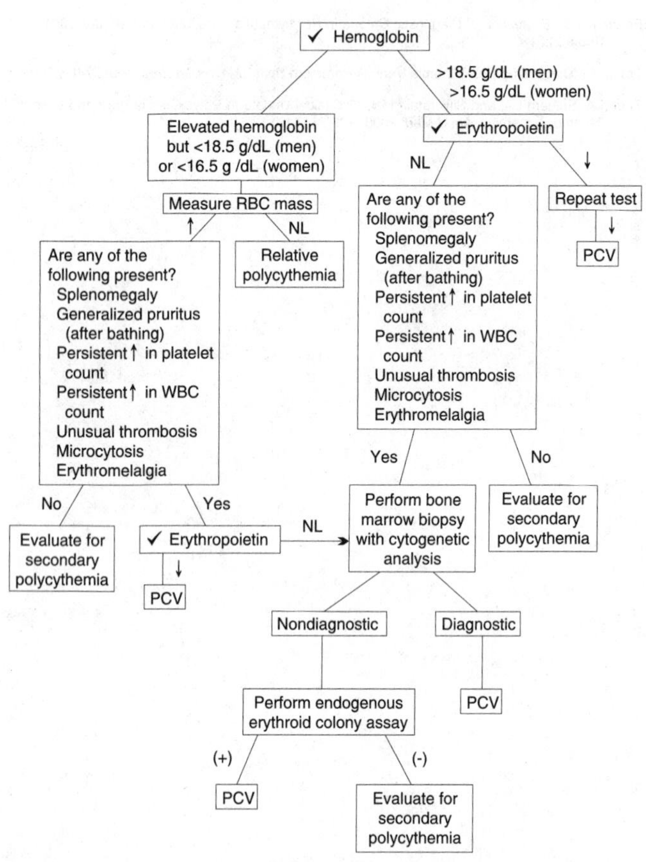

LEUKOCYTOSIS

White blood cells (leukocytes) include neutrophils, monocytes, lymphocytes, eosinophils, and basophils. An increase in any of these cell types can lead to leukocytosis. Leukocytosis is defined as a white blood cell count >11 x 10^9/L (11,000/mm^3).

Causes of Leukocytosis

Leukocytosis is a commonly encountered laboratory test abnormality. It is not sufficient to merely note the presence of leukocytosis. Rather the clinician should determine which type of blood cell is present in excess. To identify the type of white blood cell that is present in increased numbers, the clinician should examine the white blood cell differential count, which will list the percentage of each white blood cell type. These percentages are determined either by an automated electronic counter or by direct examination of the peripheral blood smear. The normal white blood cell count differential is listed in the following table.

Normal White Blood Cell Count Differential*

White Blood Cell Type	Percentage
Polymorphonuclear neutrophils	45-65
Band neutrophils	0-5
Lymphocytes	15-40
Monocytes	2-8
Eosinophils	0-5
Basophils	0-3

*The reference range for the white blood cell count may vary from laboratory to laboratory but is typically 3.5-10.5 x 10^9/L.

By examining the white blood cell differential count, the clinician can categorize the leukocytosis as follows:

- Neutrophilia
- Lymphocytosis
- Eosinophilia
- Basophilia
- Monocytosis

Neutrophilia is the most common cause of leukocytosis. However, the other types of white blood cells (eosinophils, basophils, monocytes, lymphocytes) may also be increased to such an extent that leukocytosis develops. The importance of identifying the cell type that is present in excess has to do with the fact that the causes that the clinician must consider vary with the type of leukocytosis present. In the chapters that follow, we will consider the causes of each type of leukocytosis as well as the evaluation necessary to establish the etiology of the leukocytosis.

References

Hoffman R, Benz EJ, Shattil SJ, et al, eds, *Hematology, Basic Principles and Practice*, 3rd ed, New York, NY: Churchill Livingstone, 2000.

Hoyer JD, "Leukocyte Differential," *Mayo Clin Proc*, 1993, 68(10):1027-8.

Jandl JH, *Blood, Textbook of Hematology*, 2nd ed, Boston, MA: Little, Brown and Company, 1996.

Lee GR, Forester J, Lukens J, et al, eds, *Wintrobe's Clinical Hematology*, 10th ed, Baltimore, MD: Williams and Wilkins, 1999.

Peterson L and Foucar K, "Granulocytosis and Granulocytopenia," *Hematology: Clinical and Laboratory Practice*, Bick RL, ed, St Louis, Mo: Mosby, 1993, 1137-54.

NEUTROPHILIA

Neutrophilia is the most common type of leukocytosis. Neutrophilia is defined as an absolute neutrophil count that exceeds 7.5×10^9/L. The absolute neutrophil count (ANC) is calculated by using the formula listed in the following box.

ANC = total WBC count x neutrophil %

where neutrophil percentage refers to mature and band neutrophils. Band neutrophils refer to less mature neutrophils containing band-shaped nuclei. There are significantly more mature neutrophils in the blood than band neutrophils. Mature neutrophils are also known as "segs" because of their segmented nuclei.

Causes of Neutrophilia

The causes of neutrophilia are listed in the following box.

CAUSES OF NEUTROPHILIA

- INFECTION
  - Bacterial
  - Fungal
  - Rickettsial
  - Viral
  - Parasitic
  - Spirochetal
- CONNECTIVE TISSUE DISEASE
  - Vasculitis
  - Rheumatoid arthritis
- MALIGNANCY*
  - Stomach
  - Lung
  - Uterine
  - Breast
  - Brain
  - Melanoma
  - Pancreatic
  - Renal
  - Squamous cell carcinoma
  - Hepatic
  - Non-Hodgkin's lymphoma
  - Hodgkin's disease
  - Sarcoma
- MEDICATIONS
  - Corticosteroids
  - All-trans retinoic acid
  - Epinephrine
  - Lithium
  - Growth factors (G-CSF, CM-CSF)
  - Clozapine
  - Desmopressin
- TRAUMA
  - Crush injuries
  - Extremes of temperature
  - Electric shock
- CHRONIC IDIOPATHIC NEUTROPHILIA
- CIGARETTE SMOKING
- HEMATOLOGIC DISORDERS
  - Hemolytic anemia
  - Myelodysplastic syndrome
  - Rebound from agranulocytosis
  - Postsplenectomy†
  - Myelomonocytic leukemia
  - Rebound from therapy of megaloblastic anemia
  - Recovery from marrow failure
  - Myeloproliferative disorders
    - Chronic myelogenous leukemia
    - Polycythemia vera
    - Essential thrombocytosis
    - Agnogenic myeloid metaplasia
  - Systemic mastocytosis
  - Hemolytic-uremic syndrome
  - Postneutropenia rebound
  - Sickle cell crisis
- CHEMICALS
  - Mercury poisoning
  - Lead poisoning
  - Ethylene glycol intoxication
  - Animal venom
- METABOLIC CONDITIONS
  - Lactic acidosis
  - Diabetic ketoacidosis‡
  - Thyrotoxicosis
  - Cushing's syndrome
  - Eclampsia
  - Uremia
  - Gout
- TISSUE NECROSIS
  - Myocardial infarction
  - Gangrene
  - Pulmonary infarction
  - Acute hepatic necrosis
  - Burns
  - Postoperative

CAUSES OF NEUTROPHILIA *continued*	
CHRONIC INFLAMMATORY STATES	PHYSIOLOGIC NEUTROPHILIA (pseudoneutrophilia)
Crohn's disease	Exercise
Ulcerative colitis	Epinephrine
Granulomatous infection	Pain
Bronchiectasis	Beta-agonists
Chronic hepatitis	Stress
MISCELLANEOUS	Seizures
Atheroembolic disease	Hypoxia
Acute hemorrhage	Smoking
Acute pancreatitis	Trauma
Eclampsia / preeclampsia	

*Malignancy results in neutrophilia when growth of the tumor exceeds its blood supply, leading to necrosis. Increased production of growth factors by the tumor may also play a role. Typically, the white blood cell count does not exceed 30 x 10^9 cells/L; however, in some cases, white blood cell counts approaching 100 x 10^9 cells/L have been described.

†Part of the marginal white blood cell pool resides in the spleen. The addition of these cells to the circulating pool results in the neutrophilia seen after splenectomy.

#While neutrophilia may be secondary to DKA alone, its presence should raise concern about an infectious or inflammatory disorder that may have precipitated DKA.

As shown in the above box, there are many causes of neutrophilia. In usual clinical practice, most cases of neutrophilia are due to acute or subacute infections. Infection as well as other common causes of neutrophilia will be discussed below.

Corticosteroid Therapy

It is widely known that neutrophil counts often increase with corticosteroid therapy. With intravenous administration, the increase in the white blood cell count may begin within a few hours. With oral administration, an increase may be noted within the first day of therapy. It is unusual for the white blood cell count to exceed 20 x 10^9/L and this degree of elevation should prompt consideration of another etiology superimposed on the neutrophilia of corticosteroid therapy. In addition to the neutrophilia, the WBC differential will reveal an increase in the absolute monocyte count but a fall in the absolute eosinophil and lymphocyte counts. It is important to note that corticosteroid therapy does not lead to left shift or a change in neutrophil morphology (ie, Dohle bodies, toxic granulation, vacuolization).

Bacterial Infection

The presence of neutrophilia often prompts the clinician to search for a source of infection because infection is a major cause of neutrophilia. Infection due to various microorganisms may be associated with neutrophilia. Bacterial infection is the most common infectious cause of neutrophilia. The white blood cell count typically ranges from 10-25 x 10^9 cells/L. However, some bacterial infections, such as pneumococcal pneumonia, may present with a higher white blood cell count. Classically, patients with acute bacterial infection present with leukocytosis with an increase in the percentage of mature neutrophils as well as band neutrophils. The increase in younger neutrophils, including band neutrophils, is referred to as a left shift. Accompanying the neutrophilia is a decrease in eosinophils.

It is important to realize, however, that not all bacterial infections are associated with neutrophilia. Examples include typhoid fever, paratyphoid fever, brucellosis, and glanders. In addition, bacterial infections typically presenting with neutrophilic leukocytosis may present with normal or even low white blood cell counts, particularly with advancing age, alcoholism, or overwhelming infection. In fact, leukocytosis may be absent in approximately 25% of patients with acute bacterial infection. In many of these patients, inspection of the differential white blood cell count may reveal a left shift.

Examination of the white blood cell count in patients with bacterial infection may also provide prognostic information, as shown in the following box.

WBC COUNT POOR PROGNOSTIC SIGNS
INABILITY TO DEVELOP LEUKOCYTOSIS MARKEDLY ELEVATED NEUTROPHIL COUNT SIGNIFICANT DECREASE IN LYMPHOCYTE COUNT HIGH PROPORTION OF IMMATURE CELLS

With recovery from infection, the clinician may note the findings listed in the following box.

WBC COUNT SIGNS OF RECOVERY
TRANSIENT INCREASE IN MONOCYTE COUNT INCREASED NUMBER OF EOSINOPHILS INCREASED NUMBER OF LYMPHOCYTES DECREASED NUMBER OF IMMATURE CELLS DECREASED NEUTROPHIL COUNT

Clinicians are often interested in the band neutrophil count in patients suspected of having acute bacterial infection. An elevation in the band neutrophil count is referred to as bandemia. Under normal circumstances, the neutrophils released from the bone marrow are almost all segmented. However, during stress or infection, the bone marrow may release less mature neutrophils such as band neutrophils into the circulation. When increased numbers of immature neutrophils are noted, the patient is said to have a left shift. It is important to realize that bandemia is not synonymous with acute bacterial infection. Causes of bandemia are listed in the following box.

CAUSES OF BANDEMIA
ACUTE BACTERIAL INFECTION OTHER TYPES OF INFECTION (including viral) TISSUE DAMAGE OR NECROSIS SEIZURE INTOXICATION POISONING COLLAGEN VASCULAR DISEASE GOUT ACUTE HEMORRHAGE HEMOLYSIS MEDICATIONS MYELOPROLIFERATIVE DISORDER HYPERSENSITIVITY REACTION MALIGNANCY METABOLIC DISORDER (uremia, diabetic ketoacidosis)

Viral Infection

Viral infections can present with neutrophilia but are typically associated with normal or low white blood cell counts. In viral infections, the presence of neutrophilia should prompt the clinician to consider a complication of the viral infection. Examples of such complications include meningitis in the patient with mumps and bowel perforation in the patient with typhoid fever. Nonetheless, uncomplicated viral infections, at times, may be characterized by leukocytosis. Although an increase in band forms is classically associated with bacterial infections, bandemia may also be appreciated in viral infections.

Other Infections

In tuberculosis, the white blood cell count is usually normal, but in rare instances, neutrophilia can be appreciated. Fungal and spirochetal infections can present with neutrophilia as well.

Pseudoneutrophilia (physiologic neutrophilia)

Neutrophils are found in three locations - bone marrow, peripheral blood, and the extravascular space. In the bone marrow, neutrophil precursors are present in mitotic and storage pools. Neutrophils are released into peripheral blood from the storage pool. Peripheral blood consists of circulating and marginal pools. Those neutrophils that adhere to small vessels are said to be in the marginating pool. The white blood cell count does not take into account the neutrophils that are present in the marginal pool. In response to certain stimuli, neutrophils in the marginal pool may transfer to the circulating pool in a process called demargination. When demargination results in neutrophilia, pseudoneutrophilia is said to be present. Pseudoneutrophilia, also known as physiologic neutrophilia, is defined as neutrophilia in the absence of increased granulocyte production. Stimuli that are associated with pseudoneutrophilia are listed in the following box.

STIMULI RESULTING IN PSEUDONEUTROPHILIA	
EXERCISE	STRESS
PAIN	HYPOXIA
TRAUMA	SMOKING
EPINEPHRINE	SEIZURES

Conditions causing pseudoneutrophilia usually do not lead to a white blood cell count that exceeds two times the upper limit of normal. The above conditions are not characterized by the presence of band forms or other neutrophil precursors in the peripheral blood. In pseudoneutrophilia, there is often an increase in the numbers of lymphocytes and monocytes, which is helpful in differentiating this type of neutrophilia from that due to infection. Infection characteristically presents with a decrease in the lymphocyte and monocyte counts.

Approach to the Patient With Neutrophilia

Neutrophilia is the most common type of leukocytosis. As such, it behooves the clinician to become comfortable with the evaluation of the patient presenting with neutrophilia. Because infection is a major cause of neutrophilia, initial evaluation often focuses on a search for an infectious etiology. This evaluation should begin with a thorough history and physical examination, which will often provide clues to the source of infection. Signs and symptoms of the underlying infection are usually present.

When infection is not apparent, the clinician should consider other causes of neutrophilia. The patient's clinical presentation may be consistent with a noninfectious cause of neutrophilia. Of particular importance in determining the etiology of the neutrophilia is an examination of the CBC, looking for other abnormalities, as shown in the following table.

CBC Abnormalities That May Provide Clues to the Etiology of the Neutrophilia

CBC Abnormality	Condition(s) Suggested
Anemia	Nonspecific finding that may be due to chronic infection/inflammation, malignancy, hemolytic anemia, or other condition. A review of the peripheral blood smear is warranted.
Increased hemoglobin / hematocrit	Myeloproliferative disorder, especially polycythemia vera
Thrombocytopenia	Sepsis with or without DIC TTP/HUS
Thrombocytosis	Nonspecific finding that may be due to infection, inflammation, or malignancy. Essential thrombocytosis should be a consideration.
Nucleated red blood cells	Infiltrative disease of the bone marrow Septic shock
Left shift*	Infection Myeloproliferative disorder Acute leukemia

*The left shift of infection is typically characterized by an increase in the band count, to levels exceeding 700/μL. A band count that exceeds 20% of the total white blood cell count is very specific for infection or inflammatory disease (specificity of 79%). On occasion, metamyelocytes may be appreciated on the peripheral blood smear of patients with infection. More immature neutrophils such as myelocytes, promyelocytes, and blasts are unusual findings in these patients. Their presence should prompt consideration of myeloproliferative disorders and acute leukemia.

It is particularly important to make the distinction between reactive and neoplastic neutrophilia. The term "reactive" is used to describe neutrophilia that reflects the response of a healthy bone marrow to an infectious or noninfectious stimulus. When marked reactive neutrophilia (white blood cell count >25-30 x 10^9/L) is present, the term "leukemoid reaction" is often used. When the white blood cell count is elevated to this degree or the severity of the underlying disease does not seem to correlate with the degree of white blood cell count elevation, neoplastic neutrophilia, particularly chronic myelogenous leukemia, is often considered in the differential diagnosis.

A leukemoid reaction may be the result of many disease processes including infection, hemorrhage, and trauma. In contrast to neoplastic neutrophilia, the circulating neutrophils in patients with the leukemoid reaction are not clonal in origin. In a leukemoid reaction, the elevated white blood cell count abates with treatment of the underlying disease, whereas, in the patient with chronic myelogenous leukemia, there is a progressive increase in the white blood cell count. The following table highlights the differences between reactive neutrophilia (including leukemoid reaction) and chronic myelogenous leukemia, the most common cause of neoplastic neutrophilia.

Differentiating Reactive Neutrophilia From Chronic Myelogenous Leukemia

	Reactive Neutrophilia	Chronic Myelogenous Leukemia (CML)
White blood cell count*	Usually <25-30 x 10^9L	Usually not <50 x 10^9L
Left shift	Relatively mature neutrophils: myelocytes, metamyelocytes, band forms	Mature and immature neutrophils, including blasts
Basophilia	(-)	(+)
Platelet count†	Variable	Usually increased
Platelet morphology	Normal	Abnormal (variable micromegakaryocytes)
Nucleated red blood cells	(-)	(+)
Fever‡	(+)	(-)
Splenomegaly	(-)	(+)
LAP score#	Increased	Decreased
Toxic granulations Döhle bodies Cytoplasmic vacuoles¶	(+)	(-)
Philadelphia chromosome§	(-)	(+)
bcr/abl	(-)	(+)

*On occasion, white blood cell counts >30 x 10^9/L may occur in patients with leukemoid reaction. A white blood cell count >100 x 10^9/L, however, is strongly suggestive of neoplastic neutrophilia. Growth factor therapy is also associated with neutrophilia of this degree.

†Some cases of reactive neutrophilia may be associated with reactive thrombocytosis.

‡Fever may be present if chronic myelogenous leukemia is complicated by infection.

#Leukocyte alkaline phosphatase (LAP) is an enzyme found within neutrophils. Causes of high LAP score include infection, inflammatory conditions, nonhematopoietic malignancy, stress, oral contraceptive use, medications (lithium, estrogen, growth factors, and corticosteroids), myeloproliferative disorders (other than CML), and pregnancy. Chronic myelogenous leukemia is not typically associated with an elevated LAP score. When CML is complicated by infection, however, the LAP score may rise. An elevated LAP score has also been reported in CML which has progressed to early blast crisis.

¶Toxic granulations, Döhle bodies, and cytoplasmic vacuolization are features of reactive neutrophilia, usually due to inflammation, trauma, infection, or toxin exposure. These toxic changes may also be found in the neutrophils of chronic myelogenous leukemia complicated by infection. In uncomplicated CML, toxic changes are not present.

§Presence of Philadelphia chromosome can be demonstrated by either karyotypic analysis (bone marrow) or fluorescent *in situ* hybridization (peripheral blood). It is important to note that a minority of patients with CML do not have the Philadelphia chromosome (10% to 15%).

Infectious and inflammatory causes of neutrophilia are usually associated with an outpouring of endogenous steroids. The increase in corticosteroids typically results in eosinopenia and basophilopenia. The presence of eosinophils and/or basophils argues against an inflammatory or infectious etiology. In these patients, the clinician should give serious consideration to the following:

- Coexisting adrenal insufficiency
- Malignancy associated with the secretion of GM-CSF by neoplastic cells
- Hematologic malignancy (myeloproliferative disorder, lymphoma, leukemia associated with eosinophilia, or myelodysplastic syndrome)

Bone marrow aspiration and biopsy are usually not necessary in patients with reactive neutrophilia. If performed, bone marrow examination will reveal granulocytic hyperplasia. Bone marrow aspiration and biopsy should be performed, however, whenever there is suspicion for neoplastic neutrophilia (see table above). Bone marrow biopsy may also reveal findings consistent with other bone marrow processes including myelodysplastic syndrome, acute leukemia, agnogenic myeloid metaplasia, metastatic carcinoma, and granulomatous infection of the bone marrow.

References

Ardron MJ, Westengard JC, and Dutcher TF, "Band Neutrophil Counts Are Unnecessary for the Diagnosis of Infection in Patients With Normal Total Leukocyte Counts," *Am J Clin Pathol*, 1994, 102:646-9.

Boxer L and Dale DC, "Neutropenia: Causes and Consequences," *Semin Hematol*, 2002, 39(2):75-81.

Dale DC, Bolyard AA, and Aprikyan A, "Cyclic Neutropenia," *Semin Hematol*, 2002, 39(2):89-94.

Hoffman R, Benz EJ, Shattil SJ, et al, eds, *Hematology, Basic Principles and Practice*, 3rd ed, New York, NY: Churchill Livingstone, 2000.

Jandl JH, *Blood, Textbook of Hematology*, 2nd ed, Boston, MA: Little, Brown and Company, 1996.

Lee GR, Forester J, Lukens J, et al, eds, *Wintrobe's Clinical Hematology*, 10th ed, Baltimore, MD: Williams and Wilkins, 1999.

Palmblad JE and von dem Borne AE, "Idiopathic, Immune, Infectious, and Idiosyncratic Neutropenias," *Semin Hematol*, 2002, 39(2):121-7.

Peterson L and Foucar K, "Granulocytosis and Granulocytopenia," *Hematology: Clinical and Laboratory Practice*, Bick RL, ed, St Louis, Mo: Mosby; 1993, 1137-54.

Starkebaum G, "Chronic Neutropenia Associated With Autoimmune Disease," *Semin Hematol*, 2002, 39(2):121-7.

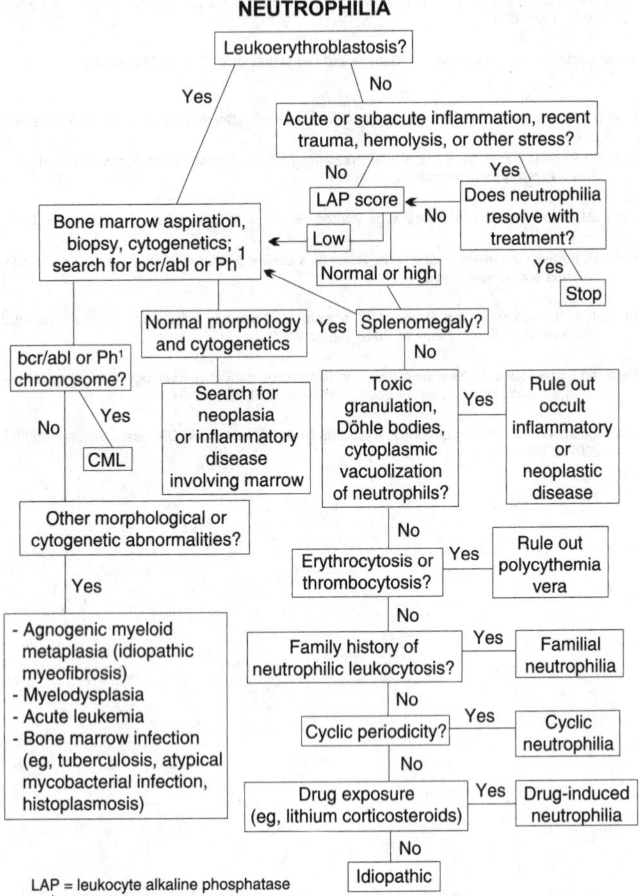

LAP = leukocyte alkaline phosphatase
Ph[1] = Philadelphia chromosome
bcr/abl = the translocation of the *c-abl* gene from chromosome 9 to the *bcr* gene on chromosome 22q
CML = chronic myelogenous leukemia

Adapted from Cecil RL, Bennett JC, and Goldman L, eds, *Cecil Textbook of Medicine*, 21st ed, Philadelphia, PA: WB Saunders Co, 1999, 931.

LYMPHOCYTOSIS

In adults, absolute lymphocytosis is said to be present if the absolute lymphocyte count exceeds 4 x 10^9 cells/L. The absolute lymphocyte count can be calculated as follows:

Absolute lymphocyte count = total WBC count x lymphocyte %

Relative lymphocytosis, defined as a lymphocyte percentage >50% in the setting of a normal absolute lymphocyte count, is more common than absolute lymphocytosis. Although relative lymphocytosis is quite common in patients with granulocytopenia (white blood cell count $<3 \times 10^9$/L), the term "relative lymphocytosis" should not be used in patients with low white blood cell counts. Because patients with granulocytopenia typically have absolute neutropenia, this term is more appropriate and the evaluation should focus on elucidating the cause of the absolute neutropenia.

Causes of Lymphocytosis

The causes of lymphocytosis are listed in the following box.

CAUSES OF LYMPHOCYTOSIS

- INFECTION
  - Viral
    - Infectious mononucleosis (Epstein-Barr virus)
    - Infectious mononucleosis-like syndrome
      - Cytomegalovirus
      - Adenovirus
      - Hepatitis (A, B, or C)
      - HIV (acute seroconversion)
      - Human herpesvirus 6
    - Other viral infection
  - Toxoplasmosis
  - Bacterial
    - Pertussis
    - Typhoid fever
    - Brucellosis
    - Rickettsial
    - Plague
    - Tuberculosis
  - Syphilis (secondary)
  - Acute infectious lymphocytosis
- DRUG REACTION
- SERUM SICKNESS
- EPINEPHRINE
- CIGARETTE SMOKING
- MALIGNANCY
  - Acute lymphoblastic leukemia (early)
  - Chronic lymphocytic leukemia (early phase)
  - Non-Hodgkin's lymphoma
  - Adult T-cell leukemia / lymphoma
  - Hodgkin's lymphoma (rare)
  - Hairy cell leukemia
  - Heavy chain diseases
  - Waldenström's macroglobulinemia
  - Mycosis fungoides / Sezary syndrome
  - Large granular lymphocytic leukemia
  - Thymoma
- TRANSIENT STRESS LYMPHOCYTOSIS
- PERSISTENT POLYCLONAL B-CELL LYMPHOCYTOSIS
- POSTSPLENECTOMY
- ENDOCRINE DISORDERS
  - Hypopituitarism
  - Graves' disease
  - Adrenal insufficiency
- EXERCISE (vigorous)
- STATUS EPILEPTICUS
- CYTOKINE ADMINISTRATION

Degree of Lymphocytosis

A total lymphocyte count >15 x 10^9 cells/L is only seen in a select number of conditions. These include the following:

- Infectious mononucleosis
- Acute infectious lymphocytosis
- Pertussis
- Chronic lymphocytic leukemia / other chronic lymphoid leukemias
- Acute lymphoblastic leukemia

Other conditions associated with lymphocytosis do not usually give rise to lymphocytosis of this magnitude. Recognize that the above conditions do not always present with this degree of lymphocytosis. In fact, it is not uncommon for mild lymphocytosis to occur in these diseases.

Reactive Lymphocytes

There is considerable variation in the diameter of peripheral blood lymphocytes. Most are small lymphocytes (10-12 micrometers) that have little in the way of cytoplasm, round or slightly indented nucleus, and condensed chromatin. Approximately 10% of the lymphocyte count consists of larger lymphocytes (12-16 micrometers) which have larger amounts of cytoplasm but less condensed nuclear chromatin. Even less common are larger lymphocytes that have more abundant cytoplasm and prominent cytoplasmic granules. These are termed large granular lymphocytes.

In response to both infectious and noninfectious stimuli, lymphocytes can undergo morphologic changes. These changes are termed "reactive." Reactive changes may consist of increased size, immaturity of the nucleus, lack of chromatin condensation, absent or indistinct nucleoli, cytoplasmic basophilia, and irregularity of the nuclear outline or lobulation.

Other terms used synonymously with the term "reactive" include "atypical," "variant," or "Downey cell." The presence of increased numbers of reactive lymphocytes in the patient with lymphocytosis should prompt consideration of the conditions listed in the following box.

CONDITIONS ASSOCIATED WITH REACTIVE LYMPHOCYTOSIS
INFECTIOUS MONONUCLEOSIS (Epstein-Barr virus)
INFECTIOUS MONONUCLEOSIS-LIKE SYNDROME
Cytomegalovirus
Toxoplasmosis
Hepatitis (A, B, or C)
HIV (acute seroconversion)
Adenovirus
Human herpesvirus 6
Rubella
OTHER VIRAL INFECTIONS
DRUG REACTION
PERTUSSIS
ACUTE INFECTIOUS LYMPHOCYTOSIS

Many of these conditions will be discussed in further detail below.

Viral Infection

Viral infection is the most common cause of lymphocytosis. Lymphocytosis seen with viral infections may be absolute or relative. Viral infection is characterized by a transient increase in the number of lymphocytes. The most common viral cause of lymphocytosis is infectious mononucleosis due to the Epstein-Barr virus. Other viral causes include cytomegalovirus, adenovirus, hepatitis (A, B, or C), HIV (acute seroconversion), human herpesvirus 6, rubella, roseola, mumps, and chickenpox.

Infectious Mononucleosis

The most common viral cause of lymphocytosis is infectious mononucleosis caused by the Epstein-Barr virus. The symptoms and signs of infectious mononucleosis are listed in the following box.

SYMPTOMS AND SIGNS OF INFECTIOUS MONONUCLEOSIS

SYMPTOMS	***SIGNS***
MALAISE (100%)	ADENOPATHY (100%)
SORE THROAT (85%)	FEVER (90%)
WARMTH, CHILLINESS (70%)	PHARYNGITIS (85%)
ANOREXIA (70%)	SPLENOMEGALY (60%)
HEADACHE (50%)	BRADYCARDIA (40%)
COUGH (40%)	PERIORBITAL EDEMA (25%)
MYALGIA (25%)	PALATAL ENANTHEM (25%)
ARTHRALGIA (5%)	JAUNDICE (10%)
SKIN RASH (5%)	
DIARRHEA (5%)	
PHOTOPHOBIA (5%)	

The hemoglobin is usually normal in most patients with infectious mononucleosis. On occasion, an autoimmune hemolytic anemia, which is usually mild, may develop. The white blood cell count is commonly increased (not always), usually to levels between 10 and 30 x 10^9/L. Rarely does the white blood cell count exceed this value. The elevation of white blood cell count may not occur until 1 week after symptom onset. After peaking during the second or third week, the white blood cell count usually returns to normal 1-2 months later. Examination of the differential white blood cell count typically reveals absolute lymphocytosis, sometimes to a significant degree (>15 x 10^9/L). A mild to moderate neutropenia is not uncommon. Thirty-three percent of infectious mononucleosis patients have mild thrombocytopenia (100-150 x 10^9/L). It is rare for the platelet count to fall to <100 x 10^9/L.

Examination of the peripheral blood smear reveals the increased numbers of reactive or atypical lymphocytes (>10 reactive lymphocytes per 100 white blood cells). It is important to realize that atypical lymphocytes are not specific for EBV and may be found in patients with other viral illnesses (see below). Immunoblasts may also be noted in infectious mononucleosis patients, particularly if the peripheral blood smear is examined early in the course of the illness. If noted, they are present in few numbers (<1% to 2% of total lymphocyte count). Other findings that may be noted include spherocytes and polychromasia in cases complicated by autoimmune hemolytic anemia. Decreased numbers of platelets may be found in 33% of patients.

The detection of serum or plasma heterophil antibodies confirms the diagnosis of infectious mononucleosis. Most laboratories use rapid tests (monospot) to detect heterophil antibodies. When heterophil antibodies are detected in the patient having the above peripheral blood smear findings, the diagnosis of infectious mononucleosis has been established.

One limitation of heterophil antibody testing is that the antibodies are often not detectable in children. Also, early in the course of the illness, heterophil antibodies may be lacking. Studies have shown, however, that heterophil antibodies are detectable in >96% of adolescents and young adults with serial testing. If initially negative, the test should be repeated after 1-2 weeks.

A minority of patients with infectious mononucleosis due to Epstein-Barr viral infection are heterophil-negative despite serial testing. When the heterophil antibody test is negative in the patient who has a clinical presentation consistent with infectious mononucleosis, the clinician may wish to obtain Epstein-Barr viral serology. The serologic profile in infectious mononucleosis is described in the following box.

EBV SEROLOGIC PROFILE IN INFECTIOUS MONONUCLEOSIS (ACUTE INFECTION)*	
+ VCA IgM	± EA IgG
+ VCA IgG	– EBNA IgG

VCA = viral capsid antigen; EA = early antigen; EBNA = Epstein-Barr nuclear antigen

*The EBV serologic findings listed in the above box only apply to patients with acute infection (0-3 months).

The diagnosis of infectious mononucleosis due to EBV is less certain in patients who are heterophil antibody positive but lack the characteristic peripheral blood smear findings. In these patients, it is reasonable to repeat the peripheral blood smear after several days to determine if reactive lymphocytes are present. Should reactive lymphocytes be present, the clinician can establish the diagnosis with more confidence. If reactive lymphocytes do not appear, it is possible that the positive heterophil antibody test was a false-positive test result. False-positive test results are rare but may be found in patients with rubella, pancreatic cancer, and leukemia. Alternatively, perhaps the patient had an infection some time ago (heterophil antibody test may remain positive for up to 1 year). In these cases, the clinician may wish to perform EBV serology.

The clinician should be aware of infectious mononucleosis-like syndromes that may mimic the presentation of infectious mononucleosis due to EBV. The causes of infectious mononucleosis-like syndromes are listed in the following box.

CAUSES OF INFECTIOUS MONONUCLEOSIS-LIKE SYNDROME	
CYTOMEGALOVIRUS	HEPATITIS (A, B, or C)
TOXOPLASMOSIS	ADENOVIRUS
ACUTE HIV INFECTION	HUMAN HERPESVIRUS 6
RUBELLA	

These illnesses should be a consideration when a patient suspected of having infectious mononucleosis due to EBV does not have serology (ie, heterophil antibody and EBV serology) supportive of the diagnosis.

Drug Reaction

A drug-induced etiology must always be considered in the patient with lymphocytosis. Among the drugs associated with lymphocytosis, phenytoin is a common offender. Absolute or relative lymphocytosis may be noted in patients with phenytoin-induced lymphocytosis. Eosinophilia and neutrophilia are not uncommon.

Pertussis

Most acute bacterial infections are characterized by neutrophilia. Pertussis due to *Bordetella pertussis* is an exception to this rule. Pertussis, also known as whooping cough, typically occurs in children who have not been vaccinated with the pertussis vaccine. The hallmarks of the infection are paroxysms of severe coughing and lymphocytosis. Absolute lymphocytosis, at times approaching 60 x 10^9/L, has been described.

Acute Infectious Lymphocytosis

Acute infectious lymphocytosis, an illness that primarily affects children, is thought to be due to viral infection. Although some patients are asymptomatic, others complain of fever, diarrhea, or abdominal pain. The symptoms, if present, usually abate within a few days. The white blood cell count is often strikingly elevated and may reach 100 x 10^9/L with a lymphocytic predominance. Examination of the peripheral blood smear reveals an abundance of morphologically mature lymphocytes. It is not unusual for the lymphocytosis to last for several weeks. Later in the illness, eosinophilia may be noted.

Approach to the Patient With Lymphocytosis

In most cases of lymphocytosis, the etiology is usually evident after a thorough history and physical examination. Transient stress-related lymphocytosis, which is an acute response to severe stress, is easily recognized if the clinician is familiar with the conditions associated with it. These conditions include acute myocardial infarction, trauma, cardiac arrest, sickle cell crisis, and obstetrical complications. Lymphocytosis may also follow exercise or the administration of epinephrine. Both of these etiologies are usually quite evident.

Quite often, the clinical presentation will be consistent with a viral infection. Viral causes of lymphocytosis are typically associated with the presence of reactive lymphocytes. The term "reactive" is used to refer to changes in the lymphocytes. In many cases of viral infection, the changes are minor, consisting of an increase in cytoplasmic basophilia or a visible nucleolus. In other cases, the reactive changes may be more impressive as is often seen in infectious mononucleosis patients. Infectious mononucleosis is characterized by the presence of atypical lymphocytes, many of which are large. These lymphocytes often have a strongly basophilic cytoplasm, large central nucleoli, and scalloped cytoplasmic margins. There is great variation, however, in the appearance of the lymphocytes in infectious mononucleosis patients. In patients suspected of having infectious mononucleosis, heterophil antibody testing should be performed. Negative test results should be followed by EBV serology. If the results (EBV serology + heterophil antibody testing) are not consistent with the diagnosis, causes of an infectious mononucleosis-like syndrome (eg, CMV, HIV, toxoplasmosis, etc) should be considered. Further evaluation of patients with viral infection includes repeating a peripheral blood smear in about 3 months to document resolution of the initial blood smear abnormalities.

When a benign condition (ie, viral infection) is not evident or lymphocytosis persists without explanation in a patient who was initially thought to have a viral cause, the clinician should consider malignant causes of lymphocytosis. If the peripheral blood smear reveals the presence of large, abnormal lymphocytes, further evaluation is necessary to exclude large granular lymphocytic leukemia. This is a form of non-Hodgkin's lymphoma, either of T-cell or natural killer cell lineage. Immunophenotyping, T-cell receptor gene rearrangement, and cytogenetic studies may need to be performed to differentiate a clonal from reactive T-cell process. Reactive T-cell large granular lymphocyte expansion has been described with viral infection (EBV, CMV, HIV) as well as other conditions.

Other types of lymphoproliferative disorders may also present with lymphocytosis. In these disorders, lymphocytosis usually reflects the presence of lymphoma cells in the peripheral blood. When lymphocytosis is due to a neoplastic cause, cytological abnormalities are often but not invariably present. These distinctive cytological features often allow these conditions to be differentiated from causes of reactive lymphyocytosis.

Two other important causes of neoplastic lymphocytosis are acute lymphoblastic leukemia (ALL) and chronic lymphocytic leukemia (CLL):

- Acute lymphoblastic leukemia

  In addition to leukocytosis with lymphocytic predominance, patients with ALL typically present with anemia and thrombocytopenia. In most benign causes of lymphocytosis, the other cell lines are typically normal in number. On occasion, however, autoimmune hemolytic anemia may develop in patients with infectious mononucleosis. Although viral infections are associated with thrombocytopenia, the decrease in platelet number is usually mild, in contrast to that seen in ALL. The peripheral blood smear plays a key role in differentiating ALL from benign causes of lymphocytosis. The hallmark of ALL is the presence of lymphoblasts. The presence of reactive lymphocytes should prompt consideration of benign causes of lymphocytosis. The definitive diagnosis of ALL requires bone marrow examination and immunophenotypic analysis.

- Chronic lymphocytic leukemia

  CLL, another neoplastic cause of lymphocytosis, deserves consideration, particularly in older individuals. As with ALL, examination of the peripheral blood smear is essential in differentiating CLL from benign causes of lymphocytosis. The lymphocytes of CLL are typically "normal appearing" and may be accompanied by smudge cells. The presence of "normal appearing" small lymphocytes in a patient who has lymphadenopathy or splenomegaly is particularly suggestive of CLL. Lymphocyte immunophenotyping using flow cytometry not only confirms clonality but also differentiates CLL from other types of chronic lymphoid leukemia that may also present with lymphocytosis.

Much information regarding the etiology of the lymphocytosis can be obtained by examining the results of the peripheral blood smear and lymphocyte immunophenotyping. Bone marrow aspiration and biopsy is also helpful in the evaluation of lymphocytosis and should be obtained in the following situations.

- The presence of immature lymphocytes (lymphoblasts) on peripheral blood smear
- Persistent lymphocytosis in the absence of acute or subacute infection
- Concomitant leukoerythroblastosis (presence of immature red blood cells and early granulocytic cells in the peripheral blood smear)

References

Hoffman R, Benz EJ, Shattil SJ, et al, eds, *Hematology, Basic Principles and Practice*, 3rd ed, New York, NY: Churchill Livingstone, 2000.

Horwitz CA, "Practical Approach to Diagnosis of Infectious Mononucleosis," *Postgrad Med*, 1979, 65:179-84.

Horwitz CA, Henle W, Henle G, et al, "Heterophil-Negative Infectious Mononucleosis and Mononucleosis-Like Illnesses: Laboratory Confirmation of 43 Cases," *Am J Med*, 1977, 63:947-57.

Jandl JH, *Blood, Textbook of Hematology*, 2nd ed, Boston, MA: Little, Brown and Company, 1996.

Lee GR, Forester J, Lukens J, et al, eds, *Wintrobe's Clinical Hematology*, 10th ed, Baltimore, MD: Williams and Wilkins, 1999.

Peterson L and Foucar K, "Granulocytosis and Granulocytopenia," *Hematology: Clinical and Laboratory Practice*, Bick RL, ed, St Louis, Mo: Mosby, 1993, 1137-54.

Peterson L and Hrisinko MA, "Benign Lymphocytosis and Reactive Neutrophilia: Laboratory Features Provide Diagnostic Clues," *Clin Lab Med*, 1993, 13:863-77.

Steeper TA, Horwitz CA, Hanson M, et al, "Heterophil-Negative Mononucleosis-Like Illnesses With Atypical Lymphocytosis in Patients Undergoing Seroconversion to the Human Immunodeficiency Virus," *Am J Clin Pathol*, 1988, 89:169-74.

MONOCYTOSIS

Monocytosis is defined as an absolute monocyte count >0.75 x 10^9/L. The absolute monocyte count may be determined as follows:

> **Absolute monocyte count** = total WBC count x monocyte %

Causes of Monocytosis

The causes of monocytosis are listed in the following box.

CAUSES OF MONOCYTOSIS

HEMATOLOGIC DISORDERS
- Acute myelogenous leukemia
  - Monocytic type
  - Myelomonocytic type
- Lymphoma
  - Hodgkin's lymphoma
  - Non-Hodgkin's lymphoma
- Chronic lymphocytic leukemia
- Myelodysplastic syndrome
- Myeloproliferative disorders
  - Chronic myelogenous leukemia
  - Polycythemia vera
- Multiple myeloma
- Hemolytic anemia
- Malignant histiocytosis
- Immune thrombocytopenic purpura

INFECTION
- Bacterial
  - Subacute bacterial endocarditis
  - Tuberculosis
- Viral
  - Infectious mononucleosis
  - CMV
  - VZV
- Syphilis
- Resolution phase of acute infection

CONNECTIVE TISSUE DISEASE
- Systemic lupus erythematosus
- Rheumatoid arthritis
- Polyarteritis nodosa
- Temporal arteritis
- Polymyositis

MISCELLANEOUS
- Sarcoidosis
- Splenectomy
- Carcinoma
- Alcoholic liver disease
- Sprue (tropical or nontropical)
- Inflammatory bowel disease
- Exogenous cytokine administration
- Parturition
- Depression
- Myocardial infarction
- Langerhan's cell histiocytosis
- Tetrachloroethane poisoning
- Glucocorticoid administration
- Chronic neutropenia
- Desmopressin administration
- Long-term hemodialysis

In one review of monocytosis, hematologic disorders accounted for over 50% of cases followed by connective tissue disease and malignancy at 10% and 8%, respectively.

Approach to the Patient With Monocytosis

Of key importance is the differentiation of reactive from neoplastic monocytosis. As indicated in the preceding box, there are many nonmalignant conditions associated with monocytosis. These causes of monocytosis are referred to as "reactive". Hematologic findings helpful in differentiating between reactive and neoplastic monocytosis are listed in the following table.

Hematologic Findings Used to Differentiate Between Reactive and Neoplastic Monocytosis

Hematologic Parameter	Reactive Monocytosis	Neoplastic Monocytosis
Peripheral blood smear	Reactive monocytes*	Immature monocytes; circulating monoblasts
Substantial left shift	Uncommon	Common
Dyspoiesis of one or more cell lines	Absent	May be present

*Vacuolated cytoplasm, mature nuclear chromatin, and indented or folded nuclei are features of reactive monocytes.

Further evaluation depends on whether the patient is thought to have reactive or neoplastic monocytosis. Patients thought to have reactive monocytosis may require blood culture or serologic studies if infection is a concern. Bone marrow examination (ie, culture) may be necessary if the infection is thought to involve the bone marrow.

In patients thought to have neoplastic monocytosis, bone marrow aspiration and biopsy is essential in not only confirming the presence of neoplastic monocytosis but also differentiating among the various causes, which include the following:

- Acute myelomonocytic leukemia
- Acute monocytic leukemia
- Myelodysplastic syndrome (chronic myelomonocytic leukemia)
- Myeloproliferative disorders (chronic myelogenous leukemia)
- Malignant histiocytosis

References

Cline MJ, "Laboratory Evaluation of Benign Quantitative Granulocyte and Monocyte Disorders," *Hematology Clinical and Laboratory Practice*, Bick RL, ed, Vol 2, St Louis, Mo: Mosby, 1993, 1155-60.

Hoffman R, Benz EJ, Shattil SJ, et al, eds, *Hematology, Basic Principles and Practice*, 3rd ed, New York, NY: Churchill Livingstone, 2000.

Jandl JH, *Blood, Textbook of Hematology*, 2nd ed, Boston, MA: Little, Brown and Company, 1996.

Lee GR, Forester J, Lukens J, et al, eds, *Wintrobe's Clinical Hematology*, 10th ed, Baltimore, MD: Williams and Wilkins, 1999.

Peterson L and Foucar K, "Granulocytosis and Granulocytopenia," *Hematology: Clinical and Laboratory Practice*, Bick RL, ed, St Louis, Mo: Mosby; 1993, 1137-54.

BASOPHILIA

Of the different types of white blood cells, basophils are present in the smallest numbers, typically accounting for <2% of the total white blood cell count.

> **Basophilia**: Absolute basophil count >0.2 x 10^9 cells/L

To calculate the absolute basophil count, use the following equation:

> **Absolute basophil count** = total WBC x basophil %

Causes of Basophilia

The causes of basophilia are listed in the following box.

CAUSES OF BASOPHILIA
CONNECTIVE TISSUE DISEASE (eg, juvenile rheumatoid arthritis)
ULCERATIVE COLITIS
ALLERGIC OR HYPERSENSITIVITY REACTIONS
ENDOCRINE DISORDERS
Diabetes mellitus
Myxedema
MEDICATIONS
Antithyroid agents
Estrogens
IRRADIATION
INFECTION (eg, smallpox, chickenpox, influenza, tuberculosis)
CHRONIC RENAL DISEASE
MYELOPROLIFERATIVE DISORDERS
Chronic myelogenous leukemia
Essential thrombocytosis
Polycythemia vera
Agnogenic myeloid metaplasia
ACUTE MYELOGENOUS LEUKEMIA
CARCINOMA
IRON DEFICIENCY
ERYTHRODERMA
IDIOPATHIC HYPEREOSINOPHILIC SYNDROME
SYSTEMIC MASTOCYTOSIS
ACUTE LYMPHOBLASTIC LEUKEMIA
BASOPHILIC LEUKEMIA
URTICARIA

Approach to the Patient With Basophilia

Reactive basophilia must be differentiated from neoplastic basophilia. The term "reactive" is used to refer to basophilia that occurs in response to a nonneoplastic condition. In patients with reactive basophilia, signs and symptoms of the underlying disease are often readily apparent. For example, the presence of urticaria should prompt consideration of an allergic or hypersensitivity reaction.

Splenomegaly is uncommonly appreciated in patients with reactive basophilia. The presence of an enlarged spleen raises concern for the possibility of a myeloproliferative disorder such as chronic myelogenous leukemia. Of note, in patients with chronic myelogenous leukemia, an increasing basophil count is a poor prognostic finding, often pointing to the development of an accelerated phase of the disease.

The degree of basophilia may provide clues to the etiology. Most causes of reactive basophilia are characterized by a modest increase in the basophil count. In contrast, neoplastic basophilia often presents with a significantly increased basophil count. Examination of the CBC is also useful in differentiating reactive from neoplastic basophilia. Anemia may be found in both types of basophilia. In reactive basophilia, it is not uncommon for patients to have the anemia of chronic disease. The platelet count is usually normal in patients with reactive basophilia whereas most patients with chronic myelogenous leukemia present with an elevated platelet count. Other findings suggestive of chronic myelogenous leukemia include leukocytosis with left shift and eosinophilia.

Examination of the peripheral blood smear typically reveals increased numbers of morphologically normal basophils in patients with reactive basophilia. Patients with myeloproliferative disorders, however, may present with a number of morphologic abnormalities.

In patients who have reactive basophilia, bone marrow aspiration and biopsy is not necessary. With appropriate treatment of the underlying disease, the basophil count will return to normal. If neoplastic basophilia is a concern (myeloproliferative disorders, acute myelogenous leukemia), bone marrow examination with cytogenetic analysis is necessary to establish the diagnosis.

References

Hoffman R, Benz EJ, Shattil SJ, et al, eds, *Hematology, Basic Principles and Practice*, 3rd ed, New York, NY: Churchill Livingstone, 2000.

Jandl JH, *Blood, Textbook of Hematology*, 2nd ed, Boston, MA: Little, Brown and Company, 1996.

Lee GR, Forester J, Lukens J, et al, eds, *Wintrobe's Clinical Hematology*, 10th ed, Baltimore, MD: Williams and Wilkins, 1999.

Peterson L and Foucar K, "Granulocytosis and Granulocytopenia," *Hematology: Clinical and Laboratory Practice*, Bick RL, ed, St Louis, Mo: Mosby, 1993, 1137-54.

EOSINOPHILIA

Absolute eosinophilia is said to be present if the eosinophil count is >0.5 x 10^9/L. The absolute eosinophil count may be calculated using the formula in the following box.

Absolute eosinophil count = total WBC x eosinophil %

It is important to realize that there is diurnal variability in the eosinophil count. The eosinophil count peaks between midnight and 4 AM. It then decreases by at least 20%, falling to a nadir during the morning hours. As a result, when following a patient with eosinophilia, the clinician should obtain eosinophil counts at roughly the same time of the day.

Causes of Eosinophilia

The causes of eosinophilia are listed in the following box.

CAUSES OF EOSINOPHILIA

- INFECTION
  - Parasitic
  - Tuberculosis
  - Scarlet fever
  - Fungal
    - Allergic bronchopulmonary aspergillosis
    - Coccidioidomycosis
- CONNECTIVE TISSUE / AUTOIMMUNE DISORDERS
  - Rheumatoid arthritis
  - Polyarteritis nodosa
  - Wegener's granulomatosis
  - Churg-Strauss syndrome
  - Eosinophilic fasciitis
  - Eosinophilia myalgia syndrome
  - Eosinophilia myositis
  - Eosinophilic gastroenteritis
  - Löffler's endocarditis
  - Ulcerative colitis
  - Regional enteritis
- ASTHMA
- ATOPIC DISORDERS
  - Seasonal allergic rhinitis
  - Chronic urticaria
  - Atopic dermatitis
- MALIGNANCY
  - Solid cancers
  - Hematologic
    - Acute eosinophilic leukemia
    - Chronic eosinophilic leukemia
    - T-lymphoblastic lymphoma
    - Acute lymphoblastic leukemia
    - Chronic myelogenous leukemia
    - Non-Hodgkin's lymphoma
    - Hodgkin's lymphoma
    - Mycosis fungoides
    - Sezary syndrome
- MYELODYSPLASTIC SYNDROME
- MYELOPROLIFERATIVE DISORDERS
- SYSTEMIC MASTOCYTOSIS
- SKIN DISEASES
  - Episodic angioedema with eosinophilia
  - Bullous pemphigoid
  - Pemphigus
  - Kimura's disease
  - Eosinophilic pustular folliculitis
- DRUG-INDUCED
- IMMUNODEFICIENCY STATES
- HYPEREOSINOPHILIC SYNDROME
- ADRENAL INSUFFICIENCY
- ATHEROEMBOLIC DISEASE
- EOSINOPHILIC PNEUMONIA (acute or chronic)

Although there are many causes of eosinophilia, when the eosinophil count exceeds 10 X 10^9/L, the clinician should consider causes of marked eosinophilia. These include parasitic infection, drug hypersensitivity, Hodgkin's lymphoma, eosinophilic leukemia, Churg-Strauss variant of polyarteritis nodosa, and the idiopathic hypereosinophilic syndrome. The major causes of eosinophilia will be discussed in further detail in the remainder of this chapter.

Parasitic Infection

Many parasitic infections are accompanied by eosinophilia. Helminthic infections usually result in significant eosinophilia. In contrast, only two protozoan infections are characterized by eosinophilia: *Isospora belli* and *Dientamoeba fragilis*. However, it is important to note that eosinophilia may be absent in some helminthic infections because of bacterial superinfection or steroid treatment. Infections that are only intraluminal may not have associated eosinophilia.

Parasitic infections characterized by encystation are usually associated with mild to no eosinophilia. This is in contrast to infections that result in tissue invasion. In these infections, very high eosinophil counts are usually seen. The degree of eosinophilia correlates rather well with the extent of tissue invasion.

If the geographic and dietary history is suggestive of possible exposure to parasitic organisms, stools should be sent for ova and parasites. With some parasitic organisms, more than three stool specimens may be needed. Because some parasitic organisms are never seen in the feces, a normal stool examination does not exclude parasitic infection. In these cases, examination of the blood or tissue biopsy of a clinically affected organ may aid in the diagnosis. In some cases, serologic and PCR-based tests may be needed to establish the diagnosis.

There are several reasons why parasitic infection should be a consideration in every patient with eosinophilia. These reasons include the following:

- Effective treatment is now available for most parasitic infections
- Administration of steroids to patients with undiagnosed parasitic infection can have untoward consequences, including fatal superinfection

Drug-Induced Eosinophilia

Drugs are the most common cause of eosinophilia; therefore, a detailed history of current and past medication use is important. Commonly implicated drugs include penicillins, cephalosporins, para-aminosalicylic acid, gold, phenytoin, hydralazine, chlorpromazine, warfarin, carbamazepine, nitrofurantoin, and sulfonamides. As clinicians become more familiar with some of the newer drugs, the list of common offenders is likely to expand. Recently, eosinophilia has been reported to occur in patients treated with IL-2/lymphocyte activated killer cells. While prescription medications are a concern, the clinician should also ask the patient about any recent use of over-the-counter or herbal medications.

While drug-induced eosinophilia may be accompanied by drug fever or organ dysfunction, in some cases, eosinophilia may be the only manifestation of a drug reaction. The finding of drug-induced eosinophilia does not always require withdrawal of the drug. In the presence of organ dysfunction, however, the medication should be discontinued. Organs that tend to be involved include lungs, kidneys, and heart. Withdrawal of the medication results in resolution of eosinophilia, but the time course to normalization is variable.

Asthma

The absolute eosinophil count may be mildly elevated in patients with uncomplicated asthma. Rarely does the count exceed 2 x 10^9/L. Eosinophil counts exceeding this value should prompt consideration of other causes of eosinophilia such as Churg-Strauss syndrome, allergic bronchopulmonary aspergillosis, Löffler's syndrome, sarcoidosis, chronic eosinophilic pneumonia, or tropical pulmonary eosinophilia.

Idiopathic Hypereosinophilic Syndrome

The hypereosinophilic syndrome is characterized by prolonged eosinophilia of unclear etiology with widespread organ dysfunction and tissue infiltration by eosinophils. To make this diagnosis, all other causes of eosinophilia must be excluded. Criteria for the diagnosis of the hypereosinophilic syndrome are listed in the following box.

CRITERIA FOR THE DIAGNOSIS OF HYPEREOSINOPHILIC SYNDROME

- Eosinophil count >1.5 x 10^9/L for >6 months or death before 6 months with signs and symptoms of the hypereosinophilic syndrome
- Absence of another etiology for the eosinophilia*
- Symptoms and signs of organ involvement

*Other causes of sustained eosinophilia with counts >1.5 x 10^9/L include Churg-Strauss syndrome, drug-induced eosinophilia, eosinophilia-myalgia syndrome, eosinophilic cellulitis, eosinophilic fasciitis, eosinophilic pneumonia, eosinophilic gastroenteritis, eosinophilic vasculitis, parasitic infection, episodic angioedema with eosinophilia, Kimura's disease, eosinophilic leukemia, bullous pemphigoid, malignancy (lymphoid or myeloid), metastatic cancer, and tropical eosinophilia.

Eosinophilia With Pulmonary Infiltrates

A number of conditions may present with eosinophilia and pulmonary infiltrates, as shown in the following box.

CONDITIONS PRESENTING WITH PULMONARY INFILTRATES AND EOSINOPHILIA

PARASITIC INFECTION
DRUG HYPERSENSITIVITY
ASTHMA
ALLERGIC BRONCHOPULMONARY ASPERGILLOSIS
INFECTION
- Tuberculosis
- Brucellosis
- Coccidioidomycosis
- Histoplasmosis
- *Pneumocystis carinii* pneumonia

CARCINOMA
HODGKIN'S LYMPHOMA
BRONCHOCENTRIC GRANULOMATOSIS
SARCOIDOSIS
EOSINOPHILIC PNEUMONIA
IDIOPATHIC HYPEREOSINOPHILIC SYNDROME
CYTOKINE ADMINISTRATION
COCAINE PNEUMONITIS
CHURG-STRAUSS DISEASE

Approach to the Patient With Eosinophilia

In many cases of eosinophilia, the cause is readily apparent. The common causes include allergic disease (eczema, hay fever), asthma, and parasitic infection (in some parts of the world). While the patient's clinical presentation usually allows the diagnosis of allergic disease to be made readily, parasitic infection can be more difficult to diagnose and it is not uncommon for eosinophilia to be the finding that prompts a thorough evaluation, ultimately leading to the diagnosis of parasitic infection. In the hospitalized patient, a new finding of eosinophilia is often due to drug allergy.

When the etiology is obscure, the clinician should assess the degree of eosinophilia. It is not uncommon to encounter patients in the outpatient setting with mild eosinophilia. These patients deserve a thorough history and physical examination in an effort to identify a cause. If no cause is apparent and the CBC is otherwise unremarkable, an extensive evaluation may not be needed.

If the eosinophilia is sustained or of greater magnitude, a more extensive evaluation is warranted. In these cases, it is important to distinguish reactive from clonal eosinophilia. The term "reactive" is used to describe eosinophilia that is due to a nonclonal disorder. Clonal eosinophilia occurs in patients with myeloproliferative disorders or other hematologic neoplasms that have an eosinophilic component.

The evaluation of patients with unexplained, sustained eosinophilia is summarized in the following box.

EVALUATION OF PATIENTS WITH IDIOPATHIC EOSINOPHILIA

FOCUSED HISTORY AND PHYSICAL EXAM
COMPLETE BLOOD COUNT AND LEUKOCYTE DIFFERENTIAL COUNT
ERYTHROCYTE SEDIMENTATION RATE
MIDSTREAM URINALYSIS AND GRAM STAIN
13-CHANNEL SERUM CHEMISTRY GROUP
VITAMIN B_{12} AND FOLATE DETERMINATIONS
QUANTITATIVE IMMUNOGLOBULIN LEVELS, INCLUDING IgE
SERUM PROTEIN ELECTROPHORESIS
SERUM INTERLEUKIN-5 DETERMINATION
AM AND PM CORTISOL LEVELS
SKIN TESTS FOR COMMON INHALANTS, MOLDS, AND FOODS
ELECTROCARDIOGRAPHY AND ECHOCARDIOGRAPHY
FRESH STOOL EXAMINATION FOR OVA AND PARASITES (x3)
PARASITE SEROLOGIC TESTS (as clinically warranted)
CT SCAN OF THE CHEST AND ABDOMEN
BONE MARROW ASPIRATE AND BIOPSY WITH CHROMOSOME STUDIES AND STAINS FOR MAST CELLS
TISSUE BIOPSY WITH STAINING FOR EOSINOPHILS AND EOSINOPHIL PROTEINS, WHEN INDICATED
MOLECULAR GENETIC STUDIES FOR B- AND T-CELL ARRANGEMENTS OF PERIPHERAL BLOOD LYMPHOCYTES
Clinical circumstances or laboratory availability may warrant or allow one or more of the following tests: urinary drug screen, rheumatoid factor, serum complement determinations, serum eosinophil protein levels, quantitation of N-methylhistamine

Adapted from Tefferi A, *Primary Hematology*, Totowa, NJ: Humana Press, 2001, 163.

The tests listed in the above box are useful in differentiating between reactive and clonal eosinophilia. A common question that arises is whether or not the patient with eosinophilia requires bone marrow aspiration and biopsy. To answer this question, the clinician should examine the peripheral blood smear. Eosinophil dyspoiesis (ie, hypogranularity, nuclear segmentation defects) may be seen in both reactive and clonal eosinophilia. However, the presence of severe eosinophil dyspoiesis or dyspoiesis in other cell lines (red blood cells, platelets, other white blood cells) is suggestive of a clonal disorder. When the peripheral blood smear reveals findings consistent with a hematologic neoplasm or myeloproliferative disorder, bone marrow aspiration and biopsy along with cytogenetic/molecular studies is indicated.

Bone marrow aspiration and biopsy is not necessary if a cause of reactive eosinophilia is apparent. In these cases, the eosinophil count should be repeated after the underlying condition has been appropriately treated. Normalization of the eosinophil count lends further support to the diagnosis of reactive eosinophilia.

References

Bain BJ, "Hypereosinophilia," *Curr Opin Hematol*, 2000, 7(1):21-5 (review).

Brigden M and Graydon C, "Eosinophilia Detected by Automated Blood Cell Counting in Ambulatory North American Outpatients: Incidence and Clinical Significance," *Arch Pathol Lab Med*, 1997, 121(9):963-7.

Brigden ML, "A Practical Workup for Eosinophilia: You Can Investigate the Most Likely Causes Right in Your Office," *Postgrad Med*, 1999, 105(3):193-210.

Brito-Babapulle F, "The Eosinophilias, Including the Idiopathic Hypereosinophilic Syndrome," *Br J Haematol*, 2003, 121(2):203-23.

Guitart J, "Idiopathic Eosinophilia," *N Engl J Med*, 2000, 342(9):659-60.

Rothenberg ME, "Eosinophilia," *N Engl J Med*, 1998, 338(22):1592-600.

NEUTROPENIA

Neutropenia is defined as an absolute neutrophil count <1.5 x 10^9/L (1500/ mm^3). The absolute neutrophil count can be calculated using the following formula:

ANC = total WBC count x neutrophil %

where neutrophil percentage refers to mature and band neutrophils.

The clinician should realize, however, that patient race has some bearing on the lower limit of the normal neutrophil count. Certain groups such as African-Americans and Yemenite Jews tend to have lower neutrophil counts. In this population, the lower limit of normal may be as low as 1 x 10^9 cells/L (1000/ mm^3). In fact, 25% of healthy black adults have an absolute neutrophil count ranging between 1000 and 1500/mm^3. Since these individuals are otherwise healthy, normal race variation is thought to explain the lower neutrophil counts appreciated in these populations.

Neutropenia must be differentiated from leukopenia, which is a term that connotes a decrease in the total white blood cell count. Although neutropenia is the major cause of leukopenia, a significant decrease in the total lymphocyte count may also present with leukopenia. Therefore, when a low white blood cell count is noted, the clinician should examine the differential white blood cell count to determine which type of white blood cell (ie, neutrophil or lymphocyte) is depressed.

Risk of Infection

Risk of infection increases as neutrophil count declines. There is also a direct correlation between infection and the degree and duration of neutropenia.

• Mild neutropenia	1.0-1.5 x 10^9 cells/L
• Moderate neutropenia	0.5-1.0 x 10^9 cells/L
• Severe neutropenia	<0.5 x 10^9 cells/L

Mild neutropenia confers little risk for infection in an otherwise healthy individual but as the neutrophil count drops below 1.0 X 10^9 cells/L, the risk of infection increases.

Causes of Neutropenia

The causes of neutropenia can be found in the following box.

CAUSES OF NEUTROPENIA

INFECTION
- Viral
- Bacterial
- Fungal
- Protozoal
- Rickettsial

DRUG-INDUCED
- Dose-dependent (predictable)
- Idiosyncratic

HYPERSPLENISM

AUTOIMMUNE / OTHER IMMUNE DISORDERS
- Systemic lupus erythematosus
- Rheumatoid arthritis
- Felty's syndrome
- Sjögren's syndrome
- Wegener's granulomatosis

BONE MARROW REPLACEMENT
- Hematologic neoplasms
- Solid cancer
- Granulomatous disease
- Myelofibrosis

MYELODYSPLASTIC SYNDROME

APLASTIC ANEMIA

MEGALOBLASTIC ANEMIA (folate or B_{12} deficiency)

CONSTITUTIONAL NEUTROPENIC DISORDERS
- Cyclic neutropenia
- Kostmann's syndrome
- Swachman-Diamond syndrome
- Immunodeficiency disorders / reticular dysgenesis
- Chediak-Higashi syndrome
- Myelokathexis
- Fanconi syndrome
- Dyskeratosis congenita

ACQUIRED IDIOPATHIC NEUTROPENIA

ACUTE ANAPHYLAXIS

HEMOPHAGOCYTIC SYNDROME

COPPER DEFICIENCY

COMPLEMENT ACTIVATION (exposure of blood to artificial membranes)

IRRADIATION

Some of the more common causes of neutropenia are discussed in further detail in the remainder of this chapter.

Drug-Induced Neutropenia

Medications are one of the more common causes of neutropenia. Drug-induced neutropenia may be predictable or idiosyncratic. Predictable drug-induced neutropenia follows the administration of cytotoxic chemotherapeutic agents.

Idiosyncratic drug-induced neutropenia may result from either decreased production or increased destruction of neutrophils. Although any medication could potentially be the cause of the neutropenia, the clinician should be particularly suspicious of medications that were recently started. This is because drug-induced neutropenia typically occurs within a few weeks of starting a medication. It may occur even sooner if the patient has received the offending medication sometime in the past. The clinician should realize, however, that neutropenia may be caused by a medication that the patient has been using on a chronic basis. In general, when considering drug-induced neutropenia in a patient on a long list of medications, the offending medication is more likely to be one that was recently started, especially if it is one that is known to be associated with neutropenia.

Common offenders are listed in the following box.

COMMON MEDICINAL CAUSES OF DRUG-INDUCED NEUTROPENIA	
CYTOTOXIC AGENTS	PHENOTHIAZINES
ANTIBIOTICS	ALPHA-METHYLDOPA
Penicillins	PENICILLAMINE
Cephalosporins	ALLOPURINOL
Sulfonamides	CIMETIDINE
Chloramphenicol	CLOZAPINE
ANTICONVULSANTS	DIURETICS
NSAIDs	Spironolactone
ANTITHYROID AGENTS	Chlorothiazide
Propylthiouracil	Ethacrynic acid
Methimazole	

After discontinuation of the offending medication, the time to recovery of the neutrophil count will vary depending upon the degree of marrow hypoplasia. One sign that indicates that the bone marrow is recovering is an increase in the blood monocyte count. Not uncommonly, the neutrophil count will overshoot, leading to the development of neutrophilia.

Infection

Viral infections are a common cause of neutropenia. The severity of neutropenia can vary from mild to severe, but because it is a transient phenomenon, co-infection with bacteria is uncommon. There are some viruses, however, that can cause a more severe, persistent neutropenia. These include Epstein-Barr virus, hepatitis B virus, parvovirus B19, and HIV.

Although some bacterial infections are typically associated with neutropenia (typhoid fever, tularemia, brucellosis), most bacterial infections are associated with neutrophilia. However, neutropenia with a shift to the left may be seen with severe bacterial infections when the peripheral utilization of neutrophils exceeds the ability of the bone marrow to produce cells. This is more likely to occur in elderly and in those who are nutritionally compromised. In the setting of septicemia, neutropenia is associated with a poor prognosis.

Nutritional Deficiency

Vitamin B_{12} and folate deficiency should always be considered in the differential diagnosis of neutropenia. Anemia is always present when neutropenia is due to vitamin B_{12} or folate deficiency. The finding of hypersegmented neutrophils is particularly supportive of the diagnosis. When present, the neutropenia is usually mild in degree. Mild neutropenia may also be noted in patients with copper deficiency.

Bone Marrow Replacement

Neutropenia may be a manifestation of bone marrow replacement by malignancy or other lesion. Both solid and hematologic tumors may present with bone marrow replacement. Nonmalignant causes include granulomatous disease as well as other conditions. Bone marrow replacement, also known as myelophthisis, should be considered, particularly when the peripheral blood smear reveals evidence of leukoerythroblastosis. The latter term refers to the presence of teardrop shaped red blood cells as well as immature red and white blood cell precursors.

Hematologic Disorders

While some hematologic disorders can cause neutropenia due to bone marrow replacement, others directly affect the neutrophil precursors in the bone marrow. Examples include leukemia, aplastic anemia, and myelodysplastic syndromes. Isolated neutropenia is unusual and most cases are characterized by the presence of anemia and/or thrombocytopenia. A disorder in which only the white blood cell line is depressed, termed pure white cell aplasia, has been described mainly in association with thymoma.

Suppressor T-Cell Induced Neutropenia

Mild-to-moderate neutropenia may be encountered in patients with suppressor T-cell induced neutropenia. This disorder, also known as large granular lymphocytic disorder (leukemia), is characterized by the presence of increased numbers of large lymphocytes with cytoplasmic granularity. Some cases are associated with splenomegaly and rheumatoid arthritis in what is termed Felty's syndrome.

Connective Tissue Disease

Neutropenia may complicate the course of a number of connective tissue diseases including systemic lupus erythematosus, rheumatoid arthritis, and Felty's syndrome. The neutropenia of connective tissue disease is thought to be due to antineutrophilic antibodies causing immune-mediated destruction. Mild-to-moderate neutropenia is the rule and, not uncommonly, there is accompanying anemia and/or thrombocytopenia.

Hypersplenism

Mild-to-moderate neutropenia is quite commonly encountered in patients with hypersplenism. In most cases, the neutropenia is accompanied by anemia and/or thrombocytopenia. Rarely will a patient with hypersplenism present with isolated neutropenia. Physical examination may reveal the presence of splenomegaly. The clinician should realize, however, that not all patients with hypersplenism will have a palpable spleen.

Cyclic Neutropenia

Although many cases of cyclic neutropenia are diagnosed in childhood, on occasion, the condition may escape diagnosis until adulthood. The classic history involves symptoms of fever, mouth sores, and fatigue which last for several days and then resolve, only to return 3-4 weeks later. In between the symptomatic episodes, patients report no complaints. The elicitation of such a history should prompt the clinician to obtain white blood cell counts twice a week for 2 months. Examination of these counts will demonstrate the periodic rise and fall in the neutrophil count characteristic of cyclic neutropenia.

Approach to the Patient With Neutropenia

Because neutropenic patients are at risk for infection, every patient with neutropenia should have a thorough history and physical examination searching for infection. The clinician should realize that infection may either be a complication of neutropenia or the cause of neutropenia. It may be difficult to identify the site of infection because the manifestations of infection are often due, in part, to the presence of substantial numbers of neutrophils at the site of infection. As a result, in neutropenic patients, the signs and symptoms of infection may be very subtle.

The evaluation of neutropenia begins with examination of the peripheral blood smear to confirm the presence of neutropenia. On occasion, pseudoneutropenia may be encountered, which will be evident on the blood film. Peripheral blood smear findings in some causes of neutropenia are listed in the following table.

Using the Peripheral Blood Smear to Elucidate the Etiology of Neutropenia

Condition	Peripheral Blood Smear Findings
B_{12} or folate deficiency	Hypersegmented neutrophils; macroovalocytes
Bone marrow replacement (myelophthisis)	Tear-drop shaped red blood cells; immature red blood cell precursors; immature white blood cell precursors
Acute myelogenous leukemia	Myeloblasts; Auer rods
Acute lymphoblastic leukemia	Lymphoblasts
Myelodysplastic syndrome	White blood cells Pseudo-Pelger-Huet change Hypogranularity Immature granulocytes Circulating myeloblasts (<5%) Platelets Large Hypogranular Micromegakaryocytes Vacuolated platelets Red blood cells Anisopoikilocytosis Basophilic stippling Nucleated red blood cells Vacuolated red blood cells

Patients suspected of having vitamin B_{12} or folate deficiency should have serum vitamin B_{12} and folate levels measured to confirm the diagnosis. If the peripheral blood smear reveals abnormalities suggestive of myelodysplastic syndrome, myelophthisis, or other clonal hematologic conditions, a bone marrow aspiration and biopsy should be obtained.

When the peripheral blood smear is unrevealing, the clinician should consider the possibility of drug-induced neutropenia The most common type of drug-induced neutropenia is that due to the use of cytotoxic agents (chemotherapy). This cause of neutropenia is readily apparent in that it occurs some time after chemotherapy administration. In other cases of drug-induced neutropenia, the cause may not be so apparent. The clinician should carefully examine the medication list, searching for common offenders. Although most cases of drug-induced neutropenia are due to medications that were recently started, even medications that have been chronically administered have been known to be causative agents. If a common offender is not identified, all nonessential medications should be discontinued and essential medications should be substituted. Resolution of the neutropenia with removal of the offending medication supports the diagnosis.

If the patient has signs and symptoms of a connective tissue disease, the clinician may wish to obtain antinuclear antibodies and rheumatoid factor. If the peripheral blood smear is unrevealing, a drug-induced etiology is unlikely, and no other cause is apparent in the asymptomatic patient with mild neutropenia, it is reasonable to follow the patient since most cases of mild neutropenia are due to benign causes. During follow-up, the absolute neutrophil count should be determined 3 times per week for a total of 8 weeks to assess for cyclic neutropenia. If the neutropenia resolves during follow-up, the cause may have been a recent infection, as postinfectious neutropenia is quite common. If the neutropenia persists after 8 weeks of observation, examination of the bone marrow is warranted along with testing for antinuclear antibodies, antineutrophil antibodies, HIV, immunoglobulins/immune evaluation, and vitamin B_{12}/folate levels. Peripheral blood immunotyping of lymphocytes may help diagnose or exclude the possibility of a large granular lymphocytic disorder.

Patients with moderate to severe neutropenia usually undergo bone marrow examination, unless the etiology is evident. If the etiology is not clear after this procedure, the tests described above for mild neutropenia that persists after 8 weeks of observation should be performed.

References

Claas FH, "Immune Mechanisms Leading to Drug-Induced Blood Dyscrasias," *Eur J Haematol Suppl*, 1996, 60:64-8.

Foucar K, Duncan MH, and Smith KJ, "Practical Approach to the Investigation of Neutropenia," *Clin Lab Med*, 1993, 13:879-94.

Peterson L and Foucar K, "Granulocytosis and Granulocytopenia," *Hematology: Clinical and Laboratory Practice*, Bick RL, ed, St Louis, Mo: Mosby, 1993, 1137-54.

Reed WW and Diehl LF, "Leukopenia, Neutropenia, and Reduced Hemoglobin Levels in Healthy American Blacks," *Arch Intern Med*, 1991, 151:501-5.

Sievers EL and Dale DC, "Nonmalignant Neutropenia," *Blood Rev*, 1996, 10:95-100.

Welte K and Boxer LA, "Severe Chronic Neutropenia: Pathophysiology and Therapy," *Semin Hematol*," 1997, 34:267-78.

NEUTROPENIA

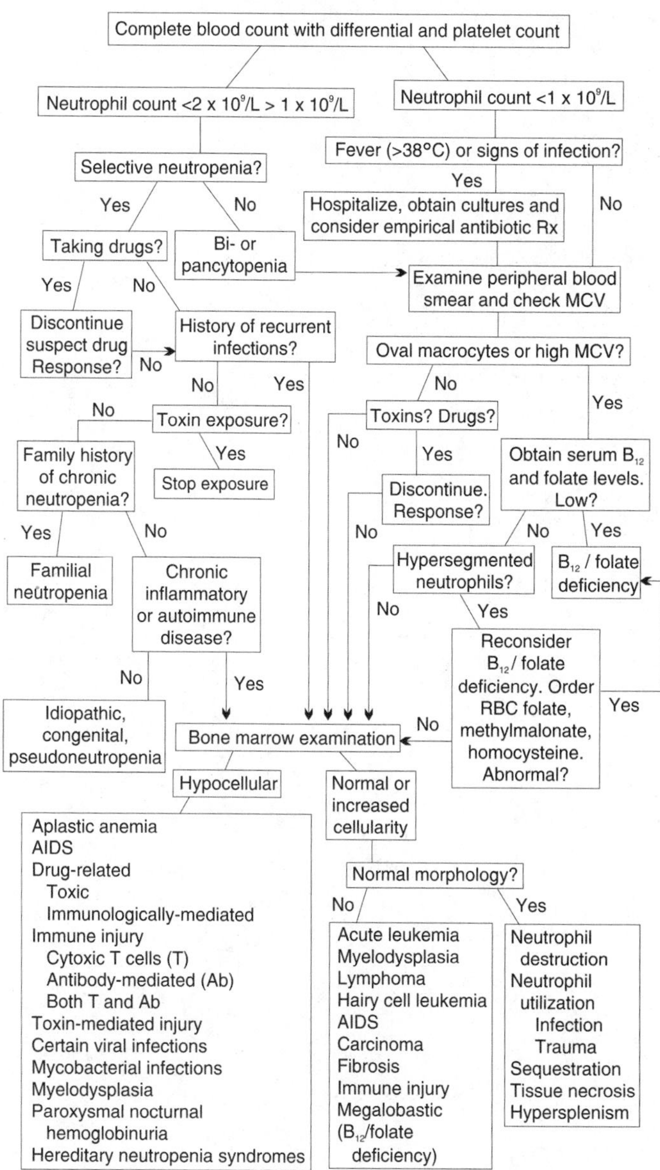

Adapted from Goldman, Bennett, et al, *Cecil Textbook of Medicine*, 21st ed, Philadelphia, PA: WB Saunders Co, 1999, 924.

THROMBOCYTOPENIA

Not all patients with thrombocytopenia present with mucosal bleeding, petechiae, or ecchymoses. The variability in the patient's clinical presentation, to some extent, has to do with the degree of thrombocytopenia, as shown in the following table.

Risk of Bleeding in Patients With Thrombocytopenia

Platelet Count	Risk of Bleeding
>100,000/µL	No abnormal bleeding even after surgery
50,000-100,000/µL	Patients may bleed longer than normal with severe trauma
20,000-50,000/µL	Bleeding occurs with minor trauma
<20,000/µL	Patients may have spontaneous bleeding

In many cases, a low platelet count is an unsuspected laboratory test abnormality, detected when a routinely ordered CBC reveals the presence of thrombocytopenia.

Causes of Thrombocytopenia

The causes of thrombocytopenia are listed in the following box.

CAUSES OF THROMBOCYTOPENIA

- SPURIOUS (pseudothrombocytopenia)
- DECREASED PRODUCTION
  - Vitamin B_{12} deficiency
  - Folate deficiency
  - Marrow replacement
    - Leukemia
    - Lymphoma
    - Metastatic tumor
    - Myelofibrosis
    - Granulomatous disease
  - Myelodysplastic syndrome
  - Aplastic anemia
  - Pure megakaryocytic aplasia
  - Medications
    - Cytotoxic (chemotherapeutic, immunosuppressive)
    - Estrogens
    - Thiazide diuretics
  - Radiation
  - Toxins
    - Alcohol
    - Cocaine
  - Infection
  - Iron deficiency
  - Congenital
    - Thrombocytopenia with absent radii syndrome
    - May-Hegglin anomaly
    - Wiskott-Aldrich syndrome
    - Bernard-Soulier syndrome
    - Gray platelet syndrome
    - Alport's syndrome

(continued)

CAUSES OF THROMBOCYTOPENIA *(continued)*

- INCREASED DESTRUCTION
  - Immune
    - Autoantibody-mediated
      - Acute immune thrombocytopenic purpura (ITP)
      - Chronic immune thrombocytopenic purpura (ITP)
      - Connective tissue disease
        - Systemic lupus erythematosus
        - Polyarteritis nodosa
      - Malignancy
        - Chronic lymphocytic leukemia
        - Lymphoma
        - Solid tumor
      - Drug-induced (including heparin)
      - Infection (EBV, CMV, HIV, hepatitis, tuberculosis)
    - Alloantibody-mediated
      - Post-transfusion purpura
      - Neonatal
  - Nonimmune
    - Hemolytic uremic syndrome (HUS)
    - Thrombotic thrombocytopenic purpura (TTP)
    - Disseminated intravascular coagulation
    - Other causes of microangiopathic hemolytic anemia (see below)
- HYPERSPLENISM
- DILUTION (massive blood transfusion)

Some of the major causes of thrombocytopenia are discussed in the remainder of this chapter.

Immune Thrombocytopenic Purpura (ITP)

Immune thrombocytopenic purpura, also known as ITP, is a condition characterized by the development of antibodies directed against platelets. The formation of these antiplatelet antibodies leads to immune-mediated thrombocytopenia. Two forms of ITP have been described: acute and chronic.

The acute form has a predilection for children, typically occurring after an individual has recovered from an infection. Most commonly, the patient reports a nonspecific viral infection although, on occasion, acute ITP has followed recovery from a bacterial infection.

Although adults may develop acute ITP, the illness more often has a gradual onset (chronic ITP). Most adults do not recall a preceding viral or bacterial infection. Approximately 90% of those affected are younger than 40 years of age. Interestingly, the chronic form of ITP has a predilection for women.

The diagnosis of ITP is one of exclusion. Every effort should be made to exclude other causes of thrombocytopenia. Since ITP is not characterized by splenomegaly, this physical examination finding should prompt consideration of another etiology. Examination of the CBC reveals no abnormality other than the depressed platelet count. The hemoglobin is typically normal unless the thrombocytopenia has led to significant bleeding. Examination of the peripheral blood smear may reveal a higher percentage of large platelets.

While bone marrow aspiration and biopsy is not needed in most cases of ITP, if performed, the bone marrow examination will reveal normal granulocytic and erythrocytic precursors. An increase in the number of megakaryocytes is consistent with the diagnosis.

Almost 75% of patients with chronic ITP have detectable platelet autoantibodies. Although antiplatelet antibodies are involved in the pathogenesis of ITP, demonstration of their presence is not necessary to establish the diagnosis of ITP. Despite the availability of antiplatelet antibody testing, they have not become a standard part of the diagnostic evaluation because of problems with sensitivity and specificity.

Thrombocytopenia During Pregnancy

Nearly 5% of women will develop thrombocytopenia during pregnancy. Many of these cases are due to gestational thrombocytopenia which needs to be differentiated from not only ITP but also other causes of pregnancy-associated thrombocytopenia such as preeclampsia, drug-induced thrombocytopenia, disseminated intravascular coagulation, HIV, and TTP/HUS. Clinical features favoring gestational thrombocytopenia over ITP include absence of thrombocytopenia history before the pregnancy as well as platelet counts >50,000/µL. If the platelet count falls to <50,000/µL, serious consideration should be given to the possibility of ITP. Criteria for the diagnosis of gestational thrombocytopenia are listed in the following box.

CRITERIA FOR THE DIAGNOSIS OF GESTATIONAL THROMBOCYTOPENIA

- Presence of mild thrombocytopenia
- Presence of asymptomatic thrombocytopenia
- No history of previous thrombocytopenia
- Development of thrombocytopenia during pregnancy
- Absence of fetal thrombocytopenia
- Thrombocytopenia resolves after delivery

For more information about the conditions that can cause thrombocytopenia during pregnancy, please refer to the chapter on preeclampsia.

Connective Tissue Disease

A variety of connective tissue diseases may be associated with immune thrombocytopenia. Thrombocytopenia has been reported in up to 26% of SLE patients. In some cases of SLE, immune thrombocytopenia may be accompanied by an autoimmune hemolytic anemia. This has been termed Evan's syndrome. Evan's syndrome has also been described in patients with no clinical features suggestive of connective tissue disease.

Infection

Viral infection is a major cause of immune thrombocytopenia. These include infectious mononucleosis, CMV, and HIV among others. In most of these cases, the patient relates a recent history of symptoms consistent with viral infection.

Thrombocytopenia seen in HIV patients may be immune or nonimmune-mediated, but most cases appear to be due to ineffective platelet production. Not uncommonly, the etiology is multifactorial. In addition to immune thrombocytopenia, thrombocytopenia in HIV patients may be due to bone marrow replacement by granulomatous disease or drug-induced. When HIV thrombocytopenia is immune-mediated, it can occur at any point in the course of the HIV infection. It may even occur when the viral load is low and the CD4 count is relatively well preserved.

In addition to viral causes, infection caused by bacteria (Gram-positive and negative), mycoplasma, syphilis, malaria, and rickettsial organisms can also be associated with thrombocytopenia.

Dilutional Thrombocytopenia

This is a common cause of thrombocytopenia in hospitalized patients who have had significant blood loss. With the aggressive administration of intravenous fluids, the platelet count falls.

Radiation

Radiation therapy can be complicated by the development of thrombocytopenia. The damage occurs in the bone marrow, affecting the megakaryocytes rather than the circulating platelets. The onset of the thrombocytopenia typically occurs 7-10 days after radiation therapy.

Alcohol

Thrombocytopenia is common in patients who drink alcohol heavily. Although the decreased platelet count may be due to alcohol-induced bone marrow suppression, two other important causes in this patient population include folate deficiency and hypersplenism secondary to chronic liver disease. The thrombocytopenia is typically mild to moderate but severe thrombocytopenia can be seen, especially when multiple factors are present (ie, folate deficiency + alcohol-induced bone marrow suppression).

Malignancy

Lymphoproliferative disorders such as chronic lymphocytic leukemia and lymphoma may also be associated with immune thrombocytopenia. More commonly, however, the thrombocytopenia is due to decreased platelet production from marrow infiltration or the effects of cancer treatment. Although immune thrombocytopenia has also been reported in patients with solid cancer, this association is rare.

Drug-Induced Thrombocytopenia

A number of different drugs have been associated with thrombocytopenia. In many cases, the thrombocytopenia is immune-mediated. In fact, over 50 drugs have been reported to cause immune thrombocytopenia. Clinicians should ask about both prescription and nonprescription drugs that the patient is taking. Common offenders are listed in the following box.

COMMON DRUG-INDUCED CAUSES OF IMMUNE THROMBOCYTOPENIA

- ANTIBIOTICS
  - Penicillin
  - Beta-lactam-containing antibiotics
  - Sulfa drugs
  - Rifampin
- ANTICONVULSANTS
  - Phenytoin
  - Valproic acid
  - Carbamazepine
- H_2 BLOCKERS
  - Cimetidine
  - Ranitidine
- ANALGESIC AGENTS
  - Acetaminophen
  - Acetylsalicylic acid
  - Ibuprofen
  - Indomethacin
  - Other NSAIDs
- MISCELLANEOUS
  - Quinine
  - Quinidine
  - Heparin
  - Digoxin
  - Amrinone
  - Alpha-methyldopa
  - Chlorthalidone
  - Furosemide
  - Gold salts
  - Interferons
  - Measles-mumps-rubella vaccine
  - Penicillamine
  - Procainamide

Most cases of drug-induced thrombocytopenia are due to medications that were recently started. In fact, the median time to the development of a low platelet count is two weeks. Despite this, cases have been reported in which the patient was taking the medication for as long as three years. The diagnosis of drug-induced thrombocytopenia is established if the platelet count returns to normal after discontinuation of the suspect medication. In most cases, thrombocytopenia usually resolves 5-7 days after withdrawal of the medication. On occasion, the thrombocytopenia is prolonged because of slow clearance of the medication or its metabolites from the body (eg, gold-induced). Although the development of thrombocytopenia with medication rechallenge provides even stronger evidence for the diagnosis, the clinician should do so with caution because rechallenge can be dangerous. Some patients have developed severe thrombocytopenia after medication rechallenge. If the medication is the culprit, rechallenge will lead to thrombocytopenia within three days of administration.

Although platelet antibody testing is available in the diagnosis of drug-induced thrombocytopenia, assays for drug-dependent antibodies are usually not obtained because the results are not often available at a time when the clinician has to make management decisions. In addition, antibody testing is cumbersome and a negative test result does not exclude the diagnosis.

Heparin-Induced Thrombocytopenia

It is important to consider heparin-induced thrombocytopenia in every patient who presents with a low platelet count because these patients are at risk for thrombosis. Thrombocytopenia due to heparin therapy may develop in 1% to 5% of patients. In most cases, the platelet count is noted to decrease within 6-10 days after starting heparin therapy. If the patient has received heparin in the past, however, thrombocytopenia may occur earlier. It is important to realize that even small doses of heparin can lead to thrombocytopenia. In fact, heparin-induced thrombocytopenia has been reported after using low doses of heparin to flush vascular catheters.

Low molecular weight heparin has been considered to be less immunogenic and to cause less thrombocytopenia relative to standard heparin. Nonetheless, immune thrombocytopenia has been reported to occur with the use of low molecular weight heparin. Because there is high cross-reactivity between the two types of heparin, it is often not possible to use low molecular weight heparin in place of standard heparin when thrombocytopenia occurs.

Although testing for heparin-induced thrombocytopenia is available, most laboratories do not routinely perform this type of testing. In addition, none of the available assays for the diagnosis of heparin-induced thrombocytopenia have a high enough sensitivity or specificity, and, therefore, the diagnosis is mainly a clinical one (see boxes below). In usual clinical practice, resolution of the thrombocytopenia with discontinuation of the heparin supports the diagnosis.

HEPARIN-INDUCED THROMBOCYTOPENIA TYPE I (Nonimmune, Nonidiosyncratic)
Episode of thrombocytopenia occurs early in exposure, generally in the first few days in naive patients and in the first few hours in previously exposed patients.
Mild thrombocytopenia: 10% to 30% decrease in platelet numbers
Clinical manifestations: None
Mechanism: Heparin-induced platelet aggregation
True incidence: Uncertain but common
Biologic issues: Episode transient; counts normalize even with continued therapy
Therapy: None
Relationship to HIT II: Unclear, but probably none

From Walenga JM, et al, *Hematol Oncol Clin N Am*, 2003, 17:265.

CLINICAL FEATURES OF HEPARIN-INDUCED THROMBOCYTOPENIA TYPE II
Usual onset at day 3-14 (median day 6)
Nadir platelet count: usually 30,000-60,000, but may be as low as 5000. The most appropriate definition is a 50% decrease in platelet numbers from the baseline values.
Risk occurs with all methods of heparin administration. Risk occurs most commonly with continuous infusion of heparin. HIT also is seen with heparin flushes (500 units/day) and with heparin-coated catheters. Risk is higher with intravenous than subcutaneous administration. Additionally, bovine heparins may induce greater risk than porcine heparins, which induce a greater risk than LMW heparins.
Can occur within hours of heparin exposure in previously heparin-treated patients
Increased incidence in patients with recent surgery (primarily venous problems)
Increased incidence in patients with pre-existing cardiovascular disease (primarily arterial)
Risks are equal in men and in women. Age is not a factor, and there is no relation to inherited deficiency or acquired defects of clotting factors.

From Walenga JM et al, *Hematol Oncol Clin N Am*, 2003, 17:261.

Thrombotic Thrombocytopenic Purpura (TTP)

TTP is characterized by the pentad of thrombocytopenia, microangiopathic hemolytic anemia (>96%), neurologic manifestations (>92%), fever (98%), and renal involvement (88%). Renal dysfunction is typically mild. Rarely does the serum creatinine level rise to >3 mg/dL. Urinalysis may reveal the presence of proteinuria, hematuria, and casts.

The clinician should realize that TTP is just one cause of microangiopathic hemolytic anemia and thrombocytopenia. The term "microangiopathic" is used to describe occlusion of small blood vessels which results in the fragmentation of red blood cells. This leads to the appearance of schistocytes and helmet cells on the peripheral blood smear. Other causes of microangiopathic hemolytic anemia and thrombocytopenia are listed in the following box.

CAUSES OF MICROANGIOPATHIC HEMOLYTIC ANEMIA AND THROMBOCYTOPENIA
THROMBOTIC THROMBOCYTOPENIC PURPURA (TTP)
HEMOLYTIC-UREMIC SYNDROME (HUS)
DISSEMINATED INTRAVASCULAR COAGULATION (DIC)
MALIGNANT HYPERTENSION
PREECLAMPSIA / ECLAMPSIA
HELLP SYNDROME*
SCLERODERMA WITH ASSOCIATED HTN AND RENAL FAILURE
VASCULITIS
CAVERNOUS HEMANGIOMA (Kasabach-Merritt syndrome)
DISSEMINATED CARCINOMA
RENAL ALLOGRAFT REJECTION
PROSTHETIC HEART VALVES (malfunctioning)

*HELLP syndrome refers to preeclampsia-associated hemolytic anemia with elevated liver enzymes and low platelets.

TTP must be differentiated from the causes listed above. In usual clinical practice, HUS and DIC are the major considerations in the differential diagnosis. The presence of coagulation abnormalities (elevated PT, PTT, and D-dimer) supports the diagnosis of DIC. TTP is not associated with coagulation abnormalities unless significant tissue necrosis occurs, in which case DIC may develop.

In contrast to TTP, HUS primarily affects children. HUS is characterized by the triad of acute renal failure, thrombocytopenia, and microangiopathic hemolytic anemia. The acute renal failure of HUS is often much more prominent than that seen in TTP. Fever and neurologic involvement are not typical features of HUS. Recently, TTP patients have been found to have deficiency of vWF-cleaving protease. This abnormality has not been noted in HUS. An assay is now available to detect this abnormality, which will be of use to clinicians in their efforts to distinguish between these two disorders. One limitation of current testing is that test results are not available at a time when treatment decisions need to be made.

In most cases of TTP, the diagnosis is fairly certain. When the diagnosis is in doubt, the clinician may choose to perform biopsy of the skin, gums, or bone marrow. Biopsy findings consistent with TTP have been reported in 40% to 60% of patients.

Hypersplenism

Hypersplenism is a fairly common cause of thrombocytopenia due to platelet pooling. Rarely does the platelet count fall to <30,000/μL in patients with hypersplenism. Platelet counts less than this should prompt a search for an additional or other etiology. Although leukopenia and/or anemia may also be present, in some cases, only thrombocytopenia may be present.

The detection of splenomegaly on physical examination supports the diagnosis. Studies, however, have shown that physical examination fails to detect many cases of splenomegaly. Therefore, in some cases, it may be necessary to assess spleen size by imaging tests.

Approach to the Patient With Thrombocytopenia

Before embarking on an evaluation of thrombocytopenia, it is wise to confirm the presence of a low platelet count. Normally 8-20 platelets are found per high-powered field under 1000 x oil magnification. One way to confirm the presence of thrombocytopenia is to count up the number of platelets in 8-10 fields (under 1000 x oil magnification) and multiply this number by 2000. If done properly, the number that is calculated should closely approximate the value reported by the automated counter.

Spurious causes of thrombocytopenia are not uncommon, occurring with an incidence of 0.09% to 0.21%. Failure to recognize spurious thrombocytopenia, also known as pseudothrombocytopenia, can lead to an extensive and unnecessary workup. In addition, failure to recognize spurious thrombocytopenia can have serious consequences for the patient if the patient is mistakenly diagnosed with another cause of thrombocytopenia. In these cases, inappropriate treatment may be given which has the potential to be detrimental to the patient's health.

For this reason, examination of the peripheral blood smear is essential in every patient with thrombocytopenia. Examination of the smear may help exclude causes of pseudothrombocytopenia, which are listed in the following box.

CAUSES OF PSEUDOTHROMBOCYTOPENIA	
IMPROPER BLOOD SAMPLING TECHNIQUE*	*EX VIVO* PLATELET CLUMPING
GIANT PLATELETS†	EDTA-dependent‡
PLATELET SATELLITISM	Other anticoagulant-dependent agglutinins
COLD AGGLUTININS	

*Careless venipuncture or the presence of inadequate amounts of anticoagulant may lead to partial clotting of the blood sample, which may result in falsely low platelet counts.

†Certain conditions (ie, myeloproliferative disorders, hereditary platelet disorders) are associated with the presence of giant platelets. Some automated blood counters may not recognize these platelets as true platelets. In these cases, the lab may incorrectly report a lower platelet count.

‡EDTA-dependent pseudothrombocytopenia is the most common cause of spurious thrombocytopenia. Examination of the peripheral blood smear may reveal platelet clumping or satellitism, which refers to platelet adherence to neutrophils. The diagnosis is supported if the platelet count is normal using another anticoagulant (ie, citrate or heparin).

Adapted from Loscalzo J and Schafer AI, *Thrombosis and Hemorrhage*, 2nd ed, Baltimore, MD: Williams and Wilkins, 1998, 462.

Pseudothrombocytopenia should be a consideration in every patient with thrombocytopenia, particularly when it occurs in individuals who have no bleeding manifestations related to thrombocytopenia. On occasion, pseudothrombocytopenia may be associated with pseudoleukocytosis. The falsely elevated white blood cell count is due to the automated blood counter counting platelet clumps as leukocytes. In other cases, pseudothrombocytopenia may be associated with pseudoleukopenia. A falsely low white blood cell count may be obtained when platelets adhere to white blood cells (satellitism). In these cases, the large masses of platelets and white blood cells may not be counted as platelets or white blood cells.

In addition to confirming the presence of true thrombocytopenia, the peripheral blood smear may provide clues to the etiology of the thrombocytopenia, as shown in the following table.

Using the Peripheral Blood Smear to Elucidate the Etiology of the Thrombocytopenia

Peripheral Blood Smear Finding	Condition Suggested
Atypical or abnormal lymphocytes	Viral etiology (ie, infectious mononucleosis) Lymphoproliferative disorder
Fragmented red blood cells (schistocytes or helmet cells)	Microangiopathic hemolytic anemia (ie, DIC, TTP, HUS)
Oval macrocytes Hypersegmented neutrophils	Vitamin B_{12} or folate deficiency
Spherocytes Increased reticulocytes	Autoimmune hemolytic anemia together with thrombocytopenia (Evan's syndrome)
Blasts	Leukemia
Dyserythropoietic features Anisopoikilocytosis Basophilic stippling Nucleated red blood cells Vacuolated red blood cells Dysgranulopoietic features Neutropenia Immature granulocytes Hypogranularity Pseudo-Pelger-Huet anomaly Myeloblasts (<5%) Dysmegakaryopoietic features Thrombocytopenia Large platelets Hypogranularity	Myelodysplastic syndrome
Leukoerythroblastosis (tear-drop shaped red blood cells along with immature red and white blood cell precursors)	Myelophthisis (bone marrow replacement or infiltration)
Left shift (bands, metamyelocytes) along with Döhle bodies and cytoplasmic vacuolization	Bacterial infection / sepsis

Further evaluation of the thrombocytopenic patient depends upon the findings noted in the peripheral blood smear. Serum folate and vitamin B_{12} levels should be obtained if hypersegmented neutrophils are found. The presence of atypical lymphocytes should prompt consideration of viral causes. A direct Coombs' test should be performed if the peripheral blood smear reveals spherocytes and reticulocytes, features suggestive of Evan's syndrome. Blood and urine cultures are indicated when bacterial sepsis is suspected. When leukoerythroblastosis, blasts, or features of myelodysplasia are noted, bone marrow examination is necessary to confirm the diagnosis.

If the peripheral blood smear reveals schistocytes and helmet cells, the clinician should search for a cause of microangiopathic hemolytic anemia. In particular, HUS, TTP, and DIC are major considerations. Laboratory tests needed to distinguish between these possibilities include PT, PTT, D-dimer, LDH, and serum creatinine. DIC can be distinguished from HUS and TTP because the former is usually associated with elevations in the PT and PTT. TTP is characterized by the pentad of microangiopathic hemolytic anemia, thrombocytopenia, fever, neurologic manifestations, and renal dysfunction but not all five features are always present. HUS is favored as the diagnosis in patients who have the triad of thrombocytopenia, microangiopathic hemolytic anemia, and acute renal failure. It is of the utmost importance that the diagnosis of HUS and TTP be established expeditiously because a delay in diagnosis and treatment can lead to a significant increase in morbidity and mortality.

Laboratory Findings in Selected Disorders Causing Thrombocytopenia

	ITP	TTP	DIC	Evan's Syndrome	HUS
Platelets	↓	↓	↓	↓	↓
PT / PTT	Normal	Normal	↑	Normal	Normal
Coombs' test	(-)	(-)	(-)	(+)	(-)
Anemia	(-)	MAHA	MAHA	AIHA	MAHA
Smear		Schistocytes	Schistocytes	Spherocytes	Schistocytes
↓Fibrinogen, ↑FSP	(-)	(-)	(+)	(-)	(-)

MAHA = microangiopathic hemolytic anemia; AIHA = autoimmune hemolytic anemia.

If the peripheral blood smear does not reveal any abnormalities suggestive of an etiology, the clinician should consider the following two causes of thrombocytopenia.

1. Drug-induced thrombocytopenia

   Drug-induced thrombocytopenia has been reported with many different medications (see above). A thorough medication history should be obtained in all thrombocytopenic patients. The development of thrombocytopenia soon after starting a medication should prompt consideration of this possibility. The clinician should realize, however, that this temporal relationship is not always present in cases of drug-induced thrombocytopenia. If drug-induced thrombocytopenia is suspected, the offending medication should be discontinued. Resolution of the thrombocytopenia after withdrawal of the suspect medication supports the diagnosis.

   The clinician should be particularly vigilant for heparin-induced thrombocytopenia because some cases may be complicated by the development of thrombotic events. Heparin-induced thrombocytopenia may occur even with small doses of heparin (ie, heparin flushes). Normalization of the platelet count after discontinuation of the heparin therapy supports the diagnosis.

2. Hypersplenism

   The presence of palpable splenomegaly should prompt consideration of hypersplenism as the cause of the thrombocytopenia. At times, however, it may be difficult to appreciate splenomegaly on physical examination. In these cases, it may be worthwhile to obtain an imaging test to assess splenic size. When the presence of splenomegaly is established, the clinician should search for an etiology. One of the most common causes of splenomegaly is chronic liver disease/cirrhosis. Other causes such as lymphoproliferative disorders (lymphoma, CLL) should also be considered.

If the etiology of the thrombocytopenia remains unclear after inspection of the peripheral blood smear and consideration of drug-induced thrombocytopenia and hypersplenism, the clinician should consider immune-mediated causes. Immune thrombocytopenia may be primary or secondary. Primary immune thrombocytopenia is also known as idiopathic thrombocytopenic purpura (ITP). ITP needs to be differentiated from secondary causes of immune thrombocytopenia (ie, associated with underlying disease). To make this distinction, the following tests may need to be obtained.

- Antinuclear antibodies (if history of serositis, skin rash, or arthritis is elicited) to assess for connective tissue disease
- CT scan of thorax/abdomen/pelvis (if examination reveals lymphadenopathy or splenomegaly) to assess for lymphoma or chronic lymphocytic leukemia
- Serologic testing for HIV

- Lupus anticoagulant/anticardiolipin antibodies (immune thrombocytopenia may be associated with the presence of antiphospholipid antibodies)

If a secondary cause of immune thrombocytopenia is not apparent, the diagnosis of ITP becomes more likely. ITP is a diagnosis of exclusion. The Practice Guidelines Panel of the American Society of Hematology has established the following criteria for the diagnosis of chronic ITP.

- Individuals must have thrombocytopenia without associated leukocyte abnormalities or anemia unless due to bleeding secondary to thrombocytopenia
- Absence of disease associated with immune thrombocytopenia such as connective tissue disease, lymphoproliferative disorders, HIV infection, etc

It is important to realize that splenomegaly is not a feature of ITP. Its presence should prompt consideration of an alternative diagnosis. Measurement of antiplatelet antibodies are not recommended at this time because these tests are lacking in both sensitivity and specificity. Bone marrow aspiration and biopsy is not needed for the diagnosis of ITP. It may be performed, however, if the clinical presentation is atypical or the patient is older than 60 years of age (to rule out myelodysplastic syndrome). Bone marrow examination will help to exclude a primary hematologic condition or a systemic disorder affecting the bone marrow. Normal or increased numbers of megakaryocytes is consistent with the diagnosis of ITP.

References

Baglin TP, "Heparin-Induced Thrombocytopenia Thrombosis (HIT/T) Syndrome: Diagnosis and Treatment," *J Clin Pathol*, 2001, 54(4):272-4.

Burrows RF, "Platelet Disorders in Pregnancy," *Curr Opin Obstet Gynecol*, 2001, 13(2):115-9.

Carey PJ, "Drug-Induced Myelosuppression: Diagnosis and Management," *Drug Saf*, 2003, 26(10):691-706.

Chong BH and Keng TB, "Advances in the Diagnosis of Idiopathic Thrombocytopenic Purpura," *Semin Hematol*, 2000, 37(3):249-60.

Cines DB and Blanchette VS, "Immune Thrombocytopenic Purpura," *N Engl J Med*, 2002, 346(13):995-1008.

Elalamy I, Lecrubier C, Horellou MH, et al, "Heparin-Induced Thrombocytopenia: Laboratory Diagnosis and Management," *Ann Med*, 2000, 321(Suppl 1):60-7.

George JN, "Idiopathic Thrombocytopenic Purpura: Current Issues for Pathogenesis, Diagnosis, and Management in Children and Adults," *Curr Hematol Rep*, 2003, 2(5):381-7.

George JN, Woolf SH, Raskob GE, et al, "Idiopathic Thrombocytopenic Purpura: A Practice Guideline Developed by Explicit Methods for the American Society of Hematology," *Blood*, 1996, 88:3-40.

Hoffman R, Benz EJ, Shattil SJ, et al, eds, *Hematology, Basic Principles and Practice*, 3rd ed, New York, NY: Churchill Livingstone, 2000.

Jandl JH, *Blood, Textbook of Hematology*, 2nd ed, Boston, MA: Little, Brown and Company, 1996.

Lee GR, Forester J, Lukens J, et al, eds, *Wintrobe's Clinical Hematology*, 10th ed, Baltimore, MD: Williams and Wilkins, 1999.

Manny N and Zelig O, "Laboratory Diagnosis of Autoimmune Cytopenias," *Curr Opin Hematol*, 2000, 7(6):414-9.

McCrae KR, "Thrombocytopenia in Pregnancy: Differential Diagnosis, Pathogenesis, and Management," *Blood Rev*, 2003, 17(1):7-14.

Moake JL, "Thrombotic Microangiopathies," *N Engl J Med*, 2002, 347(8):589-600.

Moreno A and Menke D, "Assessment of Platelet Numbers and Morphology in the Peripheral Blood Smear," *Clin Lab Med*, 2002, 22(1):193-213, vii.

Nabhan C and Kwaan HC, "Current Concepts in the Diagnosis and Management of Thrombotic Thrombocytopenic Purpura," *Hematol Oncol Clin North Am*, 2003, 17(1):177-99.

Ruggenenti P, Noris M, and Remuzzi G, "Thrombotic Microangiopathy, Hemolytic Uremic Syndrome, and Thrombotic Thrombocytopenic Purpura," *Kidney Int*, 2001, 60(3):831-46.

Scaradavou A, "HIV-Related Thrombocytopenia," *Blood Rev*, 2002 16(1):73-6.

Schwartz KA, "Gestational Thrombocytopenia and Immune Thrombocytopenias in Pregnancy," *Hematol Oncol Clin North Am*, 2000, 14(5):1101-16.

Warkentin TE and Heddle NM, "Laboratory Diagnosis of Immune Heparin-Induced Thrombocytopenia," *Curr Hematol Rep*, 2003, 2(2):148-57.

Tsai HM, "Advances in the Pathogenesis, Diagnosis, and Treatment of Thrombotic Thrombocytopenic Purpura," *J Am Soc Nephrol*, 2003, 14(4):1072-81.

Warkentin TE, "Heparin-Induced Thrombocytopenia," *Curr Hematol Rep*, 2002, 1(1):63-72.

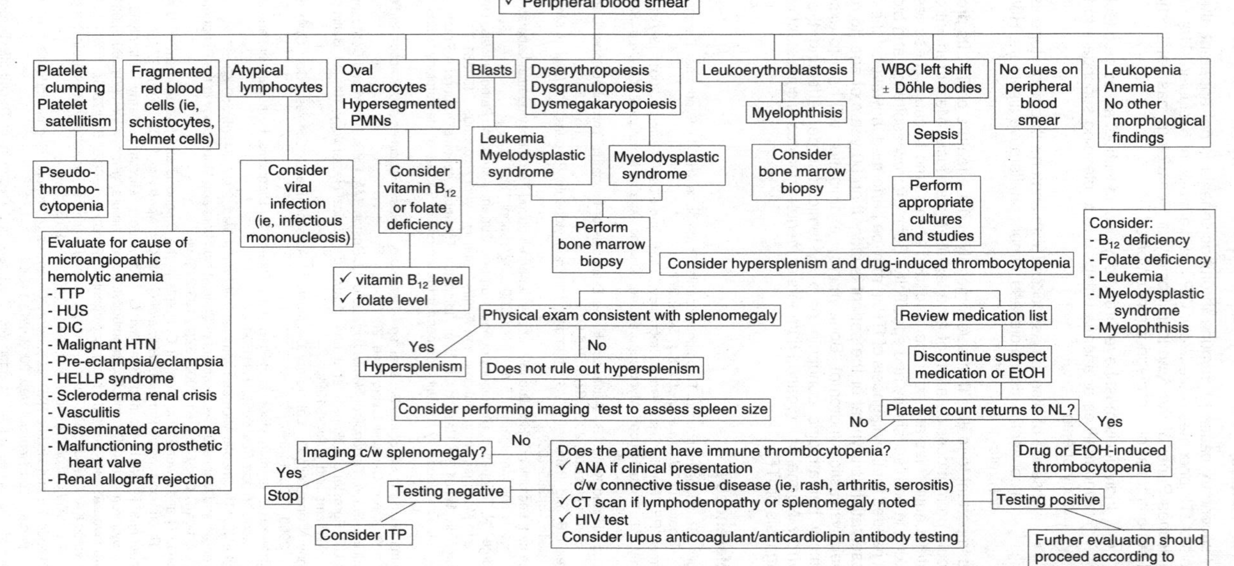
THROMBOCYTOPENIA
✓ Peripheral blood smear
Platelet clumping
Platelet satellitism
Fragmented red blood cells (ie, schistocytes, helmet cells)
Atypical lymphocytes
Oval macrocytes
Hypersegmented PMNs
Blasts
Dyserythropoiesis
Dysgranulopoiesis
Dysmegakaryopoiesis
Leukoerythroblastosis
WBC left shift ± Döhle bodies
No clues on peripheral blood smear
Leukopenia
Anemia
No other morphological findings
Pseudo-thrombo-cytopenia
Evaluate for cause of microangiopathic hemolytic anemia
- TTP
- HUS
- DIC
- Malignant HTN
- Pre-eclampsia/eclampsia
- HELLP syndrome
- Scleroderma renal crisis
- Vasculitis
- Disseminated carcinoma
- Malfunctioning prosthetic heart valve
- Renal allograft rejection
Consider viral infection (ie, infectious mononucleosis)
Consider vitamin B_{12} or folate deficiency
✓ vitamin B_{12} level
✓ folate level
Leukemia
Myelodysplastic syndrome
Myelodysplastic syndrome
Perform bone marrow biopsy
Myelophthisis
Consider bone marrow biopsy
Sepsis
Perform appropriate cultures and studies
Consider:
- B_{12} deficiency
- Folate deficiency
- Leukemia
- Myelodysplastic syndrome
- Myelophthisis
Consider hypersplenism and drug-induced thrombocytopenia
Physical exam consistent with splenomegaly
Yes
Hypersplenism
No
Does not rule out hypersplenism
Consider performing imaging test to assess spleen size
Imaging c/w splenomegaly?
Yes
Stop
No
Does the patient have immune thrombocytopenia?
✓ ANA if clinical presentation c/w connective tissue disease (ie, rash, arthritis, serositis)
✓ CT scan if lymphodenopathy or splenomegaly noted
✓ HIV test
Consider lupus anticoagulant/anticardiolipin antibody testing
Testing negative
Consider ITP
Testing positive
Further evaluation should proceed according to abnormality identified
Review medication list
Discontinue suspect medication or EtOH
Platelet count returns to NL?
Yes
Drug or EtOH-induced thrombocytopenia
No

THROMBOCYTOSIS

Thrombocytosis is defined as an increase in the platelet count. The upper limit of the normal platelet count may vary from laboratory to laboratory but usually is about 350-450 x 10^9/L. Before starting a workup to elucidate the etiology of thrombocytosis, a repeat platelet count should be obtained to verify the presence of an elevated platelet count.

Causes of Thrombocytosis

The causes of thrombocytosis may be classified as follows:

- Physiologic thrombocytosis
- Reactive (secondary) thrombocytosis
- Clonal (primary) thrombocytosis

It is important to differentiate clonal from physiologic and reactive thrombocytosis since only the former is associated with thrombotic complications. The causes of thrombocytosis are listed in the following box.

CAUSES OF THROMBOCYTOSIS
PHYSIOLOGIC
Exercise
Stress
Epinephrine
REACTIVE
Acute blood loss
Hemolytic anemia
Infection
Inflammatory disease
Iron deficiency anemia
Malignancy
Postoperative
Postsplenectomy / hyposplenism
Response to drugs (vincristine, all-trans retinoic acid, cytokines, growth factors)
Rebound thrombocytosis (recovery from thrombocytopenia)
Trauma
FAMILIAL
CLONAL
AML (acute megakaryoblastic leukemia)
Myeloproliferative disorder
Essential thrombocytosis
Polycythemia vera
Agnogenic myeloid metaplasia
Chronic myelogenous leukemia
Myelodysplastic syndrome

The causes of reactive and clonal thrombocytosis are discussed in further detail in the remainder of this chapter.

Infection

A variety of infections, both acute and chronic, have been associated with reactive thrombocytosis. These include pneumonia, pyelonephritis, pyogenic arthritis, osteomyelitis, chronic wound infection, tuberculosis, and other bacterial infections. Viral infections rarely present with thrombocytosis.

Inflammatory Disorders

Inflammatory diseases causing thrombocytosis include rheumatoid arthritis, polymyalgia rheumatica, polyarteritis nodosa, inflammatory bowel disease, nephritis, and hepatic cirrhosis. As a general rule, the degree of thrombocytosis parallels the activity of the disease. With appropriate treatment of the inflammatory disease, the platelet count returns to normal.

Iron Deficiency Anemia

An elevated platelet count is not uncommon in patients with iron deficiency anemia. On occasion, the platelet count may be >1000 x 10^9/L. With institution of iron replacement therapy, the platelet count typically returns to normal within 10 days.

Malignancy

Thrombocytosis has been reported to be associated with a wide variety of malignancies including Hodgkin's lymphoma, non-Hodgkin's lymphoma, ovarian cancer, bladder cancer, mesothelioma, lung cancer, prostate cancer, and pancreatic cancer. Ninety percent of patients with malignancy-associated reactive thrombocytosis have platelet counts between 400 and 1000 x 10^9/L.

Splenectomy

Thrombocytosis, sometimes exceeding 1000 x 10^9/L, can occur following splenectomy. The platelet count usually returns to normal over weeks to months. Persistent thrombocytosis following splenectomy should prompt consideration of an underlying myeloproliferative disorder or condition characterized by either hemolysis or ineffective erythropoiesis.

Clonal Thrombocytosis

Clonal thrombocytosis may be seen in patients with myeloproliferative and myelodysplastic disorders. The four myeloproliferative disorders include the following:

1. Essential thrombocytosis
2. Chronic myelogenous leukemia

   Two-thirds of chronic myelogenous leukemia patients have thrombocytosis at the time of diagnosis.
3. Polycythemia vera

   An elevated platelet count is noted in approximately 66% of polycythemia vera patients. Five percent have marked thrombocytosis, with platelet counts >1000 x 10^9/L.
4. Agnogenic myeloid metaplasia

   Also known as idiopathic myelofibrosis, agnogenic myeloid metaplasia is characterized by anemia and splenomegaly. Examination of the peripheral blood smear often reveals leukoerythroblastosis, defined as the presence of teardrop-shaped red blood cells as well as immature red and white blood cell precursors. Thrombocytosis is found in approximately 33% of patients but with advancing disease, thrombocytopenia is the rule.

Most myelodysplastic disorders are not characterized by thrombocytosis. In fact, a normal or decreased platelet count is much more commonly noted in these patients. One type of myelodysplastic syndrome, referred to as the "5q-syndrome," is associated with thrombocytosis in 50% of patients.

Approach to the Patient With Thrombocytosis

When thrombocytosis is first discovered, it is worthwhile to repeat the platelet count to ensure that thrombocytosis is truly present. Pseudothrombocytosis is not common but does occur in patients with cryoglobulinemia, a condition in which circulating protein precipitates are read as platelets by the automated counter. Examination of the peripheral blood smear will help exclude this possibility. Once true thrombocytosis is confirmed, further evaluation focuses on differentiating reactive from clonal thrombocytosis.

The degree of thrombocytosis does not reliably discriminate between reactive and clonal thrombocytosis. It is often thought that impressive elevations in the platelet count are more likely to be due to clonal thrombocytosis. In one study examining the causes of thrombocytosis in patients having platelet counts exceeding 1000 x 10^9/L, most of the cases were due to reactive thrombocytosis.

A thorough history and physical examination can often provide clues to aid the clinician in differentiating between reactive and clonal thrombocytosis, as shown in the following table.

Using the Clinical Presentation to Differentiate Between Reactive and Clonal Thrombocytosis

Reactive Thrombocytosis	Clonal Thrombocytosis
Platelet count recently normal (ie, before current illness known to be associated with reactive thrombocytosis)	Persistently elevated platelet count
Presence of condition known to be associated with reactive thrombocytosis	No identifiable cause of reactive thrombocytosis
No clinical features of myeloproliferative disorder present*	Clinical features suggestive of clonal thrombocytosis present*
Absence of splenomegaly	Presence of splenomegaly
No history of unusual thrombotic complications (ie, Budd-Chiari syndrome)	History of unusual thrombotic complications (ie, Budd-Chiari syndrome)

*The presence of post-bathing pruritus should prompt consideration of polycythemia vera. Erythromelalgia, which refers to painful, red, ischemic digits, may occur in patients with polycythemia vera or essential thrombocytosis. Striking plethora may be noted in some polycythemia vera patients.

Although the clinical presentation may provide clues as to whether the patient has reactive or clonal thrombocytosis, a more secure diagnosis can only be made with further evaluation. In this regard, laboratory testing plays a key role in differentiating between these two major types of thrombocytosis. Laboratory evaluation should begin with the CBC. Many of the causes of reactive thrombocytosis are associated with the anemia of inflammation. The presence of microcytic, hypochromic anemia should prompt consideration of iron deficiency anemia. An elevated hemoglobin level raises concern for the possibility of polycythemia vera but this finding may be noted in other myeloproliferative disorders.

Of key importance is examination of the peripheral blood smear, as shown in the following table.

Using the Peripheral Blood Smear to Differentiate Reactive From Clonal Thrombocytosis

Peripheral Blood Smear Finding	Condition Suggested
Leukoerythroblastosis*	Agnogenic myeloid metaplasia
Leukocytosis with marked left shift†	Chronic myelogenous leukemia
Howell-Jolly bodies	Hyposplenism
Macrocytic anemia with features of dyserythropoiesis, dysgranulopoiesis, and dysmegakaryopoiesis	Myelodysplastic syndrome

*The term "leukoerythroblastosis" refers to the presence of teardrop-shaped red blood cells, immature red blood cell precursors, and immature white blood cell precursors. Although a leukoerythroblastic peripheral blood smear is required for the diagnosis of agnogenic myeloid metaplasia, these findings may be found in other types of myeloproliferative disorders as well as stroke, trauma, or sepsis.

†The peripheral blood smear shows a characteristic left shift in the granulocytic series. Although granulocytes in all stages of maturation may be noted, most are mature cells, typically segmented neutrophils and myelocytes. Less mature cells may be present, but usually comprise a smaller percentage of the total white blood cell count. The combination of myeloblasts and promyelocytes typically does not exceed 10%, nor does the blast percentage alone exceed 5%. Increased numbers of monocytes, basophils, and eosinophils are not uncommon. Nucleated red blood cells may be seen, but the morphology of the red blood cells is usually normal. Likewise, platelet morphology is typically normal.

A normal serum ferritin level is useful in excluding iron deficiency anemia. Since many of the causes of reactive thrombocytosis are associated with inflammation, levels of C-reactive protein, an acute phase reactant, are often elevated. Elevated C-reactive protein is not a feature of clonal thrombocytosis. Other laboratory test findings suggestive of an inflammatory process include decreased levels of serum iron, TIBC, and albumin along with increased levels of fibrinogen and haptoglobin.

Some clinicians find measurement of the mean platelet volume or MPV (indicator of platelet size) and platelet distribution width (measure of platelet anisocytosis) helpful in their evaluation of thrombocytosis. In patients with clonal thrombocytosis, MPV and platelet distribution width are often elevated. In contrast, most patients with reactive thrombocytosis have normal values. Consensus, however, is lacking regarding the use of these tests in the evaluation of the thrombocytosis patient.

If the patient's clinical presentation is consistent with one of the causes of reactive thrombocytosis, the platelet count should be repeated 1 month after the underlying condition has been treated. Normalization of the platelet count provides further support for the diagnosis of reactive thrombocytosis.

If clonal thrombocytosis is suspected, further evaluation is necessary to not only confirm the presence of clonal thrombocytosis but also differentiate among the causes of clonal thrombocytosis. The evaluation of these patients may include the following.

- Bone marrow aspiration and biopsy along with cytogenetic studies

  Bone marrow aspiration and biopsy is necessary to differentiate among the causes of clonal thrombocytosis. The diagnosis of chronic myelogenous leukemia rests upon identification of the Philadelphia chromosome by cytogenetic testing. A minority of patients with chronic myelogenous leukemia do not have the Philadelphia chromosome; many of these patients are found to have the *bcr-abl* gene rearrangement with DNA-based testing. The bone marrow findings of polycythemia vera and essential thrombocytosis are similar. A major difference, however, is the absence of stainable iron stores in patients with polycythemia vera. In contrast, stainable iron is present in essential thrombocytosis patients. Significant fibrosis of the bone marrow should prompt consideration of agnogenic myeloid metaplasia.

- Red cell mass

  Measurement of red cell mass should be a consideration in patients with erythrocytosis. Red cell mass is normal in essential thrombocytosis but is increased in polycythemia vera.

- Erythropoietin level

  In patients with erythrocytosis, a low serum erythropoietin level supports the diagnosis of polycythemia vera

Essential Thrombocythemia (Essential Thrombocytosis)

The diagnosis of essential thrombocytosis is secure only when reactive causes of thrombocytosis as well as other myeloproliferative disorders have been excluded. The hematologic findings of essential thrombocytosis are listed in the following table.

Hematologic Findings of Essential Thrombocytosis

Hematologic Parameter	Abnormality
Platelet count	Elevated
Hemoglobin	Typically normal; may be low in patients with chronic bleeding
MCV	Typically normocytic; may be microcytic in patients with chronic bleeding
WBC count	Normal or increased
Peripheral blood smear	Large platelet clumps; significant variation in platelet size (giant platelets, microplatelets, abnormal granularity); normal to increased white blood cells; red blood cells usually normocytic, normochromic but may be microcytic, hypochromic due to chronic blood loss
Bone marrow examination	Predominance of megakaryocytes; normocellular to hypercellular; presence of stainable iron; no to minimal fibrosis

Criteria for the diagnosis of essential thrombocytosis are listed in the following box.

CRITERIA FOR DIAGNOSIS OF ESSENTIAL THROMBOCYTOSIS
Platelet count >600 X 10^9/L (on more than one occasion)
Absence of condition associated with reactive thrombocytosis
No evidence for myelodysplastic syndrome
No evidence for agnogenic myeloid metaplasia with myelofibrosis
Absence of Philadelphia chromosome on cytogenetic study
Absence of BCR/ABL gene rearrangement
No evidence of polycythemia vera (perform red blood cell mass if hematocrit >40%, normal iron studies)

References

Andersson BS, "Essential Thrombocythemia: Diagnosis and Treatment With Special Emphasis on the Use of Anagrelide," *Hematology*, 2002, 7(3):173-7.

Buss DH, O'Connor ML, Woodruff RD, et al, "Bone Marrow and Peripheral Blood Findings in Patients With Extreme Thrombocytosis," *Arch Pathol Lab Med*, 1991, 115:475-80.

Harrison CN and Green AR, "Essential Thrombocythemia," *Hematol Oncol Clin North Am*, 2003, 17(5):1175-90, vii.

Hoffman R, Benz EJ, Shattil SJ, et al, eds, *Hematology, Basic Principles and Practice*, 3rd ed, New York, NY: Churchill Livingstone, 2000.

Iland HJ, Laszlo J, Case DC, et al, "Differentiation Between Essential Thrombocythemia and Polycythemia Vera With Marked Thrombocytosis," *Am J Haematol*, 1987, 25:191-201.

Iland HJ, Laszlo J, Peterson P, et al, "Essential Thrombocythemia: Clinical and Laboratory Characteristics at Presentation," *Trans Assoc Am Physicians*, 1983, 96:165-74.

Jandl JH, *Blood, Textbook of Hematology*, 2nd ed, Boston, MA: Little, Brown and Company, 1996.

Lee GR, Forester J, Lukens J, et al, eds, *Wintrobe's Clinical Hematology*, 10th ed, Baltimore, MD: Williams and Wilkins, 1999.

THROMBOCYTOSIS

Is the thrombocytosis reactive or clonal*?

- Platelet count recently normal (ie, before current illness known to be associated with reactive thrombocytosis)
- Presence of condition know to be associated with reactive thrombocytosis
- No clinical features of myeloproliferative disorder†
- No splenomegaly
- No history of unusual thrombotic complications (ie, Budd-Chiari syndrome)

→ Consider reactive thrombocytosis

→ Repeat platelet count 1 month after treatment of underlying cause

→ Normalization of platelet count?

- Yes → Reactive thrombocytosis
- No → Consider clonal thrombocytosis

- Persistently elevated platelet count
- No identifiable cause of reactive thrombocytosis
- Clinical features suggestive of clonal thrombocytosis present†
- Splenomegaly
- History of unusual thrombotic complications (ie, Budd-Chiari syndrome)

→ Consider clonal thrombocytosis

→ Perform bone marrow biopsy to establish diagnosis and type of clonal thrombocytosis

*Clonal thrombocytosis occurs in patients with myeloproliferative disorders or myelodysplastic syndrome. Myeloproliferative disorders include essential thrombocytosis, CML, PCV, and agnogenic myeloid metaplasia.

†The presence of postbathing pruritus should prompt consideration of PCV. Erythromelalgia, which refers to painful, red, ischemic digits, may occur in patients with PCV or essential thrombocytosis. Striking pelthora may be noted in some PCV patients.

THROMBIN TIME

Thrombin converts fibrinogen to fibrin, which is essentially the last step in the coagulation cascade. The thrombin time is a test that is performed by adding thrombin to the patient's plasma. The time needed for clot formation to occur is known as the thrombin time. Since all the steps prior to the conversion of fibrinogen to fibrin are circumvented with the addition of thrombin, this test provides no information about the intrinsic and extrinsic pathways of coagulation. It does, however, provide useful information about any abnormalities or difficulty that may be present in the conversion of fibrinogen to fibrin. The test is said to be abnormal if the thrombin time is greater than 3 seconds over the control value.

Causes of Prolonged Thrombin Time

Causes of a prolonged thrombin time are listed in the box below.

CAUSES OF PROLONGED THROMBIN TIME
HEPARIN OR HEPARIN-LIKE COMPOUNDS
THROMBIN INHIBITORS
Hirudin
Hirulog
Argatroban
FIBRINOGEN DEFICIENCY (quantitative)
DYSFIBRINOGENEMIA
PRESENCE OF FIBRIN / FIBRINOGEN DEGRADATION PRODUCTS
HYPERFIBRINOGENEMIA (concentration >400 mg/dL)
PARAPROTEINEMIAS

It is usually not difficult to differentiate the above causes from one another. The presence of heparin, heparin-like compounds, or thrombin inhibitors is usually apparent. Heparin contamination, however, is not uncommon in specimens. If heparin contamination is suspected, thrombin time prolongation due to heparin can be excluded by performing a reptilase time. Like the thrombin time, the reptilase time also measures the conversion of fibrinogen to fibrin. In contrast, however, the reptilase time is unaffected by the presence of heparin. Therefore, a normal reptilase time in the patient with an elevated thrombin time is indicative of the presence of heparin. All other causes of thrombin time prolongation will be associated with an elevated reptilase time.

If the prolonged thrombin time is not due to heparin or other anticoagulant, fibrinogen assays (both functional and immunologic) and fibrin degradation products should be obtained. These tests will help the clinician differentiate among the remaining causes of a prolonged thrombin time.

References

Cunningham MT, Brandt JT, Laposata M, et al, "Laboratory Diagnosis of Dysfibrinogenemia," *Arch Pathol Lab Med*, 2002, 126(4):499-505.

Triplett DA, "Coagulation and Bleeding Disorders: Review and Update," *Clin Chem*, 2000, 46(8 Pt 2):1260-9.

APPROACH TO THE PATIENT WITH ELEVATED PT (NORMAL PTT)

STEP 1 – *What Are the Causes of an Elevated PT (Normal PTT)?*

The PT is a measure of the activity of the extrinsic and common pathways of coagulation. The causes of an elevated PT (normal PTT) are listed in the following box.

CAUSES OF ELEVATED PT BUT NORMAL PTT
COMMON
Liver disease (early)
Coumadin® therapy
Vitamin K deficiency (early)
UNCOMMON
DIC (early)
Factor VII deficiency
Factor VII inhibitor
Lupus anticoagulant

Proceed to Step 2.

STEP 2 – *Is the PT Falsely Prolonged?*

Before embarking on an evaluation to determine the cause of a prolonged PT, the clinician should ensure that the PT is not falsely elevated. False-positive prolongation of the PT may occur if the test tube is underfilled. It is also important to obtain the blood sample for PT determination from an arm without an intravascular line. This is because false prolongation of the PT has been described due to the mixing of intravenous fluids with blood. False prolongation of the PT may also occur in polycythemic patients (hematocrit >55%).

If there is concern that the PT may be falsely prolonged, repeat the PT taking care to avoid causes of false prolongation.

If the repeat PT is normal, ***stop here***.

If the repeat PT is elevated, ***proceed to Step 3***.

If false prolongation of the PT is not a concern, ***proceed to Step 3***.

STEP 3 – *Is the Patient Receiving Coumadin®?*

Coumadin® inhibits the gamma-carboxylation of glutamic acid residues on a number of coagulation factors integral to the PT. As a result, Coumadin® therapy is associated with an increased PT. In fact, the PT along with calculation of the international normalized ratio (INR) should be followed in every patient receiving Coumadin® therapy. Adjustments in the Coumadin® dose are based upon whether or not the INR is in the therapeutic range.

In usual clinical practice, a prolonged PT that is due to Coumadin® therapy is readily apparent by inspecting the patient's medication list. Rarely, an elevated PT may be due to the surreptitious or accidental ingestion of Coumadin®. The factitious use of Coumadin® is seen primarily in patients with major psychiatric disease. Since many of these patients repeatedly deny taking Coumadin®, factitious Coumadin® use should be suspected in any patient with unexplained

PT prolongation. A serum warfarin level may be obtained to establish the diagnosis.

If the patient is receiving Coumadin® therapy, ***stop here***.

If the patient is not receiving Coumadin® therapy, ***proceed to Step 4***.

STEP 4 – *Does the Patient Have Vitamin K Deficiency or Liver Disease?*

In the patient not receiving Coumadin® therapy, the prolonged PT is likely to be due to either vitamin K deficiency or liver disease. These will be discussed in further detail in the remainder of this step.

Vitamin K Deficiency

The normal synthesis of vitamin K-dependent coagulation factors (II, VII, IX, and X) requires an adequate supply of vitamin K. When vitamin K is lacking, these coagulation factors do not function properly and are essentially inactive. In vitamin K deficiency, the PT increases before the PTT because of the short half-life of factor VII. As the vitamin K deficiency worsens, both PT and PTT prolongation may be noted. The causes of vitamin K deficiency are listed in the following box.

CAUSES OF VITAMIN K DEFICIENCY
INADEQUATE INTAKE ANTIBIOTIC THERAPY* MALABSORPTION†

*The two main sources of vitamin K are dietary intake and synthesis of vitamin K by large intestinal bacteria. The administration of antibiotics may alter the intestinal flora to such an extent that bacterial synthesis of vitamin K is impaired, resulting in a prolonged PT. Not uncommonly, vitamin K deficiency is due to both inadequate intake and antibiotic therapy.

†Any process that affects enterohepatic circulation may result in impaired absorption of fat-soluble vitamins, including vitamin K. Examples include primary biliary cirrhosis, cholestatic hepatitis, and other disorders of cholestasis. Vitamin K is absorbed primarily in the ileum; therefore, disease of the intestine such as sprue or regional enteritis may also lead to malabsorption of vitamin K.

The clinician should also be familiar with medications or toxins that antagonize the action of vitamin K. One example is the factitious or accidental ingestion of rodenticides. Even as little as one dose can cause PT prolongation which, in some cases, persists for over a year. Similar to Coumadin®, these rodenticides increase the PT by inhibiting vitamin K action. If suspected, specific serum assays are available. Other medications that cause vitamin K deficiency-like states include aspirin (excessive doses), moxalactam, and cefamandole.

Liver Disease

Most of the coagulation factors are synthesized in the liver. Therefore, liver disease (acute hepatitis or chronic liver disease/cirrhosis) may lead to decreased production of these coagulation factors. In early or less severe forms of liver disease, this may manifest only with a prolonged PT. With progression of the liver disease or liver disease of sufficient magnitude, the PT prolongation may be accompanied by an increase in the PTT as well. The presence of liver disease is usually apparent from the patient's clinical presentation, biochemical findings, and imaging test results.

Differentiating Vitamin K Deficiency From Liver Disease

Useful in differentiating vitamin K deficiency from liver disease is the response of the PT to the administration of vitamin K. In patients with vitamin K deficiency, administration of vitamin K will result in PT normalization. In contrast, the PT will remain prolonged in patients with liver disease who are given vitamin K. The clinician should realize, however, that vitamin K deficiency may occur in the patient with liver disease, in which case, partial correction of the PT will be noted.

If the PT corrects with vitamin K replacement, the patient has vitamin K deficiency. ***Stop here.***

If the PT does not correct with vitamin K replacement, the patient is likely to have liver disease. ***Proceed to Step 5.***

STEP 5 – *Does the Patient Truly Have Liver Disease?*

When vitamin K replacement fails to correct the PT to normal, the most likely diagnosis is liver disease. In the patient who has a clinical presentation, biochemical findings, and imaging test results consistent with liver disease, no further evaluation is necessary and the PT prolongation can be attributed to the liver disease. In some cases, however, it is not clear that the patient has liver disease. It is in these patients that the clinician should consider other causes of PT prolongation that do not respond to vitamin K replacement. These rare causes of PT prolongation include the following:

- Factor VII deficiency
- Factor VII inhibitor or antibody
- Lupus anticoagulant

Proceed to Step 6.

STEP 6 – *What Are the Results of the Mixing Study?*

The mixing study, also known as the inhibitor screen, is performed by repeating the PT using a mixture of equal parts of the patient's plasma and normal pooled plasma. The mixing study will help determine if the prolonged PT is due to a factor deficiency or the presence of a factor inhibitor.

If the mixing study reveals normalization of the PT, a factor deficiency is present. Failure of the PT to correct to within the normal reference range suggests the presence of a factor inhibitor.

If the mixing study results in correction of the PT to normal, ***proceed to Step 7.***

If the mixing study does not result in normalization of the PT, ***proceed to Step 8.***

STEP 7 – *What Are the Considerations in the Patient Who Has a Prolonged PT That Normalizes With the Mixing Study?*

When the PT corrects to normal with a mixing study, the clinician should consider the following causes:

- Vitamin K deficiency (see Step 4)
- Liver disease (see Step 4)
- Factor VII deficiency

Factor VII deficiency may be inherited or acquired. Both types of factor VII deficiency are rare. If liver disease or vitamin K deficiency is not present, the clinician should obtain a factor VII level to establish the diagnosis.

End of Section.

STEP 8 – *What Are the Considerations in the Patient Who Has a Prolonged PT That Fails to Correct to Normal With the Mixing Study?*

When the PT fails to correct to normal with a mixing study, the clinician should consider the following causes:

- Factor VII inhibitor or antibody
- Lupus anticoagulant

Lupus anticoagulant is much more common than factor VII inhibitor (only four cases of the latter have been reported). Most cases of lupus anticoagulant present with an elevated PTT with or without a prolonged PT. On occasion, however, patients who have the lupus anticoagulant may present with a prolonged PT but normal PTT.

To distinguish between these two possibilities, the clinician should examine the results of the mixing study. The mixing study involves assessment of the PT immediately, as well as 2 hours after the addition of normal plasma. Lupus anticoagulant characteristically results in the immediate prolongation of the PT with a similar value obtained 2 hours later. On the other hand, factor inhibitors are characteristically time-dependent. When normal plasma is added to plasma that contains antibodies to a coagulation factor, there will be progressive prolongation of the PT. Therefore, if the PT progressively increases over 2 hours, the patient likely has a factor inhibitor.

The presence of a factor inhibitor can be confirmed by appropriate testing. When lupus anticoagulant is a consideration, the diagnosis can be established by performing the dilute Russell's viper venom test, kaolin clotting time test, or one of the other phospholipid-dependent assays.

References

Brandt JT, Triplett DA, Alving B, et al, "Criteria for the Diagnosis of Lupus Anticoagulants: An Update. On Behalf of the Subcommittee on Lupus Anticoagulant/Antiphospholipid Antibody of the Scientific and Standardization Committee of the ISTH," *Thromb Haemost*, 1995, 74(4):1185-90.

Hoffman R, Benz EJ, Shattil SJ, et al, eds, *Hematology, Basic Principles and Practice*, 3rd ed, New York, NY: Churchill Livingstone, 2000.

Jandl JH, *Blood, Textbook of Hematology*, 2nd ed, Boston, MA: Little, Brown and Company, 1996.

Lee GR, Forester J, Lukens J, et al, eds, *Wintrobe's Clinical Hematology*, 10th ed, Baltimore, MD: Williams and Wilkins, 1999.

Martin BA, Branch DW, and Rodgers GM, "Sensitivity of the Activated Partial Thromboplastin Time, the Dilute Russell's Viper Venom Time, and the Kaolin Clotting Time for the Detection of the Lupus Anticoagulant: A Direct Comparison Using Plasma Dilutions," *Blood Coag Fibrinolysis*, 1996, 7(1):31-8.

↑PT (Normal PTT)

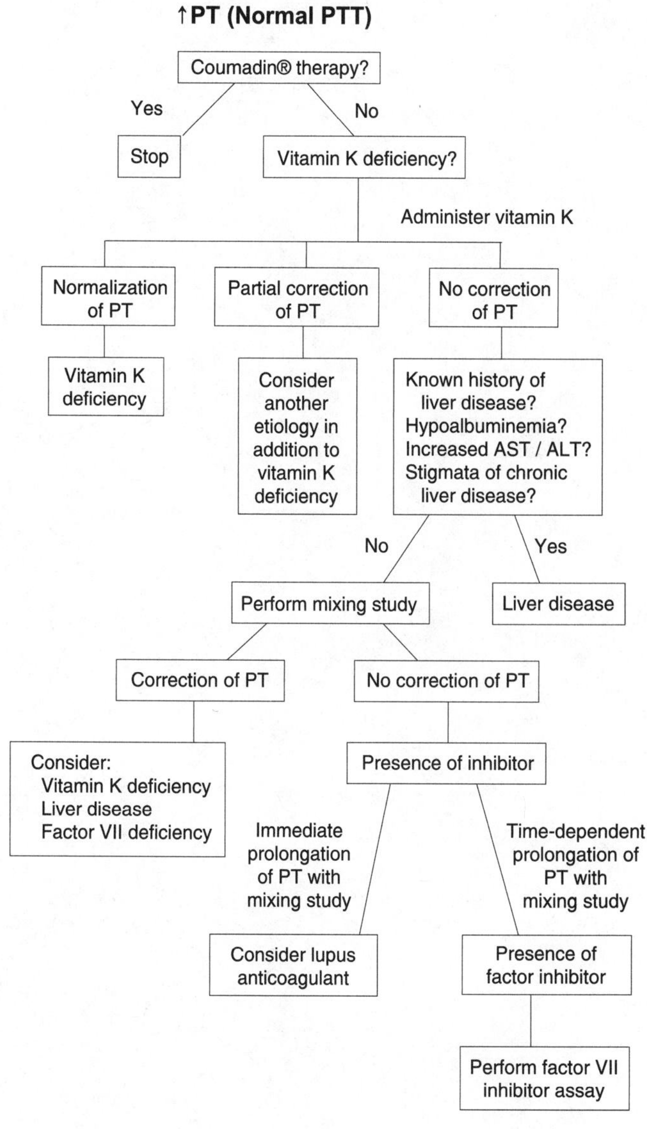

APPROACH TO THE PATIENT WITH ELEVATED PTT (NORMAL PT)

STEP 1 – *What Are the Causes of an Elevated PTT (Normal PT)?*

The PTT is a measure of the activity of the intrinsic and common pathways of coagulation. The causes of an elevated PTT (normal PT) are listed in the following box.

CAUSES OF ELEVATED PTT BUT NORMAL PT	
HEPARIN THERAPY	
FACTOR DEFICIENCY	
VIII	XII
IX	High molecular weight kininogen
XI	Prekallikrein
FACTOR INHIBITOR	
VON WILLEBRAND'S DISEASE	
LUPUS ANTICOAGULANT	

Proceed to Step 2.

STEP 2 – *Is the PTT Falsely Prolonged?*

Before embarking on an evaluation to determine the cause of a prolonged PTT, the clinician should ensure that the PTT is not falsely elevated. False-positive prolongation of the PTT may occur if the test tube is underfilled. It is also important to obtain the blood sample for PTT determination from an arm without an intravascular line. This is because false prolongation of the PTT has been described due to the mixing of intravenous fluids with blood. The causes of falsely elevated PTT measurements are listed in the following box.

CAUSES OF FALSE PROLONGATION OF THE PTT
POLYCYTHEMIA
UNDERFILLING BLOOD COLLECTION TUBE
PROLONGED STORAGE or WARMING OF SAMPLES BEFORE PROCESSING
CLOTTED SAMPLE
HEPARIN CONTAMINATION

Of the causes listed in the above box, heparin contamination deserves further mention. Heparin contamination is a common cause of falsely elevated PTT. Heparin is often used to flush intravenous lines, particularly central venous or arterial lines. When these lines are used to obtain blood specimens for PTT determination, the presence of residual heparin in these lines may lead to heparin contamination of the specimen. This will manifest as an elevated PTT. If heparin contamination is suspected, the easiest way to establish the diagnosis is to merely repeat the PTT test on a blood specimen obtained through a peripheral venipuncture. Other options available to the clinician include the following:

- Passing the plasma through a heparin-retaining filter
- Neutralizing the heparin prior to the PTT determination

- Performing thrombin time and reptilase time (prolonged thrombin time but normal reptilase time consistent with the presence of heparin)

If there is concern that the PTT may be falsely prolonged, repeat the PTT taking care to avoid causes of false prolongation.

If the repeat PTT is normal, ***stop here***.

If the repeat PTT is elevated, ***proceed to Step 3***.

If false prolongation of the PTT is not a concern, ***proceed to Step 3***.

STEP 3 – *Is the Patient Receiving Heparin?*

A common cause of isolated prolongation of the PTT is heparin therapy. Therapeutic anticoagulation with heparin causes an elevation in the PTT but does not result in a prolonged PT. When excessive doses of heparin are administered, however, both the PTT and the PT may be prolonged. In clinical practice, there is usually no difficulty in establishing the diagnosis of an elevated PTT due to heparin therapy.

If the patient is receiving heparin therapy, ***stop here***.

If the patient is not receiving heparin therapy, ***proceed to Step 4***.

STEP 4 – *What Are the Results of the Mixing Study?*

In patients who are not receiving heparin therapy, other causes of an isolated elevation of the PTT must be considered. In these patients, a mixing study should be performed to determine if the PTT elevation is due to factor deficiency or the presence of an inhibitor (factor inhibitor, lupus anticoagulant).

A mixing study involves mixing the patient's plasma with an equal volume of normal plasma. The PTT is then determined immediately and 2 hours later. The addition of normal plasma to plasma deficient in a certain factor will correct the PTT to normal values. If the PTT remains elevated despite the addition of normal plasma, an inhibitor is likely to be present. It is important for the clinician to realize that there may be some shortening of the PTT if an inhibitor is present, but there will still be a marked difference between the PTT of normal plasma and the 1:1 mixture.

If the PTT corrects with the mixing study, ***proceed to Step 5***.

If the PTT does not correct with the mixing study, ***proceed to Step 8*** *on page 143*.

STEP 5 – *Does the Patient Have a Factor Deficiency?*

Correction of the PTT when normal plasma is added to the patient's plasma suggests the presence of a factor deficiency. Since the PT is normal, the factor that is deficient has to be a part of the intrinsic pathway or involve the von Willebrand's factor (vWF).

FACTOR DEFICIENCIES CAUSING ELEVATED PTT BUT NORMAL PT	
HIGH-MOLECULAR-WEIGHT KININOGEN	FACTOR XI
PREKALLIKREIN	FACTOR XII
FACTOR VIII	VON WILLEBRAND'S FACTOR
FACTOR IX	

Of key importance in narrowing the differential diagnosis is consideration of the patient's bleeding history. Not all of the above factor deficiencies result in a bleeding disorder. In particular, deficiencies of factor XII, prekallikrein, and high molecular weight-kininogen present with an elevated PTT but a negative bleeding history.

In contrast, deficiencies of factor VIII, IX, and XI are typically associated with a significant bleeding history. In those who have severe factor deficiency, a history of delayed, prolonged bleeding into deep tissues and joints will be elicited. In those who have mild factor deficiency, hemarthroses may not occur (or may occur only with joint injury) but the patient will often relate a history of easy bruising or excessive bleeding after a dental or surgical procedure.

If the patient relates a history consistent with a bleeding disorder, ***proceed to Step 6***.

If the patient does not relate a history consistent with a bleeding disorder, ***proceed to Step 7***.

STEP 6 – *What Type of Factor Deficiency Does the Patient Have?*

When a patient with an elevated PTT due to a factor deficiency relates a history consistent with a bleeding disorder, the clinician should consider the following possibilities:

- Factor VIII deficiency
- Factor IX deficiency
- Factor XI deficiency
- von Willebrand's disease

The general approach to the evaluation of these patients is to begin by performing a factor VIII assay. If the factor VIII level is low, then the clinician should perform further testing to differentiate factor VIII deficiency from von Willebrand's disease (see below). If the factor VIII level is normal, attention should focus on deficiency of factor IX or XI. Since factor IX deficiency is more common, most clinicians measure the factor IX level first. These factor deficiencies are discussed in further detail in the remainder of this step.

Factor VIII Deficiency (Hemophilia A)

Factor VIII is one of the few clotting factors not synthesized by the liver. Synthesis is thought to take place in endothelial cells. Factor VIII deficiency, or hemophilia A, is an X-linked recessive condition. The clinical severity of hemophilia A is dependent on the factor VIII activity level, reflected as a percentage of normal.

CLASSIFICATION OF FACTOR VIII DEFICIENCY	
Severe	<1%
Moderate	1% to 5%
Mild	>5%

Severe deficiency manifests in infancy often at the time of circumcision. Patients usually suffer from repeated episodes of hemarthrosis. Moderately affected patients occasionally experience hemarthrosis. Patients with mild factor VIII deficiency usually escape diagnosis until clinically important bleeding develops following dental or surgical procedures.

To understand the laboratory findings in patients with hemophilia A, it is necessary to discuss the functions of factor VIII. Factor VIII exists in a complex with von Willebrand's factor (vWF). Factor VIII:C is the smaller portion of the complex that is responsible for the clotting activity of the factor. The larger portion of the complex is factor vWF:Ag (vWF antigen) which is responsible for von Willebrand's activity and, therefore, platelet adhesion. Patients with factor VIII deficiency will have a decrease in factor VIII:C. Factor vWF:Ag, as well as platelet function, should be normal.

von Willebrand's Disease

von Willebrand's disease is the most common inherited bleeding disorder, affecting up to 1% of the population. In this disease, there is either a quantitative of qualitative defect in the von Willebrand factor (vWF). Because vWF is important for platelet adhesion, clinical manifestations of this disease result from an inability to adhere to the subendothelial surface of the vessel wall. Although bleeding time is abnormal in patients with moderate or severe disease, it may be normal in patients with mild disease. Some subtypes of the disease present with an elevated PTT. If suspected, laboratory testing for the disease should include the following:

- Factor VIII activity level (vWF is a carrier protein for factor VIII and factor VIII activity levels can be low in some subtypes of the disease)
- vWF activity level (also known as ristocetin cofactor activity)
- vWF antigen level or activity

  vWF antigen activity may be affected by other factors. Activity may increase with acute infection, strenuous exercise, pregnancy, and hemorrhage. It is important not to discard the diagnosis of von Willebrand disease when normal levels are obtained in a patient with signs and symptoms suggestive of the disease. In these cases, it is reasonable to repeat testing at a more appropriate time.

The results of the above tests can identify patients with vWF disease and provide some information on the subtype of the disease that may be present.

Various Subtypes of von Willebrand's Disease and Expected Laboratory Tests

vWD Type	vWF Activity	vWF Antigen Activity	Factor VIII Activity
1	40% to 60%	40% to 60%	40% to 60%
3	<1%	<1%	<1%
2A	30% to 50%	70% to 150%	70% to 150%
2B	30% to 50%	70% to 150%	70% to 150%
2N	70% to 150%	70% to 150%	40% to 60%
2M	40% to 60%	40% to 60%	70% to 150%

From Taylor LJ, "Focus: Hemorrhagic Abnormalities," *Clin Lab Science*, 2003, 16(2):114.

Additional testing (ristocetin response curve, vWF multimeric analysis) may be needed to establish the precise subtype.

Factor IX Deficiency (Hemophilia B)

Factor IX deficiency, or hemophilia B, is much less common than factor VIII deficiency. Hemophilia B exhibits X-linked recessive inheritance and may present clinically with a mild to severe bleeding disorder. Severity of the disease is dependent on the level of factor IX activity. The diagnosis of factor IX deficiency is established by a specific assay for factor IX.

Factor XI Deficiency

Factor XI deficiency can present with a bleeding disorder. It exhibits autosomal recessive inheritance and has been appreciated primarily in those of Ashkenazi Jewish descent. Typically, there is little in the way of spontaneous bleeding. Patients may remain undiagnosed until the time of surgery when screening tests reveal an isolated prolongation of the PTT. The diagnosis of factor XI deficiency is established by a specific assay for factor XI. Excessive bleeding has been noted with surgical procedures.

End of Section.

STEP 7 – *Does the Patient Have a Deficiency of High Molecular Weight Kininogen, Factor XII, or Prekallikrein?*

Deficiency of high-molecular-weight kininogen, prekallikrein, or factor XII will not lead to a bleeding tendency. Since deficiencies of these factors are quite uncommon, many laboratories do not have the capability to test for these factor deficiencies. However, it is not necessary to perform specific testing as the patient with the following laboratory features can be considered to have a deficiency of one of these factors:

- Prolonged PTT
- Normal PT
- Correction of the PTT with a mixing study
- Normal levels of factors VIII, IX, and XI
- Negative bleeding history

End of Section.

STEP 8 – *What Are the Considerations in the Patient Who Has a Prolonged PTT That Fails to Correct to Normal With the Mixing Study?*

Failure of the PTT to correct to within the normal reference range after a mixing study should prompt the clinician to consider the presence of a factor inhibitor. The three major considerations include the following:

- Heparin
- Factor inhibitor
- Lupus anticoagulant

An elevated PTT due to heparin use has already been discussed in Steps 2 and 3. This step will focus on the differentiation between factor inhibitor and the lupus anticoagulant.

To distinguish between these two possibilities, the clinician should examine the results of the mixing study. The mixing study involves assessment of the PTT immediately, as well as 2 hours after the addition of normal plasma. Lupus anticoagulant characteristically results in the immediate prolongation of the PTT with a similar value obtained 2 hours later. On the other hand, factor inhibitors are characteristically time-dependent. When normal plasma is added to plasma that contains antibodies (inhibitors) to a coagulation factor, there will be progressive prolongation of the PTT. Therefore, if the PTT progressively increases over 2 hours, the patient likely has a factor inhibitor.

If the results of the mixing study are consistent with a factor inhibitor, ***proceed to Step 9***.

If the results of the mixing study are consistent with the lupus anticoagulant, ***proceed to Step 10***.

STEP 9 – *What Type of Factor Inhibitor Is Present?*

If the results of the mixing study are consistent with a factor inhibitor, appropriate testing can then be performed to identify which factor the inhibitor is directed against. In usual clinical practice, testing begins with a factor VIII antibody screening test because factor VIII inhibitor is much more common than inhibitors or antibodies directed against other factors of the intrinsic pathway. Not uncommonly, patients with factor VIII deficiency or hemophilia A develop antibodies to factor VIII, particularly after multiple infusions of factor VIII concentrates. Factor VIII antibodies may also develop in the following groups of patients:

- Previously healthy individuals
- Connective tissue disease (SLE, rheumatoid arthritis)
- Penicillin sensitivity / drug reaction
- Pregnancy / postpartum

In 50% of cases, no underlying disorder can be identified. If the results of the factor VIII antibody screening test are not consistent with the presence of a factor VIII inhibitor, the clinician should consider antibodies directed against other factors in the intrinsic pathway. Appropriate testing should be performed.

End of Section.

STEP 10 – *What Testing Should Be Performed to Confirm the Presence of the Lupus Anticoagulant?*

The term, lupus anticoagulant, is really a misnomer as it has been described in patients without SLE. Other diseases associated with the presence of lupus anticoagulant include drug-induced lupus and other autoimmune diseases. It is even seen in normal individuals. In addition, it is not usually characterized by a bleeding disorder; rather, some patients with the lupus anticoagulant are predisposed to the development of thrombosis.

The lupus anticoagulant is an antiphospholipid antibody. As such, it binds to various phospholipids. Phospholipids are required for the activation of clotting factors involved in the coagulation cascade. By binding to phospholipids, the lupus anticoagulant interferes with formation of the clot, leading to a prolonged PTT. In some cases, the PT may be prolonged as well. Diseases associated with the lupus anticoagulant are listed in the following box.

DISEASES ASSOCIATED WITH LUPUS ANTICOAGULANT

AUTOIMMUNE DISEASE
- Systemic lupus erythematosus
- Rheumatoid arthritis
- Primary antiphospholipid antibody syndrome (APS)
- Overlap syndrome

DRUG-INDUCED LUPUS
- Hydralazine
- Procainamide
- Others

LYMPHOPROLIFERATIVE DISORDERS
- Malignant lymphoma
- Hairy cell leukemia
- Waldenström's macroglobulinemia

(continued)

DISEASES ASSOCIATED WITH LUPUS ANTICOAGULANT
INFECTION
Bacterial
Viral (HIV)
Protozoal
SOLID MALIGNANCY

The presence of lupus anticoagulant is established when the following criteria are met:

- Prolonged PTT, Russell viper venom test (RVVT), or kaolin clotting time
- Failure of the above clotting tests to correct with the addition of normal plasma (mixing study)
- Normalization of the above clotting abnormalities with the use of frozen platelets (platelet neutralization procedure)

The platelet neutralization test involves the use of frozen platelets. Frozen platelets contain a significant amount of surface phospholipids. When added to the PTT test, the antiphospholipid antibodies (lupus anticoagulant) will bind to platelets. Therefore, they are not able to interfere with clotting, resulting in the normalization of PTT. This test verifies the presence of the lupus anticoagulant.

If testing for lupus anticoagulant is positive, the clinician should determine if the patient meets criteria for the diagnosis of antiphospholipid syndrome. Diagnostic criteria are listed in the following box.

PRELIMINARY CRITERIA FOR THE CLASSIFICATION OF ANTIPHOSPHOLIPID SYNDROME

Definite antiphospholipid syndrome is considered to be present if at least ONE of the following clinical criteria and at least ONE of the following laboratory criteria are met:

CLINICAL CRITERIA

Vascular thrombosis

- ≥1 clinical episodes of arterial, venous, or small-vessel thrombosis, occurring within any tissue or organ

Complications of pregnancy

- ≥1 unexplained deaths of morphologically normal fetuses at or beyond 10th week of gestation; or
- ≥1 premature births of morphologically normal neonates at or before the 34th week gestation; or
- ≥3 unexplained consecutive spontaneous abortions before 10th week of gestation, with maternal anatomic or hormonal abnormalities and paternal and maternal chromosomal excluded

LABORATORY CRITERIA

Anticardiolipin antibodies

- Anticardiolipin IgG or IgM antibodies present at moderate or high levels in the blood on ≥2 occasions, at least 6 weeks apart

Lupus anticoagulant antibodies

- Lupus anticoagulant antibodies detected in the blood on ≥2 occasions, at least 6 weeks apart, according to the guidelines of the International Society on Thrombosis and Hemostasis

From Wilson WA, Gharavi AE, Koike T, et al, "International Consensus on Preliminary Classification Criteria for Definite Antiphospholipid Syndrome: Report of an International Workshop," *Arthritis Rheum*, 1999, 42:1309.

In addition to lupus anticoagulant testing, patients suspected of having antiphospholipid syndrome should also be tested for antibodies directed against anticardiolipin and β2-glycoprotein I.

References

Brandt JT, Triplett DA, Alving B, et al, "Criteria for the Diagnosis of Lupus Anticoagulants: An Update. On Behalf of the Subcommittee on Lupus Anticoagulant/Antiphospholipid Antibody of the Scientific and Standardization Committee of the ISTH," *Thromb Haemost*, 1995, 74(4):1185-90.

Hoffman R, Benz EJ, Shattil SJ, et al, eds, *Hematology, Basic Principles and Practice*, 3rd ed, New York, NY: Churchill Livingstone, 2000.

Jandl JH, *Blood, Textbook of Hematology*, 2nd ed, Boston, MA: Little, Brown and Company, 1996.

Lee GR, Forester J, Lukens J, et al, eds, *Wintrobe's Clinical Hematology*, 10th ed, Baltimore, MD: Williams and Wilkins, 1999.

Martin BA, Branch DW, and Rodgers GM, "Sensitivity of the Activated Partial Thromboplastin Time, the Dilute Russell's Viper Venom Time, and the Kaolin Clotting Time for the Detection of the Lupus Anticoagulant: A Direct Comparison Using Plasma Dilutions," *Blood Coag Fibrinolysis*, 1996, 7(1):31-8.

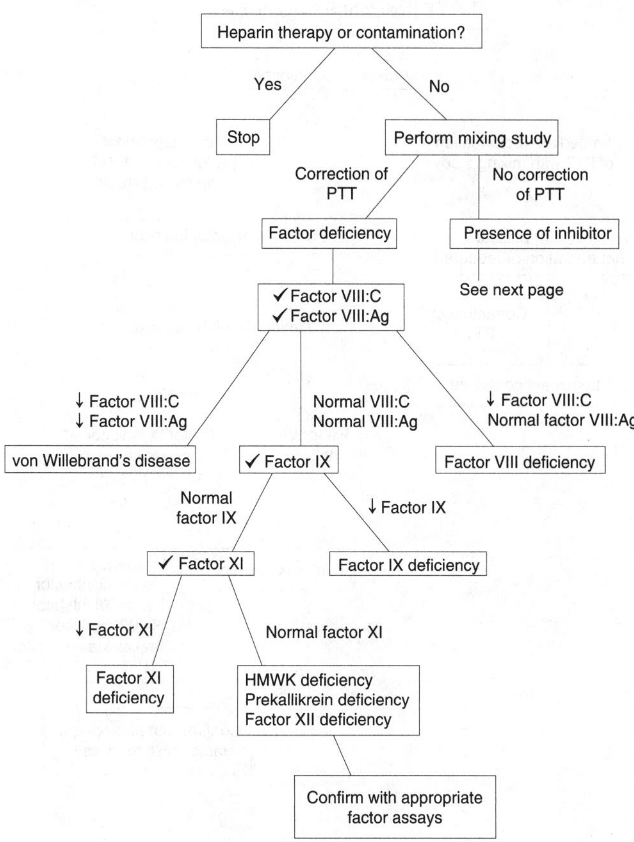
↑ PTT (Normal PT)
Heparin therapy or contamination?
Yes
No
Stop
Perform mixing study
Correction of PTT
No correction of PTT
Factor deficiency
Presence of inhibitor
See next page
✓Factor VIII:C
✓Factor VIII:Ag
↓ Factor VIII:C
↓ Factor VIII:Ag
Normal VIII:C
Normal VIII:Ag
↓ Factor VIII:C
Normal factor VIII:Ag
von Willebrand's disease
✓ Factor IX
Factor VIII deficiency
Normal factor IX
↓ Factor IX
✓ Factor XI
Factor IX deficiency
↓ Factor XI
Normal factor XI
Factor XI deficiency
HMWK deficiency
Prekallikrein deficiency
Factor XII deficiency
Confirm with appropriate factor assays

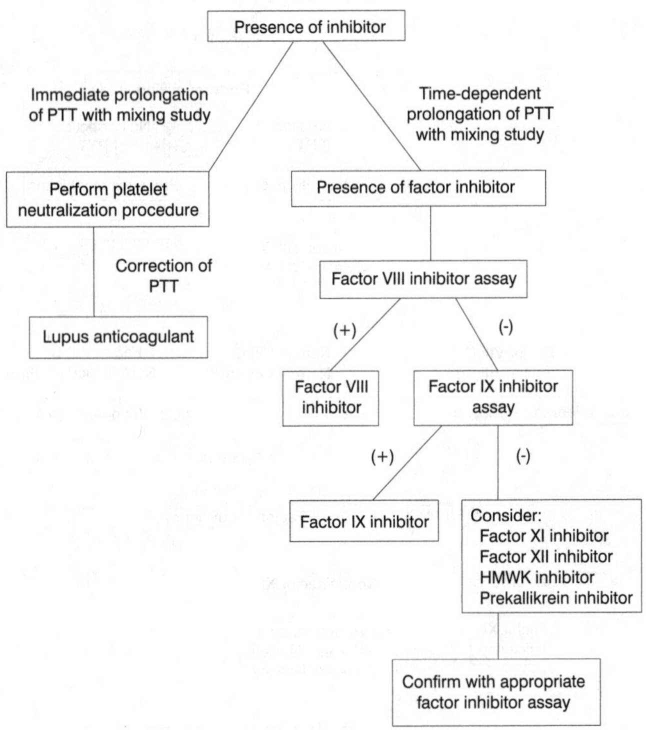
↑ PTT (Normal PT) (continued)
Presence of inhibitor
Immediate prolongation of PTT with mixing study
Time-dependent prolongation of PTT with mixing study
Perform platelet neutralization procedure
Presence of factor inhibitor
Correction of PTT
Factor VIII inhibitor assay
Lupus anticoagulant
(+)
(-)
Factor VIII inhibitor
Factor IX inhibitor assay
(+)
(-)
Factor IX inhibitor
Consider:
Factor XI inhibitor
Factor XII inhibitor
HMWK inhibitor
Prekallikrein inhibitor
Confirm with appropriate factor inhibitor assay

APPROACH TO THE PATIENT WITH ELEVATED PT AND PTT

STEP 1 – *What Are the Causes of an Elevated PT and PTT?*

A patient with an elevated PT and PTT has a coagulation abnormality in the common pathway. The differential diagnosis of an elevated PT and the PTT is listed in the following box.

ELEVATION OF PT AND PTT DIFFERENTIAL DIAGNOSIS
COMMON PATHWAY FACTOR DEFICIENCIES (I, II, V, X)
HEPARIN
COUMADIN® (warfarin) THERAPY
VITAMIN K DEFICIENCY
LIVER DISEASE
DISSEMINATED INTRAVASCULAR COAGULATION (DIC)
LUPUS ANTICOAGULANT
FACTOR INHIBITOR
PRIMARY FIBRINOLYSIS
DYSFIBRINOGENEMIA

Proceed to Step 2.

STEP 2 – *Are the PT and PTT Falsely Prolonged?*

Before embarking on an evaluation to determine the cause of the prolonged PT and PTT, the clinician should ensure that the PT and PTT are not falsely elevated. False-positive prolongation of the PT and PTT may occur if the test tube is underfilled. It is also important to obtain the blood sample for PT and PTT determination from an arm without an intravascular line. This is because false prolongation of the PT and PTT has been described due to the mixing of intravenous fluids with blood.

If there is concern that the PT and PTT may be falsely prolonged, repeat the PT and PTT taking care to avoid causes of false prolongation.

If the repeat PT and PTT are normal, ***stop here.***

If the repeat PT and PTT are prolonged, ***proceed to Step 3.***

If false prolongation of the PT and PTT are not concerns, ***proceed to Step 3.***

STEP 3 – *Is the Patient Receiving Heparin or Coumadin® Therapy?*

In patients receiving therapeutic doses of heparin, only the PTT is usually elevated. In contrast, in patients receiving therapeutic doses of Coumadin®, only the PT is usually elevated. If excessive doses of heparin or Coumadin® are taken by the patient, the PT and PTT may both be elevated. These two causes of elevated PT and PTT are discussed in further detail in the remainder of this step.

Heparin Therapy / Contamination

Heparin forms a complex with antithrombin III. This complex then inhibits factors II, IX, and X. Factors II and X are integral to the common pathway; therefore, prolongation of both PT and PTT may occur if blood levels of heparin are high enough. In usual clinical practice, heparin therapy as the cause of an elevated PT and PTT is readily apparent.

The clinician should also consider the possibility of heparin contamination as the etiology of the elevated PT and PTT. Heparin contamination typically occurs when blood is drawn through an indwelling catheter in a hospitalized patient. In these patients, heparin is often used to flush the intravenous line. If several milliliters of blood are not initially discarded before the collection of the specimen, the presence of residual heparin in the specimen will lead to an artifactual increase in the PT and PTT. To avoid this problem, the clinician can choose one of the following options:

- Passing the plasma through a heparin-retaining filter
- Neutralizing the heparin prior to the PT and PTT determination
- Performing thrombin time and reptilase time (prolonged thrombin time but normal reptilase time consistent with the presence of heparin)

Coumadin® Therapy

Coumadin® interferes with the gamma carboxylation of vitamin K-dependent factors, which include factors II, VII, IX, and X. Some of these factors are integral to both the PT and PTT. In general, patients on Coumadin® usually have an isolated PT elevation, but with excessive anticoagulation, the PTT may climb as well.

In usual clinical practice, a prolongation of the PT and PTT due to Coumadin® therapy is readily apparent by inspecting the patient's medication list. Rarely, the elevation of the PT and PTT may be due to the surreptitious or accidental ingestion of Coumadin®. The factitious use of Coumadin® is seen primarily in patients with major psychiatric disease. Since many of these patients repeatedly deny taking Coumadin®, it may be necessary to obtain a serum warfarin level if factitious Coumadin® use is a concern.

If the prolonged PT and PTT are due to heparin or Coumadin® therapy, ***stop here.***

If the prolonged PT and PTT are not due to heparin or Coumadin® therapy, ***proceed to Step 4***

STEP 4 – *Does the Patient Have Disseminated Intravascular Coagulation (DIC), Liver Disease, or Vitamin K Deficiency?*

Disseminated intravascular coagulation, liver disease, and vitamin K deficiency are major causes of prolonged PT and PTT. These causes of prolonged PT and PTT will be discussed in further detail in the remainder of this step.

Vitamin K Deficiency

The normal synthesis of vitamin K-dependent coagulation factors (II, VII, IX, and X) requires an adequate supply of vitamin K. When vitamin K is lacking, these coagulation factors do not function properly and are essentially inactive. In vitamin K deficiency, the PT increases before the PTT because of the short half-life of factor VII. As the vitamin K deficiency worsens, both PT and PTT prolongation may be noted. The causes of vitamin K deficiency are listed in the following box.

CAUSES OF VITAMIN K DEFICIENCY		
INADEQUATE INTAKE*	ANTIBIOTIC THERAPY†	MALABSORPTION‡

*Inadequate intake is typically associated with a mild degree of vitamin K deficiency.

†The two main sources of vitamin K are dietary intake and synthesis of vitamin K by large intestinal bacteria. The administration of antibiotics may alter the intestinal flora to such an extent that bacterial synthesis of vitamin K is impaired. Not uncommonly, vitamin K deficiency is due to both inadequate intake and antibiotic therapy.

‡Any process that affects enterohepatic circulation may result in impaired absorption of fat-soluble vitamins, including vitamin K. Examples include primary biliary cirrhosis, cholestatic hepatitis, and other disorders of cholestasis. Vitamin K is absorbed primarily in the ileum; therefore, disease of the intestine such as sprue or regional enteritis may also lead to malabsorption of vitamin K.

Normalization of the PT and PTT after administration of vitamin K establishes the diagnosis of vitamin K deficiency.

Liver Disease

In severe hepatitis or cirrhosis, there is a reduction in the synthesis of vitamin K-dependent factors (II, VII, IX, X). As liver disease worsens, factor V may decrease as well. Much later in the course, deficiency in fibrinogen may be noted. Indeed, except for factor VIII (not synthesized in the liver and usually normal or elevated in liver disease because of the acute phase response), all coagulation factors may be deficient in patients with liver disease, because of impairment in synthetic function. Therefore, although initially the PT alone is elevated, with worsening of the disease, there is prolongation of PTT as well.

ABNORMALITIES OF COAGULATION IN LIVER DISEASE
INCREASED PROTHROMBIN TIME
INCREASED PARTIAL THROMBOPLASTIN TIME
DECREASED PLATELETS SECONDARY TO HYPERSPLENISM
INCREASED FIBRINOLYSIS (increased fibrin degradation products)*
INCREASED BLEEDING TIME
ABNORMAL FIBRINOGEN†

*The liver is the site of antiplasmin synthesis as well as the clearance of tissue plasminogen activator (TPA). With liver disease, these processes are impaired, leading to increased fibrinolysis.

†An abnormal type of fibrinogen can be produced in patients with hepatoma and cirrhosis (dysfibrinogenemia).

At times, it may be difficult to separate DIC from liver disease. In DIC, factor VIII levels are often low, as opposed to liver disease.

Disseminated Intravascular Coagulation (DIC)

In DIC, the coagulation system is activated, leading to the consumption of coagulation factors and platelets. As a result, fibrin is deposited in many small blood vessels. The fibrinolytic system is also activated, resulting in the formation of fibrin degradation products from the breakdown of fibrin. When synthesis of coagulation factors lags behind the rate of fibrin formation, coagulation factors decrease. As a result, the PT and PTT become prolonged.

Although patients with DIC may present with clinically significant bleeding or thrombosis, bleeding manifestations are more common. Bleeding may manifest as ecchymoses, petechiae, or purpura. Postsurgical hemorrhage and trauma-related oozing should also prompt the clinician to consider the possibility of DIC. Not uncommonly, however, the manifestations of DIC may be masked by signs and symptoms of the underlying disease. Therefore, testing for DIC should be considered in every patient who presents with severe illness. If suspected, testing should include PT, PTT, platelet count, fibrinogen assay, and D-dimer assay.

The classic laboratory test abnormalities found in patients with DIC are listed in the following box.

CLASSIC LABORATORY TEST ABNORMALITIES IN DIC
PROLONGED PT*
PROLONGED PTT*
PROLONGED THROMBIN TIME
DECREASED PLATELET COUNT†
DECREASED FIBRINOGEN‡
SCHISTOCYTES ON PERIPHERAL BLOOD SMEAR§
ELEVATED FIBRIN DEGRADATION PRODUCTS (FDP)¶
ELEVATED D-DIMER#

*PT and PTT are typically elevated in patients who present with acute DIC. Although many patients with subacute or chronic DIC also have prolongation of the PT and PTT, at times, the PT and PTT may be normal.

†Although the platelet count is decreased in most patients with DIC, subacute or chronic DIC may present with a normal platelet count.

‡DIC cannot be excluded in a patient with a normal fibrinogen level. Recall that fibrinogen is an acute phase reactant and many of the underlying illnesses associated with DIC may lead to an elevation in fibrinogen level. Because of this, with the onset of DIC, the level may decrease only into the normal range and therefore, one should not exclude DIC when a normal or high level is obtained. Serial determinations of fibrinogen may be helpful in these situations. A low fibrinogen level is a very useful finding, as DIC is the most common cause of hypofibrinogenemia. Other causes of hypofibrinogenemia include congenital deficiency, severe liver disease, and primary fibrinolysis.

§The presence of schistocytes on examination of the peripheral blood smear is supportive of the diagnosis. The clinician should realize, however, that schistocytes are not found in all patients with DIC. In fact, they are not seen in approximately 50% of individuals with fulminant DIC.

¶With the lysis of formed fibrin, degradation products are released. Elevated fibrin degradation products are present in 85% to 100% of patients with DIC. However, elevated fibrin degradation products are not specific for the diagnosis since they are also found in patients with liver disease. More specific for the diagnosis of DIC is the D-dimer test. "D-dimer" is one of the fibrin degradation products released from the lysis of formed fibrin. It can be detected using specific monoclonal antibodies that are directed against it. These antibodies will not react with fibrinogen or fibrinogen degradation products.

#A positive D-dimer test signifies the presence of plasmin-cleaved, insoluble, cross-linked fibrin. Nearly 100% of patients with DIC have a positive D-dimer test, which makes it the most reliable test for the diagnosis of DIC. There are two types of D-dimer tests available; latex agglutination and ELISA. For the purposes of establishing the diagnosis of DIC, latex agglutination studies are sufficient. In recent years, D-dimer testing has been found to be useful in the diagnosis of large-vessel thrombosis such as deep venous thrombosis and pulmonary embolism. In these patients, ELISA testing is preferred.

Unfortunately, many patients do not present with the classic laboratory findings described in the above box.

Conditions associated with DIC are listed in the following box.

CONDITIONS ASSOCIATED WITH DIC	
TISSUE DAMAGE	
Asphyxia-hypoxia	Hypovolemic-hemorrhagic shock
Surgery	Hyperthermia (heat stroke)
Ischemia/infarction	Thermal injuries (burns, cold injury)
Rhabdomyolysis	Fat embolism
Physical trauma	
MALIGNANCY	
Solid tumors	Leukemia
INFECTION	
Bacterial	Protozoan (malaria)
Viral	Fungal
VASCULAR AND CIRCULATORY DISORDERS	
Pulmonary embolism	Acute myocardial infarction
Aortic aneurysm	Vasculitis
Vascular surgery	Aortic balloon pump
Intracardiac tumor	Malignant hypertension
Cardiac bypass surgery	Giant hemangioma, vascular tumors
IMMUNOLOGIC DISORDERS	
Anaphylaxis	Renal allograft rejection
Allergic reactions	Kawasaki disease
Acute hemolytic transfusion reactions	Drug (quinidine, interleukin-1)
Heparin-induced thrombocytopenia	
DIRECT ENZYME ACTIVATION	
Pancreatitis	Snake, spider venoms
OTHER DISORDERS	
Fulminant hepatic necrosis	Reye's syndrome
Cirrhosis	Le Veen shunt reinfusion
Adult respiratory distress syndrome	Hemolytic uremic syndrome
Homozygous protein C or S deficiency	Sarcoidosis
Inflammatory bowel diseases	Amyloidosis
Prothrombin-complex concentrate infusion	
Hemorrhagic shock and encephalopathy syndrome	
COMPLICATIONS OF PREGNANCY	
Abruptio placentae	Placenta accreta
Amniotic fluid embolism	Rupture of the uterus
Eclampsia and preeclampsia	Chronic tubal pregnancy
Induced (saline) abortion	Degenerating fibromyoma
Retained dead fetus or missed abortion	
NEONATAL DIC	

Two conditions that need to be distinguished from DIC include severe liver disease and fibrinogenolysis. These two conditions have laboratory findings similar to those seen in DIC.

Patients with severe liver disease may have impaired synthetic function leading to an elevation of the PT and PTT. Thrombocytopenia may be present secondary to hypersplenism that occurs because of portal hypertension. FDPs may be elevated because of fibrinogenolysis. Therefore, it can be difficult to make the distinction between severe liver disease and DIC. However, an elevated factor VIII level is usually seen in the setting of severe liver disease as opposed to DIC. The D-dimer test is probably the best test available to discriminate between the two. It will be abnormal in patients with DIC, but is typically normal in those with severe liver disease.

Primary fibrinolysis is the other condition that needs to be distinguished from DIC. Fortunately, this is a rare condition. Diseases associated with primary fibrinolysis include liver disease, acute promyelocytic leukemia, metastatic prostate cancer, and amniotic fluid embolism. Laboratory abnormalities in primary fibrinolysis include decreased fibrinogen, increased FDPs, prolonged PT, prolonged PTT, and prolonged TT. However, primary fibrinolysis is not usually characterized by abnormalities in platelet number in contrast to DIC (exception is liver disease which may present with low platelet count due to hypersplenism). The D-dimer test in primary fibrinolysis is usually normal although, on occasion, it may be mildly elevated. An abnormally short euglobulin clot lysis time is consistent with the diagnosis of primary fibrinolysis.

The coagulation test abnormalities of liver disease, vitamin K deficiency, DIC, and primary fibrinolysis are compared in the following table.

Representative Test Results for Common Bleeding Disorders in Hospitalized Patients

Test	PT	PTT	TT	Fibrinogen	Platelet Count	D-Dimer	ELT
Normal Range	**11-13.5 s**	**25-35 s**	**<30 s**	**150-450 mg/dL**	**150-350 K/μL**	**<0.5 μg/mL**	**<60 min**
Early vitamin K deficiency	18	32	21	225	250	<0.5	>60
Late vitamin K deficiency	26	58	21	225	250	<0.5	>60
Early liver disease	16	32	23	225	185	<0.5	>60
Late liver disease	22	63	45	75	60	1.0	30
Mild DIC	12.5	22	36	190	250	1.5	>60
Severe DIC	24	86	45	65	40	4.8	>60
Mild primary fibrinolysis	12.5	32	35	225	250	<0.5	15
Severe primary fibrinolysis	22	72	60	55	250	<0.5	<15

PT = prothrombin time.

PTT = partial thromboplastin time.

TT = thrombin time.

ELT = euglobulin clot lysis time.

Adapted from Goodnight SH, ed, *Disorders of Hemostasis and Thrombosis: A Clinical Guide*, 2nd ed, McGraw-Hill, 2001.

If the patient has vitamin K deficiency, liver disease, or DIC, ***stop here***.

If the patient does not have vitamin K deficiency, liver disease, or DIC, ***proceed to Step 5***.

STEP 5 – *What Are the Results of the Mixing Study?*

The mixing study, also known as the inhibitor screen, is performed by repeating the PT and PTT using a mixture of equal parts of the patient's plasma and normal pooled plasma. The mixing study will help determine if the prolonged PT and PTT are due to a factor deficiency or the presence of a factor inhibitor.

If the mixing study reveals normalization of the PT and PTT, a factor deficiency is present. Failure of the PT and PTT to correct to within the normal reference range suggests the presence of a factor inhibitor.

If the mixing study results in correction of the PT and PTT to normal, ***proceed to Step 6***.

If the mixing study does not result in normalization of the PT and PTT, ***proceed to Step 7***.

STEP 6 – *What Type of Factor Deficiency Does the Patient Have?*

If the mixing study results in correction of the PT and PTT to normal, the clinician should consider the presence of a factor deficiency. Because the PT and PTT are both elevated, the factor that is deficient must be one that they share in common. Therefore, the factor must be part of the common pathway of coagulation. Factor deficiencies that may result in prolongation of both the PT and PTT are listed in the following box.

COAGULATION FACTOR DEFICIENCIES RESULTING IN ELEVATION OF THE PT AND PTT	
FACTOR I (fibrinogen)	FACTOR V
FACTOR II (prothrombin)	FACTOR X

Of the factor deficiencies listed in the above box, fibrinogen deficiency is more commonly encountered. If results of the fibrinogen assays are normal, assays for factors II, V, and X should be obtained to identify the factor that is deficient.

End of Section.

STEP 7 – *What Type of Factor Inhibitor Does the Patient Have?*

When the PT and PTT fail to correct with a mixing study, the clinician should consider the following causes:

- Factor inhibitor
- Lupus anticoagulant

The lupus anticoagulant is a more common cause of PT and PTT prolongation than the presence of a factor inhibitor. To distinguish between these two possibilities, the clinician should examine the results of the mixing study. The mixing study involves assessment of the PT and PTT immediately, as well as 2 hours after the addition of normal plasma. Lupus anticoagulant characteristically results in the immediate prolongation of the PT and PTT with a similar value obtained 2 hours later. On the other hand, factor inhibitors are characteristically time-dependent. When normal plasma is added to plasma that contains antibodies to a coagulation factor, there will be progressive prolongation of the PT and PTT. Therefore, if the PT and PTT progressively increase over 2 hours, the patient likely has a factor inhibitor.

If the mixing study is consistent with the presence of a factor inhibitor, the clinician should perform appropriate testing for inhibitors of factor I, II, V, and X. ***Stop here***.

If the mixing study is consistent with the lupus anticoagulant, ***proceed to Step 8***.

STEP 8 – *Does the Patient Have the Lupus Anticoagulant?*

The term, lupus anticoagulant, is really a misnomer as it has been described in patients without SLE. Other diseases associated with the presence of lupus anticoagulant include drug-induced lupus and other autoimmune diseases. It is even seen in normal individuals. In addition, it is not usually characterized by a bleeding disorder; rather, some patients with the lupus anticoagulant are predisposed to the development of thrombosis. Bleeding is rare unless the lupus anticoagulant is associated with severe thrombocytopenia or factor II deficiency.

The lupus anticoagulant is an antiphospholipid antibody. As such, it binds to various phospholipids. Phospholipids are required for the activation of clotting factors involved in the coagulation cascade. By binding to phospholipids, the lupus anticoagulant interferes with formation of the clot, leading to a prolonged PTT. In some cases, the PT may be prolonged as well. Of note, the VDRL test may be falsely-positive in these patients.

DISEASES ASSOCIATED WITH LUPUS ANTICOAGULANT
IDIOPATHIC
AUTOIMMUNE DISEASE
Systemic lupus erythematosus
Rheumatoid arthritis
Primary antiphospholipid antibody syndrome (APS)
Overlap syndrome
DRUG-INDUCED LUPUS
Hydralazine
Procainamide
Chlorpromazine
Quinidine
Others
LYMPHOPROLIFERATIVE DISORDERS
Malignant lymphoma
Hairy cell leukemia
Waldenström's macroglobulinemia
INFECTION
Bacterial
Viral (HIV)
Protozoal
SOLID MALIGNANCY
PREGNANCY

The presence of lupus anticoagulant is established when the following criteria are met:

- Prolonged PTT, Russell viper venom test (RVVT), or kaolin clotting time
- Failure of the above clotting tests to correct with the addition of normal plasma (mixing study)
- Normalization of the above clotting abnormalities with the use of frozen platelets (platelet neutralization procedure)

The platelet neutralization test involves the use of frozen platelets. Frozen platelets contain a significant amount of surface phospholipids. When added to the PTT test, the antiphospholipid antibodies (lupus anticoagulant) will bind to platelets. Therefore, they are not able to interfere with clotting, resulting in the normalization of PTT. This test verifies the presence of the lupus anticoagulant. For more information about lupus anticoagulant testing and the diagnosis of the antiphospholipid syndrome, please refer to step 10 of the chapter ***Approach to the Patient With Elevated PTT (Normal PT)*** *on page 144.*

References

Brandt JT, Triplett DA, Alving B, et al, "Criteria for the Diagnosis of Lupus Anticoagulants: An Update. On Behalf of the Subcommittee on Lupus Anticoagulant/Antiphospholipid Antibody of the Scientific and Standardization Committee of the ISTH," *Thromb Haemost*, 1995, 74(4):1185-90.

Carey MJ and Rodgers GM, "Disseminated Intravascular Coagulation: Clinical and Laboratory Aspects," *Am J Hematol*, 1998, 59(1):65-73 (review).

Hoffman R, Benz EJ, Shattil SJ, et al, eds, *Hematology, Basic Principles and Practice*, 3rd ed, New York, NY: Churchill Livingstone, 2000.

Jandl JH, *Blood, Textbook of Hematology*, 2nd ed, Boston, MA: Little, Brown and Company, 1996.

Lee GR, Forester J, Lukens J, et al, eds, *Wintrobe's Clinical Hematology*, 10th ed, Baltimore, MD: Williams and Wilkins, 1999.

Martin BA, Branch DW, and Rodgers GM, "Sensitivity of the Activated Partial Thromboplastin Time, the Dilute Russell's Viper Venom Time, and the Kaolin Clotting Time for the Detection of the Lupus Anticoagulant: A Direct Comparison Using Plasma Dilutions," *Blood Coag Fibrinolysis*, 1996, 7(1):31-8.

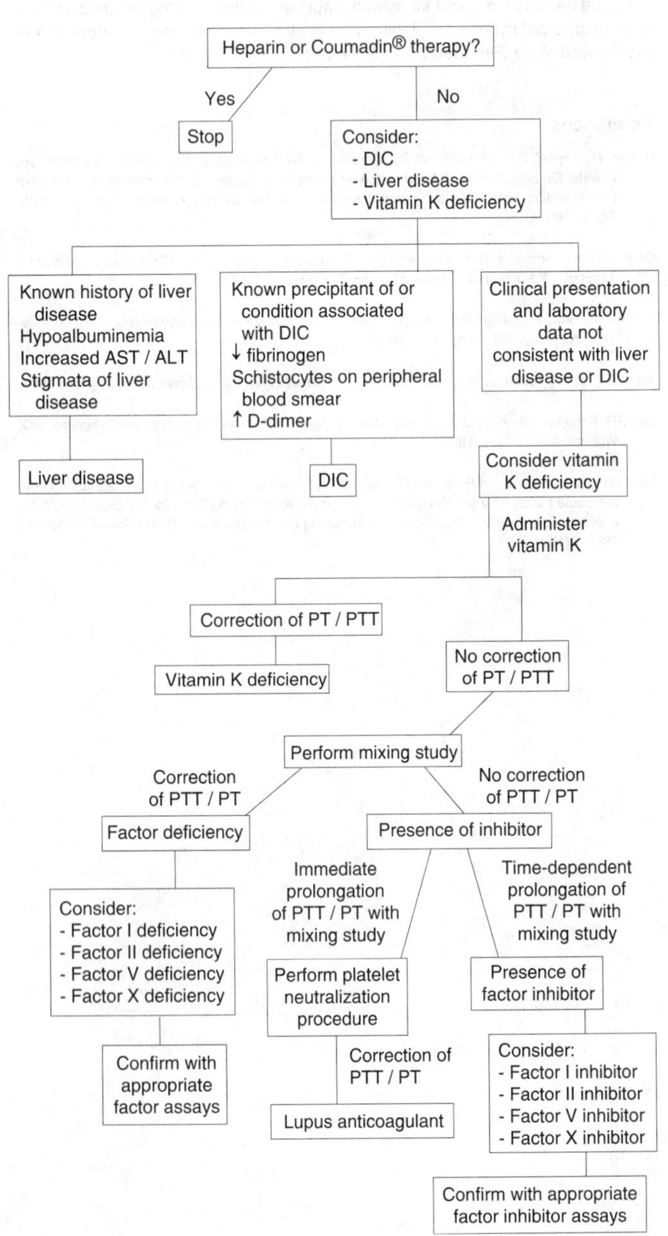
↑ PT / ↑ PTT
Heparin or Coumadin® therapy?
Yes
No
Stop
Consider:
- DIC
- Liver disease
- Vitamin K deficiency
Known history of liver disease
Hypoalbuminemia
Increased AST / ALT
Stigmata of liver disease
Known precipitant of or condition associated with DIC
↓ fibrinogen
Schistocytes on peripheral blood smear
↑ D-dimer
Clinical presentation and laboratory data not consistent with liver disease or DIC
Liver disease
DIC
Consider vitamin K deficiency
Administer vitamin K
Correction of PT / PTT
Vitamin K deficiency
No correction of PT / PTT
Perform mixing study
Correction of PTT / PT
No correction of PTT / PT
Factor deficiency
Presence of inhibitor
Immediate prolongation of PTT / PT with mixing study
Time-dependent prolongation of PTT / PT with mixing study
Consider:
- Factor I deficiency
- Factor II deficiency
- Factor V deficiency
- Factor X deficiency
Perform platelet neutralization procedure
Presence of factor inhibitor
Confirm with appropriate factor assays
Correction of PTT / PT
Lupus anticoagulant
Consider:
- Factor I inhibitor
- Factor II inhibitor
- Factor V inhibitor
- Factor X inhibitor
Confirm with appropriate factor inhibitor assays

HYPERCOAGULABLE STATES

APPROACH TO THE PATIENT WITH VENOUS THROMBOSIS

There are a number of conditions that predispose to the development of venous thrombosis. These conditions may be categorized as inherited or acquired. Acquired risk factors for venous thrombosis are much more common than inherited risk factors. These risk factors are listed in the following box.

RISK FACTORS FOR VENOUS THROMBOSIS
ACQUIRED
PREGNANCY
MORBID OBESITY
TRAUMA
MALIGNANCY
IMMOBILIZATION
ORTHOPEDIC SURGERY OF LOWER EXTREMITIES
SMOKING
AGE
NEPHROTIC SYNDROME
HEPARIN-INDUCED THROMBOCYTOPENIA
HORMONE REPLACEMENT
ORAL CONTRACEPTIVES
ANTIPHOSPHOLIPID ANTIBODY SYNDROME
MYELOPROLIFERATIVE DISORDERS
HYPERHOMOCYSTEINEMIA
INHERITED
RESISTANCE TO ACTIVATED PROTEIN C
ANTITHROMBIN III DEFICIENCY
PROTEIN C DEFICIENCY
PROTEIN S DEFICIENCY
PROTHROMBIN GENE MUTATION
DYSFIBRINOGENEMIA
HYPERHOMOCYSTEINEMIA
THROMBOMODULIN ABNORMALITIES

Since the acquired risk factors for venous thrombosis are much more common, a thorough evaluation should be performed in order to identify the predisposing condition. If an etiology is not apparent, then the clinician should consider the possibility of an inherited disorder. The inherited disorders should only be evaluated if acquired disorders are not present or if one or more of the following holds true:

- Thrombosis at an early age (<45 years)
- Recurrent thrombosis
- Family history of thrombosis
- Thrombosis in an unusual site (mesenteric, axillary, hepatic, sagittal sinus)
- Heparin resistance (consider AT III deficiency)
- Coumadin® skin necrosis (consider protein C or S deficiency)

When an inherited cause of venous thrombosis is suspected, appropriate testing is required to establish the diagnosis. In general, it is preferable to perform testing months after the thrombotic event. In addition, testing should be delayed until the patient has been off of anticoagulant therapy for at least 2 weeks. The interpretation of many of these tests can be difficult in the setting of acute thrombosis or while the patient is receiving anticoagulant therapy. The clinician should realize, however, that some tests may be able to be performed because they are not affected by acute thrombosis or anticoagulant therapy (ie, DNA-based tests to identify factor V Leiden or prothrombin gene mutation). If it is not possible to wait before performing testing, one option available to the clinician is to test asymptomatic family members for the inherited disorder under consideration.

It is important to realize that a considerable percentage of patients having a hypercoagulable state will have no apparent etiology. In these patients, it is likely that an uncharacterized predisposition to venous thrombosis, acquired or inherited, exists. In the remainder of this chapter, we will discuss some of the more common inherited disorders in more detail.

ACTIVATED PROTEIN C RESISTANCE (APCR)

Protein C is a vitamin K-dependent factor that inactivates activated factors V and VIII. As a result, protein C has an important role in the inhibition of coagulation. Activated protein C resistance exists when there is a mutation in factor V that renders it resistant to inactivation. The mutation results in prolonged procoagulant factor V activity, which predisposes the patient to the development of thrombosis. Although a number of different mutations have been described, factor V Leiden is the most common, accounting for >95% of cases. Activated protein C resistance is the most common genetic disorder predisposing patients to venous thrombosis. In patients who have the factor V Leiden mutation, the risk for venous thrombosis differs depending upon whether the patient is homozygous or heterozygous for the mutation. Homozygous patients have an 80-fold increase in risk while those that are heterozygous may have up to a seven-fold increase in risk.

Prevalence

The prevalence of APCR varies depending upon the population studied. In the white population, the prevalence ranges between 5% and 7%. The prevalence of APCR is much lower in individuals of Asian or African-American descent.

Clinical Presentation

Although APCR is associated with a propensity for venous thrombosis, not all patients will develop venous thromboembolism. Studies have shown that about 10% of patients with APCR will develop venous thrombosis over the following 10 years. In those that do develop venous thromboembolism, other risk factors (usually acquired rather than inherited) are often present.

Establishing the Diagnosis

Establishing the diagnosis of APCR requires performing a PTT-based test. Initially, a routine PTT test is performed. The PTT test is then repeated after activated protein C (APC) is added. This will allow the clinician to calculate the following ratio:

(PTT + APC) / PTT (without APC)

Healthy individuals usually have a ratio >2.0 while patients with factor V Leiden typically have a ratio <2.0. This original PTT-based test is not useful in patients treated with anticoagulants and in those who have an elevated PTT due to other coagulation abnormalities.

The sensitivity and specificity of this test can be increased by initially diluting the patient's plasma with factor V-deficient plasma. In fact, studies have shown that this modified PTT-based test has a sensitivity and specificity that is close to 100%. This modified PTT-based test can be performed in patients who are being treated with anticoagulants as well as in those who have an abnormal PTT due to other coagulation abnormalities.

The gold standard test for the detection of the factor V Leiden mutation is DNA testing (PCR). Because other mutations can also cause APCR, negative results of DNA analysis do not exclude the diagnosis of APCR; it merely rules out the presence of factor V Leiden.

PROTEIN C DEFICIENCY

Protein C is activated when it binds to the thrombomodulin-thrombin complex. Activated protein C inactivates factors V and VIII. Therefore, protein C plays an important role in the inhibition of coagulation. As a result, protein C deficiency predisposes patients to the development of venous thrombosis. Genetic protein C deficiency has been noted to be present in 0.14% to 0.5% of the general population.

Clinical Presentation

Approximately 50% of patients with protein C deficiency present with venous thrombosis before 40 years of age. In most of these patients, the thrombosis is spontaneous. In nearly 33%, however, another risk factor may be identified. The development of skin necrosis following warfarin therapy should also prompt consideration of protein C deficiency. It is important to realize that patients may be heterozygous or homozygous for protein C deficiency. Homozygous protein C deficiency presents at birth with purpura fulminans and disseminated intravascular coagulation.

Establishing the Diagnosis

Protein C deficiency can be divided into two types. Type I refers to a quantitative deficiency in which reduced levels of properly functioning protein C are synthesized. Type II is a qualitative deficiency characterized by normal levels of poorly functioning protein C.

Two different assays are available to establish the diagnosis of protein C deficiency. The antigenic assay determines the amount of protein C. On the other hand, the functional assay measures the function of protein C. In type I deficiency, the antigenic and functional assays will be abnormal. In type II deficiency, the antigenic assay will be normal but the functional assay will be abnormal. Therefore, performing only an antigenic assay will not diagnose those patients having a type II deficiency. As a result, the functional assay is the test of choice for initial screening. If this assay is abnormal, the antigenic assay can be performed to differentiate between type I and II deficiency.

Of note, clot-based functional assays may not be accurate in patients who have abnormal coagulation times due to elevated factor VIII levels or the lupus anticoagulant. Chromogenic assays are not affected by the presence of other coagulation abnormalities.

Differentiating Inherited From Acquired Protein C Deficiency

Certain conditions are characterized by acquired rather than inherited protein C deficiency. The clinician needs to be aware of these conditions.

ACQUIRED PROTEIN C DEFICIENCY DIFFERENTIAL DIAGNOSIS
LIVER DISEASE
ORAL ANTICOAGULANTS
VITAMIN K DEFICIENCY
RECENT OR ACTIVE THROMBOSIS
SURGICAL PROCEDURES
DISSEMINATED INTRAVASCULAR COAGULATION
L-ASPARAGINASE THERAPY
SEVERE INFECTION / SEPTIC SHOCK
HUS / TTP
ACUTE RESPIRATORY DISTRESS SYNDROME

When interpreting the results of the protein C assay, it is important to ensure that none of the above conditions are present. Although the presence of an acquired cause of protein C deficiency is usually apparent, it is essential to obtain a DIC panel and liver function tests to exclude DIC and liver disease, respectively. If one of the above conditions exists, the assay for protein C should be repeated when the underlying condition has been treated.

Measurement of a protein C level is not recommended in a patient on oral anticoagulant therapy. While some maintain that testing can be done, the diagnostic accuracy is not clear. If it is necessary to test a patient receiving Coumadin® therapy for protein C deficiency, oral anticoagulation therapy should be discontinued at least 1 week before testing. During this time, the patient may be maintained on heparin therapy without concern that the test results will be affected. Family studies can also be performed to help establish the diagnosis.

The protein C level may decrease after a thrombotic event, because of consumption. Not recognizing this important point may lead the clinician into falsely labeling the patient with protein C deficiency.

PROTEIN S DEFICIENCY

Remember that activated protein C inactivates factors V and VIII. Protein S is an important cofactor of protein C. Hereditary deficiency of protein S has been found in 0.7% of the general population.

Clinical Presentation

Protein S deficiency can be divided into heterozygous and homozygous forms. As in protein C deficiency, homozygous protein S deficiency presents shortly after birth as purpura fulminans and DIC. About 50% of patients with protein S deficiency will develop venous thrombosis before the age of 45 years. As with protein C deficiency and activated resistance to protein C, the presence of other risk factors for thrombosis increases the risk of a thrombotic event. Protein S deficiency should also be a consideration when a patient treated with Coumadin® develops skin necrosis.

Establishing the Diagnosis

Both antigenic and functional assays are available. In type I deficiency, both assays will be abnormal. The functional assay will be abnormal but the antigenic assay will be normal in patients with type II deficiency. Therefore, the functional assay is recommended as the screening test of choice in the diagnosis of protein S deficiency. If the functional assay is abnormal, the antigenic assay should be performed to distinguish type I from type II deficiency. Patients with type II deficiency can be further subdivided into types IIa and IIb based upon measurement of the free and total protein S level.

False-positive test results may be obtained if the functional assay is used in patients with activated protein C resistance. As a result, patients deemed to be protein S deficient from the functional assay should have additional testing to exclude the diagnosis of activated protein C resistance. Of note, clot-based functional assays may not be accurate in patients who have abnormal coagulation times due to elevated factor VIII levels or the lupus anticoagulant.

Differentiating Inherited From Acquired Protein S Deficiency

The causes of acquired protein S deficiency are listed in the following box.

ACQUIRED PROTEIN S DEFICIENCY DIFFERENTIAL DIAGNOSIS
ORAL ANTICOAGULANTS
VITAMIN K DEFICIENCY
LIVER DISEASE
DIABETES MELLITUS
ESSENTIAL THROMBOCYTHEMIA
ACTIVE OR RECENT THROMBOSIS
SURGICAL PROCEDURES
DISSEMINATED INTRAVASCULAR COAGULATION
L-ASPARAGINASE THERAPY
ESTROGEN THERAPY
Oral contraceptives
Replacement therapy
Pregnancy
HIV
NEPHROTIC SYNDROME

It is important for the clinician to be aware of the conditions that can cause acquired protein S deficiency. Although the presence of acquired causes of protein S deficiency are usually apparent, the clinician should obtain a DIC panel and liver function tests to exclude DIC and liver disease, respectively. In addition, a urinalysis should be performed to exclude the nephrotic syndrome. If the patient has one of the above disorders, it is best to perform tests for protein S deficiency after the underlying condition has been treated.

Measurement of a protein S level is not recommended in a patient on oral anticoagulant therapy. While some maintain that testing can be done, the diagnostic accuracy is not clear. If it is necessary to test a patient receiving Coumadin® therapy for protein S deficiency, oral anticoagulation therapy should be discontinued at least 10 days before testing. During this time, the patient may be maintained on heparin therapy without concern that the test results will be affected.

The protein S level may decrease after a thrombotic event, because of consumption. Not recognizing this important point may lead the clinician into falsely labeling the patient as being protein S deficient. A normal level, however, suggests that protein S deficiency does not exist.

ANTITHROMBIN III DEFICIENCY

As its name suggests, antithrombin III inhibits thrombin but it also inhibits factors IX, X, XI, and XII.

Clinical Presentation

Antithrombin III deficiency can be homozygous or heterozygous. Homozygous deficiency is not compatible with life. Heterozygous deficiency is associated with an increased risk of venous thrombosis.

Establishing the Diagnosis

There may be quantitative or qualitative defects in antithrombin III. In type I deficiency, decreased levels of properly functioning antithrombin III are present. Patients with type II deficiency have normal levels of a poorly functioning antithrombin III.

Both functional and antigenic assays are available. Type I deficiency is characterized by abnormal results of both assays. Type II deficiency, however, is associated with an abnormal result of the functional assay but a normal antigenic assay. Therefore, the initial screening test of choice in patients suspected of having antithrombin III deficiency is the functional assay, as the antigenic assay will not diagnose type II deficiency. If the result of the functional assay is abnormal, the antigenic assay should be performed to differentiate between type I and II deficiency.

Differentiating Inherited From Acquired Antithrombin III Deficiency

The causes of acquired antithrombin III deficiency are listed in the following box.

ACQUIRED ANTITHROMBIN III DEFICIENCY DIFFERENTIAL DIAGNOSIS
LIVER DISEASE
ACTIVE OR RECENT THROMBOSIS
SURGICAL PROCEDURES
DISSEMINATED INTRAVASCULAR COAGULATION
L-ASPARAGINASE THERAPY
HEPARIN THERAPY
NEPHROTIC SYNDROME
ESTROGEN THERAPY
Oral contraceptives
Pregnancy

It is essential to exclude the acquired causes of antithrombin III deficiency before establishing a diagnosis of inherited antithrombin III deficiency. Acquired causes are usually apparent. Nevertheless, every patient should have a DIC panel, liver function tests, and a urinalysis for protein to exclude DIC, liver disease, and the nephrotic syndrome, respectively.

Heparin therapy can lead to a decreased antithrombin III level. It is not possible to separate heparin therapy from inherited antithrombin III deficiency based on the functional antithrombin III assay.

The antithrombin III level may be measured while on Coumadin® with one caveat. In a minority of patients, Coumadin® may actually increase the antithrombin III level.

PROTHROMBIN GENE MUTATION (Factor II G20210A)

An increased risk of venous thromboembolism has been found in patients who have a mutation in the prothrombin gene at position 20210. The only reliable test available to establish the diagnosis of the prothrombin gene mutation is DNA testing.

HYPERHOMOCYSTEINEMIA

Elevated levels of homocysteine have been associated with an increased risk of arterial and venous thrombosis. Studies have shown that an elevated homocysteine level is a strong, independent risk factor for atherosclerosis in the coronary, aortic, carotid, and peripheral vasculature.

Hyperhomocysteinemia may be inherited or acquired. Homozygous deficiencies of the enzymes integral to the metabolic pathway lead to homocystinuria, a childhood condition characterized by arterial or venous thrombosis by the age of 30 in approximately 50% of patients. These patients also have mental retardation, lens dislocation, as well as other problems.

About 5% to 15% of the population is homozygous for the thermolabile variant of the enzyme, 5,10-methylenetetrahydrofolatereductase (MTHFR). This condition, which is characterized by elevated homocysteine levels, usually is silent until the patient presents with venous or arterial thrombosis. Heterozygous forms of the thermolabile variant are asymptomatic. PCR-based tests are available to establish the diagnosis.

Acquired causes of hyperhomocysteinemia are listed in the following box.

ACQUIRED CAUSES OF HYPERHOMOCYSTEINEMIA
RENAL FAILURE
HYPOTHYROIDISM
MALIGNANCY
MEDICATIONS
Corticosteroids
Phenytoin
Cyclosporine
Methotrexate
Trimethoprim
Niacin
VITAMIN DEFICIENCY
B_{12}
B_6
Folate
Riboflavin

Testing begins with a fasting serum homocysteine level. Fasting levels are recommended because the ingestion of protein can increase the homocysteine level. The clinician should realize, however, that up to 40% of patients with hyperhomocysteinemia may not be identified by routine fasting serum homocysteine levels alone. In these patients, the measurement of serum homocysteine levels before and after oral methionine loading is recommended to establish the diagnosis.

References

Bertina RM, Koeleman BP, Koster T, et al, "Mutation in Blood Coagulation Factor V Associated With Resistance to Activated Protein C," *Nature*, 1994, 369(6475):64-7.

Comp PC, "Measurement of the Natural Anticoagulant Protein S: How and When," *Am J Clin Pathol*, 1990, 94(2):242-3.

Deitcher SR and Gomes MP, "Hypercoagulable State Testing and Malignancy Screening Following Venous Thromboembolic Events," *Vasc Med*, 2003, 8(1):33-46.

de Ronde H and Bertina RM, "Laboratory Diagnosis of APC-Resistance: A Critical Evaluation of the Test and the Development of Diagnostic Criteria," *Thromb Haemost*, 1994, 72(6):880-6.

Hirsh J, "Congenital Antithrombin III Deficiency: Incidence and Clinical Features," *Am J Med*, 1989, 87(Suppl 3B):34S-8S (review).

Jennings I and Cooper P, "Screening for Thrombophilia: A Laboratory Perspective," *Br J Biomed Sci*, 2003, 60(1):39-51.

Key NS and McGlennen RC, "Hyperhomocyst(e)inemia and Thrombophilia," *Arch Pathol Lab Med*, 2002, 126(11):1367-75.

Lee R and Frenkel EP, "Hyperhomocysteinemia and Thrombosis," *Hematol Oncol Clin North Am*, 2003, 17(1):85-102.

Marlar RA and Adcock DM, "Clinical Evaluation of Protein C: A Comparative Review of Antigenic and Functional Assays," *Hum Pathol*, 1989, 20(11):1040-7 (review).

Nicolaes GA and Dahlback B, "Activated Protein C Resistance (FV(Leiden)) and thrombosis: Factor V Mutations Causing Hypercoagulable States," *Hematol Oncol Clin North Am*, 2003, 17(1):37-61, vi.

Rees MM and Rodgers GM, "Homocysteinemia: Association of a Metabolic Disorder With Vascular Disease and Thrombosis," *Thromb Res*, 1993, 71(5):337-59 (review).

Rodgers GM and Chandler WL, "Laboratory and Clinical Aspects of Inherited Thrombotic Disorders," *Am J Hematol*, 1992, 41(2):113-22 (review).

Ueland PM, Refsum H, Stabler SP, et al, "Total Homocysteine in Plasma or Serum: Methods and Clinical Applications," *Clin Chem*, 1993, 39(9):1764-79 (review).

Van Cott EM, Soderberg BL, and Laposata M, "Activated Protein C Resistance, the Factor V Leiden Mutation, and a Laboratory Testing Algorithm," *Arch Pathol Lab Med*, 2002, 126(5):577-82.

Van Cott EM, Soderberg BL, and Laposata M, "Hypercoagulability Test Strategies in the Protein C and Protein S Pathway," *Clin Lab Med*, 2002, 22(2):391-403.

HEMATOLOGIC MALIGNANCIES

CHRONIC LYMPHOCYTIC LEUKEMIA (CLL)

Chronic lymphocytic leukemia (CLL) is a lymphoproliferative neoplasm that is characterized by the proliferation and accumulation of lymphocytes in the blood, bone marrow, and lymphatic organs. In CLL, there is clonal expansion of mature appearing B-cells. The clinician should realize, however, that CLL is only one type of B-cell lineage hematologic malignancy. In this section on CLL, we will discuss how the diagnosis of CLL is established as well as how it is differentiated from other types of B-cell lineage neoplasms.

Clinical Presentation

CLL is a B-cell neoplasm that has a predilection for older individuals. Rarely is CLL found in a person younger than 30 years of age. Most patients are asymptomatic when the disease is diagnosed with the disease coming to clinical attention after a routine CBC demonstrates absolute lymphocytosis. Some patients, however, present with symptoms of weakness, weight loss, malaise, and fatigue. With disease progression, patients are susceptible to infection. In these patients, fever or frequent viral and bacterial infections may be the initial manifestation of CLL. Although physical examination may be unremarkable, the presence of lymphadenopathy or splenomegaly should prompt consideration of CLL.

Laboratory Testing

The laboratory features of CLL are listed in the following box.

CHRONIC LYMPHOCYTIC LEUKEMIA - LABORATORY FEATURES	
LYMPHOCYTOSIS (>5-10 x 10^9 cells/L)*	BONE MARROW§
ANEMIA†	Hypercellular
THROMBOCYTOPENIA‡	Lymphocytic infiltration
MONOCLONAL GAMMOPATHY¶	HYPOGAMMAGLOBULINEMIA++
ELEVATED β-2 MICROGLOBULIN**	ELEVATED LDH**

*Examination of the peripheral blood smear in patients with CLL typically reveals increased numbers of mature appearing lymphocytes, usually >10 x 10^9 cells/L. While the white blood cell count may approach 200 x 10^9 cells/L, 66% of patients with CLL have counts <30 x 10^9 cells/L at the time of diagnosis. Larger cells may be appreciated, some of which have prominent nucleoli, but this is an uncommon finding. Morphologic abnormalities may occur secondary to preparation of the blood smear; so-called "smudge cells" may appear. Increased susceptibility of leukocytes to the mechanical shearing forces *in vitro* is thought to explain the presence of these cells.

†Anemia may be noted at the time of CLL diagnosis but, if present, is typically mild. A hemoglobin level <11 g/dL is a poor prognostic finding. The direct Coombs' test is positive in up to 35% of cases but autoimmune hemolytic anemia only occurs in 10% to 15% of patients. When hemolysis occurs, spherocytes and reticulocytes may be appreciated on the blood film. Anemia due to pure red cell aplasia may also occur in CLL patients.

‡While the platelet number and morphology are usually normal at the time of diagnosis, some patients may present with thrombocytopenia. A platelet count <100,000/microliter is considered a poor prognostic finding. Autoimmune thrombocytopenia may occur, in which case, large platelets may be observed. While autoimmune hemolytic anemia and thrombocytopenia are important concerns, most CLL patients have other reasons for a decline in hemoglobin and platelets. Other causes of thrombocytopenia and anemia include bone marrow replacement and hypersplenism. In these cases, the reticulocyte count is usually normal.

§Bone marrow examination is usually hypercellular and always reveals infiltration of the marrow by lymphocytes. Recall that four patterns may be recognized; the most important distinction is between diffuse and nondiffuse types with the former being associated with a worse prognosis.

¶A monoclonal protein is identified in up to 5% of cases.

++At the time of diagnosis, hypogammaglobulinemia may be noted in up to 10% of patients. As the disease progresses, hypogammaglobulinemia becomes more common.

**Elevated levels of serum LDH and β-2 microglobulin are commonly found in CLL patients.

Bone Marrow Examination

A bone marrow examination is not required in the initial diagnosis of CLL, especially in cases where there is significant lymphocytosis (lymphocyte count >30 x 10^9 cells/L), and where monoclonality of the lymphocytes is established by cell surface marker studies. While the bone marrow examination does not play a role in staging CLL, it does provide prognostic information. Patterns of marrow involvement are listed in the following box.

PATTERNS OF BONE MARROW INVOLVEMENT IN CLL
DIFFUSE*
INTERSTITIAL
NODULAR
MIXED INTERSTITIAL-NODULAR
MIXED INTERSTITIAL-NODULAR-DIFFUSE

*Differentiating the diffuse form from the other types is essential. Diffuse involvement is associated with advanced stage and poor survival, as compared to the other types of involvement.

Criteria for Diagnosis

The diagnostic criteria for CLL are listed in the following box.

DIAGNOSTIC CRITERIA FOR CLL*
1) Sustained peripheral blood lymphocytosis >10 x 10^9 cells/L†
2) Normocellular to hypercellular bone marrow aspirate with >30% lymphocytes
3) Monoclonal B cells in peripheral blood

*Diagnosis is established if criteria 1+ 2 or 1+ 3 are present. If the lymphocyte count is <10 x 10^9 cells/L, then criteria 2 and 3 must be present.

†Mainly mature appearing lymphocytes are appreciated on the peripheral smear.

Staging

Important prognostic information is gained from staging patients with CLL. Two staging systems that are currently used in CLL include the Rai and Binet staging systems.

Rai Staging System

Stage	Clinical Features	Median Survival (y)
0	Lymphocytosis alone	14.5
I	Lymphocytosis Lymphadenopathy	7.5
II	Lymphocytosis Spleen or liver enlargement or both Lymphadenopathy may be present	7.5
III	Lymphocytosis Anemia (Hgb <11 g/dL) Lymphadenopathy, splenomegaly, or hepatomegaly may be present	2.5
IV	Lymphocytosis Thrombocytopenia (platelet <100,000/mm^3) Anemia and organomegaly may be present	2.5

Binet Staging System

Stage	Clinical Features	Median Survival (y)
A	Hemoglobin >10 g/dL Platelets >100,000/mm^3 <3 node-bearing regions involved*	14
B	Hemoglobin >10 g/dL Platelets >100,000/mm^3 ≥3 node-bearing regions involved*	5
C	Anemia (Hgb <10 g/dL) Thrombocytopenia (platelet <100,000/mm^3) Or both	2.5

*The five lymph node-bearing regions that are assessed in the Binet staging system include the following: Cervical, axillary, inguino-femoral, spleen, and liver.

Other laboratory test results that are considered poor prognostic findings include elevated levels of IL-6, IL-10, LDH, β-2 microglobulin, and TNF-alpha.

Differentiating CLL From Reactive Lymphocytosis

When confronted with a patient with lymphocytosis, many features help to distinguish reactive (benign) lymphocytosis from CLL. The following points should be kept in mind.

1. Reactive lymphocytosis is transient in nature while the lymphocytosis of CLL is sustained.
2. The history may reveal evidence of a benign disorder (ie, infectious mononucleosis) supporting the diagnosis of reactive lymphocytosis. Patients with infectious mononucleosis are typically younger and present with acute symptoms including fever.
3. Many cases of infectious lymphocytosis are characterized by the presence of large lymphocytes. The lymphocytes of CLL are usually small. As the disease progresses, however, larger cells may be appreciated.
4. At times, however, the distinction is not straightforward or an expedient diagnosis is necessary. In these cases, cell surface marker studies (immunophenotyping) will distinguish between the two. Recall that reactive lymphocytosis is characterized by its T-cell lineage and polyclonality, whereas the great majority of CLL cases are B cell in nature with monoclonality.

Comparison of CLL and Reactive Lymphocytosis

	Reactive Lymphocytosis	CLL
Duration	Transient	Sustained
History of infection	(+)	(-)
Size / shape of lymphocytes	Large/irregular	Small/round*
Type of lymphocyte	T-cell	Usually B cell, occasionally T-cell

*As the disease progresses, larger cells may be appreciated.

Immunophenotyping

Cell surface marker studies or immunophenotyping is used to confirm the diagnosis of CLL. It establishes the monoclonality of the disorder by identifying light chain restriction. This is particularly important in patients with mild degrees of lymphocytosis (<10 x 10^9 cells/L). Immunophenotyping can be performed on peripheral blood, cell suspensions from bone marrow, or other tissues (ie, lymph node). Immunophenotyping is not only useful in confirming the diagnosis but allows the clinician to distinguish CLL from other chronic lymphoproliferative disorders (see below).

Differentiating CLL From Other Lymphoproliferative Disorders

It is important to realize that CLL is only one type of B-cell lineage neoplasm. Although it is the most common type, it still needs to be differentiated from other B-cell malignancies. The B-cell lymphoproliferative disorders that need to be differentiated from CLL are listed in the following box.

LYMPHOPROLIFERATIVE DISORDERS TO BE DIFFERENTIATED FROM CLL
B-CELL PROLYMPHOCYTIC LEUKEMIA LEUKEMIC PHASE OF NON-HODGKIN'S LYMPHOMA HAIRY CELL LEUKEMIA WALDENSTRÖM'S MACROGLOBULINEMIA

B-cell prolymphocytic leukemia is characterized by marked lymphocytosis, often >100 x 10^9 cells/L, and splenomegaly. Lymphadenopathy is usually absent. Anemia, thrombocytopenia, and neutropenia are common at the time of diagnosis. The diagnosis is established by the cell's particular morphology and is substantiated by the results of cell surface marker studies. The prolymphocytes are large in size, contain large amounts of cytoplasm, are relatively free of cytoplasmic granules, and display prominent nucleoli. To satisfy the diagnosis, >55% of the circulating blood lymphocytes must have this morphology. In >75% of patients, the B-cell marker phenotype allows differentiation between CLL and B-cell prolymphocytic leukemia (see below).

On occasion, lymphoma cells may circulate in the bloodstream in patients with follicular or diffuse small cleaved cell lymphoma. One can differentiate between the leukemic phase of NHL and CLL by the results of cell surface marker studies (see below).

Hairy cell leukemia typically presents with cytopenia, bicytopenia, or pancytopenia. However, some patients may present with leukocytosis characterized by malignant cells circulating in the blood stream. These cases can be particularly difficult to distinguish from CLL, especially when splenomegaly is present. Features that support hairy cell leukemia are found in the following box.

HAIRY CELL LEUKEMIA LABORATORY FEATURES
PANCYTOPENIA (80%) NEUTROPENIA (80%) THROMBOCYTOPENIA (75%) ANEMIA (75%) MONOCYTOPENIA (98%) LEUKOCYTOSIS (15%) PERIPHERAL BLOOD HAIRY CELLS (85%)* BONE MARROW† Hairy cells (99%) "Dry tap" INCREASED ALKALINE PHOSPHATASE (20%) TARTRATE RESISTANT ACID PHOSPHATASE ACTIVITY‡

*These cells are characterized by the presence of cytoplasmic "hairy" projections and the presence of a large amount of cytoplasm.

†Bone marrow biopsy is essential for diagnosis. A dry tap is characteristic of the bone marrow aspiration. However, core biopsy will demonstrate variable degrees of infiltration by hairy cells. Reticulin fibrosis is nearly always present in varying degrees.

‡TRAP is a cytochemical stain used to confirm the diagnosis of hairy cell leukemia and is usually done on the peripheral blood smear or bone marrow aspirate smears.

Adapted from Fraffoldati A, Lamparelli T, Frederico M, et al "Hairy Cell Leukemia: A Clinical Review Based on 725 Cases of the Italian Cooperative Group (ICGHCL)," *Leuk Lymph*, 1994, 13:307-16.

Immunophenotyping plays a key role in differentiating CLL from these other lymphoproliferative disorders, as shown in the following table.

Immunophenotype of B-Cell Chronic Lymphoproliferative Disorders

Antigen	CLL	B-Cell PLL	HCL	SMZL	FL	MCL
SIg	+(dim)	(+)	(+)	(+)	(+)	(+)
CD19	(+)	(+)	(+)	(+)	(+)	(+)
CD20	+(dim)	(+)	(+)	(+)	(+)	(+)
CD22	(±)	(+)	(+)	(+)	(+)	(+)
CD23	(+)	(±)	(–)	(±)	(±)	(–)
CD25	(±)	(–)	(+)	(–)	(–)	(–)
CD5	(+)	(–)	(–)	(–)	(–)	(+)
FMC7	(–)	(+)	(+)	(+)	(+)	(+)
CD11c	(±)	(–)	(+)	(±)	(–)	(–)
CD103	(–)	(–)	(+)	(–)	(–)	(–)
CD10	(–)	(–)	(–)	(–)	(+)	(–)
CD79b	(–)	(+)	(±)	(+)	(+)	(+)

SIg = surface immunoglobulin; CLL = chronic lymphocytic leukemia; PLL = prolymphocytic leukemia; HCL = hairy cell leukemia; SMZL = splenic marginal zone lymphoma; FL = follicular lymphoma; MCL = mantle cell lymphoma.

(+) = Most cases are positive for this antigen.

(–) = Most cases are negative.

(±) = Cases are variably positive.

Adapted from Kjeldsberg C, *Practical Diagnosis of Hematologic Disorders*, 3rd ed, Chicago, IL: American Society of Clinical Pathologists, 2000, 540.

Richter's Syndrome

Richter's syndrome (transformation to diffuse large B-cell lymphoma) occurs in up to 15% of patients with CLL. Of the patients developing this transformation, most will manifest with signs and symptoms between 24-48 months after the diagnosis of CLL. Unfortunately, there are no predictors available to discern the population who will develop this complication. The transformation is often heralded by the abrupt onset of fever, weight loss, and rapidly enlarging masses in the lymph nodes. Laboratory results are usually not helpful in separating the two conditions, although increasing LDH levels may be a subtle clue reflecting the increasing proliferation of cells. To establish the diagnosis, a lymph node biopsy is required.

CHRONIC MYELOGENOUS LEUKEMIA (CML)

CML is a clonal disorder characterized by the proliferation of hematopoietic elements of the blood. The disease can be divided into phases, although patients may present in any phase. Initially, the course, as its name suggests, is slowly progressive or chronic. In fact, 85% of CML patients are diagnosed during the chronic phase. This is followed by an accelerated phase, which ultimately culminates in blast crisis. The blast crisis resembles acute leukemia. While patients may present with signs and symptoms related to the proliferation of granulocytes and/or platelets, an increasing number of patients are diagnosed when an elevated white blood cell count is noted on routine blood work.

Leukemic cells in patients with CML usually contain a cytogenetic abnormality known as the Philadelphia chromosome. It refers to a balanced translocation involving chromosomes 9 and 22. As a result of this translocation, a specific fusion gene *bcr-abl* is produced. Nearly 5% of patients, however, lack the Philadelphia chromosome but can be shown to have the fusion gene. These patients behave similarly to CML patients with the Philadelphia chromosome. There exists, however, a subset of patients with CML that are Philadelphia chromosome and *bcr-abl* negative who have a distinct clinical course.

Laboratory Test Findings

Laboratory features of the chronic phase of CML are listed in the following box.

CHRONIC PHASE OF CML LABORATORY FEATURES
INCREASED WBC COUNT
NORMOCYTIC NORMOCHROMIC ANEMIA (Hgb may be normal)
NORMAL / INCREASED PLATELET COUNT*
DECREASED / ABSENT LAP SCORE (90%)†
INCREASED VITAMIN B_{12} LEVEL
INCREASED URIC ACID LEVEL
INCREASED LACTATE DEHYDROGENASE

*It is rare to encounter a chronic phase CML patient with thrombocytopenia. A low platelet count in this setting should prompt consideration of possible disease progression to the accelerated or blast phase.

†The LAP score is quite helpful in differentiating CML from a leukemoid reaction, as well as other myeloproliferative disorders. LAP scores may return to normal in patients achieving remission. Levels may increase in CML patients who develop concurrent inflammation or infection. The LAP score often rises as the disease progresses from the chronic to the accelerated or blastic phase.

Peripheral Blood Smear Findings (Chronic Phase)

The peripheral blood smear shows a characteristic left shift in the granulocytic series. Granulocytes in all stages of maturation may be noted. However, most of the granulocytes are more mature cells, typically segmented neutrophils and myelocytes. Less mature cells may be present, but comprise a smaller percentage of the total white blood cell count. The combination of myeloblasts and promyelocytes usually does not exceed 10%, nor does the blast percentage alone exceed 5%. Increased numbers of monocytes, basophils, and eosinophils are commonly appreciated. Nucleated red blood cells may be seen, but the morphology of red blood cells is usually normal. Likewise, platelet morphology is normal.

Bone Marrow Examination

While peripheral blood smear findings may be quite characteristic in patients with CML, bone marrow aspirate and biopsy are usually performed to confirm the diagnosis. Hypercellular marrow is usually found with a myeloid to erythroid ratio >10:1 (a normal M:E ratio is 3:1). A left shift in granulocytic cells of the bone marrow is seen and tends to be more striking than that appreciated in the peripheral blood smear. The blast percentage does not exceed 5% to 10%. Megakaryocytic hyperplasia is commonly noted. There may be a slight increase in reticulin staining when compared to normal, but considerable marrow fibrosis is not common at the time of presentation. Fibrosis is more common as the disease progresses. In these cases, it may be difficult to differentiate CML from myeloid metaplasia with myelofibrosis.

Although these findings are supportive of the diagnosis, the key to the diagnosis is cytogenetic and molecular studies of the bone marrow specimen to demonstrate the presence of the Philadelphia chromosome and *bcr-abl* gene rearrangement, respectively. Although bone marrow tissue is preferable for demonstration of the Philadelphia chromosome, on occasion, a buffy coat of the peripheral blood may suffice. The Philadelphia chromosome is present in >95% of CML patients. When the Philadelphia chromosome is not present in patients suspected of having CML, the clinician should perform molecular studies to demonstrate the presence of the *bcr-abl* gene rearrangement. Southern blot hybridization and fluorescent *in situ* hybridization are two molecular techniques available to the clinician. For both techniques, bone marrow tissue is preferable for testing but, on occasion, the testing may be performed on peripheral blood.

Differentiating CML From Leukemoid Reaction

Recall that a leukemoid reaction is defined as neutrophilia >30 x 10^9 cells/L. As opposed to CML, the circulating neutrophils present in patients with leukemoid reaction are not clonal in origin. In leukemoid reaction, the proliferation of nonclonal neutrophils is a response to a disease process such as infection, inflammation, hemorrhage, or severe hemolysis.

Comparison of Leukemoid Reaction and CML

	Leukemoid Reaction	CML
Fever	(+)	(-)
Splenomegaly	(-)	(+)
Eosinophilia	(-)	(+)
Basophilia	(-)	(+)
LAP score*	High	Low
Philadelphia chromosome	(-)	(+)
WBC maturity	Mature / occasionally immature	Commonly immature blasts / promyelocytes
Toxic granulations, Döhle bodies, Cytoplasmic vacuoles	(+)	(-)

*Leukocyte alkaline phosphatase (LAP score) elevation is more consistent with the diagnosis of leukemoid reaction. It is important to realize, however, that the LAP score may be normal or high in CML patients who develop infection or progress to the accelerated or blastic phase of their illness. Other causes of an elevated LAP score include pregnancy, oral contraceptive use, other myeloproliferative disorders (polycythemia vera, essential thrombocytosis, myelofibrosis), Hodgkin's disease, and growth factor therapy. Low LAP scores are not synonymous with CML as they may also be seen in patients with paroxysmal nocturnal hemoglobinuria, myeloma, myelodysplastic syndrome, infectious mononucleosis, ITP, hypophosphatemia, and pernicious anemia.

Course of CML

Approximately 2-3 years after diagnosis, most patients with CML will progress to an accelerated phase of the disease. The accelerated phase of the disease usually precedes the blastic phase. However, up to 33% of patients may develop blast crisis without an antecedent accelerated phase.

Accelerated Phase of CML

Progression to the accelerated phase should be suspected when one or more of the features in the following box are noted.

FEATURES OF ACCELERATED PHASE OF CML (WHO DIAGNOSTIC CRITERIA)

PERIPHERAL BLOOD OR BONE MARROW BLASTS 10% to 19%
PERIPHERAL BLOOD BASOPHILS ≥20%
PLATELETS <100,000/μL, UNRELATED TO THERAPY
CYTOGENETIC EVOLUTION
PLATELETS >1,000,000/μL UNRESPONSIVE TO THERAPY
PROGRESSIVE SPLENOMEGALY AND INCREASED WBC UNRESPONSIVE TO THERAPY

Vardiman JW, Harris NL, and Brunning RD, "The World Health Organization (WHO) Classification of the Myeloid Neoplasms," *Blood*, 2002, 100(7):2292-302 (review).

Blastic Phase of CML

The blastic phase of CML is diagnosed if the patient meets one or more of the following criteria:

- ≥20% blasts in the peripheral blood
- ≥30% blasts in the bone marrow
- Presence of extramedullary blastic infiltrates
- Bone marrow revealing presence of clusters of blasts

As discussed earlier, approximately 33% of CML patients will develop blast crisis without an antecedent accelerated phase. The clinical presentation of these patients is similar to acute leukemia. The CBC may reveal pancytopenia. Basophilia may be impressive. In close to 70% of patients, the blast crisis is myeloid in nature. Most of the remaining patients will have a lymphoid blast crisis. Rarely, megakaryocytic or erythrocytic blast crisis may occur.

ACUTE MYELOGENOUS LEUKEMIA (AML)

AML refers to the proliferation of immature cells of granulocytic or monocytic lineage. The proliferation of myeloblasts and other immature myeloid cells in the bone marrow as well as other tissues (ie, lymph nodes, spleen, liver) are responsible for the manifestations of AML.

Laboratory Test Findings

Laboratory test findings of AML are listed in the following box.

ACUTE MYELOGENOUS LEUKEMIA LABORATORY FEATURES
INCREASED WBC COUNT*
DECREASED PLATELET COUNT
ANEMIA†
INCREASED URIC ACID
INCREASED LACTATE DEHYDROGENASE
SPURIOUS HYPERKALEMIA‡
HYPOKALEMIA§
SPURIOUSLY DECREASED ARTERIAL pO_2 LEVELS
INCREASED SERUM / URINE MURAMIDASE IN MONOCYTIC LEUKEMIA (M5)
DISSEMINATED INTRAVASCULAR COAGULATION (AML M3)

*The leukocyte count varies from low to markedly high, at times exceeding 100×10^9 cells/L. Approximately 20% of patients have white blood cell counts exceeding 100×10^9/L. The increase in the white blood cell count reflects the expansion and proliferation of myeloblasts and other immature myeloid cells. Over 50% of patients have a low or normal white blood cell count at the time of presentation.

†Normocytic normochromic anemia is appreciated in most patients with AML. Rarely, macrocytic anemia is encountered.

‡The hyperkalemia encountered in AML patients is often spurious, due to the release of potassium from the white blood cells during clotting. The clinician should realize, however, that true hyperkalemia does occur in these patients which is why spurious hyperkalemia should be a diagnosis of exclusion.

§Hypokalemia is not uncommon, especially in patients with monocytic leukemias, and is thought to be due to renal potassium loss caused by lysozyme-induced tubular damage.

Peripheral Blood Smear Findings

It is best to discuss the findings on the peripheral blood smear as they relate to red blood cells, platelets, and white blood cells.

- Red blood cells

  The degree of anisocytosis and poikilocytosis is variable. Nucleated red blood cells are found in many patients.

- Platelets

  Most AML patients are thrombocytopenic, but a small percentage have a normal or even elevated platelet count. Hypogranular platelets and giant forms are commonly appreciated.

- White blood cells

  Although the white blood cell count can vary from low to high, the presence of blasts in the peripheral blood smear should prompt consideration of AML. At times, blasts may comprise >90% of the total white cell count. The circulating blasts may be myeloblasts, monoblasts, or megakaryoblasts. At times, there may be a mixed population of blasts. The clinician should realize, however, that the absence of blasts does not exclude the diagnosis. While it is often difficult to distinguish myeloid from lymphoid blast cells on the peripheral blood smear, the presence of Auer rods is diagnostic of AML. Additionally, there may be a relative increase in the number of monocytes, eosinophils, or basophils. Neutropenia is quite common, but in some patients, neutrophilia may be present. Mature neutrophils may have dysplastic features.

Although examination of the peripheral blood smear may reveal findings consistent with AML, confirmation of the diagnosis requires bone marrow aspiration and biopsy.

Bone Marrow Examination

Definitive diagnosis of AML is established by bone marrow aspirate and biopsy. Marrow aspirate allows for evaluation of morphology, cytochemistry, immunophenotyping, and cytogenetic analysis.

Biopsy is also necessary to establish the degree of marrow cellularity (hypercellular in most cases). Recall that not all patients with leukemia have leukocytosis. A substantial number have normal or low white blood cell counts. Leukopenic patients with AML often have no evidence of blasts on examination of the peripheral blood smear, but may reveal striking numbers of blasts on examination of the bone marrow. In fact, to satisfy the definition of leukemia established by the FAB classification, blasts must exceed 30% of nonerythroid nucleated cells. It is not unusual for the blast count to approach 100%. Dysplastic features of varying degrees are noted to affect all cell lines in the bone marrow.

Differentiating AML From ALL

Determining if blast cells are myeloid or lymphoid in lineage requires the following studies:

- Morphology

  Morphologic characteristics that are useful in differentiating myeloid from lymphoid blasts include those listed in the following table.

Morphologic Features of AML vs ALL

	Myeloid Blast Cells	Lymphoid Blast Cells
Auer rods	Present	Absent
Size of blast cell	Larger	Smaller
Nuclear chromatin pattern	Fine and reticulated	Dense
Presence of nucleoli	Multiple and distinct	Indistinct
Amount of cytoplasm	Moderate	Small

Of these morphologic differences, only the presence of Auer rods allows AML to be distinguished from ALL. Auer rods are azurophilic rod-like structures in the cytoplasm of blast cells. Their presence is pathognomic for AML. Unfortunately, Auer rods are found in <50% of cases. For this reason, additional studies are needed to make this distinction.

- Cytochemistry

  A number of stains can be used to differentiate not only myeloid from lymphoid blasts, but also the different subtypes of myeloid blasts defined by the FAB classification. Most often used are the following cytochemical reactions:

  – Myeloperoxidase (MPO)

    MPO testing is performed to confirm the presence of granulocytic differentiation. When positive, it essentially excludes lymphoid disease. However, negative test results may be found in certain types of AML (M5, 6, 7).

  – Sudan Black B (SBB)

    SBB testing is performed to confirm the presence of granulocytic differentiation. A positive test result is supportive of AML. However, it is not as specific as MPO testing. Some cases of ALL will also yield positive results with SBB testing.

  – Nonspecific esterase

    One type of nonspecific esterase that is commonly used is alpha-naphthyl acetate esterase (ANAE). This esterase is used to confirm the presence of monocytic differentiation. ANAE testing of leukemic granulocytes will be negative or weakly reactive. The test may be positive in some T-cell ALL cases.

  Although cytochemistry is still performed, in recent years, flow cytometry and immunophenotypic marker testing has assumed a greater role in establishing the diagnosis and differentiating myeloid from lymphoid blasts (see below).

- Immunophenotyping

  Immunophenotyping is particularly useful in cases where lineage cannot be assigned based on cytochemical staining and morphology. In addition, immunophenotyping is useful in the subtyping and prognostication of patients with AML. In almost all cases, proper cell lineage (myeloid vs lymphoid) can be determined using monoclonal antibodies directed against cell surface antigens. Surface marker immunophenotyping can be performed peripheral blood, bone marrow tissue, or other tissues. It is usually performed by flow cytometric techniques.

Comparison of the Monoclonal Antibodies Found in AML, B-ALL, and T-ALL

	CD33	CD13	CD65	CD19	CD10	CD24	CD7	CD2
AML	(+)	(+)	(+)	(–)	(–)	(–)	(–)	(–)
B-ALL	(–)	(–)	(–)	(+)	(+)	(+)	(–)	(–)
T-ALL	(–)	(–)	(–)	(–)	(–)	(–)	(+)	(+)

Using a limited number of monoclonal antibodies, >90% of leukemias can be identified as myeloid or lymphoid in nature. Furthermore, ALL can be divided into T-ALL and B-ALL. Additional monoclonal antibodies can then be used to subdivide AML into granulocytic, monocytic, erythrocytic, and megakaryocytic forms as defined by the FAB classification system. This is beyond the scope of this section and the reader is referred to a specialized hematology text for further information.

- Cytogenetic analysis

  Many patients with AML have abnormal karyotypes. While patients with CML have a characteristic cytogenetic abnormality, namely, the Philadelphia chromosome, there are a number of different karyotype abnormalities in patients with AML. Over 50% of AML patients have cytogenetic abnormalities. Often these cytogenetic abnormalities provide prognostic information.

Cytogenetic Abnormalities in AML as a Predictor of Prognosis

	Chromosomal Abnormality	Prognosis
M2	t(8;21)	Favorable prognosis
M3	t(15;17)	Intermediate prognosis
M4E	Inversion 16	Favorable prognosis
Chemotherapy-related leukemia	5q-/7q-	Unfavorable prognosis

French-American-British Cooperative Group Classification of AML

The French-American-British (FAB) system is used to classify AML. Seven subtypes of AML have been defined by this classification system based on cell morphology, cytochemistry, and immunophenotyping.

ACUTE MYELOGENOUS LEUKEMIA FAB CLASSIFICATION	
M0	AML with minimal differentiation
M1	AML without maturation
M2	AML with maturation
M3	Acute promyelocytic leukemia
M4	Acute myelomonocytic leukemia
M5	Acute monocytic leukemia
M6	Acute erythroleukemia
M7	Acute megakaryoblastic leukemia

Recently, the WHO classification of acute myeloid leukemia was developed and it is quite possible that this new system will gain increasing acceptance. One of the major differences between the FAB and WHO classification systems is that the former required that the marrow blast cell percentage be at least 30% for the diagnosis of AML while the latter has defined a count of at least 20% as being diagnostic.

ACUTE LYMPHOBLASTIC LEUKEMIA (ALL)

Acute lymphoblastic leukemia (ALL) is a hematological malignancy characterized by the proliferation of lymphoblasts in the bone marrow and/or the blood. While the disease can be appreciated in individuals of all ages, its highest incidence occurs in children. It accounts for up to 20% of all cases of acute leukemia in adults.

Laboratory Test Findings

Laboratory test findings of ALL are listed in the following box.

ACUTE LYMPHOBLASTIC LEUKEMIA LABORATORY FEATURES	
DECREASED HEMOGLOBIN (75%)	PERIPHERAL LYMPHOBLASTS†
DECREASED PLATELETS (75%)	INCREASED URIC ACID
INCREASED WBC COUNT (50%)*	INCREASED LACTATE DEHYDROGENASE

*Ten percent of ALL patients have white blood cell counts >100 x 10^9/L. Despite high WBC counts, many patients with ALL have neutropenia.

†While lymphoblasts may be readily apparent in peripheral blood smears of patients with high WBC counts, they may be difficult to detect in patients with low WBC counts. Occasionally, lymphoblasts are not appreciated, despite extensive bone marrow involvement.

French-American-British Cooperative Group Classification of ALL

The French-American-British study group has classified ALL based on the morphologic appearance of the lymphoblasts.

FAB Classification for ALL

	L1	L2	L3
Size	Small	Large, heterogeneous	Large, homogeneous
Nuclei	Regular	Irregular	Irregular
Nucleoli	Small, solitary	Multiple	Multiple
Cytoplasm	Scant	Variable, often abundant	Abundant
Cytoplasmic vacuolization	Variable	Variable	Usually prominent
Cytoplasmic basophilia	Slight or moderate	Variable, sometimes intense	Very intense

Based on the above morphological features, the diagnosis of ALL L3 is usually not difficult. At times, however, the differentiation of L1 from L2 may be difficult. While scoring systems have been devised to aid in making this distinction, most laboratories now use cell marker and cytogenetic studies to classify ALL.

Bone Marrow Examination

ALL is characterized by a hypercellular bone marrow with leukemic replacement of normal marrow elements. In contrast to AML, myeloid and erythroid precursors appear morphologically normal. Megakaryocytes are decreased or absent. Bone marrow biopsy also provides cells for cytochemistry, immunophenotyping, and cytogenetic analysis.

Cytochemistry

Cytochemistry can be quite useful in differentiating ALL from AML. Most often used are the following cytochemical reactions:

- Myeloperoxidase (MPO)

  ALL is characteristically MPO negative, in contrast to most cases of AML
- Sudan Black B (SBB)

  ALL is characteristically SBB negative, in contrast to most cases of AML

- Nonspecific esterase

  Nonspecific esterase testing is usually negative in ALL

Although cytochemistry is still performed, in recent years, flow cytometry and immunophenotypic marker testing has assumed a greater role in establishing the diagnosis and differentiating lymphoid from myeloid blasts (see below).

Immunophenotyping

The diagnosis of ALL can be confirmed by immunophenotyping. Immunophenotyping allows the clinician to differentiate ALL from AML and other lymphoproliferative disorders. Furthermore, lymphoblasts can be divided into B- and T-cell lineage. About 70% of ALL cases are of B-cell lineage. The remaining cases are of T-cell lineage.

Once B- or T-cell lineage is established, the monoclonal antibody panel may be expanded to further characterize ALL. Specifically, maturation of the blast can be determined. This is important in that it provides prognostic information.

When acute leukemia is suspected, the specimen of choice for immunophenotypic testing is bone marrow. Peripheral blood may also be used but adequate numbers of circulating leukemic cells must be present.

Cytogenetic Testing

Cytogenetic studies of the bone marrow provide information regarding prognosis. Approximately 80% of patients with ALL have bone marrow chromosome abnormalities.

References

Bennett JM, Catovsky D, Daniel MT, et al, "Proposals for the Classification of Chronic (Mature) B and T Lymphoid Leukemias. French-American-British (FAB) Cooperative Group," *J Clin Pathol*, 1989, 42(6):567-84.

Bennett JM, Catovsky D, Daniel MT, et al, "Proposals for the Classification of the Acute Leukaemias. French-American-British (FAB) Cooperative Group," *Br J Haematol*, 1976, 33(4):451-8.

Bennett JM, Catovsky D, Daniel MT, et al, "Proposed Revised Criteria for the Classification of Acute Myeloid Leukemia. A Report of the French-American-British (FAB) Cooperative Group," *Ann Intern Med*, 1985, 103(4):620-5.

Bennett JM, Catovsky D, Daniel MT, et al, "The Chronic Myeloid Leukaemias: Guidelines for Distinguishing Chronic Granulocytic, Atypical Chronic Myeloid, and Chronic Myelomonocytic Leukaemia. Proposals by the French-American-British Cooperative Leukaemia Group," *Br J Haematol*, 1994, 87(4):746-54.

Bennett JM, Catovsky D, Daniel MT, et al, "The Morphological Classification of Acute Lymphoblastic Leukaemia: Concordance Among Observers and Clinical Correlations," *Br J Haematol*, 1981, 47(4):553-61.

Bitter MA, LeBeau MM, Rowley JD, et al, "Associations Between Morphology, Karyotype, and Clinical Features in Myeloid Leukemias," *Hum Pathol*, 1987, 18(3):211-25 (review).

Faderl S, Kantarjian HM, Talpaz M, et al, "Clinical Significance of Cytogenetic Abnormalities in Adult Acute Lymphoblastic Leukemia," *Blood*, 1998, 91(11):3995-4019 (review).

Harris NL, Jaffe ES, Diebold J, et al, "The World Health Organization Classification of Hematological Malignancies Report of the Clinical Advisory Committee Meeting, Airlie House, Virginia, November 1997," *Mod Pathol*, 2000, 13(2):193-207.

Hernandez JA, Land J, and McKenna RW, "Leukemias, Myeloma, and Other Lymphoreticular Neoplasms," *Cancer*, 1995, 75(1 Suppl):381-94.

Hoffman R, Benz EJ, Shattil SJ, et al, eds, *Hematology. Basic Principles and Practice*, 3rd ed, New York, NY: Churchill Livingstone, 2000.

Jandl JH, *Blood. Textbook of Hematology*, 2nd ed, Boston, MA: Little, Brown and Company, 1996.

Lee GR, Forester J, Lukens J, et al, eds, *Wintrobe's Clinical Hematology*, 10th ed, Baltimore, MD: Williams and Wilkins, 1999.

McKenna RW, "A Multifaceted Approach to Diagnosis and Classification of Acute Leukemia," *Arch Pathol Lab Med*, 1991, 115(4):328-30.

Rowley JD, "The Philadelphia Chromosome Translocation: A Paradigm for Understanding Leukemia," *Cancer*, 1990, 65(10):2178-84 (review).

Rozman C and Montserrat E, "Chronic Lymphocytic Leukemia," *N Engl J Med*, 1995, 333(16):1052-7 (review).

Sawyers CL, "Chronic Myeloid Leukemia," *N Engl J Med*, 1999, 340(17):1330-40 (review).

MONOCLONAL GAMMOPATHY

STEP 1 – *What Is a Monoclonal Gammopathy?*

The term monoclonal gammopathy refers to a group of disorders characterized by the production of immunoglobulin or its components by a clone of plasma cells.

The different types of monoclonal gammopathies are included in the following box.

TYPES OF MONOCLONAL GAMMOPATHIES
MYELOMA Solitary plasmacytoma Asymptomatic myeloma (smoldering myeloma) Multiple myeloma POEMS syndrome* WALDENSTRÖM'S MACROGLOBULINEMIA HEAVY-CHAIN DISEASES IMMUNOGLOBULIN DEPOSITION DISEASES AMYLOIDOSIS (AL type) MONOCLONAL GAMMOPATHY OF UNDETERMINED SIGNIFICANCE

*The syndrome is characterized by polyneuropathy, organomegaly, endocrinopathy, monoclonal protein, and skin changes.

Proceed to Step 2.

STEP 2 – *What Clinical Clues Should Lead the Clinician to Suspect a Monoclonal Gammopathy?*

The clinical manifestations of multiple myeloma are included in the following box.

MULTIPLE MYELOMA CLINICAL MANIFESTATIONS
UNEXPLAINED WEAKNESS OR FATIGUE ANEMIA BACK PAIN OSTEOPOROSIS OSTEOLYTIC LESIONS SPONTANEOUS FRACTURE INCREASED ERYTHROCYTE SEDIMENTATION RATE HYPERCALCEMIA RENAL INSUFFICIENCY IMMUNOGLOBULIN DEFICIENCY RECURRENT INFECTIONS

The clinical manifestations of Waldenström's macroglobulinemia are included in the following box.

WALDENSTRÖM'S MACROGLOBULINEMIA CLINICAL MANIFESTATIONS
LYMPHADENOPATHY
SPLENOMEGALY
ANEMIA SECONDARY TO BONE MARROW INFILTRATION
HYPERVISCOSITY SYNDROME
CRYOGLOBULINEMIA WITH RAYNAUD'S SYNDROME AND VASCULITIS
COLD AGGLUTININ HEMOLYTIC ANEMIA
BLEEDING
PERIPHERAL NEUROPATHY WITH SYMMETRICAL SENSORIMOTOR DEFICITS

The clinical manifestations of amyloidosis (AL type) are included in the following box.

AMYLOIDOSIS (AL TYPE) CLINICAL MANIFESTATIONS
SENSORIMOTOR PERIPHERAL NEUROPATHY
CARPAL TUNNEL SYNDROME
REFRACTORY CONGESTIVE HEART FAILURE
NEPHROTIC SYNDROME
ORTHOSTATIC HYPOTENSION
MALABSORPTION

When any of these clinical manifestations are present, alone or in combination, the clinician should consider the presence of a monoclonal gammopathy.

Proceed to Step 3.

STEP 3 – *What Are the Results of the Serum Protein Electrophoresis?*

Every patient suspected of having a monoclonal gammopathy should have a serum protein electrophoresis (SPEP). It is preferable to perform high resolution electrophoresis, if possible. The SPEP should be performed to assess for the presence of a monoclonal immunoglobulin.

If present, a monoclonal protein (M-protein) will be noted either as a discrete band on the agarose gel or as a tall, narrow peak on the densitometer tracing (M-spike). This differs from a polyclonal gammopathy, in which there is a broad band or broad-based peak on inspection of the gel or densitometer tracing, respectively. See the following figure.

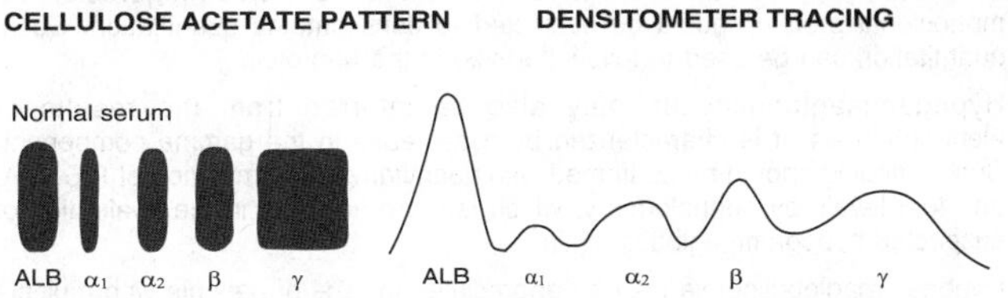

Figure 1.

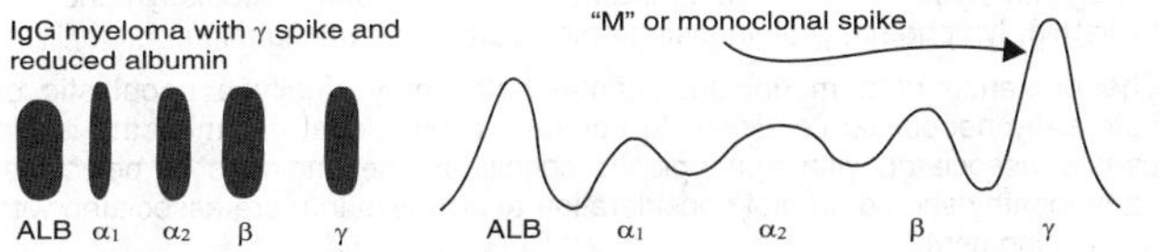

Figure 2.

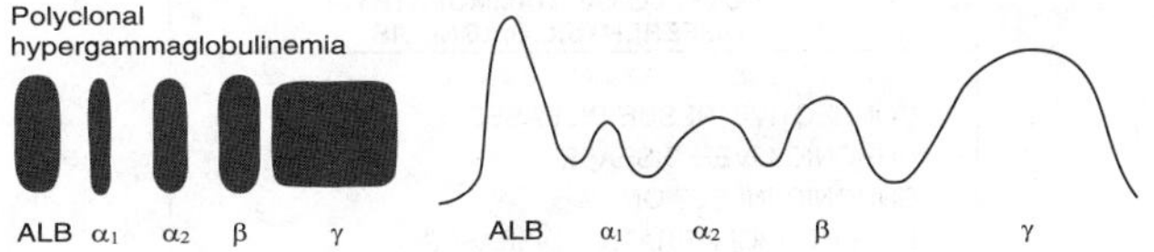

Figure 3.

Figures 1-3. Patterns of serum protein electrophoresis showing characteristic patterns of normal serum, monoclonal M spike, and polyclonal antibody production.

Adapted from Harmening DM, *Clinical Hematology and Fundamentals of Hemostasis*, 2nd ed, Philadelphia, PA: FA Davis Company, 1992.

Not all narrow peaks on the densitometer tracing represent a monoclonal protein. The differential diagnosis of a narrow peak found on a densitometer tracing is found in the following box.

NARROW PEAK ON DENSITOMETER DIFFERENTIAL DIAGNOSIS
MONOCLONAL PROTEIN FREE HEMOGLOBIN-HAPTOGLOBIN COMPLEXES* LARGE AMOUNTS OF TRANSFERRIN† PRESENCE OF FIBRINOGEN

*Free hemoglobin-haptoglobin complexes from hemolysis will be noted in the α_2 globulin region.

†This is often seen in patients with iron deficiency anemia and is noted in the β region.

While most M-proteins are detected in the gamma region of the densitometer tracing (corresponding to the gamma globulin fraction of circulating proteins), at times, a peak may be noted in the β or α_2 region. In most cases, one monoclonal protein is present, however, two monoclonal proteins may be present in up to 4% of patients (biclonal gammopathy).

When an M-spike is noted on the serum protein electrophoresis, the monoclonal protein should be subjected to densitometric quantitation. Serial quantitation can be used to follow the size of the M-protein.

Hypogammaglobulinemia may also be inferred from the results of electrophoresis. It is characterized by a decrease in the gamma component. Such a finding should be confirmed with quantitative determination of IgG, IgA, and IgM levels by nephelometry, which is more accurate in the evaluation of suspected hypogammaglobulinemia.

Hypogammaglobulinemia may be appreciated in 10% of patients with multiple myeloma and 20% of patients with primary amyloidosis. The majority of these patients have a significant amount of urinary light chain excretion (Bence Jones proteinuria) as detected by urine protein electrophoresis. Other causes of hypogammaglobulinemia include the nephrotic syndrome, chronic lymphocytic leukemia, lymphoma, protein losing enteropathy, and malnutrition.

The presence of a monoclonal gammopathy may signify a neoplastic or potentially neoplastic condition. In contrast, a polyclonal gammopathy is not usually associated with a neoplastic condition. The finding of a polyclonal gammopathy should prompt consideration of diseases that are associated with its development.

The causes of polyclonal gammopathy are listed in the following box.

POLYCLONAL GAMMOPATHY DIFFERENTIAL DIAGNOSIS
CONNECTIVE TISSUE DISEASES CHRONIC LIVER DISEASE CHRONIC INFECTION LYMPHOPROLIFERATIVE DISEASES

If a monoclonal protein is identified on the serum protein electrophoresis, ***proceed to Step 4***.

If a monoclonal protein is not identified on the serum protein electrophoresis, but suspicion remains, ***proceed to Step 5***.

STEP 4 – *What Are the Results of the Urine Protein Electrophoresis?*

Urine protein electrophoresis should be performed on every patient with a large monoclonal serum protein. The first step is to determine the total amount of protein excreted in the urine in a 24-hour period. After this, a urine protein electrophoresis should be performed on an aliquot of the urine collected. A urinary monoclonal protein will be identified as a dense band on the gel, and a tall narrow peak on the densitometer tracing. Information obtained from the 24-hour urine collection and electrophoresis can be used to calculate the amount of urinary monoclonal protein using the following formula:

CALCULATION OF URINARY MONOCLONAL PROTEIN
Urinary monoclonal protein = (size of spike on densitometer tracing) x (protein g/24 hours)

This value is important in following the course of the patient's illness since it reflects disease burden.

Proceed to Step 7.

STEP 5 – *What Are the Results of the Urine Protein Electrophoresis?*

It is important to also perform urine protein electrophoresis in these patients because some individuals with a monoclonal gammopathy, who have a normal serum protein electrophoresis, will demonstrate monoclonal light chains (ie, Bence Jones proteinuria) in the urine.

If the urine protein electrophoresis is negative, ***proceed to Step 6***.

If the urine protein electrophoresis is positive, ***proceed to Step 7.***

STEP 6 – *What Are the Results of the Serum and Urine Immunofixation Study?*

Every patient suspected of having a monoclonal gammopathy should have immunofixation testing of the serum and urine, even with a negative serum and urine protein electrophoresis.

Serum immunofixation may reveal the presence of a monoclonal protein in low concentrations (<0.2 g/dL). Such levels are below the sensitivity of the serum protein electrophoresis.

Urine immunofixation testing may detect the presence of a monoclonal protein even when the urine protein electrophoresis is normal.

If serum and urine immunofixation studies are negative, ***stop here***.

If serum and/or urine immunofixation studies are positive, ***proceed to Step 8.***

STEP 7 – *What Are the Results of the Serum and Urine Immunofixation Studies?*

These studies confirm the presence of the monoclonal protein and determine the heavy chain class and light chain type. It should be performed whenever a monoclonal protein is demonstrated on the serum and/or urine electrophoresis.

Proceed to Step 8.

STEP 8 – *What Are the Results of Nephelometry?*

A rate nephelometer may be used to quantitate immunoglobulin concentrations. It can be used to confirm a positive immunofixation test, by demonstrating high levels of one component, along with low or normal levels of other components. In adults, normal immunoglobulin concentrations are as follows.

Immunoglobulin	Concentration (mg/dL)
IgG	800-1200
IgA	180-480
IgM	50-150
IgD	3
IgE	0.3

Nephelometric measurement of immunoglobulins should never be relied on alone to screen patients for a monoclonal protein, because a monoclonal protein can be present despite normal quantitative immunoglobulin levels.

Proceed to Step 9.

STEP 9 – *What Is the Size of the M Protein?*

When a monoclonal protein is identified, the next step is to determine the type of monoclonal gammopathy present. Of all the monoclonal gammopathies described in Step 1, monoclonal gammopathy of undetermined significance (MGUS) is the most common, affecting 1% of the population older than 50 years of age. MGUS is said to be present when a monoclonal protein is identified in the serum and/or urine of a patient who has no features consistent with multiple myeloma, Waldenström's macroglobulinemia, or other monoclonal gammopathy. While some patients with MGUS progress to develop a malignant lymphoproliferative disorder such as multiple myeloma, Waldenström's macroglobulinemia, amyloidosis, or another lymphoproliferative disorder, most do not.

As a result, it is imperative to distinguish benign MGUS from a malignant lymphoproliferative disorder. This is often difficult to do. Monoclonal protein size may be helpful in this regard. Monoclonal protein levels >3 g/dL are more supportive of the diagnosis of a malignant lymphoproliferative disorder than of MGUS.

If the serum M-spike is <3 g/dL, ***proceed to Step 10***.

If the serum M-spike is >3 g/dL, ***proceed to Step 11.***

STEP 10 – *Does the Patient Have MGUS?*

The traditional criteria for the diagnosis of MGUS are listed in the following box.

MGUS TRADITIONAL DIAGNOSTIC CRITERIA
SERUM MONOCLONAL PROTEIN <3 g/dL
<10% PLASMA CELLS IN THE BONE MARROW
ABSENCE OR SMALL AMOUNT OF BENCE JONES PROTEINURIA
ABSENCE OF LYTIC BONE LESIONS
ABSENCE OF ANEMIA
ABSENCE OF HYPERCALCEMIA
ABSENCE OF RENAL INSUFFICIENCY

Not all patients with MGUS will go on to develop multiple myeloma, Waldenström's macroglobulinemia, or another type of monoclonal gammopathy. Because it is difficult to predict which patients with MGUS will go on to develop multiple myeloma, Waldenström's macroglobulinemia, or another type of monoclonal gammopathy, all patients with MGUS must be followed on a regular basis. During these periodic evaluations, the clinician should measure the serum monoclonal protein concentration. Although the serum monoclonal protein concentration may be measured by nephelometry or densitometric quantitation, only one of these techniques should be consistently performed in the serial follow-up of these patients.

In addition, a thorough history and physical examination should be performed searching for any signs or symptoms of multiple myeloma, Waldenström's macroglobulinemia, or other lymphoproliferative disorder. The patient should be referred to an oncologist if signs and symptoms of these disorders are present or if an increase in the monoclonal protein concentration is noted. These developments would argue strongly against a diagnosis of MGUS.

If the patient has signs and symptoms of multiple myeloma (and the monoclonal immunoglobulin is not IgM), ***proceed to Step 11***.

If the patient has signs and symptoms of Waldenström's macroglobulinemia (monoclonal immunoglobulin is IgM), ***proceed to Step 13*** *on page 191.*

If the patient has signs and symptoms of amyloidosis, ***proceed to the section on Amyloidosis*** *on page 839.*

If the patient has MGUS, perform serial measurements of the monoclonal protein concentration and periodic evaluations (thorough history and physical examination) to assess for any change suggestive of the development of a lymphoproliferative disorder. ***Stop here.***

STEP 11 – *What Type of Immunoglobulin Is the Monoclonal Protein?*

If the patient has a monoclonal increase in IgM, ***proceed to Step 13*** *on page 191.*

When the monoclonal protein level is >3 g/dL and the immunoglobulin involved is not IgM, the clinician should consider the diagnosis of multiple myeloma. When multiple myeloma is suspected, the tests in the following box are recommended.

SUGGESTED TESTS FOR PATIENTS IN WHOM MULTIPLE MYELOMA IS SUSPECTED
Complete history and physical examination
Complete blood count and differential; peripheral blood smear
Chemistry screen (including calcium and creatinine determinations)
Serum protein electrophoresis, immunofixation, quantitation of immunoglobulins
Serum viscosity if IgG value is >6 g/dL or IgA value is >5 g/dL, or symptoms of hyperviscosity are present
Routine urinalysis, 24-hour urine collection for electrophoresis and immunofixation
Bone marrow aspiration, biopsy, plasma cell labeling index, and cytogenetics
Metastatic bone survey, including single views of humeri and femurs
Peripheral blood labeling index
β_2-microglobulin, C-reactive protein, and lactate dehydrogenase determinations

Adapted from Kyle RA, "Multiple Myeloma, Macroglobulinemia, and the Monoclonal Gammopathies," *Current Practice of Medicine*, Bone RC, ed, Volume 3, New York, NY: Churchill Livingstone, 1996, 19.1-19.6.

Classic Triad of Multiple Myeloma

The diagnostic triad of multiple myeloma is listed in the following box.

TRIAD OF DIAGNOSTIC FINDINGS IN MULTIPLE MYELOMA
1) Bone marrow plasmacytosis >10%
2) Lytic bone lesions
3) Serum and/or urine monoclonal component

In 80% of patients with multiple myeloma, the serum protein electrophoresis demonstrates a peak or band. In the remaining 20% of patients, 50% will be found to have hypogammaglobulinemia and the other 50% will have no abnormality identified. Urine electrophoresis will show a peak or band in about 80% of patients as well. However, 15% to 20% of patients have a normal urine electrophoresis. Approximately 98% of patients with multiple myeloma will have a monoclonal protein identified in the serum and/or urine.

Monoclonal Components Found in Multiple Myeloma

Monoclonal Component	Percentage
IgG	55%
IgA	22%
Light chains only	18%
IgD	2%
Biclonal	1%

Criteria for Diagnosis of Multiple Myeloma

Many patients with multiple myeloma do not have the classic diagnostic triad. One example is the patient with extensive bone marrow infiltration, but a normal skeletal survey. Investigators have therefore established the following criteria for the diagnosis of multiple myeloma.

MULTIPLE MYELOMA – DIAGNOSTIC CRITERIA

MAJOR CRITERIA	***MINOR CRITERIA***
PLASMACYTOMA ON TISSUE BIOPSY	MARROW PLASMACYTOSIS 10% TO 29%*
MARROW PLASMACYTOSIS ≥30%*	PRESENCE OF MONOCLONAL PROTEIN AT LEVELS BELOW THOSE DIAGNOSTIC OF MULTIPLE MYELOMA
MONOCLONAL PROTEIN IgG >3.5 g/dL IgA >2 g/dL Bence Jones ≥1 g/24 hours	LYTIC BONE LESIONS
	DECREASE IN UNINVOLVED IMMUNOGLOBULINS IgM <50 mg/dL IgA <100 mg/dL IgG <600 mg/dL

*Examination of the bone marrow aspirate and biopsy is necessary to confirm the diagnosis. Since the disease may sometimes be focal, the clinician may need to perform aspiration and biopsy at several sites. Although marrow usually contains >10% plasma cells, cases have been reported in which the percentage of marrow cells was <5%. Immunoperoxidase staining is quite useful in establishing the diagnosis. With the use of this technique, the plasma cells of multiple myeloma will show cytoplasmic staining for either kappa or lambda light chains, which is consistent with a monoclonal process. In patients with reactive plasmacytosis, however, immunoperoxidase staining will demonstrate both light chain types.

To fulfill the diagnosis of multiple myeloma, at least one major and one minor criteria, or at least three minor criteria, must be present.

Differentiating Multiple Myeloma From MGUS

Multiple myeloma must be differentiated from monoclonal gammopathy of undetermined significance (MGUS). MGUS is much more common than multiple myeloma, affecting 1% of the population older than 50 years of age. The criteria for MGUS are listed in the following box.

MGUS – DIAGNOSTIC CRITERIA

SERUM MONOCLONAL PROTEIN <3 g/dL	ABSENCE OF ANEMIA
<10% PLASMA CELLS IN THE BONE MARROW	ABSENCE OF HYPERCALCEMIA
ABSENCE OR SMALL AMOUNT OF BENCE JONES PROTEINURIA	ABSENCE OF RENAL INSUFFICIENCY
ABSENCE OF LYTIC BONE LESIONS	STABILITY OF THE MONOCLONAL PROTEIN OVER TIME
	NORMAL PLASMA CELL LABELING INDEX*

*The plasma cell labeling index is one test that can be used to help differentiate multiple myeloma from MGUS. This test, which is performed on bone marrow tissue, is normal in MGUS patients but typically elevated in those with multiple myeloma. The clinician should realize, however, that up to 35% of multiple myeloma patients may have normal values.

Of patients found to have a monoclonal gammopathy, the majority will have MGUS. In various studies, only 10% to 25% progress to multiple myeloma. At the present time, no single test is available to differentiate all cases of multiple myeloma from MGUS. The most useful feature supporting MGUS is stability of the monoclonal protein concentration over time.

Laboratory Test Findings in Multiple Myeloma

The laboratory features of multiple myeloma are included in the following box.

MULTIPLE MYELOMA – LABORATORY FEATURES	
ANEMIA*	RENAL INSUFFICIENCY§
ROULEAUX FORMATION ON PERIPHERAL BLOOD SMEAR	URINE DIPSTICK NEGATIVE FOR PROTEIN¶
THROMBOCYTOPENIA / THROMBOCYTOSIS†	HYPERCALCEMIA#
	HYPERVISCOSITY**
LEUKOPENIA†	DECREASED ANION GAP
HYPOGAMMAGLOBULINEMIA‡	INCREASED ESR

*Normocytic, normochromic anemia is commonly present in patients with multiple myeloma (66% of patients at diagnosis). Even in patients who do not have anemia at the time of presentation, it will occur in almost all patients as the disease progresses. The etiology is multifactorial and includes the following possibilities: bone marrow infiltration by plasma cells, anemia of chronic disease, renal insufficiency, and chemotherapy.

†Anemia may occur alone; however, in some patients, leukopenia or thrombocytopenia, or both, accompany anemia. The decrease in these cell lines is thought to be due to bone marrow infiltration and chemotherapy. In a minority of patients, thrombocytosis may be appreciated.

‡Hypogammaglobulinemia is characterized by a decrease in the gamma component. When electrophoresis supports hypogammaglobulinemia, a quantitative determination of immunoglobulin levels should be performed for confirmation. Hypogammaglobulinemia has been described in approximately 10% of multiple myeloma patients. The majority of these individuals show significant Bence Jones proteinuria. Increased susceptibility to infection is mainly due to the characteristic hypogammaglobulinemia.

§Renal insufficiency is present in nearly 50% of patients at the time of diagnosis. In fact, 25% of multiple myeloma patients will have a serum creatinine level exceeding 2 mg/dL when first diagnosed. Not uncommonly, renal failure is the initial presentation of the disease. The two major causes of renal insufficiency are myeloma kidney and hypercalcemia. Myeloma kidney should be a consideration in an older patient with renal failure (acute or subacute). Characteristic features of myeloma kidney include a bland urinary sediment and a negative urine dipstick for protein. Other factors that may contribute to the renal insufficiency include hyperuricemia, dehydration, amyloidosis, NSAIDs, kidney infiltration by plasma cells, increased serum viscosity, and radiocontrast administration.

¶Many patients with multiple myeloma excrete light chains in the urine but because the urine dipstick test mainly detects albumin, urine dipstick testing is usually negative. Urine light chains may be detected by sulfosalicylic acid testing or by performing a 24-hour urine collection for electrophoresis and immunofixation.

#Hypercalcemia is present in up to 40% of multiple myeloma patients. Its presence usually signifies a large tumor burden. It is not uncommon for symptoms of hypercalcemia to be the presenting feature of multiple myeloma.

**Symptoms of hyperviscosity are more commonly encountered in Waldenström's macroglobulinemia, but do occur in multiple myeloma (<10%). Hyperviscosity occurs more commonly in patients with IgA and IgG subclass 3 myeloma. The diagnosis is established by measuring serum viscosity.

Proceed to Step 12.

STEP 12 – *What Laboratory Tests Are Useful as Prognostic Factors in Patients With Multiple Myeloma?*

The Durie and Salmon clinical staging system employs various factors in estimating survival and is outlined in the following box.

DURIE AND SALMON CLINICAL STAGING SYSTEM* FOR MULTIPLE MYELOMA

STAGE 1: LOW TUMOR MASS†

- Hemoglobin >10 g/dL
- Myeloma protein
  - IgG <5 g/dL
  - IgA <3 g/dL
  - Bence Jones <4 g/24 hours
- Normal calcium level
- 0-1 lytic bone lesion

STAGE II: INTERMEDIATE TUMOR MASS

- Not fitting stage I or III

STAGE III: HIGH TUMOR MASS‡

- Hemoglobin <8.5 g/dL
- Myeloma protein
  - IgG >7 g/dL
  - IgA >5 g/dL
  - Bence Jones >12 g/24 hours
- Calcium level >12 mg/dL (adjusted for albumin)
- Multiple lytic lesions

*Each of the stages can be further divided into A or B depending on the creatinine level. A represents a creatinine <2 mg/dL and B represents a creatinine ≥2 mg/dL.

†For a patient to be deemed stage I, all of the criteria must be fulfilled.

‡For a patient to be deemed stage III, only one of the criteria needs to be present.

Durie and Salmon Staging System: A Prognostic Indicator of Survival in Multiple Myeloma

Stage	Median Survival (mo)
I	60
III	15

Other laboratory values that are helpful in determining prognosis include the following.

- Plasma cell labeling index (PCLI)

  The plasma cell labeling index (PCLI) is the major prognostic factor for patients treated with conventional chemotherapy.

- β_2-microglobulin

  β_2-microglobulin levels predict survival independent of renal function and tumor load.

- C-reactive protein (CRP)

  The CRP level predicts survival independent of the β_2-microglobulin level.

  The combined parameters can be used to further stratify risk as demonstrated in the following table.

β_2-Microglobulin	CRP	Risk
<6 mg/L	<6 mg/L	Low
>6 mg/L	<6 mg/L	Intermediate
<6 mg/L	>6 mg/L	Intermediate
>6 mg/L	>6 mg/L	High

Proceed to Step 14.

STEP 13 – *Does the Patient Have Waldenström's Macroglobulinemia?*

If the monoclonal protein consists of IgM, the clinician should consider the possibility of Waldenström's macroglobulinemia. This disease is characterized by infiltration of bone marrow with lymphoplasmacytoid cells, along with a high concentration of IgM in the peripheral blood.

The clinical manifestations of Waldenström's macroglobulinemia are listed in the following box.

WALDENSTRÖM'S MACROGLOBULINEMIA
CLINICAL MANIFESTATIONS

LYMPHADENOPATHY
SPLENOMEGALY
ANEMIA SECONDARY TO BONE MARROW INFILTRATION
HYPERVISCOSITY SYNDROME
CRYOGLOBULINEMIA WITH RAYNAUD'S SYNDROME AND VASCULITIS
COLD AGGLUTININ HEMOLYTIC ANEMIA
BLEEDING
PERIPHERAL NEUROPATHY WITH SYMMETRICAL SENSORIMOTOR DEFICITS

The laboratory features of Waldenström's macroglobulinemia are listed in the following box.

WALDENSTRÖM'S MACROGLOBULINEMIA
LABORATORY FEATURES

ANEMIA*
BENCE JONES PROTEINURIA (seldom >1 g/24 hours)
MILD LYMPHOCYTOSIS / MONOCYTOSIS
INCREASED β_2-MICROGLOBULIN (33% of patients)
INCREASED C-REACTIVE PROTEIN (66% of patients)
INCREASED ERYTHROCYTE SEDIMENTATION RATE
INCREASED SERUM VISCOSITY†
INCREASED CRYOGLOBULINS
COLD AGGLUTININ HEMOLYTIC ANEMIA (10% patients)‡
INCREASED BLEEDING TIME

*Anemia is present in almost patients. At times, there may be spurious lowering of hemoglobin secondary to increased plasma volume. Increased plasma volume results from the presence of large amounts of monoclonal protein. In many patients, Rouleaux formation is striking.

†Serum viscosity is increased in most patients, but only 20% have symptoms. Those having a serum viscosity >4 times that of water are at higher risk of becoming symptomatic.

‡The cold agglutinin titer is often >1:1000 in these patients.

Proceed to Step 14.

STEP 14 – *Does the Patient Have the Hyperviscosity Syndrome?*

While Waldenström's macroglobulinemia is the most common cause of hyperviscosity, it may also occur in patients with multiple myeloma who have high levels of monoclonal IgG or IgA. Serum viscosity should therefore be measured in the following situations.

INDICATIONS FOR MEASURING SERUM VISCOSITY	
CLINICAL MANIFESTATIONS OF HYPERVISCOSITY	
Blurring or loss of vision	Diplopia
Oronasal bleeding	Congestive heart failure
Headache	Somnolence
Vertigo	Stupor
Nystagmus	Coma
Decreased hearing	Dilation of retinal veins
Ataxia	Flame-shaped retinal hemorrhage
Paresthesia	
MONOCLONAL IgM PROTEIN >4 g/dL	
MONOCLONAL IgA PROTEIN >6 g/dL	
MONOCLONAL IgG PROTEIN >6 g/dL	

It is important to always correlate the patient's signs and symptoms with the serum viscosity. It is unusual for symptoms of hyperviscosity to occur when the serum viscosity is <4 centipoises. There have been reports, however, of patients who are free of symptoms at 10 centipoises. As a result, the clinician should manage the patient based on the combination of clinical findings and serum viscosity, with more importance placed on the clinical presentation. When a diagnosis of hyperviscosity syndrome is established, the patient may require emergent plasmapheresis.

Proceed to Step 15.

STEP 15 – *Does the Patient Have Cryoglobulinemia?*

In the patient with a monoclonal gammopathy, testing for cryoglobulins is recommended only when there are signs and symptoms of cryoglobulinemia.

CRYOGLOBULINEMIA CLINICAL FEATURES	
SKIN LESIONS*	RAYNAUD'S PHENOMENON
LIVER DISEASE	NEUROLOGIC MANIFESTATIONS
RENAL DISEASE	ACROCYANOSIS
ARTHRALGIA / ARTHRITIS	HEMORRHAGE

*Skin manifestations include palpable purpura, changes in pigmentation, petechiae, telangiectasia, urticaria, livedo, and leg ulcers.

For more information regarding cryoglobulinemia, refer to the Rheumatology section.

End of Section.

References

Aguzzi F, Bergami MR, Gesparro C, et al, "Occurrence of Monoclonal Components in General Practice: Clinical Implications," *Eur J Haematol*, 1992, 48:192-5.

Anderson KC, "Multiple Myeloma: How Far Have We Come?" *Mayo Clin Proc*, 2003, 78(1):15-7.

Dimopoulos MA and Alexanian R, "Waldenström's Macroglobulinemia," *Blood*, 1994, 83:1452-9.

Ghobrial IM, Gertz MA, and Fonseca R, "Waldenström Macroglobulinaemia," *Lancet Oncol*, 2003, 4(11):679-85.

Greipp PR, "Advances in the Diagnosis and Management of Myeloma," *Semin Hematol*, 1992, 29:24-45.

Johnson SA, Oscier DG, and Leblond V, "Waldenstroöm's Macroglobulinaemia" *Blood Rev*, 2002, 16(3):175-84.

Keren DF, "Procedures for the Evaluation of Monoclonal Immunoglobulins," *Arch Pathol Lab Med*, 1999, 123:126-32.

Keren DF, Alexanian R, Goeken JA, et al, "Guidelines for Clinical and Laboratory Evaluation of Patients With Monoclonal Gammopathies," *Arch Pathol Lab Med*, 1999, 123:106-7.

Kyle RA, "Monoclonal Gammopathy of Undetermined Significance and Solitary Plasmacytoma: Implications for Progression to Overt Multiple Myeloma," *Hematol Oncol Clin North Am*, 1997, 11:71-87.

Kyle RA, "Monoclonal Gammopathy of Undetermined Significance and Solitary Plasmacytoma: Implications for Progression to Overt Multiple Myeloma," *Hematol Oncol Clin North Am*, 1997, 11:71-87.

Kyle RA and Greipp PR, "Plasma Cell Dyscrasias: Current Status," *Crit Rev Oncol Hematol*, 1988, 8:93-152.

Kyle RA and Rajkumar SV, "Monoclonal Gammopathies of Undetermined Significance," *Rev Clin Exp Hematol*, 2002, 6(3):225-52.

Rajkumar SV, Kyle RA, and Gertz MA, "Myeloma and the Newly Diagnosed Patient: A Focus on Treatment and Management," *Semin Oncol*, 2002, 29(6 Suppl 17):5-10.

Stone MJ, "Myeloma and Macroglobulinemia: What Are the Criteria for Diagnosis?" *Clin Lymphoma*, 2002, 3(1):23-5.

PART II:

FLUIDS, ELECTROLYTES, AND ACID-BASE

HYPONATREMIA

STEP 1 – *Does the Patient Have Hyponatremia?*

Normal plasma or serum sodium concentration is 136-145 mmol/L. Hyponatremia is said to be present when the sodium concentration is <136 mmol/L. Hyponatremia is a commonly encountered electrolyte abnormality in hospitalized patients. In fact, mild to moderate hyponatremia (126-135 mmol/L) has been noted in 14% of hospitalized patients. Severe hyponatremia, defined as a serum sodium concentration ≤125 mmol/L, is seen in 1% of such patients.

Although hyponatremia can occur at any age, it is clearly more common with increasing age. One study found that 7% of community-residing individuals over age 65 had a plasma sodium concentration <137 mmol/L. Of note, this study examined a population that was free of acute illness. In patients of this age who have acute illness requiring hospitalization, the incidence of hyponatremia is even higher.

Proceed to Step 2.

STEP 2 – *What Are the Causes of Hyponatremia?*

The causes of hyponatremia are listed in the following box.

CAUSES OF HYPONATREMIA

SPURIOUS HYPONATREMIA
- "Drip-arm" hyponatremia
- "Dead-space" hyponatremia

ISOTONIC HYPONATREMIA
- Pseudohyponatremia (hyperlipidemia, hyperproteinemia)

HYPERTONIC HYPONATREMIA
- Hyperglycemia
- Mannitol administration
- Glycine
- Maltose

HYPOTONIC HYPONATREMIA
- Hypovolemic
  - Extrarenal
    - Gastrointestinal fluid loss (vomiting, diarrhea, blood loss)
    - Skin losses of fluid (excessive sweating)
    - Third-space fluid loss (bowel obstruction, pancreatitis, peritonitis, burns, muscle trauma)
  - Renal
    - Salt-losing nephropathies
    - Diuretic therapy
    - Osmotic diuresis (glucose, urea, mannitol)
    - Mineralocorticoid deficiency
    - Ketonuria
    - Bicarbonaturia
    - Cerebral salt-wasting syndrome

(continued)

CAUSES OF HYPONATREMIA *(continued)*
HYPOTONIC HYPONATREMIA *(continued)*
Euvolemic
Syndrome of inappropriate antidiuretic hormone (SIADH)
Adrenal insufficiency
Hypothyroidism
Thiazide diuretics
Primary polydipsia
Decreased intake of solutes (beer drinkers' potomania, tea-and-toast diet)
Hypervolemic
Congestive heart failure
Cirrhosis
Nephrotic syndrome
Acute renal failure
Chronic renal failure

Proceed to Step 3.

STEP 3 – *Do All Patients With Hyponatremia Need to Be Evaluated?*

Mild hyponatremia, defined as a serum or plasma sodium concentration between 130 and 136 mmol/L, is quite common. Because this degree of hyponatremia is often transient, no further evaluation is usually necessary. Hyponatremia that is more marked, however, does require further evaluation as does hyponatremia that is prolonged, irrespective of the degree of the hyponatremia.

If the patient has mild hyponatremia that is transient, ***stop here***.

If the patient has mild hyponatremia that is persistent, ***proceed to Step 4***.

If the patient has mild hyponatremia that worsens in severity (ie, serum or plasma sodium concentration <131 mmol/L), ***proceed to Step 4***.

STEP 4 – *Does the Patient Have Spurious Hyponatremia?*

Before embarking on an extensive evaluation to elucidate the etiology of the hyponatremia, the clinician should ensure that the patient does not have spurious hyponatremia. One type of spurious hyponatremia, termed "drip arm" hyponatremia, occurs when the sodium concentration is measured from a blood sample taken upstream from an intravenous infusion of hypotonic fluid. Performing a venipuncture in the antecubital fossa of an arm that is receiving an intravenous infusion of glucose through one of the hand veins is the classic setting in which "drip arm" hyponatremia occurs.

"Dead-space" hyponatremia is another type of spurious hyponatremia. This type of hyponatremia typically occurs when blood is taken from a central venous line. If the dead space in the central venous line is not discarded, the dead space, which usually consists of heparin solution, will result in a falsely low sodium concentration. It is important to consider these causes of spurious hyponatremia because recognition of their presence can obviate an unnecessary workup of hyponatremia. One other type of hyponatremia, termed pseudohyponatremia, can also be considered a form of spurious hyponatremia. Pseudohyponatremia will be discussed shortly.

If the patient has spurious hyponatremia, ***stop here***.

If the patient does not have spurious hyponatremia, ***proceed to Step 5***.

STEP 5 – *What Is the Plasma Osmolality?*

Once spurious hyponatremia has been excluded, the clinician should then measure the plasma osmolality. The patient may be categorized into one of three groups based on the measurement of the plasma osmolality.

1. Hypotonic hyponatremia (plasma osmolality <280 mOsm/kg)
2. Hypertonic hyponatremia (plasma osmolality >295 mOsm/kg)
3. Isotonic hyponatremia (plasma osmolality between 280 and 295 mOsm/kg)

If the patient has hypertonic hyponatremia, ***proceed to Step 6.***

If the patient has isotonic hyponatremia, ***proceed to Step 7.***

If the patient has hypotonic hyponatremia, ***proceed to Step 8.***

STEP 6 – *What Is Hypertonic Hyponatremia?*

A plasma osmolality that exceeds 295 mOsm/kg is consistent with hypertonic hyponatremia. This is usually seen with hyperglycemia or with the administration of other osmotically active solutes, such as mannitol or glycerol.

The high concentration of glucose in the extracellular fluid (ECF) draws water out of the intracellular fluid (ICF), thereby diluting sodium in the ECF. A useful calculation to remember is that for every 100 mg/dL increase in the glucose concentration >100 mg/dL, the serum sodium level falls by 1.6 mmol/L. This calculation should be done for every hyperglycemic patient with hyponatremia. If the plasma sodium level corrects, then no other process leading to hyponatremia is present. The absence of correction suggests the presence of an additional etiology for the hyponatremia. Recently, several studies have suggested that the decrease in the serum sodium concentration should be closer to 2.4 mmol/L as the glucose level reaches and exceeds 400 mg/dL.

FORMULA FOR THE CORRECTION OF SODIUM IN THE PRESENCE OF HYPERGLYCEMIA
$Na^+_{corrected} = Na^+_{measured} + \frac{1.6\ mEq/L\ (glucose_{measured} - 100)}{100}$

Hypertonic hyponatremia may also occur with the administration of hypertonic mannitol. This typically occurs in patients receiving an infusion of mannitol to reduce cerebral edema. Hypertonic hyponatremia has also been described after administration of IgG solutions containing maltose.

End of Section.

STEP 7 – *What Is Isotonic Hyponatremia?*

The major cause of isotonic hyponatremia is pseudohyponatremia, which is defined as a falsely low serum sodium concentration. Pseudohyponatremia only occurs in patients with extreme hyperlipidemia or hyperproteinemia. Not all laboratory methods available in the measurement of the sodium concentration, however, will give spurious results in the setting of hyperlipidemia or hyperproteinemia. The laboratory that measures the sodium concentration by direct reading potentiometry using a sodium-selective electrode will give the true sodium concentration, irrespective of the presence of hyperlipidemia or hyperproteinemia. In contrast, falsely low serum sodium concentrations may be obtained if flame emission spectrophotometry (flame photometry) is used.

Of major importance for the clinician is to determine what technique is being used by the laboratory. In recent years, pseudohyponatremia is infrequently encountered as labs are using ion-selective electrodes rather than flame photometry to measure the serum sodium concentration. In fact, the widespread use of ion-selective electrodes has all but eliminated pseudohyponatremia.

Nevertheless, it still behooves the clinician to know exactly what methodology is being employed at his/her particular laboratory. If the clinician learns that the older technique of flame photometry is still being used, then it should prompt the clinician to consider pseudohyponatremia, particularly when a low serum sodium concentration is obtained in the setting of a normal serum osmolality. By considering this possibility, the clinician can avoid making errors in patient management that have the potential to be life-threatening.

End of Section.

STEP 8 – *What Is the Patient's Volume Status?*

Hypotonic hyponatremia is present when plasma osmolality is <280 mOsm/kg. Once the presence of hypotonic hyponatremia has been established, the next step involves assessment of the patient's volume status. History and physical examination can help classify the patient into one of the following categories.

- Hypovolemic hypotonic hyponatremia
- Hypervolemic hypotonic hyponatremia
- Euvolemic hypotonic hyponatremia

The following table lists the physical exam findings that help to differentiate between the three types of hypotonic hyponatremia.

Physical Exam Findings Used to Assess Volume Status

Findings in the Physical Exam	Volume Status
Orthostatic changes in blood pressure and heart rate Dry mucous membranes Poor skin turgor Flat jugular veins Absence of axillary sweat	Hypovolemic
Peripheral edema Elevated jugular venous pressure Ascites Other signs of congestive heart failure, cirrhosis, or nephrotic syndrome	Hypervolemic
Absence of physical exam findings consistent with hypervolemia or hypovolemia	Euvolemic

If the patient has hypovolemic hypotonic hyponatremia, ***proceed to Step 9.***

If the patient has hypervolemic hypotonic hyponatremia, ***proceed to Step 10.***

If the patient has euvolemic hypotonic hyponatremia, ***proceed to Step 11.***

STEP 9 – *What Is the Approach to the Patient With Hypovolemic Hypotonic Hyponatremia?*

In hypovolemic hyponatremia, volume depletion becomes an important stimulus for ADH secretion. Decreased volume leads to increased secretion of ADH which results in water retention and a decrease in serum sodium concentration as water ingestion continues. The causes of hypovolemic hyponatremia are listed in the following box.

CAUSES OF HYPOVOLEMIC HYPOTONIC HYPONATREMIA	
EXTRARENAL	***RENAL***
Gastrointestinal fluid loss	Salt-losing nephropathies
(vomiting, diarrhea, blood loss)	Diuretic therapy (usually thiazides)
Skin losses of fluid	Osmotic diuresis
(excessive sweating)*	(glucose, urea, mannitol)
Third-space fluid loss	Mineralocorticoid deficiency
(bowel obstruction, ileus,	Ketonuria
pancreatitis, peritonitis, burns,	Bicarbonaturia
muscle trauma)	Cerebral salt-wasting syndrome

*Excessive sweating is an uncommon cause of hypovolemic hyponatremia. It is most commonly seen in endurance athletes who exercise for extended periods of time (usually >6 hours). These athletes are prone to significant losses of sodium and water. Hyponatremia can ensue if these losses are replaced by large amounts of tap water.

As indicated in the above box, hypovolemic hyponatremia can be divided into renal and extrarenal causes. The history can often establish whether a renal or extrarenal cause is present. When the etiology is not clear, a urine sodium concentration may be helpful in differentiating between the two.

If the urine sodium is <20 mEq/L, consider the following extrarenal possibilities:

- Vomiting
- Diarrhea
- Third space losses
- Skin fluid losses (excessive sweating)

If the urine sodium is >20 mEq/L, consider the following renal causes:

- Diuretic use
- Mineralocorticoid deficiency
- Salt-losing nephropathies
- Ketonuria
- Bicarbonaturia
- Osmotic diuresis
- Cerebral salt-wasting syndrome

Brief mention should be made here of the cerebral salt-wasting syndrome. The cerebral salt-wasting syndrome may occur in patients who have suffered a cerebral insult. Precipitants of this syndrome include head injury/trauma, subarachnoid hemorrhage, brain tumors, or CNS infection. Although it was initially described before SIADH, later it was thought that the cerebral salt-wasting syndrome was a form of SIADH. Experts now feel that it is its own entity, having characteristics that differentiate it from SIADH. These characteristics are listed in the following table.

Differentiating Cerebral Salt-Wasting Syndrome From SIADH

	Cerebral Salt-Wasting Syndrome	SIADH
Plasma sodium	Decreased	Decreased
Blood urea nitrogen	Increased	Low or normal
Serum albumin	Increased	Normal
Hematocrit	Increased	Normal
Blood pressure	Low or postural hypotension	Normal
Central venous pressure	Decreased	Normal

Differentiating Cerebral Salt-Wasting Syndrome From SIADH *(continued)*

	Cerebral Salt-Wasting Syndrome	SIADH
Urine sodium concentration	Increased	Increased
Urinary volume	Increased	Decreased
Thirst	Increased	Normal

The cerebral salt-wasting syndrome usually resolves spontaneously 3-4 weeks after the cerebral insult. The pathogenesis of the syndrome has not been fully elucidated but several studies have shown increased levels of atrial natriuretic peptide. In neurosurgical settings, the cerebral salt-wasting syndrome has been found to be more common than SIADH. It is important to differentiate between the two because the treatment of hyponatremia differs in these two conditions. The hyponatremia of the cerebral salt-wasting syndrome responds readily to intravenous saline. This is in contrast to SIADH in which intravenous saline may not improve the sodium concentration and may even worsen the hyponatremia.

End of Section.

STEP 10 – *What Is the Approach to the Patient With Hypervolemic Hypotonic Hyponatremia?*

The causes of hypervolemic hyponatremia are listed in the following box.

CAUSES OF HYPERVOLEMIC HYPOTONIC HYPONATREMIA	
CONGESTIVE HEART FAILURE	ACUTE RENAL FAILURE
CIRRHOSIS	CHRONIC RENAL FAILURE
NEPHROTIC SYNDROME	

CHF, cirrhosis, and nephrotic syndrome result in decreased effective arterial blood volume, which results in the nonosmotic release of ADH, ultimately leading to hyponatremia. In patients with CHF or cirrhosis, the degree of the hyponatremia usually correlates with the severity of the underlying disease. Hypervolemic hypotonic hyponatremia is also appreciated in patients with acute or chronic renal failure. The pathophysiology involves a decrease in the number of functioning nephrons. Even though the remaining nephrons can dilute urine appropriately, there is an inability to excrete all of the free water because not enough functioning nephrons remain.

The etiology can be established by information gathered from the history and physical examination. When the etiology remains unclear, a urine sodium concentration may be helpful.

A urine sodium level <20 mEq/L is consistent with:

- Congestive heart failure
- Cirrhosis
- Nephrotic syndrome

The clinician should realize, however, that the urine sodium level may exceed 20 mEq/L in patients with CHF, cirrhosis, and nephrotic syndrome if diuretic therapy is part of the treatment regimen.

A urine sodium level >20 mEq/L is consistent with:

- Acute renal failure
- Chronic renal failure

End of Section.

STEP 11 – *What Is the Approach to the Patient With Euvolemic Hypotonic Hyponatremia?*

Euvolemic hypotonic hyponatremia is the most common cause of hyponatremia in hospitalized patients. The causes are listed in the following box.

CAUSES OF EUVOLEMIC HYPOTONIC HYPONATREMIA	
SYNDROME OF INAPPROPRIATE ANTIDIURETIC HORMONE (SIADH)	PRIMARY POLYDIPSIA
HYPOTHYROIDISM	THIAZIDE DIURETICS
ADRENAL INSUFFICIENCY	DECREASED INTAKE OF SOLUTES (beer drinkers' potomania, tea-and-toast diet)

The major causes of euvolemic hyponatremia will be further discussed in the remainder of this step.

SYNDROME OF INAPPROPRIATE ANTIDIURETIC HORMONE (SIADH)

SIADH is the most common cause of euvolemic hypotonic hyponatremia. This disorder occurs when ADH secretion is the result of nonphysiologic stimuli. Remember that the major physiologic stimuli for ADH secretion are increasing osmolality and decreasing volume.

SIADH is diagnosed when criteria in the following box are met.

ESSENTIAL CRITERIA FOR SIADH	
NORMAL ACID-BASE BALANCE	INAPPROPRIATE URINARY CONCENTRATION (urine osmolality >100 mOsm/kg)
NORMAL ADRENAL FUNCTION	EUVOLEMIC VOLUME STATUS
NORMAL RENAL FUNCTION	URINE SODIUM >40 mEq/L
NORMAL THYROID FUNCTION	
PLASMA OSMOLALITY <270 mOsm/kg	

Remember that a patient with hypo-osmolality should respond with excretion of maximally dilute urine. Urine osmolality between 50 and 100 mOsm/kg corresponds to maximally dilute urine. If urine osmolality exceeds this, then ADH is inappropriately high. Urine osmolality does not need to be higher than serum osmolality for SIADH to be present.

Differentiating SIADH From Hypovolemic Hypotonic Hyponatremia

One may ask why this question is here in this section since presumably this distinction has been made with the assessment of volume status in Step 8. The reason is because it can be very difficult, at times, to separate hypovolemic hyponatremia from SIADH by history and physical examination. This is particularly true in patients with mild volume depletion. In these difficult cases, laboratory testing may help make the distinction (see following table). In SIADH, as described above, the urine sodium concentration is usually >40 mEq/L whereas, in hypovolemia, it is typically <20 mEq/L. SIADH is often characterized by low or low-normal uric acid levels, as opposed to hypovolemia which often has a normal or even high level. The BUN:creatinine ratio is characteristically low in SIADH, in contrast to hypovolemia. Remember that urine osmolality may be greater than serum osmolality in both conditions.

	SIADH	Hypovolemic Hypotonic Hyponatremia
Urine sodium	>40 mEq/L	<20 mEq/L*
Uric acid	Low / low-normal	Normal / high
BUN:creatinine	Low	High

*This applies to nonrenal causes only (see below).

Urine sodium concentration is very helpful in separating SIADH from hypovolemic hyponatremia when the hypovolemia is from a nonrenal condition. Recall in the section on hypovolemic hypotonic hyponatremia, that renal conditions can lead to this state as well. Renal conditions are characterized by urine sodium concentration >20 mEq/L and, thus, may overlap with the urine sodium level found in SIADH. A useful diagnostic and therapeutic maneuver in these cases is to observe the response to water restriction. When water ingestion is restricted to about 700 mL/day, patients with SIADH will lose weight, usually 2-3 kg over the next 2-3 days. An increase in urine sodium will accompany the decrease in weight. However, if this maneuver is unsuccessful in increasing the urine sodium level, SIADH is unlikely. A renal disorder, particularly a disorder of renal salt wasting, should then be considered.

Differentiating SIADH From the Cerebral Salt-Wasting Syndrome

The cerebral salt-wasting syndrome may occur in patients who have suffered a cerebral insult. Precipitants of this syndrome include head injury/trauma, subarachnoid hemorrhage, brain tumors, or CNS infection. Although it was initially described before SIADH, later it was thought that the cerebral salt-wasting syndrome was a form of SIADH. Experts now feel that it is its own entity, having characteristics that differentiate it from SIADH. These characteristics are listed in the following table.

Differentiating Cerebral Salt-Wasting Syndrome From SIADH

	Cerebral Salt-Wasting Syndrome	SIADH
Plasma sodium	Decreased	Decreased
Blood urea nitrogen	Increased	Low or normal
Blood pressure	Low or postural hypotension	Normal
Central venous pressure	Decreased	Normal
Urine sodium concentration	Increased	Increased
Urinary volume	Increased	Decreased
Thirst	Increased	Normal

The cerebral salt-wasting syndrome usually resolves spontaneously 3-4 weeks after the cerebral insult. The pathogenesis of the syndrome has not been fully elucidated but several studies have shown increased levels of atrial natriuretic peptide. In neurosurgical settings, the cerebral salt-wasting syndrome has been found to be more common than SIADH. It is important to differentiate between the two because the treatment of hyponatremia differs in these two conditions. The hyponatremia of the cerebral salt-wasting syndrome responds readily to intravenous saline. This is in contrast to SIADH in which intravenous saline may not improve the sodium concentration and may even worsen the hyponatremia.

Causes of SIADH

A thorough history and physical examination will often provide clues regarding the etiology of the SIADH. Further workup should be individualized depending upon the clues elicited in the history and physical examination. A chest radiograph is an essential part of the evaluation given the fact there are many pulmonary conditions associated with SIADH. A normal chest radiograph should prompt consideration of CT scan of the thorax to exclude retrocardiac or retrosternal tumors. In addition, CT scan of the brain or abdomen may also be indicated, depending upon the patient's clinical presentation.

SIADH DIFFERENTIAL DIAGNOSIS	
LUNG DISEASE	MEDICATIONS
Abscess	Chlorpropamide
Chronic obstructive pulmonary disease	Cyclophosphamide
Pneumonia (viral, bacterial)	Opiates
Tuberculosis	Tegretol
Aspergillosis	Tricyclic antidepressants
Acute bronchial asthma	Vincristine / Vinblastine
Bronchiectasis	SSRIs
Empyema	Oxytocin
Cystic fibrosis	Ifosfamide
Pneumothorax	Desmopressin
CNS CONDITIONS	Lysine vasopressin
Brain tumor	Clofibrate
Cerebrovascular accident	Prostaglandin synthesis inhibitors
Encephalitis	Nicotine
Meningitis	Antipsychotics
Subarachnoid hemorrhage	Acetaminophen
Subdural hematoma	NSAIDs
Acute psychosis	MALIGNANCY
Head trauma	Lymphoma
Brain abscess	Pancreatic cancer
Cavernous sinus thrombosis	Small cell cancer of lung
Multiple sclerosis	Pharyngeal carcinoma
Acute intermittent porphyria	Duodenal cancer
Guillan-Barré syndrome	Thymoma
Delirium tremens	Mesothelioma
Hydrocephalus	Bladder carcinoma
POSITIVE PRESSURE VENTILATION	Prostate cancer
STRESS / PAIN	Reticulum cell sarcoma
	Ureteric cancer
	Endometrial cancer
	MDMA / ECSTASY
	MISCELLANEOUS
	Postoperative state
	Severe nausea
	HIV infection

Adrenal Insufficiency

Adrenal insufficiency is characterized by secretion of ADH secondary to volume depletion. ADH is also cosecreted with ACTH in response to increased corticotropin-releasing factor in these patients. Mineralocorticoid deficiency may contribute to hyponatremia as well. Not all patients with adrenal insufficiency will present with the classic electrolyte abnormalities of hyponatremia and hyperkalemia. Therefore, the absence of hyperkalemia should not prompt the clinician to discard the diagnosis of adrenal insufficiency. The elderly, in particular, are more prone to present with nonspecific symptoms of adrenal insufficiency along with chronic hyponatremia. The cosyntropin stimulation test can be used to establish the diagnosis of adrenal insufficiency.

Hypothyroidism

Hypothyroidism, through a decrease in cardiac output and GFR as well as an increase in ADH, leads to hyponatremia. Laboratory testing will reveal characteristic abnormalities in thyroid function.

Primary Polydipsia

Primary polydipsia is characterized by compulsive water drinking in amounts that exceed renal excretory ability (4-25 L/day). Patients often have psychiatric problems, particularly schizophrenia. Many are taking phenothiazines which may lead to dry mouth, a further impetus for water ingestion. Urine osmolality is appropriately low, usually <100 mOsm/kg. The hyponatremia may wax and wane with exacerbations and remissions of the underlying psychogenic disorder.

Diuretic-Induced Hyponatremia

Although diuretic-induced hyponatremia has been reported with a number of different diuretic medications, thiazide diuretics are the most common offenders. In one large review, 73% of cases were due thiazide diuretics. The elderly are at increased risk of developing hyponatremia after starting diuretic therapy. Interestingly, there seems to be a female preponderance, with 80% of those affected being women. It typically occurs within the first few weeks of therapy in contrast to furosemide-induced hyponatremia which usually occurs after a longer interval. Thiazide-induced hyponatremia is clearly reproducible and cases where hyponatremia recurred after a single dose have been reported.

While one would expect that diuretic-induced hyponatremia would present with hypovolemic hyponatremia, in reality, these patients are a heterogeneous group. While there are some that clearly present with hypovolemic hyponatremia, there are others who present with apparent euvolemia. The difference in volume status is likely to be related to the magnitude of sodium loss and water retention.

Beer Drinker's Potomania

Beer drinkers' potomania results from the ingestion of large amounts of beer. Binge beer drinkers with poor dietary intake is the classic profile of the patient who is prone to develop beer drinkers' potomania. In contrast to SIADH, these patients present with urine that is dilute. In addition, their hyponatremia responds readily to the administration of isotonic saline.

References

Adrogue HJ and Madias NE, "Hyponatremia," *N Engl J Med*, 2000, 342(21):1581-9 (review).

Al-Salman J, Kemp D, and Randall D, "Hyponatremia,"*West J Med*, 2002, 176(3):173-6.

Fall PJ, "Hyponatremia and Hypernatremia. A Systematic Approach to Causes and Their Correction," *Postgrad Med*, 2000, 107(5):75-82; quiz 179 (review).

Greenberg A, "Diuretic Complications," *Am J Med Sci*, 2000, 319(1):10-24 (review).

Harrigan MR, "Cerebral Salt Wasting Syndrome," *Crit Care Clin*, 2001, 17(1):125-38.

Kugler JP and Hustead T, "Hyponatremia and Hypernatremia in the Elderly," *Am Fam Physician*, 2000, 61(12):3623-30.

Kumar S and Berl T, "Sodium," *Lancet*, 1998, 352(9123):220-8.

Milionis HJ, Liamis GL, and Elisaf MS, "The Hyponatremic Patient: A Systematic Approach to Laboratory Diagnosis,"*CMAJ*, 2002, 166(8):1056-62.

Miller M, "Syndromes of Excess Antidiuretic Hormone Release," *Crit Care Clin*, 2001, 17(1):11-23, v.

Oh MS, "Pathogenesis and Diagnosis of Hyponatremia,"*Nephron*, 2002, 92(Suppl 1):2-8.

Oiso Y, "Hyponatremia: How to Approach This Confusing Abnormality,"*Intern Med*, 1998, 37(11):907-8 (review).

Smith DM, McKenna K, and Thompson CJ, "Hyponatraemia," *Clin Endocrinol (Oxf)*, 2000, 52(6):667-78.

Spital A, "Diuretic-Induced Hyponatremia," *Am J Nephrol*, 1999, 19(4):447-52 (review).

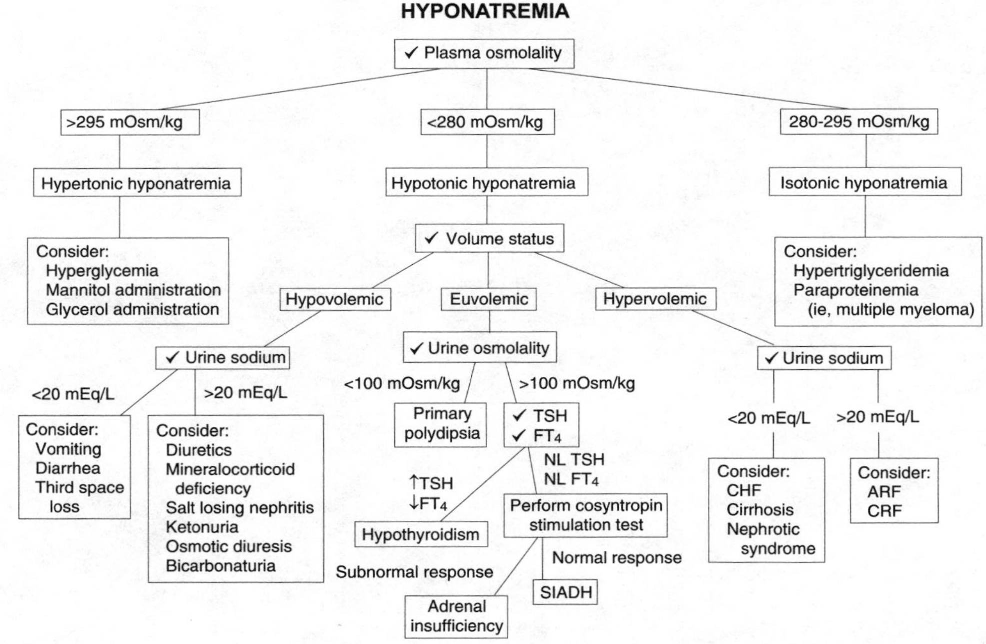
HYPONATREMIA
✓ Plasma osmolality
>295 mOsm/kg
<280 mOsm/kg
280-295 mOsm/kg
Hypertonic hyponatremia
Hypotonic hyponatremia
Isotonic hyponatremia
Consider: Hyperglycemia Mannitol administration Glycerol administration
✓ Volume status
Consider: Hypertriglyceridemia Paraproteinemia (ie, multiple myeloma)
Hypovolemic
Euvolemic
Hypervolemic
✓ Urine sodium
<20 mEq/L
>20 mEq/L
Consider: Vomiting Diarrhea Third space loss
Consider: Diuretics Mineralocorticoid deficiency Salt losing nephritis Ketonuria Osmotic diuresis Bicarbonaturia
✓ Urine osmolality
<100 mOsm/kg
>100 mOsm/kg
Primary polydipsia
✓ TSH ✓ FT_4
↑TSH ↓FT_4
Hypothyroidism
NL TSH NL FT_4
Perform cosyntropin stimulation test
Subnormal response
Normal response
Adrenal insufficiency
SIADH
✓ Urine sodium
<20 mEq/L
>20 mEq/L
Consider: CHF Cirrhosis Nephrotic syndrome
Consider: ARF CRF

HYPERNATREMIA

STEP 1 – *What Are the Causes of Hypernatremia?*

The normal serum or plasma sodium concentration is 136-145 mmol/L. Hypernatremia is defined as a rise in sodium concentration to a level >145 mmol/L.

Hypernatremia results whenever there is a deficit of water relative to sodium in the body. Hypernatremia can only result if there is net water loss or hypertonic sodium gain. In the great majority of cases, hypernatremia occurs because of free water loss. In hospitalized patients, the prevalence of hypernatremia is between 0.5% and 2%.

The causes of hypernatremia are listed in the following box.

CAUSES OF HYPERNATREMIA

HYPOVOLEMIC HYPERNATREMIA

Extrarenal losses	Renal losses
Skin losses (burns, increased sweating secondary to fever, increased sweating from exercise, increased sweating from exposure to high temperatures)	Chronic renal insufficiency
Gastrointestinal losses (diarrhea, vomiting, nasogastric tube drainage, enterocutaneous fistula)	Diuretics (usually loop)
	Osmotic diuresis (glucose, urea, mannitol)
	Polyuric phase of acute tubular necrosis
	Postobstructive diuresis

EUVOLEMIC HYPERNATREMIA

Diabetes insipidus	Hypodipsia
Central (neurogenic)	Unreplaced insensible losses (dermal and respiratory)
Nephrogenic	

HYPERVOLEMIC HYPERNATREMIA

Hypertonic sodium bicarbonate infusion	Hypertonic sodium chloride infusion
Hypertonic feeding preparation	Hypertonic dialysis
Ingestion of sea water	Hypertonic saline enemas
Sodium chloride-rich emetics	Cushing's syndrome
Ingestion of sodium chloride	Primary hyperaldosteronism

Proceed to Step 2.

STEP 2 – *What Is the Volume Status of the Patient?*

The first step in elucidating the etiology of hypernatremia is an assessment of the patient's volume status. Based on the history and physical examination, patients can be divided into the following categories:

- Hypovolemic hypernatremia
- Hypervolemic hypernatremia
- Euvolemic hypernatremia

Findings on the physical exam that help differentiate between the three types of hypernatremia are listed in the following table.

Physical Exam Findings Used to Assess Volume Status

Findings in the Physical Exam	Volume Status
Orthostatic changes in blood pressure and heart rate and/or blood pressure Dry mucous membranes Poor skin turgor Flat jugular veins Absence of axillary sweat	Hypovolemic
Peripheral edema Elevated jugular venous pressure	Hypervolemic
No findings consistent with hypervolemic or hypovolemic hypernatremia	Euvolemic

If the patient has hypovolemic hypernatremia, ***proceed to Step 3***.

If the patient has hypervolemic hypernatremia, ***proceed to Step 4***.

If the patient has euvolemic hypernatremia, ***proceed to Step 5***.

STEP 3 – *What Is the Approach to the Patient With Hypovolemic Hypernatremia?*

The causes of hypovolemic hypernatremia are included in the following box.

CAUSES OF HYPOVOLEMIC HYPERNATREMIA	
EXTRARENAL LOSSES	***RENAL LOSSES***
SKIN LOSSES (burns; increased sweating due to fever, exercise, or exposure to high temperatures)	CHRONIC RENAL INSUFFICIENCY
GASTROINTESTINAL LOSSES (diarrhea, vomiting, nasogastric tube drainage, enterocutaneous fistula)	DIURETICS (usually loop)
	OSMOTIC DIURESIS (glucose, mannitol, urea)
	POLYURIC PHASE OF ACUTE TUBULAR NECROSIS
	POSTOBSTRUCTIVE DIURESIS

The etiology of hypernatremia is usually apparent after a thorough history and physical examination. If necessary, a urine sodium level may be helpful in separating a renal disorder from an extrarenal disorder. Urine sodium concentration >20 mEq/L is consistent with renal causation. When the urine sodium level is <20 mEq/L, consideration should be given to extrarenal etiologies. The urine osmolality may also provide some important information. In extrarenal conditions, urine osmolality will be >800 mOsm/kg as the kidney produces a maximally concentrated urine. In renal disorders, the urine is less than maximally concentrated.

End of Section.

STEP 4 – *What Are the Causes of Hypervolemic Hypernatremia?*

Hypervolemic hypernatremia, the least common type of hypernatremia, is likely to be present when the physical examination provides evidence of volume overload. The causes of hypervolemic hypernatremia are listed in the following box.

CAUSES OF HYPERVOLEMIC HYPERNATREMIA	
HYPERTONIC SODIUM BICARBONATE INFUSION	HYPERTONIC SODIUM CHLORIDE INFUSION
HYPERTONIC FEEDING PREPARATION	HYPERTONIC DIALYSIS
INGESTION OF SEA WATER	HYPERTONIC SALINE ENEMAS
SODIUM CHLORIDE-RICH EMETICS	CUSHING'S SYNDROME
INGESTION OF SODIUM CHLORIDE	PRIMARY HYPERALDOSTERONISM

Although hypervolemic hypernatremia can occur with the accidental intake of large amounts of sodium salts, it more commonly occurs as an iatrogenic phenomenon. The etiology is usually apparent, with urine sodium levels typically exceeding 20 mEq/L.

End of Section.

STEP 5 – *What Is the Approach to the Patient With Euvolemic Hypernatremia?*

The causes of euvolemic hypernatremia are listed in the following box.

CAUSES OF EUVOLEMIC HYPERNATREMIA	
DIABETES INSIPIDUS Central (neurogenic) Nephrogenic	HYPODIPSIA UNREPLACED INSENSIBLE LOSSES (dermal and respiratory)

The first step in elucidating the etiology of euvolemic hypernatremia involves the measurement of urine osmolality. If the urine osmolality is >700 mOsm/kg, then the patient has unreplaced insensible losses as the etiology for hypernatremia. If the urine osmolality is <700 mOsm/kg, the diagnosis of diabetes insipidus should be considered. The reminder of this step will focus exclusively on diabetes insipidus.

Diabetes Insipidus

In central diabetes insipidus, there is a defect in the secretion of ADH. In nephrogenic diabetes insipidus, the secretion of ADH remains intact but there is a defect in its action at the level of the kidney. The causes of central diabetes insipidus are listed in the following box.

CAUSES OF CENTRAL (NEUROGENIC) DIABETES INSIPIDUS	
GRANULOMATOUS DISEASE	POST-TRAUMATIC
Histiocytosis	CYSTS
Sarcoidosis	CEREBROVASCULAR DISEASE
Wegener's granulomatosis	Hypoxic or ischemic encephalopathy
Tuberculosis	(cardiopulmonary arrest, shock,
IDIOPATHIC*	Sheehan's syndrome)
INFECTION	Aneurysm
Encephalitis	Cerebrovascular accident
Meningitis	Cavernous sinus thrombosis
Syphilis	MALIGNANCY
Tuberculosis	Craniopharyngioma
Toxoplasmosis	Leukemia
MISCELLANEOUS	Metastatic cancer (breast, lung)
Anorexia nervosa	Lymphoma
Guillan-Barré syndrome	Pinealoma
PITUITARY SURGERY	Pituitary tumor

*Idiopathic diabetes insipidus accounts for approximately ~30% of all cases of central diabetes insipidus. On occasion, the idiopathic form is familial, exhibiting autosomal dominant inheritance.

The causes of nephrogenic diabetes insipidus are listed in the following box.

CAUSES OF NEPHROGENIC DIABETES INSIPIDUS		
CONGENITAL*		
ACQUIRED		
Medications		
Amphotericin B	Foscarnet	Ethacrynic acid
Demeclocycline	Ifosfamide	Phenytoin
Lithium†	Propoxyphene (overdose)	Acetohexamide
Methoxyflurane	Colchicine	Tolazamide
Streptozotocin	Gentamicin	Glyburide
Vasopressin	Methicillin	Norepinephrine
V_2-receptor antagonist	Furosemide	Vinblastine
Electrolyte disorders		
Hypercalcemia‡	Hypokalemia§	
Renal disease		
Obstructive uropathy	Sickle cell nephropathy	Sarcoidosis
Medullary cystic disease	Analgesic nephropathy	Polycystic kidney disease
Sjögren's syndrome	Systemic lupus erythematosus	Multiple myeloma
Amyloidosis		

*Congenital nephrogenic diabetes insipidus is rare. Cases with autosomal recessive and X-linked recessive inheritance have been described.

†Lithium therapy is a major cause of nephrogenic diabetes insipidus, occurring in up to 20% of patients. It can occur as early as 8-12 weeks after the institution of therapy but is usually reversible with discontinuation of the medication. However, in some cases, the defect in ADH action may be permanent, particularly when patients have been receiving lithium therapy over a prolonged period of time.

‡Hypercalcemia is a well known cause of nephrogenic diabetes insipidus. It is usually reversible, with resolution of the diabetes insipidus occurring within 1-2 weeks after correction of the serum calcium level. Mild degrees of hypercalcemia (<11 mg/dL) are not usually associated with nephrogenic diabetes insipidus.

§Hypokalemia usually does not cause nephrogenic diabetes insipidus unless significant potassium depletion is present (serum potassium <3 mEq/L).

Polyuria and polydipsia are the major clinical manifestations of both central and nephrogenic diabetes insipidus. Polyuria results from the fall in renal water reabsorption occurring because of failure in the secretion or action of ADH. It is important to realize that most of these patients maintain water balance with a normal or near-normal plasma sodium concentration. This is true so long as the thirst mechanism is intact. If the thirst mechanism or mental status is impaired or if the patient does not have adequate access to water, then hypernatremia will ensue. Distinguishing central from nephrogenic diabetes insipidus requires performance of a water deprivation test. Details regarding performance and interpretation of the water deprivation test are included in the following table.

Water Deprivation Test

Test procedure: Water intake is restricted until the patient loses 3% to 5% body weight or until three consecutive hourly determinations of urinary osmolality are within 10% of each other. (Caution must be exercised to ensure that the patient does not become excessively dehydrated.) Aqueous vasopressin (5U subcutaneously) is given and urinary osmolality is measured after 60 minutes. Expected responses follow.

Condition	Urine osmolality with water deprivation (mOsm/kg H_2O)	Plasma vasopressin after dehydration (ng/L)	Increase in urinary osmolality with exogenous vasopressin
Normal	>800	>2	Little or no increase
Complete central diabetes insipidus	<300	Undetectable	Substantially increased
Partial central diabetes insipidus	300-800	<1.5	Increase >10% of urinary osmolality after water deprivation
Nephrogenic diabetes insipidus	<300-500	>5	Little or no increase
Primary polydipsia	>500	<5	Little or no increase

Adapted from Johnson R, *Comprehensive Clinical Nephrology*, Philadelphia, PA: Mosby, Inc, 2000, 3.9.16.

References

Adrogue HJ and Madias NE, "Hypernatremia," *N Engl J Med*, 2000, 342(20):1493-9.

Andreoli TE, "Water: Normal Balance, Hyponatremia, and Hypernatremia," *Ren Fail*, 2000, 22(6):711-35.

Fall PJ, "Hyponatremia and Hypernatremia. A Systematic Approach to Causes and Their Correction," *Postgrad Med*, 2000, 107(5):75-82.

Kang S, Kim W, and Oh MS, "Pathogenesis and Treatment of Hypernatremia," *Nephron*, 2002, 92(Suppl 1):14-7.

Kugler JP and Hustead T, "Hyponatremia and Hypernatremia in the Elderly," *Am Fam Physician*, 2000, 61(12):3623-30.

Kumar S and Berl T, "Sodium," *Lancet*, 1998, 352(9123):220-8.

Palevsky PM, "Hypernatremia," *Semin Nephrol*, 1998, 18(1):20-30.

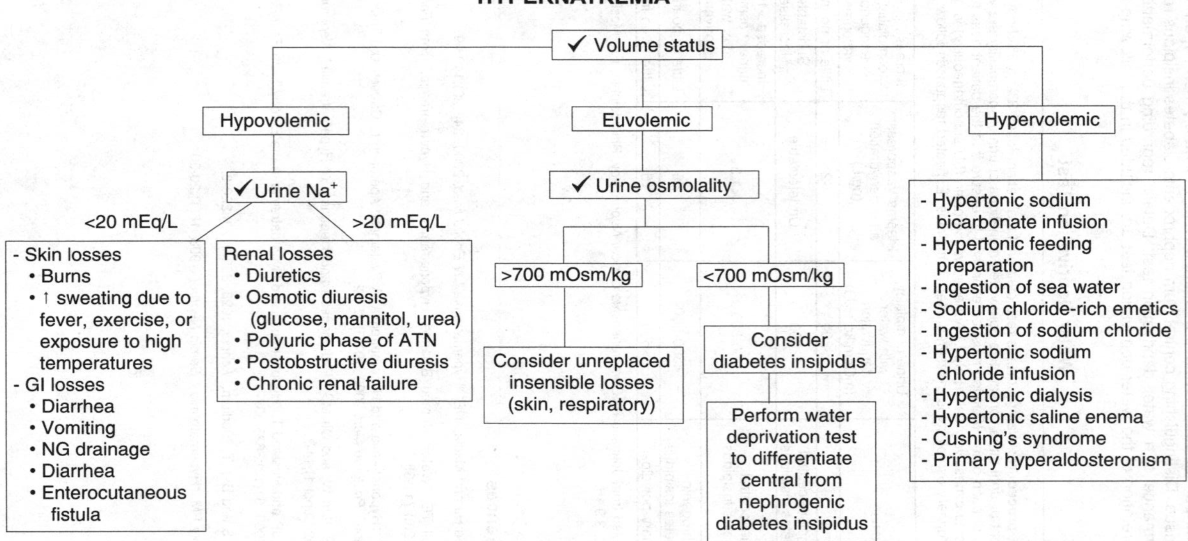
HYPERNATREMIA
✔ Volume status
Hypovolemic
Euvolemic
Hypervolemic
✔ Urine Na+
<20 mEq/L
>20 mEq/L
- Skin losses
• Burns
• ↑ sweating due to fever, exercise, or exposure to high temperatures
- GI losses
• Diarrhea
• Vomiting
• NG drainage
• Diarrhea
• Enterocutaneous fistula
Renal losses
• Diuretics
• Osmotic diuresis (glucose, mannitol, urea)
• Polyuric phase of ATN
• Postobstructive diuresis
• Chronic renal failure
✔ Urine osmolality
>700 mOsm/kg
<700 mOsm/kg
Consider unreplaced insensible losses (skin, respiratory)
Consider diabetes insipidus
Perform water deprivation test to differentiate central from nephrogenic diabetes insipidus
- Hypertonic sodium bicarbonate infusion
- Hypertonic feeding preparation
- Ingestion of sea water
- Sodium chloride-rich emetics
- Ingestion of sodium chloride
- Hypertonic sodium chloride infusion
- Hypertonic dialysis
- Hypertonic saline enema
- Cushing's syndrome
- Primary hyperaldosteronism

HYPOKALEMIA

STEP 1 – *What Are the Causes of Hypokalemia?*

Hypokalemia is said to be present when the potassium concentration falls to <3.5 mmol/L. It is one of the most common electrolyte disorders, occurring in >20% of hospitalized patients. Although most of these patients have potassium levels between 3.0-3.5 mmol/L, approximately 25% have a potassium concentration <3.0 mmol/L. The causes of hypokalemia are listed in the following box.

CAUSES OF HYPOKALEMIA

- PSEUDOHYPOKALEMIA
- DECREASED POTASSIUM INTAKE
- REDISTRIBUTION
  - Alkalemia
  - Insulin administration
  - β_2-adrenergic agonist
  - Anabolic states
    - Therapy of pernicious anemia
    - Growth factor therapy
    - Rapidly growing leukemias / lymphomas
    - Response to total parenteral nutrition
    - Refeeding syndrome
  - Hypokalemic periodic paralysis
  - Theophylline overdose
  - Barium salt poisoning
  - Increased endogenous catecholamine release
    - Myocardial infarction
    - Delirium tremens
    - Head trauma
    - Cardiac surgery
    - Other stressful illnesses
  - Hypothermia
  - Multiple transfusions of frozen, washed RBCs
  - Acute chloroquine intoxication
- EXCESS POTASSIUM LOSS
  - Gastrointestinal – vomiting, diarrhea, fistula
  - Skin
    - Excessive exercise in hot climates
    - Burns (extensive)
  - Renal – associated with hypertension
    - Malignant hypertension
    - Renin-secreting tumor
    - Renovascular hypertension
    - Glucocorticoid suppressible aldosteronism
    - Primary hyperaldosteronism
    - Congenital adrenal hyperplasia
    - Cushing's syndrome
    - 11-β-hydroxysteroid dehydrogenase inhibition
    - Syndrome of apparent mineralocorticoid excess
    - Liddle's syndrome
    - Diuretic therapy

(continued)

CAUSES OF HYPOKALEMIA *(continued)*
Renal – not associated with hypertension
Renal tubular acidosis
Proximal (type II)
Distal (type I)
Diuretic therapy
Bartter's syndrome
Gitelman's syndrome
Vomiting / nasogastric drainage
Antibiotic use
Penicillin
Amphotericin B
Aminoglycosides
Hypomagnesemia
Lysozymuria

Proceed to Step 2.

STEP 2 – *Does the Patient Have Pseudohypokalemia?*

Before embarking on a workup for hypokalemia, it is essential to exclude pseudohypokalemia. Pseudohypokalemia has been well described in acute myelogenous leukemia with markedly elevated white blood cell counts (>50,000-100,000 cells/mm^3). In this condition, the malignant cells, which continue to remain metabolically active after the blood is drawn, take up the extracellular potassium if the blood is stored for a prolonged period of time at room temperature. The low potassium concentration that is seen in pseudohypokalemia does not reflect true potassium depletion and is merely an artifact of the storage procedure.

Pseudohypokalemia can be avoided if the serum or plasma is expeditiously separated from the cells or if the specimen is stored at 4°C. It should be noted, however, that true hypokalemia can occur in acute myelogenous leukemia. The mechanism of the true hypokalemia is thought to be increased urinary loss of potassium due to lysozymuria (see Step 10 *on page 222*).

If pseudohypokalemia is the cause of the low potassium level, ***stop here.***

If pseudohypokalemia is not present, ***proceed to Step 3.***

STEP 3 – *Is the Hypokalemia Secondary to Decreased Potassium Intake?*

Decreased potassium intake is a rare cause of potassium deficiency because potassium is widely available in many foods. In addition, the kidneys can adapt to decreased potassium intake by conservation of potassium. If intake is severely limited, however, hypokalemia can occur. More commonly, diminished intake is a contributing factor in the development of hypokalemia, often exacerbating hypokalemia due to other causes.

Causes of hypokalemia secondary to decreased intake include:

- Anorexia nervosa / bulimia
- Starvation (tea and toast diet)
- Prolonged fasting

Another condition, known as geophagia, deserves mention here. Geophagia, most commonly seen in African-American women living in the Southeast, refers to the chronic ingestion of clay. The ingested clay binds dietary potassium and impairs its absorption, resulting in hypokalemia. The clay can also bind dietary iron leading to the development of iron deficiency anemia. The combination of hypokalemia and iron deficiency anemia should, at least, prompt consideration of geophagia as the etiology of the hypokalemia. It is important to realize, however, that not all types of clay ingestion will lead to hypokalemia. Red clay, for example, contains large amounts of potassium. As such, hypokalemia is not likely to occur with the ingestion of red clay. In fact, hyperkalemia has been noted in patients ingesting red clay, particularly in those who have advanced renal failure.

If the patient has hypokalemia secondary to decreased intake, ***stop here***.

If decreased intake of potassium is likely to be contributing to the hypokalemia but is not the sole cause of the hypokalemia, ***proceed to Step 4***.

If the patient does not have hypokalemia secondary to decreased intake, ***proceed to Step 4***.

STEP 4 – *Is the Hypokalemia Secondary to Redistribution of Potassium?*

Hypokalemia may result from redistribution, that is, the movement of potassium from the extracellular fluid to the intracellular fluid as in the following situations.

- Alkalemia (primarily metabolic)

  It is useful to remember that plasma potassium falls 0.4 mEq/L for every 0.1 increase in pH. As such, the hypokalemia that accompanies metabolic alkalosis is typically mild. It should be noted, however, that some conditions associated with alkalosis may cause hypokalemia not only because of the alkalosis, but because of increased urinary potassium loss (ie, primary hyperaldosteronism, diuretic therapy). In these conditions, the hypokalemia may be more marked.

- Insulin therapy

  In patients with diabetic ketoacidosis, potassium levels fall after the administration of insulin. Initially, patients with diabetic ketoacidosis or markedly elevated blood glucose may present with normal or even high potassium levels. This is a reflection of the insulin deficiency and hyperosmolality that is present, leading to the movement of potassium into the extracellular fluid. In these patients, the potassium depletion that is present will become more apparent with the administration of insulin.

  A similar decline in potassium concentration may be noted after intravenous dextrose is administered to the nondiabetic patient (secondary to endogenous insulin release). For example, intravenous potassium chloride may be given in a dextrose solution to correct hypokalemia. The dextrose that is given may stimulate endogenous insulin release, leading to a further fall in the potassium concentration (usually transient).

- β_2-adrenergic agonist

  β_2-agonists increase the uptake of potassium into cells. This effect can be appreciated in the asthmatic patient receiving nebulized β-agonists. Potassium may decline 0.3-1.5 mEq/L if particularly large doses are used. This effect lasts for about 1 hour. This may also be appreciated in patients given terbutaline to abort premature labor. Treatment with dobutamine, dopamine, pseudoephedrine, or ritodrine may also result in hypokalemia due to increased uptake of potassium into cells. Significant hypokalemia has been reported to occur in patients who take large amounts of cough medication that contains pseudoephedrine, ephedrine, chlorpheniramines, and promethazine.

- Anabolic states

  In these states, there is rapid growth leading to uptake of potassium into the cell at a rate that exceeds ingestion. Examples of this include:

  - Therapy for pernicious anemia

    Hypokalemia is frequently encountered during treatment of pernicious anemia. It tends to be most pronounced during the first 48 hours of therapy, with levels, at times, falling to <3 mEq/L.

  - Growth factor therapy

    The administration of GM-CSF to correct neutropenia has been complicated with hypokalemia, which can be profound (potassium levels <2 mEq/L).

  - Rapidly growing leukemias/lymphomas
  - Response to total parenteral nutrition
  - Refeeding syndrome – when a patient suffering from prolonged starvation is suddenly fed, insulin is secreted causing potassium to shift into the cell

- Hypokalemic periodic paralysis

  Hypokalemic periodic paralysis is a rare condition characterized by episodes of muscle weakness or paralysis. If the respiratory muscles are involved, the condition can be fatal. Two forms of hypokalemic periodic paralysis have been described. One form develops between the ages of 10 and 20 and is inherited in an autosomal dominant fashion. The acquired form has a predilection for Asians (particularly Chinese males), manifesting between the ages of 30 and 40, and is associated with thyrotoxicosis. Typically, patients have attacks of muscle weakness precipitated by rest after vigorous exercise, alcohol, stress, carbohydrate-rich meals, or insulin administration. There is a rapid movement of potassium into the intracellular fluid with a corresponding decrease in the potassium concentration to levels as low as 1.5-2.5 mEq/L. Not uncommonly, the hypokalemia is accompanied by other electrolyte abnormalities, such as hypomagnesemia and hypophosphatemia. Left untreated, the muscle weakness abates after 6-48 hours as potassium shifts back into the extracellular fluid.

- Theophylline overdose

  Hypokalemia occurs in most patients with acute theophylline intoxication.

- Barium salt poisoning

  The egress of potassium from cells is blocked by barium which may lead to profound hypokalemia. Patients are not at risk with radiologic procedures because the barium used is not absorbed into the circulation. Barium salt poisoning also leads to vomiting and diarrhea, two other contributing factors to the hypokalemia seen in these patients.

- Increased endogenous catecholamine release

  Conditions such as myocardial infarction, delirium tremens, head trauma, cardiac surgery, hypoglycemia, postcardiopulmonary resuscitation, and other stressful illnesses can lead to an outpouring of endogenous catecholamines. These catecholamines can then cause a shift of potassium into cells.

- Multiple transfusion with frozen, washed red blood cells

  Hypokalemia, with potassium levels <3 mEq/L, may also occur after the administration of multiple transfusions with frozen, washed red blood cells. During the storage of these red blood cells, up to 50% of the intracellular potassium may be lost. When transfused, extracellular potassium in the recipient moves quickly into the cells to replace that which was lost during storage. This does not occur when red blood cells are stored in acid-citrate-dextran solution.

- Hypothermia

  Potassium levels <3 mEq/L have been reported in patients presenting with hypothermia. The potassium level rapidly corrects with rewarming. The clinician should be vigilant for overshoot hyperkalemia, especially in cases where potassium was given to correct the hypokalemia.

- Acute chloroquine intoxication

  Hypokalemia, sometimes profound (<2 mEq/L), is common with acute chloroquine intoxication.

If the patient has hypokalemia secondary to redistribution, ***stop here***.

If the patient does not have hypokalemia secondary to redistribution, ***proceed to Step 5***.

STEP 5 – *Is the Hypokalemia Secondary to Excess Potassium Loss?*

Increased losses of potassium may be appreciated in both renal and nonrenal conditions. Nonrenal conditions leading to hypokalemia include the following.

- Gastrointestinal losses

  Vomiting – In patients with vomiting, hypokalemia may be marked. Most potassium loss occurs at the level of the kidney. Potassium in gastric fluid is too low in concentration to account for the degree of deficiency seen with vomiting. Bicarbonaturia occurs with vomiting because of developing alkalosis. In combination with hyperaldosteronism due to volume depletion, this leads to kaliuresis.

  Diarrhea – Diarrhea can lead to gastrointestinal loss of potassium as well. In particular, secretory diarrheas (eg, villous adenoma) can lead to a profound loss. Secondary hyperaldosteronism that occurs in diarrheal states exacerbates hypokalemia by increasing colonic potassium secretion.

  Surreptitious use of laxatives should be considered in hypokalemic patients, particularly women, who seem overly concerned about abdominal symptoms. A positive urine or stool phenolphthalein test supports this diagnosis. With anthracene laxatives (senna, cascara, aloe), melanosis coli may develop that can be detected on sigmoidoscopic exam. Magnesium or phosphate-containing cathartics can be detected by direct measurement of these compounds in the stool.

- Skin

  Excessive sweating does not usually lead to hypokalemia since low concentrations of potassium are present in sweat fluid (5-10 mEq/L). In individuals exercising in hot climates, however, production of sweat fluid can be in excess of 10 liters. In these situations, significant amounts of potassium may be lost if intake is not increased.

  Skin losses of potassium may may also be appreciated in patients who have sustained extensive burns.

If nonrenal conditions are not apparent, the patient most likely has a renal etiology for potassium deficiency. If there is uncertainty, a 24-hour urine collection for potassium can be performed. If the potassium excreted over the 24-hour time period exceeds 25-30 mEq, then the patient should be evaluated for a renal loss of potassium. If the value obtained is less than 25-30 mEq, then nonrenal etiologies should be considered. Instead of performing the 24-hour urine collection for potassium, the clinician may wish to obtain a random urine specimen for measurement of the potassium concentration.

Measurement of the potassium concentration in a random urine specimen can also help differentiate renal from nonrenal causes of hypokalemia. However, it may be less accurate than the 24-hour urine collection. Potassium levels <15 mEq/L are consistent with a nonrenal cause. Levels higher than this usually signify a renal etiology. Of note, vomiting is the one nonrenal condition that may be characterized by a high urine potassium concentration.

Another important point to recognize is that renal potassium loss may be masked in patients who have volume depletion. This is due to a decrease in the amount of salt and water that is presented to the distal tubules/collecting ducts, the site where potassium secretion takes place. Masking of renal potassium wasting should not be a concern if the amount of sodium excreted in the urine exceeds 30-40 mEq/day. The clinician should also realize that the kidney may require up to 72 hours to fully decrease urinary potassium excretion in patients with nonrenal causes of hypokalemia.

If the patient has hypokalemia secondary to a nonrenal condition, ***stop here***.

If hypokalemia is not due to one of the conditions above, then the cause is likely renal in origin. ***Proceed to Step 6.***

STEP 6 – *What Is the Blood Pressure?*

It is helpful to consider the renal causes of hypokalemia in the context of the patient's blood pressure.

If the blood pressure is normal, ***proceed to Step 7.***
If the blood pressure is elevated, ***proceed to Step 11.***

STEP 7 – *What Is the pH?*

The renal causes of hypokalemia not associated with hypertension are listed in the following box.

RENAL CAUSES OF HYPOKALEMIA IN THE NORMOTENSIVE PATIENT	
RENAL TUBULAR ACIDOSIS	ANTIBIOTIC USE
Proximal (type II)	Penicillin
Distal (type I)	Amphotericin B
TOLUENE EXPOSURE	Aminoglycosides
DIURETIC THERAPY	HYPOMAGNESEMIA
BARTTER'S SYNDROME	CISPLATIN
GITELMAN'S SYNDROME	LYSOZYMURIA
VOMITING / NASOGASTRIC DRAINAGE	

These disorders can be further classified based on the blood pH.

If the patient is acidemic, ***proceed to Step 8.***

If the patient is alkalemic, ***proceed to Step 9.***
If the pH is normal, ***proceed to Step 10.***

STEP 8 – *What Is the Differential Diagnosis of Metabolic Acidosis and Hypokalemia in the Normotensive Patient?*

The differential diagnosis of metabolic acidosis and hypokalemia in the normotensive patient includes the following:

- Proximal (type II) renal tubular acidosis (RTA)

- Distal (type I) RTA
- Toluene exposure

These conditions are discussed in further detail in the remainder of this step.

Proximal RTA

Patients having proximal renal tubular acidosis present with a normal anion gap metabolic acidosis. This may occur with other defects of proximal tubular function in what is known as the Fanconi syndrome. The Fanconi syndrome is characterized by bicarbonaturia, uricosuria, glycosuria, aminoaciduria, and phosphaturia.

Distal RTA

In distal RTA, the kidney is not able to lower urine pH in the normal fashion. Hypokalemia accompanies a normal anion gap metabolic acidosis. A urine pH >5.5 in the presence of a normal anion gap metabolic acidosis should raise suspicion for this condition.

For more information regarding the approach to patients with renal tubular acidosis, please refer to the chapter, Approach to the Patient With a Normal Anion Gap Metabolic Acidosis *on page 299*.

Toluene Exposure

Toluene exposure, which can occur from sniffing paint or glue vapors, has also been associated with hypokalemia due to renal losses of potassium. These patients often present with metabolic acidosis.

End of Section.

STEP 9 – *What Is the Urine Chloride Level?*

The differential diagnosis of metabolic alkalosis and hypokalemia in the normotensive patient is listed in the following box.

METABOLIC ALKALOSIS AND HYPOKALEMIA IN THE NORMOTENSIVE PATIENT DIFFERENTIAL DIAGNOSIS
BARTTER'S SYNDROME
GITELMAN'S SYNDROME
DIURETICS
GI LOSS
Chloride-losing diarrhea
Nasogastric drainage
Vomiting

In many cases, the etiology is apparent from the history. If there is any uncertainty, a urine chloride level can be obtained.

A urine chloride level <10 mEq/day suggests one of the following.

- Vomiting – Often apparent from the history; however, surreptitious vomiting may be difficult to diagnose. The following findings should prompt the clinician to consider this possibility.
  - Ulcers, calluses, or scars on the dorsum of the hand
  - Dental erosions due to chronic exposure to gastric acid
  - Puffy cheeks from salivary gland hypertrophy

- Nasogastric drainage
- Chloride-losing diarrhea (villous adenoma)
- Diuretic use (remote use) – When the urine chloride concentration is determined after the diuretic's time-period of action, it may be low. Surreptitious diuretic use is a real concern, especially when another etiology is not apparent. A urinary assay for specific diuretic drugs may be necessary to confirm the diagnosis.

A urine chloride >10 mEq/day is consistent with the following.

- Bartter's syndrome – Rare condition which is characterized by growth and mental retardation, muscle weakness, muscle cramps, polyuria, and polydipsia. Usually diagnosed during childhood, the characteristic features include hypokalemia, normomagnesemia (occasional hypomagnesemia), hypercalciuria, metabolic alkalosis, decreased urinary concentration ability, and high levels of renin and aldosterone. Urinary excretion of prostaglandin E2 is also increased. These patients are not able to properly reabsorb sodium and chloride in the thick ascending limp of the loop of henle.
- Gitelman's syndrome – Rare disorder that tends to be more benign than Bartter's syndrome. Forms of Gitelman's syndrome exhibiting both autosomal recessive and dominant inheritance have been described. Like Bartter's syndrome, it may be diagnosed in childhood but, in contrast to Bartter's syndrome, the diagnosis is often established later in childhood. Not uncommonly, the diagnosis is not made until adulthood. The syndrome presents with metabolic alkalosis and hypokalemia in the setting of a normal blood pressure. Plasma renin activity and aldosterone levels are elevated. Features favoring a diagnosis of Gitelman's syndrome over Bartter's syndrome include hypomagnesemia, low urine calcium excretion, intact urinary concentrating ability, and normal urinary prostaglandin excretion.

Comparison of Bartter's Syndrome and Gitelman's Syndrome

Bartter's Syndrome	Gitelman's Syndrome
Salt wasting	Salt wasting
Hypokalemia / alkalosis	Hypokalemia / alkalosis
Childhood	Adulthood
Hypercalciuria	Hypocalciuria
Increased PRA / aldosterone	Increased PRA / aldosterone
Na / K / Cl mutation	Na / Cl mutation

- Diuretic use (recent use) – When the urine chloride concentration is determined during the diuretic's time of action, the level will be high. Most of the biochemical and hormonal findings seen in Bartter's and Gitelman's syndromes can be seen with diuretic use. Although diuretic use is apparent in most patients, some patients may be surreptitiously taking diuretic medication. It is best to entertain diagnoses of Bartter's and Gitelman's syndrome only after surreptitious diuretic use has been excluded.

End of Section.

STEP 10 – *What Is the Differential Diagnosis of Hypokalemia in the Normotensive Patient With a Normal Serum pH?*

The differential diagnosis of hypokalemia in the normotensive patient with a normal serum pH includes the following.

- Antibiotics – There are several different mechanisms by which antibiotics can lead to potassium loss. High doses of penicillin, carbenicillin, ampicillin, and oxacillin increase the delivery of nonreabsorbable anions to the distal tubule, thereby increasing urinary potassium excretion. Amphotericin B increases potassium excretion by altering permeability in distal tubular cells. It is thought that gentamicin causes hypokalemia through the depletion of magnesium.

- Cisplatin / ifosfamide therapy
- Hypomagnesemia – Hypokalemia and hypomagnesemia commonly occur together. In fact, hypomagnesemia is present in up to 40% of hypokalemic patients. In some cases, both the hypokalemia and hypomagnesemia are manifestations of the underlying disease. Examples include primary hyperaldosteronism, diuretic use, and cisplatin therapy. In other cases, the hypokalemia may be caused by the hypomagnesemia. Hypomagnesemia, due to any cause, can lead to hypokalemia by increasing potassium loss in stool and urine. Treatment of the hypokalemia can be difficult in the setting of hypomagnesemia. For this reason, magnesium replacement should precede potassium replacement. When administering magnesium in patients with both hypokalemia and hypomagnesemia, it is preferable to treat with magnesium chloride or lactate rather than magnesium sulfate. This is because treatment with magnesium sulfate may initially increase urinary potassium loss because sulfate can act as a nonreabsorbable anion.
- Acute myelocytic or myelomonocytic leukemia – Severe renal potassium wasting has been described in several types of leukemia. The mechanism of the hypokalemia is not quite clear, but has been attributed to lysozymuria.

End of Section.

STEP 11 – *What Is the Differential Diagnosis of Hypokalemia in the Hypertensive Patient?*

The differential diagnosis of hypokalemia in the hypertensive patient is listed in the following box.

HYPOKALEMIA AND HYPERTENSION DIFFERENTIAL DIAGNOSIS
MALIGNANT HYPERTENSION
RENIN-SECRETING TUMORS
RENOVASCULAR HYPERTENSION
GLUCOCORTICOID SUPPRESSIBLE ALDOSTERONISM
PRIMARY HYPERALDOSTERONISM
CONGENITAL ADRENAL HYPERPLASIA
CUSHING'S SYNDROME
11-β-HYDROXYSTEROID DEHYDROGENASE INHIBITION
LIDDLE'S SYNDROME
DIURETIC THERAPY
SYNDROME OF APPARENT MINERALOCORTICOID EXCESS

Proceed to Step 12.

STEP 12 – *Is the Patient on a Diuretic?*

Hypokalemia is a commonly encountered electrolyte abnormality in patients receiving diuretic therapy. It has been reported with thiazide and loop diuretics as well as carbonic anhydrase inhibitors. Studies have shown that the incidence of hypokalemia in patients receiving hydrochlorothiazide increases with higher doses of the medication. In patients receiving 50 mg of hydrochlorothiazide per day, the average fall in the potassium level is about 0.5 mEq/L. With the increasing realization that low doses of hydrochlorothiazide (12.5 mg) produce a similar blood pressure lowering effect as high doses (50 mg), hydrochlorothiazide-induced hypokalemia may become less of a problem.

There is no doubt that the combination of hypertension and hypokalemia is most often due to diuretic therapy. However, this combination should also prompt consideration of other conditions, particularly secondary causes of hypertension (see box in Step 11) such as primary hyperaldosteronism and renal artery stenosis. It can be difficult to determine if hypokalemia in the hypertensive patient is a complication of diuretic therapy or a reflection of an underlying problem associated with hypertension and hypokalemia such as primary hyperaldosteronism. The evaluation of the potassium level after discontinuation of the diuretic medication can be quite helpful in these cases.

If the patient is on a diuretic, remove the diuretic. ***Proceed to Step 13.***

If the patient is not on a diuretic, ***proceed to Step 14.***

STEP 13 – *Is the Patient Still Hypokalemic Despite Discontinuing the Diuretic?*

Persistence of hypokalemia after withdrawal of the diuretic medication raises concern for one of the conditions associated with hypertension and hypokalemia (see box in Step 11).

Normalization of the potassium level after discontinuation of the diuretic medication supports diuretic-induced hypokalemia. It is important to realize, however, that there is a subset of patients with primary hyperaldosteronism who present with normokalemia. The potassium level in these patients is usually between 3.5 and 4 mmol/L.

Most patients with normalization of the potassium level after withdrawal of the diuretic medication do not have primary hyperaldosteronism. Therefore, it is not cost-effective to test all of these patients for this condition. In those who have features of secondary hypertension (difficult to control hypertension, hypertension requiring multiple medications for control of blood pressure, etc), however, it is reasonable to perform testing for primary hyperaldosteronism. This testing is best done with the patient off of diuretic therapy.

If the patient is no longer hypokalemic and suspicion for primary hyperaldosteronism is low, then the hypokalemia was due to the diuretic. ***Stop here.***

If the patient is no longer hypokalemic, but suspicion for primary aldosteronism is present, then ***proceed to Step 14.***

If the patient remains hypokalemic despite discontinuation of the diuretic, ***proceed to Step 14.***

STEP 14 – *What Are the Results of the Plasma Renin Activity and Plasma Aldosterone Measurements?*

When diuretic therapy is not thought to be the cause of the hypokalemia in the hypertensive patient, the next step involves measurement of the plasma renin activity and aldosterone. These patients may be divided into one of the following groups based upon the results of these laboratory tests, as shown in the following table.

Lab Test Finding	Condition Suggested	Proceed to...
Elevated PRA Elevated aldosterone Aldosterone:PRA ratio <10	Renovascular hypertension Renin-secreting tumor Malignant hypertension Diuretic therapy	Step 15
Decreased PRA Decreased aldosterone	Exogenous mineralocorticoid therapy Congenital adrenal hyperplasia Liddle's syndrome 11-β-hydroxysteroid dehydrogenase inhibition Syndrome of apparent mineralocorticoid excess	Step 16
Normal PRA Normal aldosterone	Consider Cushing's syndrome	Step 17
Decreased PRA Elevated aldosterone Aldosterone:PRA ratio >20	Primary hyperaldosteronism Glucocorticoid-suppressible aldosteronism	Step 18

STEP 15 – *What Are the Causes of an Elevated PRA and Aldosterone in the Hypertensive Patient With Hypokalemia?*

The causes of an elevated PRA and aldosterone in the hypertensive patient with hypokalemia are listed in the following box.

CAUSES OF ELEVATED PRA AND ALDOSTERONE IN THE HYPOKALEMIC PATIENT WITH HYPERTENSION

MALIGNANT HYPERTENSION
RENOVASCULAR HYPERTENSION
RENIN-SECRETING TUMORS
DIURETIC THERAPY

These conditions will be discussed in further detail in the remainder of this step.

Malignant Hypertension

Malignant hypertension is defined as an elevated blood pressure in association with grade 3 and 4 retinopathy. The complications of malignant hypertension include renal damage, retinopathy, cardiac ischemia or infarction, hypertensive heart failure, or other hypertensive emergencies.

Renal abnormalities of malignant hypertension include a fairly rapid increase in creatinine, hematuria, proteinuria, as well as red and white blood cell casts in the urinary sediment. Because of activation of the renin system, there may be hypokalemic metabolic alkalosis early in the course. In fact, 50% of patients with malignant hypertension are hypokalemic. As renal insufficiency worsens, metabolic acidosis and hyperkalemia may ensue. A peripheral blood smear will reveal schistocytes consistent with a microangiopathic hemolytic anemia.

Renovascular Hypertension (Renal Artery Stenosis)

Approximately 80% of cases of renovascular hypertension are due to atherosclerosis. Of the remaining cases, nearly 15% are due to fibromuscular dysplasia. Patients with atherosclerotic renal artery stenosis tend to be older individuals, who have evidence of atherosclerotic disease elsewhere (carotid, coronary, peripheral vascular disease). Most are heavy cigarette smokers.

Although atherosclerotic renal artery stenosis has a predilection for whites, African-Americans can also develop renovascular hypertension. In contrast to atherosclerotic renal artery stenosis, fibromuscular dysplasia tends to affect young white women.

The clinical characteristics associated with renovascular hypertension are listed in the following box.

CLINICAL CHARACTERISTICS ASSOCIATED WITH RENOVASCULAR HYPERTENSION
MALIGNANT OR ACCELERATED HYPERTENSION
ABDOMINAL OR FLANK BRUIT
PROGRESSION IN THE SEVERITY OF CHRONIC HYPERTENSION
ONSET EARLY (AGE <25 YEARS) OR LATE (>60 YEARS)
HYPOTENSION OR RENAL FAILURE WITH ACE INHIBITOR
SEVERE OR DIFFICULT TO CONTROL HYPERTENSION
RECENT ONSET OF HYPERTENSION
MODERATE HYPERTENSION AND DIFFUSE VASCULAR DISEASE
NEW ONSET OF HYPERTENSION FOLLOWING RENAL TRANSPLANTATION

Adapted from *Primer on Kidney Diseases,* 2nd ed, Greenberg A, ed, San Diego, CA: Academic Press, 1998, 502.

A number of radiologic tests are available for the evaluation of renovascular hypertension. The sensitivity and specificity of these tests are listed in the following table.

Radiologic Tests for Evaluation of Renovascular Hypertension

Diagnostic Test	Sensitivity (%)	Specificity (%)
Renal artery arteriography	99	99
Magnetic resonance angiography	97	95
Captopril renal scan	93	95
Renal artery duplex sonography	86	93
Intravenous digital subtraction angiography	88	89
Rapid sequence intravenous pyelography	74	86

Adapted from Crawford MH and DiMarco JP, *Cardiology,* St Louis: CV Mosby, 2001, 3.10.7.

Renin-Secreting Tumor

Renin-secreting tumors are very uncommon causes of hypokalemia. These tumors usually present in the third or fourth decade of life. Renal cell carcinoma, juxtaglomerular tumors, and ovarian carcinomas are the most common malignancies associated with renin secretion. Renal arteriography usually establishes the diagnosis when the renin secretion is due to a renal tumor. Even with renal arteriography, however, small renin-secreting tumors may be missed. In these difficult cases, the clinician may need to perform selective venography or renal vein renin sampling to detect the tumor. When renal arteriography is unremarkable, consideration should also be given to the possibility of an extrarenal renin-secreting tumor.

End of Section.

STEP 16 – *What Are the Causes of a Low PRA and Aldosterone in the Hypertensive Patient With Hypokalemia?*

The causes of a low PRA and aldosterone level in the hypertensive patient with hypokalemia are listed in the following box.

CAUSES OF A LOW PRA AND ALDOSTERONE LEVEL IN THE HYPOKALEMIC PATIENT WITH HYPERTENSION
11-β-HYDROXYSTEROID DEHYDROGENASE INHIBITION CONGENITAL ADRENAL HYPERPLASIA LIDDLE'S SYNDROME SYNDROME OF APPARENT MINERALOCORTICOID EXCESS EXOGENOUS MINERALOCORTICOID USE

These conditions will be discussed in further detail in the remainder of this step.

Exogenous Mineralocorticoid Use

The chronic ingestion of exogenous mineralocorticoids can lead to hypokalemia. For example, hypokalemia has been seen in patients treated with fludrocortisone, a synthetic mineralocorticoid used in the treatment of hypoaldosteronism.

11-β-Hydroxysteroid Dehydrogenase Inhibition

Under normal circumstances, cortisol is present in serum at sufficient concentrations to bind to mineralocorticoid receptors and promote sodium reabsorption and potassium secretion. However, cortisol is converted locally by the enzyme, 11-β-hydroxysteroid dehydrogenase, to metabolites such as cortisone which do not have mineralocorticoid activity.

This enzyme may be inhibited, however, by glycyrrhetinic acid, a steroid present in licorice. While small quantities of licorice are not likely to be clinically significant, the chronic ingestion of large amounts of licorice (licorice-containing chewing tobacco or gum) can impair the ability of this enzyme to convert cortisol to cortisone. The cortisol can then act as a mineralocorticoid leading to the development of hypokalemia. The competitive inhibition of 11-β-hydroxysteroid dehydrogenase has also been described in patients treated with carbenoxolone, an antiulcer agent used mainly in Europe.

Syndrome of Apparent Mineralocorticoid Excess

In this condition, there is a mutation in the 11-β-hydroxysteroid dehydrogenase gene, which results in a marked decrease in enzyme activity. This mutation allows cortisol to act as an endogenous mineralocorticoid with the subsequent development of hypokalemia.

Congenital Adrenal Hyperplasia

Two forms of congenital adrenal hyperplasia are associated with hypokalemia; 11-β-hydroxylase deficiency and 17-α-hydroxylase deficiency. The hypertension seen in these two forms of congenital adrenal hyperplasia is thought to be secondary to the accumulation of deoxycorticosterone and other steroids that possess mineralocorticoid activity. 11-β-hydroxylase deficiency is more common than 17-α-hydroxylase deficiency, occurring with a prevalence of 1/100,000. In contrast to 11-β-hydroxylase deficiency which is associated with androgen excess, patients with 17-α-hydroxylase deficiency are unable to make sex steroids.

Liddle's Syndrome

Liddle's syndrome, a rare syndrome with autosomal dominant transmittance, is thought to be the result of a mutation in the sodium channel, resulting in hyperabsorption of sodium at the level of the collecting duct. It is characterized by hypertension, hypokalemia, metabolic alkalosis, and low levels of renin and aldosterone.

End of Section.

STEP 17 – *Is Cushing's Syndrome the Cause of the Hypokalemia?*

Normal PRA and aldosterone levels in the hypertensive patient with hypokalemia should prompt consideration of Cushing's syndrome. The PRA is usually normal because the mechanism of hypertension in Cushing's syndrome is not directly related to sodium retention and volume expansion. The signs and symptoms of Cushing's syndrome are listed in the following box.

SIGNS AND SYMPTOMS OF CUSHING'S SYNDROME

CENTRAL OBESITY	SPONTANEOUS ECCHYMOSES
PROXIMAL MUSCLE WEAKNESS	FACIAL PLETHORA
HYPERTENSION	ACNE
PSYCHIATRIC DISORDERS	HYPERPIGMENTATION
WIDE PURPLE STRIAE	HIRSUTISM

Oversecretion of cortisol is thought to be the mechanism of the hypokalemia in these patients. Although cortisol normally binds to the mineralocorticoid receptor as avidly as aldosterone, it exerts little mineralocorticoid activity. This is because cortisol is converted to the inactive metabolite, cortisone, by the action of the enzyme, 11-β-hydroxysteroid dehydrogenase. In Cushing's syndrome, the marked hypersecretion of cortisol can overwhelm the ability of the enzyme to inactivate it, thereby allowing it to function as a mineralocorticoid.

The evaluation of Cushing's syndrome begins with a 24-hour urine collection for cortisol to determine if hypercortisolism is truly present. The hypokalemia of Cushing's syndrome is more commonly seen in patients with ectopic ACTH secretion. For more information, the reader is referred to the chapter, Cushing's Syndrome *on page 387*.

End of Section.

STEP 18 – *What Are the Causes of a Decreased PRA and an Elevated Aldosterone Level in the Hypertensive Patient With Hypokalemia?*

The causes of a decreased PRA but elevated aldosterone level in the hypertensive patient with hypokalemia is listed in the following box.

CAUSES OF AN ELEVATED ALDOSTERONE LEVEL BUT LOW PRA IN THE HYPOKALEMIC PATIENT WITH HYPERTENSION

PRIMARY HYPERALDOSTERONISM
GLUCOCORTICOID SUPPRESSIBLE ALDOSTERONISM

These conditions will be discussed in further detail in the remainder of this step.

Primary Hyperaldosteronism

Primary hyperaldosteronism is said to be present when there is autonomous secretion of aldosterone. Primary hyperaldosteronism was first described by Conn who reported a patient with an aldosterone-producing adrenal adenoma. This is the most common cause of primary hyperaldosteronism (65%) followed by bilateral adrenal hyperplasia. In rare cases, adrenal carcinoma has been implicated. Laboratory findings reveal mild hypernatremia and metabolic alkalosis. The diagnosis should be suspected in the patient with persistent hypokalemia in the absence of diuretic therapy. If the patient is on a diuretic, the diuretic should be stopped and the patient should be given potassium supplements. A potassium level that remains low after 1-2 weeks is concerning for hyperaldosteronism. A subset of patients with primary hyperaldosteronism, however, have normal potassium levels ranging from 3.5-4.0 mEq/L. These patients also deserve an evaluation for primary hyperaldosteronism, particularly if they have features suggestive of secondary hypertension.

The reader is referred to the Endocrine Section for further information regarding the evaluation of primary hyperaldosteronism.

Glucocorticoid Suppressible Aldosteronism

This is a condition that involves the fusion of the 11-β-hydroxylase gene promoter to the aldosterone synthase coding sequence. The gene promoter is under the influence of ACTH, and as a result, aldosterone synthase is regulated by ACTH. Remember that under normal circumstances, aldosterone secretion depends on the renin system and potassium level, but not on ACTH. It should be suspected when a positive family history is obtained (autosomal dominant inheritance) in a patient who develops hypertension before the age of 21. Treatment of this condition includes steroids to blunt ACTH levels and hence aldosterone secretion. The diagnosis can be established with genetic testing. Elevated levels of 18-hydroxycortisol and 18-oxocortisol are supportive of the diagnosis.

References

Bartholow C, Whittier FC, and Rutecki GW, "Hypokalemia and Metabolic Alkalosis: Algorithms for Combined Clinical Problem Solving," *Compr Ther*, 2000, 26(2):114-20.

Brown CA, Bouldin MJ, Blackston JW, et al, "Hyperaldosteronism: The Internist's Hypertensive Disease," *Am J Med Sci*, 2002, 324(4):227-31

Fardella CE and Mosso L, "Primary Aldosteronism," *Clin Lab*, 2002, 48(3-4)181-90.

Frey FJ, "The Hypertensive Patient With Hypokalaemia: The Search for Hyperaldosteronism," *Nephrol Dial Transplant*, 2001, 16(6):1112-6.

Gennari FJ, "Disorders of Potassium Homeostasis. Hypokalemia and Hyperkalemia," *Crit Care Clin*, 2002, 18(2):273-88, vi.

Gennari FJ, "Hypokalemia," *N Engl J Med*, 1998, 339(7):451-8.

Greenberg A, "Diuretic Complications," *Am J Med Sci*, 2000, 319(1):10-24.

Halperrin ML and Kamel KS, "Potassium," *Lancet*, 1998, 352(9122):135-40.

Mandal AK, "Hypokalemia and Hyperkalemia," *Med Clin North Am*, 1997, 81(3):611-39.

Nussberger J, "Investigating the Mineralocorticoid Hypertension," *J Hypertens Suppl*, 2003, 21(Suppl 2):S25-30.

Wheeler MH and Harris DA, "Diagnosis and management of Primary Aldosteronism," *World J Surg*, 2003, 27(6):627-31.

Young WF Jr, "Minireview: Primary Aldosteronism -Changing Concepts in Diagnosis and Treatment," *Endocrinology*, 2003, 144(6):2208-13.

HYPOKALEMIA

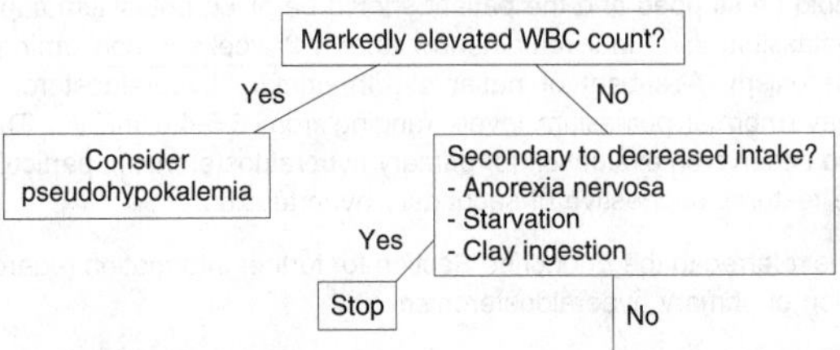

Secondary to cellular redistribution?
- Alkalemia
- Insulin therapy
- β-agonist
- Anabolic states
  - Therapy for pernicious anemia
  - Growth factor therapy
  - Rapidly growing leukemia / lymphoma
  - Response to TPN
  - Refeeding syndrome
- Hypokalemic periodic paralysis
- Theophylline overdose
- Barium salt poisoning
- ↑ endogenous catecholamine release
- Transfusion with frozen, washed red blood cells
- Hypothermia
- Acute chloroquine intoxication

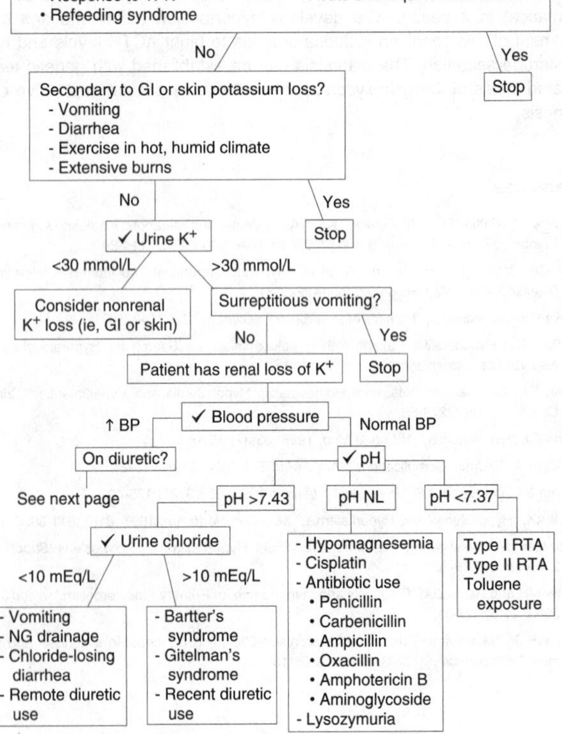

HYPOKALEMIA (*continued*)

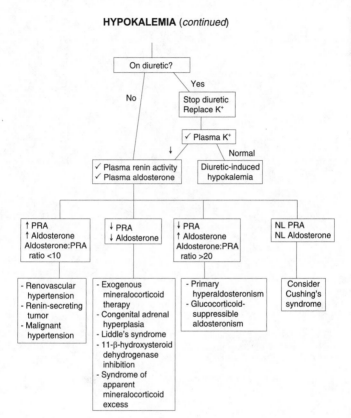

On diuretic?

- Yes → Stop diuretic; Replace K^+ → ✓ Plasma K^+
  - Normal → Diuretic-induced hypokalemia
  - ↓ → ✓ Plasma renin activity; ✓ Plasma aldosterone
- No → ✓ Plasma renin activity; ✓ Plasma aldosterone

✓ Plasma renin activity
✓ Plasma aldosterone

- ↑ PRA; ↑ Aldosterone; Aldosterone:PRA ratio <10
  - Renovascular hypertension
  - Renin-secreting tumor
  - Malignant hypertension
- ↓ PRA; ↓ Aldosterone
  - Exogenous mineralocorticoid therapy
  - Congenital adrenal hyperplasia
  - Liddle's syndrome
  - 11-β-hydroxysteroid dehydrogenase inhibition
  - Syndrome of apparent mineralocorticoid excess
- ↓ PRA; ↑ Aldosterone; Aldosterone:PRA ratio >20
  - Primary hyperaldosteronism
  - Glucocorticoid-suppressible aldosteronism
- NL PRA; NL Aldosterone
  - Consider Cushing's syndrome

HYPERKALEMIA

STEP 1 – *What Are the Causes of Hyperkalemia?*

Hyperkalemia is a commonly encountered electrolyte abnormality. In several large series of hospitalized patients, potassium levels >6.0 mEq/L were found in 1.2% to 1.4% of all patients at the time of admission. Levels >5.3 mEq/L were found in approximately 10% at some point during the hospitalization. The causes of hyperkalemia are listed in the following box.

CAUSES OF HYPERKALEMIA

PSEUDOHYPERKALEMIA

INCREASED POTASSIUM INTAKE

REDISTRIBUTION
- Metabolic acidosis
- Insulin deficiency
- Hyperosmolality
- Succinylcholine
- Arginine hydrochloride
- Somatostatin
- Hyperkalemic periodic paralysis
- β_2-receptor blocker
- Tissue catabolism
- Digoxin overdose
- Severe exercise
- Cardiac surgery

DECREASED URINARY EXCRETION
- Renal failure (acute / chronic)
- Hypoaldosteronism
  - Hyporeninemic hypoaldosteronism
  - Gordon's syndrome
  - Adrenal insufficiency
  - Congenital adrenal hyperplasia
  - Medications
    - Heparin
    - Cyclosporine
    - ACE inhibitors
    - Angiotensin II receptor antagonists
    - NSAIDs
- Aldosterone resistance
  - Potassium-sparing diuretics
    - Spironolactone
    - Triamterene
    - Amiloride
  - Trimethoprim
  - Pentamide
  - Renal tubular disorders
    - Systemic lupus erythematosus
    - Obstructive uropathy
    - Amyloidosis
    - Renal transplant
    - Sickle cell disease
    - Medullary cystic disease
    - Lead nephropathy
    - Idiopathic interstitial nephritis

Proceed to Step 2.

STEP 2 – *Is There Evidence of Pseudohyperkalemia?*

At times, the clinician may encounter an elevated potassium level that does not reflect true hyperkalemia. This has been termed pseudohyperkalemia. In pseudohyperkalemia, the potassium level is artificially high, caused by the movement of potassium out of cells either during or after the drawing of the blood specimen. It is essential to exclude pseudohyperkalemia before embarking on an extensive evaluation of hyperkalemia. The danger in not recognizing pseudohyperkalemia is that treatment to lower the potassium level may be instituted, which may result in hypokalemia. Conditions leading to pseudohyperkalemia include the following.

- Hemolysis

  The most common cause of pseudohyperkalemia is hemolysis. This does not reflect true hemolysis occurring within the body but represents damage to the red blood cells either during or after the blood draw. One cause of hemolysis may be encountered when centrifugation of the blood specimen is performed prior to complete formation of the clot. This will lead to red blood cell damage with subsequent release of potassium from the cells.

  Potassium may also be released from cells when blood is drawn in an exercising extremity. For example, it is not uncommon for patients to clench and unclench the fist in an effort to make the veins more apparent. This repeated clenching and unclenching of the fist can lead to the release of potassium from the cells, raising the potassium concentration by as much as 2 mEq/L. Hemolysis is usually easily recognized by the lab as the release of hemoglobin from the red blood cells will leave the specimen with a red tint or pink tinge. Careful repeat venipuncture (to avoid hemolysis) can be performed to exclude this cause of pseudohyperkalemia.

- Familial pseudohyperkalemia

  Familial pseudohyperkalemia is a rare condition in which potassium leaks out of abnormally permeable red blood cells. Within the body, hyperkalemia is not seen because the excess potassium is excreted in the urine. After a blood draw, however, hyperkalemia may be noted. If suspected, rapid centrifugation to separate the red blood cells from plasma can be performed to prevent the *in vitro* leakage of potassium out of cells.

- Leukocytosis / thrombocytosis

  Under normal circumstances, potassium is released from white blood cells and platelets when cell lysis occurs after a blood specimen clots. This explains why the serum potassium is 0.2-0.4 mEq/L higher than the plasma potassium. With leukocytosis >100,000 cells/mm^3 and thrombocytosis >400,000 cells/mm^3, much more potassium is released. The spuriously elevated potassium levels seen in patients with marked leukocytosis or thrombocytosis may approach 9 mEq/L. In general, the degree of elevation of the potassium concentration is directly related to the severity of the leukocytosis or thrombocytosis. If this is suspected, a simultaneous plasma and serum potassium level should be obtained. When the serum potassium concentration exceeds the plasma potassium concentration by >0.3 mEq/L, pseudohyperkalemia is present. In these cases, further potassium measurements should be made on plasma rather than serum.

If the patient has pseudohyperkalemia, ***stop here.***

If the patient does not have pseudohyperkalemia, ***proceed to Step 3.***

STEP 3 – *Is the Hyperkalemia Due to Increased Intake of Potassium?*

An increased intake of potassium seldom leads to hyperkalemia in the absence of other contributing factors. When increased intake of potassium occurs in a patient who has a condition that is impairing urinary excretion of potassium, dangerously high potassium levels may ensue.

Even in patients with normal renal function, an acute potassium load can significantly increase the plasma potassium concentration. The ingestion of 135-160 mEq of oral potassium, for example, can increase the plasma potassium concentration by as much as 2.5-3.5 mEq/L. This transient rise in plasma potassium concentration is usually well tolerated. When an individual ingests >160 mEq, however, the plasma potassium concentration may rise to levels that are fatal (>8 mEq/L). Very high levels of potassium may also occur in patients who have been given intravenous potassium too rapidly.

In patients who have decreased urinary excretion of potassium (irrespective of cause), it is wise to counsel the patient on avoiding too much dietary potassium as the combination of increased potassium intake in the setting of decreased urinary potassium excretion can lead to substantial elevations in the plasma potassium concentration. In studies involving both inpatients and outpatients, >50% of hyperkalemia cases were iatrogenically caused by the administration of potassium supplements. The majority of these cases occurred in the setting of some other predisposition to hyperkalemia such as concomitant use of medications that increase potassium or intrinsic renal disease, in which the urinary excretion of potassium was impaired. Potassium supplements are just one source of exogenous potassium but certainly not the only one. Salt substitutes, high-dose penicillin administration, and citrate salts all contain considerable amounts of potassium. A complete medication history is essential because patients may not report the use of salt substitutes, which are readily available over-the-counter. The potassium that is given with enteral nutritional support or hyperalimentation can also cause hyperkalemia, especially in patients with renal insufficiency.

If the hyperkalemia is solely due to increased intake of potassium, ***stop here.***

If the hyperkalemia is partly due to increased intake of potassium, but another cause is likely to be present, ***proceed to Step 4.***

If the hyperkalemia is not due to increased intake of potassium, ***proceed to Step 4.***

STEP 4 – *Is the Hyperkalemia Secondary to Redistribution of Potassium?*

Redistribution refers to the movement of potassium from the intracellular to extracellular fluid. Causes of hyperkalemia secondary to the redistribution of potassium are listed in the following box.

CAUSES OF HYPERKALEMIA DUE TO REDISTRIBUTION	
CARDIAC SURGERY*	HYPERTONICITY‡
β-ADRENERGIC ANTAGONISTS†	MEDICATIONS
TISSUE DAMAGE	Digitalis intoxication
Hemolysis	Succinylcholine§
Rhabdomyolysis	HEAVY EXERCISE¶
Trauma	HYPERKALEMIC PERIODIC PARALYSIS**
Burns	SOMATOSTATIN
Tumor lysis syndrome	ARGININE HYDROCHLORIDE
METABOLIC ACIDOSIS#	

*A mildly elevated plasma potassium concentration may be noted in patients on cardiac bypass. It may be multifactorial with β-blocker use and rewarming both playing roles. Cardiac surgery is performed under hypothermic conditions. Hypothermia is a stimulus for potassium movement into cells. With rewarming, an overshoot hyperkalemia may occur, particularly if potassium was administered during the period of hypothermia.

†The hyperkalemia seen with β-blocker use is typically mild. Rarely does the rise in the plasma potassium concentration exceed 0.5 mEq/L.

#Hyperkalemia is commonly seen in patients with metabolic acidosis due to mineral acids (hydrochloric acid or ammonium chloride). It is not seen with metabolic acidosis due to organic acids such as β-hydroxybutyrate or lactic acid. The plasma pH may rise 0.2-1.7 mEq/L for every 0.1 unit decrease in the pH.

‡In poorly controlled diabetes, it is insulin deficiency along with hyperosmolality that results in the development of hyperkalemia. However, the patient is usually total-body-potassium depleted because of increased potassium losses in the urine. Hyperkalemia due to hyperosmolality may also occur with the administration of intravenous mannitol.

§In healthy individuals, the administration of succinylcholine may cause an elevation in the plasma potassium concentration. Rarely does the rise exceed .5 mEq/L. In certain situations (burns, tetanus, neuromuscular disease, extensive trauma), however, substantial elevations in the plasma potassium concentration (as much as 6 mEq/L) can occur, which can be fatal.

¶With exercise, potassium is normally released from cells. How much the potassium concentration rises is directly related to the degree of exercise. It is not unusual to see 0.3-0.4 mEq/L increase in the plasma potassium concentration with slow walking. With more exertion (marathon runners), the rise in plasma potassium concentration may reach 1.2 mEq/L. In individuals who have exerted themselves to exhaustion, the plasma potassium concentration may increase by as much as 2 mEq/L. Although the rise in plasma potassium concentration is transient, there are those who believe that hyperkalemia may be a contributing factor for some cases of sudden death that have occurred during exercise.

**This is a rare disorder characterized by muscle weakness precipitated by any stimulus that can lead to hyperkalemia (eg, exercise, ingestion of potassium). The hyperkalemia is typically mild but cases where the plasma potassium concentration exceeds 7 mEq/L have been reported. Hyperkalemic periodic paralysis, which exhibits autosomal dominant inheritance, should be suspected when a history of recurrent episodic attacks of muscle weakness can be elicited (personal and family history) in the setting of an elevated plasma potassium concentration. The diagnosis can be confirmed if muscle weakness and hyperkalemia are induced with oral potassium (0.5-1.0 mEq/kg).

If redistribution is the cause of the hyperkalemia, ***stop here.***

If redistribution is not the cause of the hyperkalemia, ***proceed to Step 5.***

STEP 5 – *Is the Hyperkalemia Secondary to Decreased Renal Excretion of Potassium?*

Conditions causing hyperkalemia due to decreased renal excretion of potassium are listed in the following box.

HYPERKALEMIA DUE TO DECREASED RENAL EXCRETION OF POTASSIUM	
RENAL FAILURE (acute / chronic)	ALDOSTERONE RESISTANCE
HYPOALDOSTERONISM	Potassium-sparing diuretics
Hyporeninemic hypoaldosteronism	Amiloride
Medications	Spironolactone
ACE inhibitors	Triamterene
Angiotensin II receptor antagonists	Cyclosporine
Heparin	Trimethoprim
Cyclosporine	Pentamidine
Tacrolimus	Renal tubular disorders
NSAIDs	Systemic lupus erythematosus
Adrenal insufficiency (primary)	Obstructive uropathy
Congenital adrenal hyperplasia	Amyloidosis
	Renal transplant
	Sickle cell disease
	Medullary cystic disease
	Lead nephropathy
	Idiopathic interstitial nephritis
	Pseudohypoaldosteronism
	Type I
	Type II (Gordon's syndrome)

Proceed to Step 6.

STEP 6 – *Is the Patient's Hyperkalemia Secondary to Renal Failure?*

Hyperkalemia may be appreciated in both acute and chronic renal failure. In acute renal failure, there are a number of reasons why patients may be predisposed to the development of hyperkalemia. Impaired renal function leads to a decrease in potassium excretion. Hyperkalemia is much more common in oliguric rather than nonoliguric acute renal failure. Other contributing factors to the hyperkalemia include acidosis and the catabolic state that frequently accompanies acute renal failure.

As renal failure progresses in patients with chronic renal insufficiency, the remaining nephrons increase potassium secretion. Also, there is increased potassium secretion at the level of the colon. When the GFR falls to <10-15 mL/minute, these adaptations may no longer be effective in maintaining normokalemia, and hyperkalemia may result. Hyperkalemia can, however, occur in chronic renal failure patients who have a GFR >10-15 mL/minute if they have hypoaldosteronism or aldosterone resistance (see box above).

If acute or chronic renal failure is the cause of the hyperkalemia, ***stop here.***

If acute or chronic renal failure is not the cause of the hyperkalemia, ***proceed to Step 7.***

STEP 7 – *Are There Any Clues in the Patient's Clinical Presentation That Point to the Etiology of the Hyperkalemia?*

Once acute and chronic renal failure have been excluded, many of the other causes of hyperkalemia listed in the box in Step 5 can be differentiated from one another by performing a thorough history and physical exam. These causes will be discussed in further detail in the remainder of this step.

MEDICATION-INDUCED

A careful medication history will reveal if the patient is taking any medication known to cause hyperkalemia (potassium-sparing diuretics, NSAIDs, heparin, trimethoprim, pentamidine, cyclosporine, ACE inhibitor). NSAID use may lead to decreased renal potassium excretion by inhibiting the production of prostaglandins. Impaired prostaglandin production can inhibit renin release and decrease the glomerular filtration rate.

Unfractionated and low molecular weight heparins inhibit the synthesis of aldosterone by a direct action on the adrenal gland. By itself, heparin therapy rarely causes hyperkalemia. There are certain groups of patients, however, who are predisposed to serious hyperkalemia after beginning heparin therapy. These include the elderly, diabetics, and patients receiving NSAIDs, ACE inhibitors, or potassium-sparing diuretics.

Angiotensin-converting enzyme inhibitors (ACE inhibitors) produce hypoaldosteronism and thus hyperkalemia by decreasing levels of angiotensin II (AGII). Recall that the cascade of events leading to the production of aldosterone starts with renin. Renin, produced by the juxtaglomerular cells of the kidney, converts angiotensinogen to angiotensin I. Angiotensin I is then converted to angiotensin II by the angiotensin-converting enzyme. Angiotensin II then stimulates the production of aldosterone. Thus, if AGII production is blocked by an ACE inhibitor and aldosterone is not produced, hyperkalemia may ensue. Those at highest risk of developing hyperkalemia during ACE inhibitor therapy include the following:

- Advanced age
- Underlying renal disease
- Concomitant therapy with β-adrenergic antagonists
- Concomitant use of potassium-sparing diuretics
- Concomitant use of potassium supplements
- Renal artery stenosis
- Congestive heart failure

In recent years, the use of angiotensin type II receptor blockers has increased. Like the ACE inhibitors, angiotensin type II receptor blockers can also cause significant hyperkalemia.

Spironolactone is a competitive mineralocorticoid receptor antagonist which inhibits sodium reabsorption and potassium secretion in the distal nephron. Triamterene and amiloride exert their effects independent of the mineralocorticoid receptor. Both interfere with proper functioning of the sodium channel in the cortical collecting duct. Trimethoprim and pentamidine block sodium reabsorption in the distal tubule as well. Trimethoprim-induced hyperkalemia was initially reported in AIDS patients given high doses for the treatment of *Pneumocystis carinii* pneumonia. It is now recognized that treatment with lower doses of trimethoprim may also be complicated by hyperkalemia. Potassium levels have been found to increase by as much as 1.2 mEq/L in patients treated with standard doses of trimethoprim / sulfamethoxazole (320 mg/day), even if renal function is normal. Advancing age and renal insufficiency are risk factors for the development of significant hyperkalemia in patients receiving trimethoprim. Hyperkalemia has also been noted in AIDS patients with *Pneumocystis carinii* pneumonia who are receiving pentamidine. Most of these patients also have a hyperchloremic metabolic acidosis. Cyclosporine A, an immunosuppressive agent, can produce hyperkalemia by inhibiting renin secretion and/or decreasing renal excretion of potassium (tubular injury, decreased glomerular filtration rate).

In patients with hyperkalemia, any potentially offending medication should be discontinued. The potassium level should then be repeated to ensure normalization of the potassium concentration after discontinuation of the medication. No further evaluation is necessary if the potassium concentration returns to normal after withdrawal of the medication. Persistence of the hyperkalemia after removal of the suspect medication warrants further investigation.

ADRENAL INSUFFICIENCY (Primary)

In primary adrenal insufficiency, there is diminished production of glucocorticoids and mineralocorticoids by the adrenal gland. The lack of mineralocorticoid production leads to hyperkalemia. Patients with secondary (pituitary) or tertiary (hypothalamic) adrenal insufficiency have diminished production of glucocorticoids but intact production of mineralocorticoids. As a result, hyperkalemia is not seen in these forms of adrenal insufficiency.

Signs and symptoms of adrenal insufficiency are often nonspecific. They may include weakness, malaise, fatigue, weight loss, anorexia, diarrhea, constipation, abdominal pain, and dizziness with standing. Physical exam may reveal orthostatic changes in heart rate and blood pressure as well as hyperpigmentation. These as well as other clinical features of Addison's disease (autoimmune disease of the adrenal glands), one of the major causes of primary adrenal insufficiency, are listed in the following table.

Clinical Features of Addison's Disease

Clinical Feature	Percentage
Weakness and fatigue	100
Weight loss	100
Anorexia	100
Hyperpigmentation	92
Hypotension	88
Gastrointestinal symptoms	56
Nervousness and mental symptoms	50
Hypoglycemic symptoms	50
Loss of axillary and pubic hair	30
Postural dizziness	12
Muscle pains	6

Adapted from *The Kidney: Physiology and Pathophysiology,* 3rd ed, Seldin DW and Giebisch G, eds, Philadelphia, PA: Lippincott Williams and Wilkins, 2000, 1664.

Laboratory test abnormalities include hyponatremia, hyperchloremic metabolic acidosis, and hypoglycemia. These as well as other laboratory features of Addison's disease are listed in the following table.

Laboratory Features of Addison's Disease

Laboratory Feature	Percentage
Hyponatremia	88
Eosinophilia	70-80
Neutropenia	70-80
Lymphocytosis	70-80
Azotemia	70-80
Hyperkalemia	64
Hypoglycemia	50
Hyperchloremic metabolic acidosis	30-50
Hypercalcemia	6

Adapted from *The Kidney: Physiology and Pathophysiology,* 3rd ed, Seldin DW and Giebisch G, eds, Philadelphia, PA: Lippincott Williams and Wilkins, 2000, 1664.

The diagnosis can be established with the use of a cosyntropin stimulation test. The reader is referred to the chapter, ***Adrenal Insufficiency*** *on page 379* for further information.

HYPORENINEMIC HYPOALDOSTERONISM

In patients who do not have significant renal failure (oliguric acute renal failure, chronic renal failure with GFR <10-15 mL/minute) or medication-induced hyperkalemia, the most likely etiology of the hyperkalemia is the syndrome of hyporeninemic hypoaldosteronism. DeFronzo, et al, was the first to review hyporeninemic hypoaldosteronism in 1980. In that report, he described the clinical and laboratory features of 81 patients with hyporeninemic hypoaldosteronism. These features are listed in the following box.

CLINICAL AND LABORATORY CHARACTERISTICS IN 81 PATIENT WITH SYNDROME OF SELECTIVE HYPOALDOSTERONISM
Mean age, 64 years; 32-82 years
Findings at presentation
Asymptomatic hyperkalemia (75%)
Muscle weakness (25%)
Cardiac arrhythmia (25%)
Hyperchloremic acidosis (approximately 50%)
Salt wasting (unusual)
Normal glucocorticoid function
Mild to moderate renal insufficiency, 70% of patients
Diabetes mellitus, 49% of patients
Low or low-normal baseline plasma aldosterone levels; all patients had a subnormal increase after volume contraction
Normal baseline and/or stimulated plasma renin levels, 18% of patients

Adapted from DeFronzo RA, "Hyperkalemia and Hyporeninemic Hypoaldosteronism," *Kidney Int*, 1980, 17(10):118-34.

The typical patient with hyporeninemic hypoaldosteronism has the following profile.

- Older age
- Unexplained, chronic, usually asymptomatic hyperkalemia
- Mild to moderate chronic renal insufficiency (creatinine clearance 15-20 to 70 mL/minute)
- Diabetes mellitus (approximately 50% of patients)

Seventy percent of patients have mild-to-moderate chronic renal insufficiency. Many different types of renal disease have been described in patients with hyporeninemic hypoaldosteronism, as shown in the following table.

Causes of Renal Disease in 57 Patients With the Syndrome of Hypoaldosteronism

Cause of Renal Disease	Number of Patients (Total of 57)
Diabetes mellitus	25
Interstitial nephritis (unknown etiology)	7
Hypertension	7
Gout	6
Glomerulonephritis	3
Nephrolithiasis	2
Analgesic nephropathy	1
Urinary tract obstruction	1
Mixed cryoglobulinemia	1
Unknown	4
Obstructive uropathy	8
Sickle cell disease	5

Hypoaldosteronism has been described in a number of other types of renal diseases including lead nephropathy, amyloidosis, medullary cystic disease, and allergic interstitial nephritis.

NSAIDs are a common cause of hyporeninemic hypoaldosteronism. Renin release is dependent on prostaglandin stimulation. NSAIDs inhibit prostaglandin synthesis, resulting in hyporeninemia. These agents may cause clinically-significant hyperkalemia even in the absence of any renal dysfunction.

RENAL TUBULAR DISORDER

A variety of renal tubular disorders may present with hyperkalemia. These disorders may present with hyperkalemia along with hyperchloremic metabolic acidosis in what has been termed hyperkalemic distal renal tubular acidosis (type IV RTA). It is most often seen in patients with obstructive uropathy or sickle cell disease. Renal tubular disorders that may present with hyperkalemia are listed in the following box.

RENAL TUBULAR DISORDERS CAUSING HYPERKALEMIA	
AMYLOIDOSIS	MEDULLARY CYSTIC DISEASE
OBSTRUCTIVE UROPATHY	LEAD NEPHROPATHY
SYSTEMIC LUPUS ERYTHEMATOSUS	SICKLE CELL DISEASE
RENAL TRANSPLANT	IDIOPATHIC INTERSTITIAL NEPHRITIS

The renal tubular disorders listed above cause hyperkalemia because of renal resistance to the effects of aldosterone. When end-organ resistance to aldosterone is present, the patient is said to have "pseudohypoaldosteronism." While pseudohypoaldosteronism can be drug-induced (potassium-sparing diuretics) or due to one of the renal tubular disorders listed above, it can also be idiopathic. Idiopathic pseudohypoaldosteronism is uncommon and has been divided into two forms. Type I disease is diagnosed in children while type II pseudohypoaldosteronism, also known as Gordon's syndrome, can be seen in adults.

References

Gennari FJ, "Disorders of Potassium Homeostasis. Hypokalemia and Hyperkalemia," *Crit Care Clin*, 2002, 18(2):273-88, vi.

Greenberg A, "Diuretic Complications," *Am J Med Sci*, 2000, 319(1):10-24.

Halperrin ML and Kamel KS, "Potassium," *Lancet*, 1998, 352(9122):135-40.

Mandal AK, "Hypokalemia and Hyperkalemia," *Med Clin North Am*, 1997, 81(3):611-39.

Perazella MA, "Drug-Induced Hyperkalemia: Old Culprits and New Offenders," *Am J Med*, 2000, 109(4):307-14.

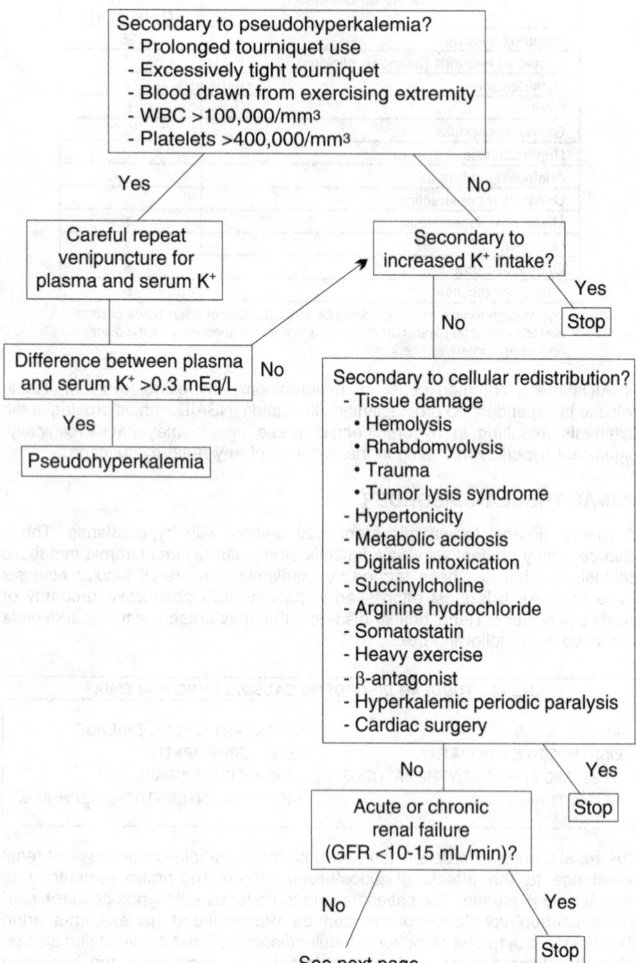
HYPERKALEMIA
Secondary to pseudohyperkalemia?
- Prolonged tourniquet use
- Excessively tight tourniquet
- Blood drawn from exercising extremity
- WBC >100,000/mm3
- Platelets >400,000/mm3
Yes
No
Careful repeat venipuncture for plasma and serum K+
Difference between plasma and serum K+ >0.3 mEq/L
Yes
Pseudohyperkalemia
No
Secondary to increased K+ intake?
Yes
Stop
No
Secondary to cellular redistribution?
- Tissue damage
• Hemolysis
• Rhabdomyolysis
• Trauma
• Tumor lysis syndrome
- Hypertonicity
- Metabolic acidosis
- Digitalis intoxication
- Succinylcholine
- Arginine hydrochloride
- Somatostatin
- Heavy exercise
- β-antagonist
- Hyperkalemic periodic paralysis
- Cardiac surgery
Yes
Stop
No
Acute or chronic renal failure (GFR <10-15 mL/min)?
Yes
Stop
No
See next page

HYPERKALEMIA *(continued)*

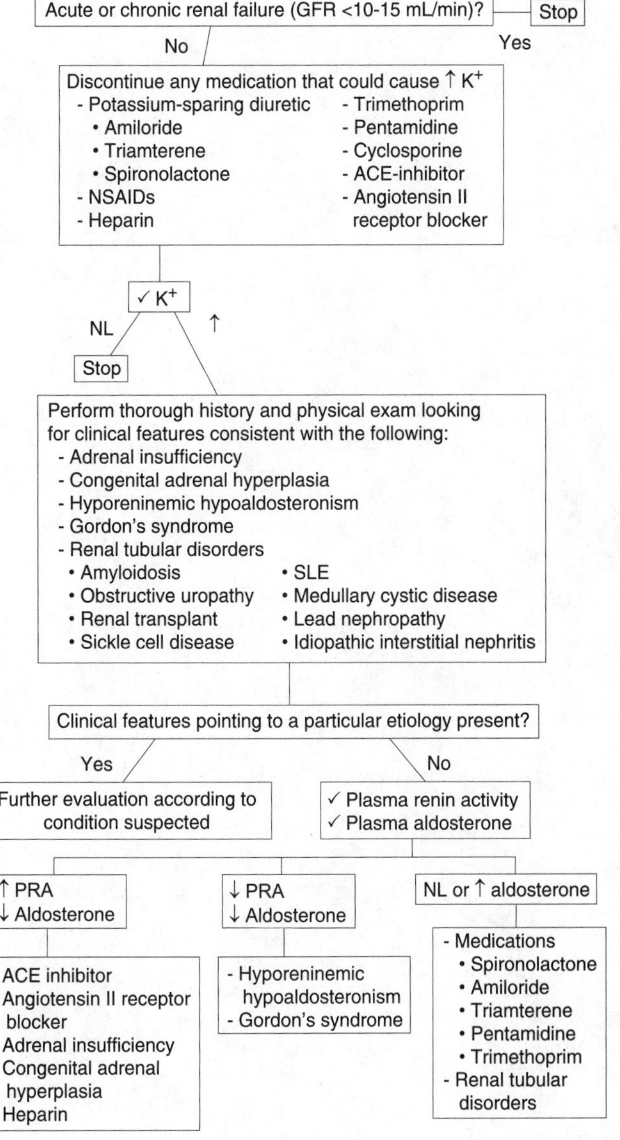
Acute or chronic renal failure (GFR <10-15 mL/min)?
Yes
Stop
No
Discontinue any medication that could cause ↑ K+
- Potassium-sparing diuretic
• Amiloride
• Triamterene
• Spironolactone
- NSAIDs
- Heparin
- Trimethoprim
- Pentamidine
- Cyclosporine
- ACE-inhibitor
- Angiotensin II receptor blocker
✓ K+
NL
Stop
↑
Perform thorough history and physical exam looking for clinical features consistent with the following:
- Adrenal insufficiency
- Congenital adrenal hyperplasia
- Hyporeninemic hypoaldosteronism
- Gordon's syndrome
- Renal tubular disorders
• Amyloidosis
• Obstructive uropathy
• Renal transplant
• Sickle cell disease
• SLE
• Medullary cystic disease
• Lead nephropathy
• Idiopathic interstitial nephritis
Clinical features pointing to a particular etiology present?
Yes
Further evaluation according to condition suspected
No
✓ Plasma renin activity
✓ Plasma aldosterone
↑ PRA
↓ Aldosterone
- ACE inhibitor
- Angiotensin II receptor blocker
- Adrenal insufficiency
- Congenital adrenal hyperplasia
- Heparin
↓ PRA
↓ Aldosterone
- Hyporeninemic hypoaldosteronism
- Gordon's syndrome
NL or ↑ aldosterone
- Medications
• Spironolactone
• Amiloride
• Triamterene
• Pentamidine
• Trimethoprim
- Renal tubular disorders

HYPOMAGNESEMIA

The prevalence of hypomagnesemia varies depending upon the clinical setting. Depending upon the study, hypomagnesemia has been reported in 7% to 12% of hospitalized patients. The incidence increases, however, in the intensive care unit where approximately 60% of patients have hypomagnesemia. Usually, the signs and symptoms of magnesium deficiency are not evident until serum magnesium levels fall below 1 mEq/L.

Serum Magnesium Level

Approximately 99% of the body's magnesium stores are found intracellularly, located mainly in muscle and bone. Extracellular magnesium accounts for about 1% of the body's total magnesium stores. Extracellular magnesium is present in one of three forms:

1. Protein-bound magnesium, accounting for 30% of extracellular magnesium (mostly bound to albumin)
2. Magnesium chelated to various anions, accounting for 15% of extracellular magnesium
3. Ionized or free magnesium, accounting for 55% of extracellular magnesium

Because most of the body's magnesium stores are present intracellularly, the serum magnesium level may not be a reliable measure of body magnesium stores. In most cases, however, a low serum magnesium level reflects a total body magnesium deficit. The clinician should realize, however, that cases of magnesium deficiency have been described in which patients had signs and symptoms of magnesium deficiency in the setting of a normal serum magnesium level. In these patients, magnesium deficiency was diagnosed by more sophisticated testing including measurement of intracellular magnesium stores. In these patients, the signs and symptoms of magnesium deficiency did, in fact, resolve with magnesium supplementation.

Quite often, clinicians use the terms "hypomagnesemia" and "magnesium deficiency" interchangeably. However, it is important to understand that these two terms are not synonymous. As stated above, magnesium deficiency can be present in patients with normomagnesemia (normal serum magnesium level) and a low serum magnesium level does not always mean that the patient is magnesium deficient. Clearly, these are some of the limitations of the serum magnesium level but at the present time, a better test for determining the body's magnesium stores is not available. Until such a test is developed clinicians will continue to rely on the serum magnesium level even if it is a relatively insensitive measure of magnesium deficiency.

Most techniques used to determine the serum magnesium level measure the total magnesium concentration, which includes free magnesium and that bound to albumin. A decreased serum magnesium level is common in hypoalbuminemic states because of a decrease in the protein-bound fraction. This situation is analogous to that seen with hypocalcemia. Unlike hypocalcemia, a formula to correct the serum magnesium level in the hypoalbuminemic patient is not available. In general, slightly low serum magnesium levels in the hypoalbuminemic patient can be attributed to the hypoalbuminemia.

Measurement of Intracellular Magnesium

Because testing to determine intracellular magnesium is difficult to perform, it is seldom done. In the event that there is strong suspicion of magnesium deficiency in the setting of a normal serum magnesium level, a magnesium retention test, which is a measure of intracellular magnesium stores, may be performed. In patients with magnesium deficiency, the retention of a significant proportion of injected magnesium supports the diagnosis.

Causes of Hypomagnesemia

Conditions causing hypomagnesemia may do so through one of the three major mechanisms:

- Decreased intake of magnesium
- Redistribution
- Increased loss (renal or gastrointestinal)

In the following box, the causes of hypomagnesemia are grouped under the above mechanisms.

CAUSES OF HYPOMAGNESEMIA

DECREASED MAGNESIUM INTAKE

PROTEIN-CALORIE MALNUTRITION
TOTAL PARENTERAL NUTRITION
ALCOHOLISM
MAGNESIUM-FREE INTRAVENOUS FLUIDS

REDISTRIBUTION

INCREASED CIRCULATING CATECHOLAMINES
β-ADRENERGIC AGONISTS
SYSTEMIC ACIDOSIS (after correction)
MASSIVE BLOOD TRANSFUSION
GLUCOSE INFUSION
AMINO ACID INFUSION
INSULIN INFUSION
REFEEDING SYNDROME

INCREASED LOSS

GASTROINTESTINAL
- Malabsorption syndromes
- Diarrhea (acute or chronic)
- Intestinal fistula
- Short bowel syndrome
- Intestinal resection
- Jejunoileal bypass
- Pancreatitis
- Laxative abuse
- Emesis
- Prolonged nasogastric suction
- Steatorrheic states
- Primary intestinal hypomagnesemia

INCREASED LOSS

RENAL
- Medications
  - Diuretics (loop, thiazide, osmotic)
  - Cisplatin
  - Foscarnet
  - Aminoglycosides
  - Pentamidine
  - Cyclosporine
  - Tacrolimus
  - Amphotericin B
- Acute tubular necrosis (recovery phase)
- Volume expansion
- Alcoholism / alcohol withdrawal
- Endocrine disorders
  - Hyperparathyroidism
  - Hyperthyroidism
  - Hyperaldosteronism (primary or secondary)
  - Inappropriate ADH secretion
  - Hypercalcemia
  - Diabetes mellitus
  - Ketoacidosis
- Postrenal transplantation
- Postobstructive diuresis
- Tubulinterstitial nephropathies
- Genetic conditions
  - Bartter's syndrome
  - Gitelman's syndrome
  - Primary renal magnesium wasting

MISCELLANEOUS

SEVERE BURNS
CARDIOPULMONARY BYPASS
EXCESSIVE SWEATING
EXCESSIVE LACTATION
PREGNANCY (last trimester)
HYPOALBUMINEMIA
HUNGRY BONE SYNDROME
INTENSE EXERCISE

Approach to the Patient With Hypomagnesemia

A serum magnesium level is usually not routinely measured when a patient is admitted to the hospital. It should be assessed if the patient has any of the following:

- Condition predisposing to the development of hypomagnesemia (ie, chronic diarrhea)
- Signs and symptoms of hypomagnesemia

- Cardiac condition in which hypomagnesemia may be dangerous to the patient (ventricular ectopy, congestive heart failure, digoxin use)
- Presence of other electrolyte abnormalities (hypocalcemia or hypokalemia) since these electrolyte disorders are quite common in the hypomagnesemic patient

The finding of a low serum magnesium level in any of the above settings is sufficient evidence to support the presence of magnesium deficiency. Since serum magnesium levels correlate poorly with body stores, the finding of a low serum magnesium level in the absence of any of the above settings may or may not reflect true deficiency. However, most clinicians would treat with magnesium supplementation in either case.

In most cases of hypomagnesemia, the etiology is evident. If the cause is not clear, some measure of urinary magnesium excretion should be obtained to differentiate renal magnesium loss from extrarenal causes of hypomagnesemia. Tests that can be obtained include the urine magnesium concentration, 24-hour urine magnesium level, fractional excretion of magnesium, or urine magnesium to creatinine ratio. The table below provides more information about the use of these tests in the evaluation of hypomagnesemia.

RELATIVE MERITS OF DIFFERENT INDICES OF URINARY MAGNESIUM EXCRETION

	Criteria for renal magnesium wasting	Advantages	Disadvantages
Urine magnesium concentration	>1.6 mg/dL	Can be measured in a spot urine	Varies with the urine concentration
Fractional excretion of magnesium*	>1%	Can be measured in a spot urine Adjusted for filtered load	Not well validated in the literature
Urine magnesium to creatinine ratio	>0.02 (mg/mg)	Can be measured in a spot urine	Varies with gender and muscle mass
24-hour urine magnesium level	>24 mg	Normal and abnormal values widely available in published studies of hypomagnesemia	Requires 24-hour urine collection

*The fractional excretion of magnesium (%) = [(urine magnesium X plasma creatinine) / (.7 X plasma magnesium X urine creatinine)] X 100

From Brenner and Rector's *The Kidney*, 6th ed, Philadelphia, PA: WB Saunders Co, 2000, 1059.

These tests will help differentiate gastrointestinal (or poor dietary intake) from renal etiologies of hypomagnesemia. In patients with an extrarenal etiology, the kidney should respond by increasing renal magnesium reabsorption. In disorders associated with increased renal magnesium loss, this is not possible. Of the tests described above, the one that is most widely used is the 24-hour urine magnesium level. When performing this test, it is important to also obtain a creatinine measurement to ensure that the collection was complete. A 24-hour urine magnesium level <24 mg supports an extrarenal etiology while a level that exceeds 24 mg is consistent with a renal cause.

References

Agus ZS, "Hypomagnesemia," *J Am Soc Nephrol*, 1999, 10(7):1616-22.

Dacey MJ, "Hypomagnesemic Disorders," *Crit Care Clin*, 2001, 17(1):155-73, viii.

Greenberg A, "Diuretic Complications," *Am J Med Sci*, 2000, 319(1):10-24.

Kelepouris E and Agus ZS, "Hypomagnesemia: Renal Magnesium Handling," *Semin Nephrol*, 1998, 18(1):58-73.

Sanders GT, Huijgen HJ, and Sanders R, "Magnesium in Disease: A Review With Special Emphasis on the Serum Ionized Magnesium," *Clin Chem Lab Med*, 1999, 37(11-12):1011-33.

Topf JM and Murray PT, "Hypomagnesemia and Hypermagnesemia," *Rev Endocr Metab Disord*, 2003, 4(2):195-206.

Whang R, "Clinical Disorders of Magnesium Metabolism," *Compr Ther*, 1997, 23(3):168-73.

HYPERMAGNESEMIA

Hypermagnesemia is more commonly encountered in patients with renal failure, particularly when large amounts of magnesium-containing medications are given (ie, antacids or laxatives). The causes of hypermagnesemia are listed in the following box.

CAUSES OF HYPERMAGNESEMIA

INCREASED INTAKE*
- Magnesium-containing cathartics
- Magnesium-containing antacids
- Rectal administration of magnesium salts
- Magnesium sulfate infusion (eclampsia)
- Urethral irrigation with hemiacidrin
- Swallowing sea water during near-drowning in Dead Sea

RENAL FAILURE
- Acute renal failure (oliguric phase)†
- Chronic renal failure‡

ADRENAL INSUFFICIENCY
FAMILIAL HYPOCALCIURIC HYPERCALCEMIA
PRIMARY HYPERPARATHYROIDISM
TUMOR LYSIS SYNDROME
MILD-ALKALI SYNDROME
LITHIUM THERAPY
POSTOPERATIVE
DEHYDRATION
ACUTE ACIDOSIS

*The increased intake of magnesium usually in and of itself does not lead to significant hypermagnesemia unless massive ingestion has taken place. Not uncommonly, however, increased intake of magnesium plays a major role in the development of significant hypermagnesemia in patients with another predisposition to hypermagnesemia (ie, renal failure).

†Hypermagnesemia is not uncommon during acute renal failure, particularly in the oliguric phase. Although usually mild in degree, severe degrees of hypermagnesemia may be encountered, especially if magnesium-containing medications are given.

‡The serum magnesium level is usually normal in patients with chronic renal failure until the GFR falls to <30 mL/minute. Hypermagnesemia is usually mild in degree unless the patient becomes oliguric or is given large amounts of magnesium-containing medications such as enemas, laxatives, antacids, phosphate binders, or dialysis fluids. Most patients with end-stage renal disease have serum magnesium levels between 2 and 3 mEq/L.

References

Fung MC, Weintraub M, and Bowen DL, "Hypermagnesemia. Elderly Over-the-Counter Drug Users at Risk," *Arch Fam Med*, 1995, 4(8):718-23.

Sanders GT, Huijgen HJ, and Sanders R, "Magnesium in Disease: A Review With Special Emphasis on the Serum Ionized Magnesium," *Clin Chem Lab Med*, 1999, 37(11-12):1011-33.

Topf JM and Murray PT, "Hypomagnesemia and Hypermagnesemia," *Rev Endocr Metab Disord*, 2003, 4(2):195-206.

Van Hook JW, "Endocrine Crisis. Hypermagnesemia," *Crit Care Clin*, 1991, 7(1):215-23.

Whang R, "Clinical Disorders of Magnesium Metabolism," *Compr Ther*, 1997, 23(3):168-73.

HYPOPHOSPHATEMIA

Hypophosphatemia, defined as a low serum phosphate level, is a commonly encountered electrolyte abnormality. The incidence of hypophosphatemia differs depending upon the patient population studied. In one study, hypophosphatemia was noted in approximately 50% of patients admitted to a VA hospital. In other series, the incidence of hypophosphatemia has ranged from 0.24% to 2.15%. The higher incidence reported in the VA study was thought to be due to the higher incidence of alcoholism among these patients.

The incidence of hypophosphatemia also varies depending upon when the serum phosphate level is measured during the hospitalization. Measurement of the serum phosphate level on the first day often underestimates the incidence of this electrolyte abnormality. Many patients with initially normal serum phosphate levels have a decrease in the serum phosphate concentration over several days of the hospitalization. It is clear that hypophosphatemia is not recognized in many of these patients, including some who have severe hypophosphatemia.

It is important to realize, however, that a low serum phosphate level is not synonymous with phosphate depletion or deficiency. In some cases, a low serum phosphate level may merely reflect redistribution (movement of phosphate from extracellular to intracellular fluid). Phosphorus deficiency can occur in the setting of low, normal, or even high serum phosphate levels.

Causes of Hypophosphatemia

The causes of hypophosphatemia are listed in the following box.

CAUSES OF HYPOPHOSPHATEMIA

SPURIOUS
- IgG interference (multiple myeloma)
- Mannitol interference
- Lipemia
- Macroglobulinemia
- Bilirubin >3 mg/dL (assay-dependent)

DECREASED DIETARY INTAKE

DECREASED INTESTINAL ABSORPTION
- Vitamin D deficiency
- Malabsorption
- Steatorrhea
- Secretory diarrhea
- Vomiting
- Cushing's syndrome
- Corticosteroids
- Phosphate-binding antacids
  - Calcium acetate
  - Calcium carbonate
  - Aluminum hydroxide
  - Sodium ferrous citrate
  - Magnesium-containing

REDISTRIBUTION
- Respiratory alkalosis
- Hormonal effects
  - Insulin
  - Glucagon
  - Epinephrine
  - Androgens
  - Cortisol
  - Anovulatory hormones
- Nutrient effects
  - Glucose
  - Fructose
  - Glycerol
  - Lactate
  - Amino acids
  - Xylitol
- Cellular uptake syndromes
  - Recovery from hypothermia
  - Burkitt's lymphoma
  - Histiocytic lymphoma
  - Acute myelomonocytic leukemia
  - Acute myelogenous leukemia
  - Treatment of pernicious anemia
  - Treatment of iron deficiency with intravenous saccharated iron oxide
  - Erythropoietin therapy
  - Hungry bone syndrome

(continued)

CAUSES OF HYPOPHOSPHATEMIA *(continued)*
INCREASED RENAL EXCRETION
Primary hyperparathyroidism
Tumor-induced osteomalacia
Renal tubular defects
Nonacidotic and hypercalciuric proximal tubulopathy
Multiple myeloma
Renal rickets
Oncogenic osteomalacia
Chinese crude drugs
Polyostotic fibrous dysplasia
Following renal transplantation
Maleic acid
Ifosfamide
Suramin
Aldosteronism
Licorice ingestion
Volume expansion
Inappropriate secretion of ADH
Mineralocorticoid administration
Corticosteroid therapy
Magnesium deficiency
Diuretics
Diphosphonates
Foscarnet
Bartter's syndrome
Gitelman's syndrome
Cushing's syndrome

Adapted from Seldin DW and Giebisch G, *The Kidney: Physiology and Pathophysiology*, Philadelphia, PA: Lippincott Williams & Wilkins, 2000, 1906.

Causes of Severe Hypophosphatemia

Severe hypophosphatemia is said to be present if the serum phosphate concentration is <1.5 mg/dL. This degree of hypophosphatemia can be caused by a limited number of conditions. The causes of severe hypophosphatemia are listed in the following box.

CAUSES OF SEVERE HYPOPHOSPHATEMIA	
CHRONIC ALCOHOLISM	RECOVERY FROM EXHAUSTIVE EXERCISE
ALCOHOL WITHDRAWAL	ACUTE PANIC DISORDER
SEVERE THERMAL BURNS	ACUTE RENAL FAILURE
RECOVERY FROM DIABETIC KETOACIDOSIS	MULTIPLE MYELOMA
HYPERALIMENTATION	AFTER MAJOR SURGERY
NUTRITIONAL RECOVERY SYNDROME	ACUTE MALARIA
RESPIRATORY ALKALOSIS	MEDICATIONS (ifosfamide, cisplatin)
FOLLOWING RENAL TRANSPLANTATION	ACETAMINOPHEN INTOXICATION
THERAPEUTIC HYPERTHERMIA	CYTOKINE INFUSION (TNF, IL-2)
NEUROLEPTIC MALIGNANT SYNDROME	PERIODIC PARALYSIS
	REYE SYNDROME

Adapted from Seldin DW and Giebisch G, *The Kidney: Physiology and Pathophysiology*, Philadelphia, PA: Lippincott Williams & Wilkins, 2000, 1910.

Approach to the Patient With Hypophosphatemia

Serum phosphate levels exhibit diurnal variability with the nadir being at 11 AM and the peak at 12:30 AM. Levels also fluctuate because of meals. These are reasons why it is preferable to obtain serum phosphate levels in the fasting state, preferably in the morning.

Once hypophosphatemia is detected, the etiology needs to be established. The etiology is often apparent from the history and physical examination. If the cause is unclear, a test that measures phosphate excretion should be determined, either through a 24-hour urine collection for phosphate or by calculating the fractional excretion of phosphate. The fractional excretion of phosphate, which can be performed on a spot urine specimen, can be calculated using the following formula:

FRACTIONAL EXCRETION OF PHOSPHATE
$$FE_{PO_4^{-3}} (\%) = \frac{urine_{PO_4^{-3}} \times plasma_{Cr}}{0.7 \times plasma_{PO_4^{-3}} \times urine_{Cr}} \times 100$$
Normal = 5% to 20%

When hypophosphatemia is due to a nonrenal condition, the kidneys are able to respond by decreasing urinary phosphate excretion. In these cases, less than 100 mg of phosphate should be excreted over a 24-hour period. Similarly, the fractional excretion of phosphate should be low (<5%). These patients should be evaluated for hypophosphatemia due to redistribution or decreased intestinal absorption. Common causes include glucose or insulin infusion, respiratory alkalosis, vitamin D deficiency, chronic antacid use, and chronic diarrhea.

If the fractional excretion of phosphate is >5% or the 24-hour urine phosphate is >100 mg, then the patient is likely to have renal phosphate wasting, the causes of which are listed in the previous box.

References

Crook M, "Importance of Plasma Phosphate Determination," *J Int Fed Clin Chem*, 1997, 9(3):110-3, 116-7.

Crook M and Swaminathan R, "Disorders of Plasma Phosphate and Indications for Its Measurement," *Ann Clin Biochem*, 1996, 33(Pt 5):376-96.

DiMeglio LA, White KE, and Econs MJ, "Disorders of Phosphate Metabolism," *Endocrinol Metab Clin North Am*, 2000, 29(3):591-609.

Shiber JR and Mattu A, "Serum Phosphate Abnormalities in the Emergency Department," *J Emerg Med*, 2002, 23(4):395-400.

Subramanian R and Khardori R, "Severe Hypophosphatemia. Pathophysiologic Implications, Clinical Presentations, and Treatment," *Medicine (Baltimore)*, 2000, 79(1):1-8.

Weisinger JR and Bellorin-Font E, "Magnesium and Phosphorus," *Lancet*, 1998, 352(9125):391-6.

HYPERPHOSPHATEMIA

Causes of Hyperphosphatemia

Causes of hyperphosphatemia are listed in the following box.

CAUSES OF HYPERPHOSPHATEMIA

SPURIOUS
- Thrombocytosis
- Hyperlipidemia
- Myeloma paraproteins
- Stored blood
- Mannitol

INCREASED INTAKE / EXOGENOUS LOAD
- Cow's milk
- Vitamin D intoxication
- Phosphorus-containing laxatives / enema
- Intravenous phosphorus administration
- White phosphorus burns

INCREASED ENDOGENOUS LOAD
- Tumor lysis syndrome
- Rhabdomyolysis
- Malignant hyperthermia
- Heat stroke
- Lactic acidosis
- Ketoacidosis
- Respiratory acidosis
- Respiratory alkalosis (chronic)
- Bowel infarction

DECREASED EXCRETION
- Renal insufficiency*
- Hypoparathyroidism
- Bisphosphonates
- Growth hormone / acromegaly
- Insulin-like growth factor I
- Vitamin D intoxication
- Vitamin A intoxication
- Tumoral calcinosis
- Pseudohypoparathyroidism
- Steroid withdrawal

MISCELLANEOUS
- Verapamil
- β-blockers
- Fluoride poisoning
- Hemorrhagic shock
- Sleep deprivation

*In patients with chronic renal failure, plasma phosphate levels are usually within the normal range until the GFR falls below 25 mL/minute. Acute renal failure may also be associated with hyperphosphatemia, especially in patients who have infection or rhabdomyolysis.

References

Crook M, "Importance of Plasma Phosphate Determination," *J Int Fed Clin Chem*, 1997, 9(3):110-3, 116-7.

DiMeglio LA, White KE, and Econs MJ, "Disorders of Phosphate Metabolism," *Endocrinol Metab Clin North Am*, 2000, 29(3):591-609.

Llach F, "Hyperphosphatemia in End-Stage Renal Disease Patients: Pathophysiological Consequences," *Kidney Int Suppl*, 1999, 73:S31-7.

Malluche HH and Monier-Faugere MC, "Understanding and Managing Hyperphosphatemia in Patients With Chronic Renal Disease," *Clin Nephrol*, 1999, 52(5):267-77.

Shiber JR and Mattu A, "Serum Phosphate Abnormalities in the Emergency Department," *J Emerg Med*, 2002, 23(4):395-400.

Weisinger JR and Bellorin-Font E, "Magnesium and Phosphorus," *Lancet*, 1998, 352(9125):391-6.

HYPOCALCEMIA

STEP 1 – *Does the Patient Have True Hypocalcemia?*

Prior to embarking on what, at times, can be an extensive workup for hypocalcemia, the clinician should ensure that the patient has true hypocalcemia. True hypocalcemia needs to be differentiated from false hypocalcemia, which is seen in patients with hypoalbuminemia.

A decrease in albumin concentration will lead to a decrease in albumin-bound calcium and, therefore, total calcium. In patients with hypoalbuminemia, the measured total calcium concentration may not be an accurate marker of the patient's calcium status. Formulas have been devised to correct the total calcium in the setting of hypoalbuminemia. One that is widely used clinically is to add 0.8 mg/dL to the total serum calcium concentration for every 1 g/dL the serum albumin is <4 g/dL

or

Corrected Ca^{2+} = measured Ca^{2+} + 0.8 (4 - serum albumin)

False hypocalcemia due to hypoalbuminemia can also be excluded by measuring the ionized calcium level. Ionized calcium is the fraction of the total serum calcium that is physiologically active. Patients who have a low total calcium level due to hypoalbuminemia will have a normal ionized calcium concentration.

If the serum calcium level corrects to the normal range using the above formula or the ionized calcium level is normal, the patient has false hypocalcemia and ***no further evaluation is necessary***.

If the serum calcium level is low despite correction for albumin or if the ionized calcium level is low, the patient has true hypocalcemia and requires further evaluation. ***Proceed to Step 2.***

STEP 2 – *What Are the Causes of Hypocalcemia?*

Once false hypocalcemia due to hypoalbuminemia has been excluded, the clinician can focus on elucidating the cause of the hypocalcemia. The causes of hypocalcemia are listed in the following box.

CAUSES OF HYPOCALCEMIA

HYPOPARATHYROIDISM
PTH RESISTANCE
- Pseudohypoparathyroidism
- Hypomagnesemia

VITAMIN D DEFICIENCY
1-α HYDROXYLASE DEFICIENCY (vitamin D-dependent rickets type I)
VITAMIN D RESISTANCE (vitamin D-dependent rickets type II)
MALIGNANCY
- Osteoblastic metastases
- Tumor lysis syndrome

SEPSIS

(continued)

CAUSES OF HYPOCALCEMIA *(continued)*	
HUNGRY BONE SYNDROME	
RHABDOMYOLYSIS	
MEDICATIONS	
Plicamycin	Citrated blood
Calcitonin	Radiographic contrast dyes
Bisphosphonates	Fluoride
Phosphate	Foscarnet
Phenobarbital	Pentamidine
ACUTE PANCREATITIS	
TOXIC SHOCK SYNDROME	

Proceed to Step 3.

STEP 3 – *What Is the Serum Phosphate Level?*

The differential diagnosis of hypocalcemia can be narrowed further with consideration of the serum phosphate concentration. Causes of hypocalcemia that present with an elevated serum phosphate level are listed in the following box.

CAUSES OF HYPOCALCEMIA ASSOCIATED WITH AN ELEVATED SERUM PHOSPHATE LEVEL
HYPOPARATHYROIDISM
PSEUDOHYPOPARATHYROIDISM TYPE I OR II
CHRONIC RENAL FAILURE
RHABDOMYOLYSIS
TUMOR LYSIS SYNDROME
ACUTE RENAL FAILURE (oligoanuric stage)

Causes of hypocalcemia that present with a low or normal serum phosphate level are listed in the following box.

CAUSES OF HYPOCALCEMIA ASSOCIATED WITH LOW OR NORMAL SERUM PHOSPHATE
VITAMIN D DEFICIENCY
DECREASED 25-HYDROXYVITAMIN D GENERATION
Liver disease
Anticonvulsants
DECREASED CALCITRIOL FORMATION
Vitamin D-dependent rickets type I
RESISTANCE TO CALCITRIOL (vitamin D-dependent rickets type II)
ACUTE PANCREATITIS
HYPOMAGNESEMIA
HUNGRY BONE SYNDROME

Although the serum phosphate level may provide a clue as to the etiology of the hypocalcemia, the serum phosphate level may be affected by many factors. For this reason, further evaluation is usually necessary to establish the etiology of the hypocalcemia.

Proceed to Step 4.

STEP 4 – *Is the Cause of the Hypocalcemia Readily Apparent?*

Some of the causes of hypocalcemia are readily apparent after a thorough history and physical examination. Causes of hypocalcemia that are readily apparent include the following.

- Acute pancreatitis

  Acute pancreatitis results in both hypomagnesemia and hypocalcemia, secondary to saponification of magnesium and calcium in necrotic fat. A thorough history, physical exam, and an amylase level will be helpful in establishing the diagnosis.

- Sepsis

  Hypocalcemia has been appreciated in 80% of patients in the intensive care unit setting. This is usually due to a decrease in albumin and therefore is not true hypocalcemia. However, in some septic patients, true hypocalcemia may be observed.

- Medications

  Hypocalcemia may be seen with a number of medications, many of which are used in the treatment of hypercalcemia.

MEDICATIONS CAUSING HYPOCALCEMIA	
CALCITONIN	CITRATED BLOOD
MITHRAMYCIN	FOSCARNET
BISPHOSPHONATES	PENTAMIDINE
PHOSPHATE (oral or intravenous)	RADIOGRAPHIC CONTRAST DYES
PHENYTOIN	FLUORIDE
PHENOBARBITAL	

- Hungry bone syndrome

  The "hungry bone syndrome" occurs in patients having surgery to correct primary or secondary hyperparathyroidism. With successful surgery, there is a rapid fall in the PTH which leads to a significant decrease in bone resorption in the wake of ongoing mineralization.

- Tumor lysis syndrome

  The tumor lysis syndrome occurs in patients receiving chemotherapy for hematologic or solid malignancies. Rarely, it can occur without chemotherapy in patients with cancer. Destruction of the tumor results in hyperuricemia, hyperphosphatemia, hypocalcemia, and hyperkalemia. Hypocalcemia is the result of the precipitation of calcium phosphate in the extravascular tissues.

- Osteoblastic metastases

  Hypocalcemia may occur due to osteoblastic metastases. In these patients, growth factors produced by tumor cells in bone stimulate osteoblastic bone formation. This stimulation of bone formation requires increased calcium entry into the skeleton. The diagnosis is usually readily apparent because patients with osteoblastic metastases typically have widespread disease and markedly increased alkaline phosphatase level. The malignancies most commonly associated with hypocalcemia due to osteoblastic metastases include carcinoma of the breast and prostate.

- Rhabdomyolysis

  Rhabdomyolysis refers to the breakdown of muscle. There are many causes of rhabdomyolysis. Laboratory features include an elevated CK, hyperkalemia, hyperphosphatemia, and hypocalcemia. Hypocalcemia is the result of precipitation of calcium phosphate in the extravascular tissues.

- Chronic renal failure

  As chronic renal insufficiency progresses, there are derangements in calcium and phosphorus metabolism. One of the earliest is the development of hyperphosphatemia. The kidney is also the site of hydroxylation of vitamin D at the 1 position, converting 25-hydroxyvitamin D to 1,25-dihydroxyvitamin D, the physiologically active form of vitamin D necessary for calcium absorption. With worsening renal insufficiency, the activity of this enzyme is impaired. These changes, among others, predispose the patient to the development of hypocalcemia.

- Hypomagnesemia

  Hypomagnesemia can lead to hypocalcemia. Magnesium deficiency impairs the action of PTH at the level of bone. It also leads to the impaired release of PTH from the parathyroid glands.

If the patient has one of the above causes of hypocalcemia, ***stop here***.

If the patient does not have one of the above causes of hypocalcemia, ***proceed to Step 5***.

STEP 5 – *What Is the PTH Level?*

The remaining causes of hypocalcemia can be narrowed further by consideration of the serum PTH level.

If the patient has a low PTH level, ***proceed to Step 6***.

If the patient has a high PTH level, ***proceed to Step 7***.

STEP 6 – *Does the Patient Have Hypoparathyroidism?*

In the absence of hypomagnesemia, a low PTH level is consistent with the diagnosis of hypoparathyroidism. The causes of hypoparathyroidism are listed in the following box.

CAUSES OF HYPOPARATHYROIDISM
IDIOPATHIC DiGeorge's syndrome Congenital absence of parathyroids Associated with polyglandular autoimmune disorders* Isolated late onset POSTSURGICAL† TRANSIENT SUPPRESSION INFILTRATIVE DISEASE‡ IRRADIATION#

*Hypoparathyroidism, occurring as part of the polyglandular autoimmune disorder type I, is the most common type of idiopathic hypoparathyroidism. In this disorder, hypoparathyroidism is typically associated with chronic mucocutaneous candidiasis and primary adrenal insufficiency. Other autoimmune disorders, such as pernicious anemia, diabetes mellitus, vitiligo, primary hypogonadism, and thyroid disease, have also been described in these patients.

†Postsurgical hypoparathyroidism usually occurs in patients who have had extensive thyroid surgery (ie, near-total thyroidectomy for thyroid cancer). Inadvertent removal of the parathyroid glands results in the onset of hypocalcemia within 24 hours of surgery. These patients have permanent hypocalcemia. In other patients, the hypocalcemia may be transient, lasting anywhere from 2 weeks to 6 months. In transient cases, the hypocalcemia is likely to be due to trauma or ischemia during the surgery.

‡There are infiltrative diseases as well that can lead to hypoparathyroidism and hypocalcemia. Wilson's disease, hemochromatosis, granulomatous diseases, and metastasis are some examples.

#Hypoparathyroidism can result from external radiation to the neck. It has also occurred following low dose radioactive iodine therapy for Graves' disease.

End of Section.

STEP 7 – *What Are the Considerations in the Patient With a High Serum PTH Level?*

High serum PTH levels should prompt the clinician to consider the following causes:

- Vitamin D deficiency
- Vitamin D-dependent rickets type I and II
- Pseudohypoparathyroidism
- Severe liver disease
- Chronic renal failure
- Nephrotic syndrome
- Hypomagnesemia

The clinical presentation often allows the clinician to differentiate among the above conditions. If necessary, biochemical testing can be performed to confirm the diagnosis. As shown in the following table, measurement of the serum phosphate level and vitamin D metabolites are the tests needed to establish the diagnosis. Vitamin D metabolites that should be obtained include 25-hydroxyvitamin D, also known as 25(OH)D, and 1,25 dihydroxyvitamin D, also known as 1,25$(OH)_2$D3.

Biochemical Findings in Hypocalcemic Conditions Associated With Increased PTH

Diagnosis	Phosphate	PTH	25(OH)D	$1,25(OH)_2D3$
Vitamin D deficiency	Decreased	Increased	Decreased	Decreased, normal, increased
Severe liver disease	Decreased	Increased	Decreased	Decreased, normal, increased
Chronic renal failure	Increased	Increased	Normal	Decreased
Nephrotic syndrome	Decreased	Increased	Decreased	Decreased, normal
Pseudo-hypoparathyroidism	Increased	Increased	Normal	Decreased
Vitamin D-dependent rickets type I	Decreased	Increased	Normal, increased	Decreased
Vitamin D-dependent rickets type II	Decreased	Increased	Normal, increased	Increased

Some of the above causes are discussed in further detail in the remainder of this step.

Vitamin D Deficiency

Vitamin D is either ingested or produced by the skin after exposure to ultraviolet irradiation. The causes of vitamin D deficiency are listed in the following box.

CAUSES OF VITAMIN D DEFICIENCY

DECREASED INTAKE
IMPAIRED ABSORPTION*
LACK OF SUNLIGHT
INCREASED LOSS (nephrotic syndrome)
MEDICATION EFFECT (anticonvulsants)†
DECREASED PRODUCTION (liver disease, chronic renal failure)

*Conditions associated with the malabsorption of fat can result in vitamin D deficiency. Examples of fat malabsorptive states include chronic pancreatitis, primary biliary cirrhosis, short bowel syndrome, celiac disease, sprue, ingestion of cathartics, and gastrectomy.

†The mechanism of vitamin D deficiency secondary to anticonvulsant therapy is not clear.

In the United States, dietary deficiency of vitamin D is rarely encountered because milk products and other foods are supplemented with vitamin D. It can occur, however, in the elderly and in malnourished alcoholics, particularly when decreased intake is combined with lack of sunlight. Immigrants from the Middle East who migrate to northern latitudes are also susceptible to vitamin D deficiency. These immigrants have decreased exposure to sunlight because they continue to wear traditional clothing.

Chronic Renal Failure

As chronic renal insufficiency progresses, there are derangements in calcium and phosphorus metabolism. One of the earliest is the development of hyperphosphatemia. The kidney is also the site of hydroxylation of vitamin D at the 1 position, converting 25-hydroxyvitamin D to 1,25-dihydroxyvitamin D, the physiologically active form of vitamin D necessary for calcium absorption. With worsening renal insufficiency, the activity of this enzyme is impaired. These changes, among others, predispose the patient to the development of hypocalcemia. In chronic renal failure, the 25(OH)D level will be normal and the 1,25$(OH)_2$D3 level will be decreased.

Severe Liver Disease

In patients with severe liver disease, 25 hydroxylation of vitamin D may be impaired. This will lead to low 25(OH)D levels.

References

Body JJ and Bouillon R, "Emergencies of Calcium Homeostasis," *Rev Endocr Metab Disord*, 2003, 4(2):167-75.

Bushinsky DA and Monk RD, "Calcium," *Lancet*, 1998, 352(9124):306-11.

Carlstedt F and Lind L, "Hypocalcemic Syndromes," *Crit Care Clin*, 2001, 17(1):139-53, vii-viii.

Fukugawa M and Kurokawa K, "Calcium Homeostasis and Imbalance," *Nephron*, 2002, 92(Suppl 1):41-5.

Marx SJ, "Hyperparathyroid and Hypoparathyroid Disorders," *N Engl J Med*, 2000, 343(25):1863-75.

Thomas MK and Demay MB, "Vitamin D Deficiency and Disorders of Vitamin D Metabolism," *Endocrinol Metab Clin North Am*, 2000, 29(3):611-27, viii.

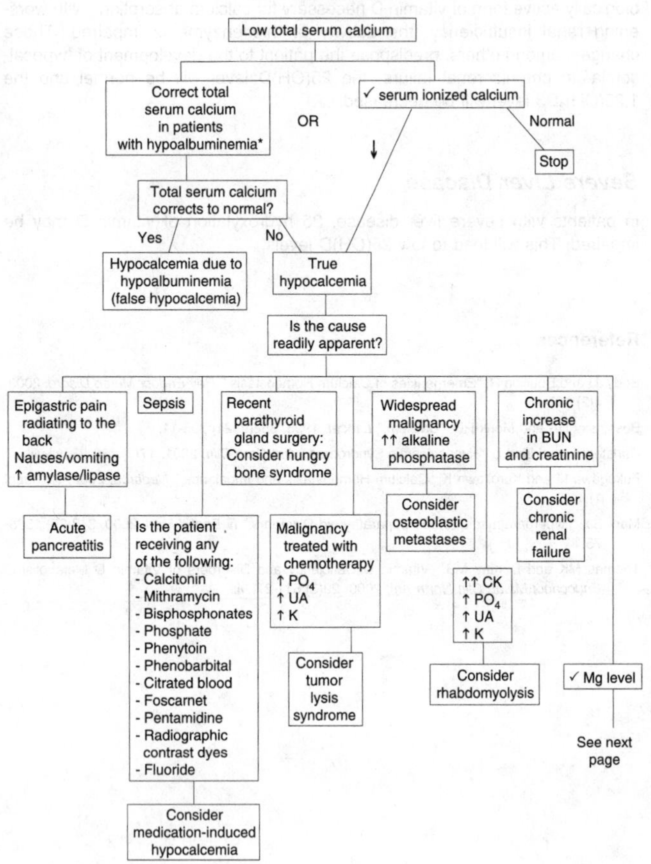
HYPOCALCEMIA
Low total serum calcium
Correct total serum calcium in patients with hypoalbuminemia*
OR
✓ serum ionized calcium
↓
Normal
Stop
Total serum calcium corrects to normal?
Yes
No
Hypocalcemia due to hypoalbuminemia (false hypocalcemia)
True hypocalcemia
Is the cause readily apparent?
Epigastric pain radiating to the back
Nauses/vomiting
↑ amylase/lipase
Acute pancreatitis
Sepsis
Is the patient receiving any of the following:
- Calcitonin
- Mithramycin
- Bisphosphonates
- Phosphate
- Phenytoin
- Phenobarbital
- Citrated blood
- Foscarnet
- Pentamidine
- Radiographic contrast dyes
- Fluoride
Consider medication-induced hypocalcemia
Recent parathyroid gland surgery: Consider hungry bone syndrome
Malignancy treated with chemotherapy
↑ PO4
↑ UA
↑ K
Consider tumor lysis syndrome
Widespread malignancy
↑↑ alkaline phosphatase
Consider osteoblastic metastases
↑↑ CK
↑ PO4
↑ UA
↑ K
Consider rhabdomyolysis
Chronic increase in BUN and creatinine
Consider chronic renal failure
✓ Mg level
See next page

*Corrected calcium = measured calcium + 0.8 (4 - patient's albumin)

HYPOCALCEMIA *(continued)*

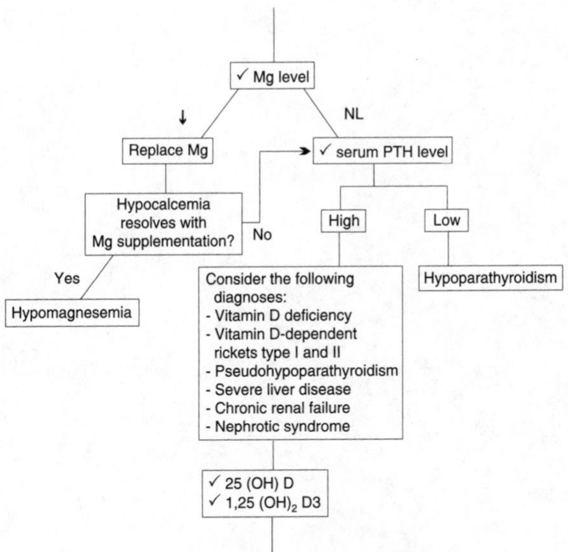

See table "Biochemical Findings in Hypocalcemic Conditions Associated With Increased pH," in this chapter

HYPERCALCEMIA

STEP 1 – *Does the Patient Have Hypercalcemia?*

The normal range for total serum calcium is 8.5-10.5 mg/dL. Hypercalcemia, which is defined as a total serum calcium level above the upper limit of normal, is reported in about 0.1% of the general population.

Forty percent of the total serum calcium is protein-bound. Because of this, changes in the serum albumin or globulin concentration can affect the total serum calcium level. Every 1 g/dL increase in the serum albumin concentration above 4 g/dL will increase the total serum calcium level by 0.8 mg/dL. An increase in the serum globulin level by 1 g/dL will increase the serum calcium concentration by 0.16 mg/dL. When an increase in the total serum calcium concentration is due to an increase in the serum albumin or globulin level, no further evaluation is necessary because changes in protein concentration do not affect free calcium. Only increases in free calcium can result in the clinical manifestations of hypercalcemia.

The clinician should also realize that a decrease in the serum albumin concentration can lead to a decrease in the total serum calcium level. This may mask the presence of hypercalcemia if the clinician does not correct the total serum calcium concentration for the degree of hypoalbuminemia, using the following formula:

$$\text{Calcium (corrected)} = \text{Calcium (measured)} + [(4.0 - \text{albumin}) \times 0.8]$$

Dehydration or hemoconcentration during venipuncture may result in a falsely elevated total serum calcium level. Gross hemolysis can also falsely elevate the total serum calcium concentration.

When an elevated total serum calcium concentration is obtained, it should be repeated to confirm the presence of hypercalcemia. If necessary, the clinician may choose to measure the serum ionized calcium level to confirm the presence of true hypercalcemia. This is a measure of the physiologically active calcium present in the serum. It will be normal in patients who have falsely elevated total serum calcium levels and in those who have increased serum calcium levels due to an increase in the serum albumin or globulin concentration.

If the patient has true hypercalcemia, ***proceed to Step 2.***

If the patient does not have true hypercalcemia, ***stop here.***

STEP 2 – *What Are the Causes of Hypercalcemia?*

The causes of hypercalcemia are listed in the following box.

PTH-DEPENDENT HYPERCALCEMIA	
Primary hyperparathyroidism	Lithium therapy
Familial hypocalciuric hypercalcemia	Secondary / tertiary hyperparathyroidism
PTH-INDEPENDENT HYPERCALCEMIA	
Malignancy	Milk-alkali syndrome
Vitamin A / D intoxication	Acute renal failure (diuretic phase)
Endocrine disorders	Medication-induced
Hyperthyroidism	Calcium supplements
Adrenal insufficiency	Vitamin D administration
Acromegaly	Theophylline
Pancreatic islet cell tumors	Thiazide diuretics
Pheochromocytoma	Antiestrogens
Granulomatous disease	(in treatment of breast cancer)
Immobilization	Paget's disease
	Parenteral nutrition

Although there are many causes of hypercalcemia, primary hyperparathyroidism and malignancy account for 80% to 90% of cases.

Proceed to Step 3.

STEP 3 – *What Is the Serum Phosphate Level?*

The serum phosphate level may provide a clue to the diagnosis, as shown in the following table.

USING THE SERUM PHOSPHATE LEVEL AS A CLUE TO THE DIAGNOSIS OF HYPERCALCEMIA

If the serum phosphate level is low, consider...	If the serum phosphate level is normal or high, consider...
Primary hyperparathyroidism	Granulomatous disease
Humoral hypercalcemia of malignancy (mediated by PTHrP)	Vitamin D intoxication
	Thyrotoxicosis
	Milk alkali syndrome
	Malignancy (metastatic bone disease)
	Immobilization

Although the serum phosphate level may provide a clue to the diagnosis, in and of itself, it cannot be used to establish the cause of the hypercalcemia with certainty.

Proceed to Step 4.

STEP 4 – *What Is the Serum PTH Level?*

Knowledge of the serum PTH level can help divide patients with hypercalcemia into PTH-dependent and PTH-independent causes (see box above). Remember that hypercalcemia should result in a low or undetectable serum PTH level through a negative-feedback system. This will occur if the hypercalcemia is mediated through a PTH-independent mechanism. The serum PTH will be high if the hypercalcemia is PTH-dependent. When measuring the serum PTH level, it is important to ensure that the lab is using an immunoradiometric assay, which is more sensitive and specific than previous assays.

If the serum PTH is high, ***proceed to Step 5.***

If the serum PTH is low, ***proceed to Step 7.***

STEP 5 – *What Are the Causes of PTH-Dependent Hypercalcemia?*

Patients who have an elevated serum PTH level are said to have PTH-dependent hypercalcemia, the causes of which are listed in the following box.

CAUSES OF PTH-DEPENDENT HYPERCALCEMIA
PRIMARY HYPERPARATHYROIDISM
FAMILIAL HYPOCALCIURIC HYPERCALCEMIA
LITHIUM THERAPY
SECONDARY / TERTIARY HYPERPARATHYROIDISM

Proceed to Step 6.

STEP 6 – *What Type of PTH-Dependent Hypercalcemia Does the Patient Have?*

The different types of PTH-dependent hypercalcemia are discussed in the remainder of this step.

Primary Hyperparathyroidism

Primary hyperparathyroidism, which is the most common cause of hypercalcemia in otherwise healthy outpatients, results from the inappropriate secretion of PTH by parathyroid adenoma, hyperplasia, or carcinoma. Eight-five percent of primary hyperparathyroidism cases are due to parathyroid adenoma while multiple adenomas and hyperplasia account for 5% and 10% of cases, respectively. Parathyroid carcinoma accounts for <1% of cases.

As plasma calcium is part of various biochemical panels, most patients with primary hyperparathyroidism are diagnosed when they are asymptomatic. The hallmarks of primary hyperparathyroidism are hypercalcemia and an elevated serum PTH level. Other laboratory test findings that support this diagnosis are included in the following box.

PRIMARY HYPERPARATHYROIDISM LABORATORY FEATURES
ELEVATED SERUM CALCIUM
ELEVATED SERUM CHLORIDE
SERUM CHLORIDE / PHOSPHATE RATIO >33
ELEVATED URINARY pH
ELEVATED PARATHYROID HORMONE
ELEVATED URINE CALCIUM
NORMAL OR DECREASED SERUM PHOSPHATE
ELEVATED ALKALINE PHOSPHATASE*
HYPERCHLOREMIC METABOLIC ACIDOSIS†
ELEVATED URINE cAMP
ELEVATED BUN / CREATININE‡

*This occurs only in the setting of bone disease associated with primary hyperparathyroidism.

†This occurs secondary to the effects of increased parathyroid hormone on acid-base balance at the level of the kidney.

‡Most patients with primary hyperparathyroidism do not have renal insufficiency. However, renal insufficiency may develop if hypercalcemia is of prolonged duration and sufficient severity.

The clinician should realize that not all patients with primary hyperparathyroidism will have an elevated serum PTH level. In fact, 10% to 20% will present with high-normal levels. In these patients, the key to the diagnosis is to realize that a high-normal serum PTH level is inappropriate in the patient with hypercalcemia. An appropriate response is suppression of the serum PTH level.

Although parathyroidectomy is the only definitive treatment for primary hyperparathyroidism, not all patients need to be referred for surgery. Listed below are the general indications for parathyroidectomy. Some of the indications are based on specific laboratory testing.

INDICATIONS FOR PARATHYROIDECTOMY IN PRIMARY HYPERPARATHYROIDISM
SYMPTOMATIC HYPERCALCEMIA
TOTAL SERUM CALCIUM CONCENTRATION >1.0 mg/dL ABOVE THE UPPER LIMIT OF NORMAL
24-HOUR URINARY CALCIUM EXCRETION >400 mg
DECREASING CREATININE CLEARANCE (<70% OF NORMAL)
DECREASED AND DECREASING BONE DENSITY (>2 SD)
AGE <50 YEARS WITH MILD HYPERCALCEMIA
CALCIUM NEPHROLITHIASIS
PATIENT PREFERENCE FOR SURGERY
INABILITY TO UNDERGO PROLONGED FOLLOW-UP

Primary hyperparathyroidism patients who do not meet criteria for surgery should be followed carefully. An NIH consensus conference has recommended initial follow-up on a semiannual basis. For patients who remain stable, follow-up at longer intervals is reasonable. During follow-up, patients should be assessed for symptoms of hypercalcemia. In addition, measurement of the serum/urine calcium and creatinine levels are required to assess for the development of hypercalcemia, hypercalciuria, and decreasing creatinine clearance, all of which are indications for surgical treatment. Abdominal radiographs should be ordered every year and bone densitometry should be performed at 1- to 2-year intervals.

Secondary / Tertiary Hyperparathyroidism

In contrast to primary hyperparathyroidism in which there is autonomous secretion of excessive PTH, excessive PTH secretion in secondary hyperparathyroidism is a normal response to hypocalcemia, hyperphosphatemia, or low calcitriol levels. The latter three abnormalities are all seen in patients with chronic renal failure, which is the most common cause of secondary hyperparathyroidism. The excessive PTH secretion is an attempt to bring the total serum calcium concentration back into the normal range.

In patients with secondary hyperparathyroidism, prolonged hypocalcemia may eventually result in autonomous production and secretion of PTH. When this occurs, the patient is said to have progressed from secondary to tertiary hyperparathyroidism. Serum PTH levels are often >10-20 times normal.

Lithium Therapy

Many patients treated with lithium for bipolar affective disorders have an increase in the serum calcium concentration. Quite often, this increase is mild and does not exceed the normal reference range. On occasion, hypercalcemia may be encountered. If the hypercalcemia is mild and the patient is asymptomatic, lithium therapy is often continued. If severe or the patient is symptomatic, lithium therapy should be stopped. When lithium therapy is discontinued, in most cases, the serum calcium level returns to normal. In some patients, however, hypercalcemia persists. Surgical treatment should be considered in these patients using the same guidelines that have been developed for primary hyperparathyroidism patients. When the parathyroid glands are examined at the time of surgery, parathyroid hyperplasia is most commonly noted.

Familial Hypocalciuric Hypercalcemia

This is an autosomal dominant condition characterized by a gene mutation affecting the calcium-sensing receptor. As a result of the mutation, the parathyroid glands cannot recognize the actual extracellular calcium concentration, which then leads to excessive production of PTH.

Patients with familial hypocalciuric hypercalcemia have mild to moderate hypercalcemia. It can be difficult to distinguish these patients from those with mild primary hyperparathyroidism. The distinction is an important one, however, since patients with familial hypocalciuric hypercalcemia, in contrast to primary hyperparathyroidism, are not cured of their disease if taken for parathyroidectomy. No laboratory testing is 100% reliable in differentiating between these two conditions. The clinical picture and laboratory profile taken together, however, usually allows the clinician to make the distinction in the majority of cases.

Symptomatic hypercalcemia is not a feature of this condition and if symptoms are present, the clinician should search for another etiology. Serum PTH levels are normal or mildly elevated. Clues to the diagnosis are a family history of hypercalcemia, lack of symptoms, and low urinary calcium excretion (urinary calcium to creatinine clearance ratio <0.01). The latter feature is particularly useful in distinguishing familial hypocalciuric hypercalcemia from primary hyperparathyroidism (>0.02 in primary hyperparathyroidism). The clinician should realize that familial hypocalciuric hypercalcemia is not the only cause of hypercalcemia that presents with hypocalciuria. Two other considerations include thiazide diuretic use and the milk-alkali syndrome.

End of Section.

STEP 7 – *What Are the Causes of PTH-Independent Hypercalcemia?*

A low or low-normal serum PTH level should prompt the clinician to consider the causes of PTH-independent hypercalcemia, the causes of which are listed in the following box.

CAUSES OF PTH-INDEPENDENT HYPERCALCEMIA	
MALIGNANCY	MEDICATION-INDUCED
VITAMIN A / D INTOXICATION	Calcium supplements
ENDOCRINE DISORDERS	Vitamin D administration
Hyperthyroidism	Theophylline
Adrenal insufficiency	Thiazide diuretics
Acromegaly	Antiestrogens (in treatment
Pancreatic islet cell tumors	of breast cancer)
Pheochromocytoma	PAGET'S DISEASE
GRANULOMATOUS DISEASE	PARENTERAL NUTRITION
IMMOBILIZATION	
MILK-ALKALI SYNDROME	
ACUTE RENAL FAILURE (diuretic phase)	

Although there are many causes of PTH-independent hypercalcemia, malignancy is the most common cause.

Proceed to Step 8.

STEP 8 – *Does the Patient Have Malignancy?*

Hypercalcemia of malignancy is the most common cause of hypercalcemia in hospitalized patients. Among outpatients, it is the second most common cause of hypercalcemia. Most patients with malignancy-associated hypercalcemia present after the diagnosis of malignancy has been made. However, hypercalcemia can be an occult manifestation of malignancy. When malignancy is not clinically evident, the evaluation often includes mammography, chest radiography, chest CT, abdominal CT, and serum/urine immunoelectrophoresis in an effort to identify the occult malignancy.

The finding of an elevated serum calcium concentration for more than 6 months argues against the diagnosis of malignancy-associated hypercalcemia, because most patients with malignancy-associated hypercalcemia succumb to their disease within months. In one study, the mean time to death after the development of hypercalcemia of malignancy was 4-6 weeks.

If the patient does not have a malignancy, ***proceed to Step 9.***

If the patient has a malignancy, ***see below.***

Hypercalcemia may be a complication of both solid and hematologic malignancies but the former accounts for 80% to 90% of malignancy-associated hypercalcemia. For years, it was thought that hypercalcemia was simply secondary to invasion of bone with subsequent bony destruction. While this does play a role in some types of malignancy, it is now know that tumors can secrete humoral mediators that lead to the development of hypercalcemia. The four types of malignancy-associated hypercalcemia are described in the following box.

MALIGNANCY-ASSOCIATED HYPERCALCEMIA: MECHANISTIC CLASSIFICATION AND COMMONLY ASSOCIATED TUMOR TYPES
HUMORAL HYPERCALCEMIA OF MALIGNANCY*
Squamous cell carcinoma (eg, lung, cervix, head and neck, esophagus)
Renal carcinoma
Bladder carcinoma
Ovarian carcinoma
Breast carcinoma
HTLV-1 lymphoma leukemia
LOCAL OSTEOLYTIC HYPERCALCEMIA#
Breast carcinoma
Multiple myeloma
Lymphoma leukemia
1,25 (OH)2 VITAMIN D-PRODUCING TUMORS+
Lymphoma
ECTOPIC PARATHYROID HORMONE SECRETION

*The humoral hypercalcemia of malignancy is the most common type of malignancy-associated hypercalcemia. In these patients, there is little or no skeletal metastatic involvement. The mechanism of the hypercalcemia with these malignancies involves the production and secretion of parathyroid hormone related peptide (PTH-rp), which was discovered in 1987 and has been found to be responsible for approximately 75% of hypercalcemia encountered in patients with malignancy. PTH-rp shares some degree of homology with PTH, thereby explaining some of the biochemical similarities between patients with primary hyperparathyroidism and the humoral hypercalcemia of malignancy. The diagnosis can be confirmed by demonstrating an elevated concentration of serum PTH-rp (two-site assays using radioimmunometric, immunofluorometric, or immunochemiluminescence techniques are the more sensitive and specific PTH-rp tests). In usual clinical practice, however, this test is not often performed because most patients have clinically evident malignancy. Testing should be considered if a hypercalcemic patient is suspected of having malignancy but an extensive evaluation fails to detect the underlying malignancy.

#Local osteolytic hypercalcemia is the mechanism in about 20% of malignancy-associated hypercalcemia cases. Multiple myeloma, breast cancer, lymphoma, and leukemia are examples of malignancies that present in this fashion. In these cases, tumor cells invade the bone marrow and produce cytokines which activate osteoclasts, leading to bone resorption with subsequent hypercalcemia. In these patients, bone scans usually reveal extensive skeletal metastatic involvement.

+Some patients with lymphoma have been found to have elevated levels of 1,25-dihydroxyvitamin D (or calcitriol). The mechanism seems to be similar to that observed with granulomatous diseases. The malignant lymphocytes are able to convert 25-hydroxyvitamin D to 1,25-dihydroxyvitamin D.

Adapted from Kinder BK and Stewart AF, "Hypercalcemia," *Curr Probl Surg*, 2002, 39(4):382.

End of Section.

STEP 9 – *What Causes of Hypercalcemia Should Be Considered in Patients With Low Serum PTH Levels Who Do Not Have Malignancy-Associated Hypercalcemia?*

Malignancy is the most common cause of hypercalcemia presenting with low serum PTH levels. If malignancy-associated hypercalcemia is not present, the clinician should consider the other causes of hypercalcemia, which are discussed in the remainder of this step.

Sarcoidosis / Other Granulomatous Disease

Hypercalcemia has been reported in approximately 10% of patients with sarcoidosis. This results from macrophages converting 25-hydroxyvitamin D to 1,25-dihydroxyvitamin D in the granulomas because of overexpression of the enzyme 1-α-hydroxylase. Other granulomatous diseases associated with hypercalcemia include tuberculosis, histoplasmosis, coccidioidomycosis, cryptococcus, blastomycosis, nocardiosis, cat-scratch disease, disseminated candidiasis, silicon-induced granulomatosis, leprosy, berylliosis, Wegener's granulomatosis, and borreliosis. An elevated 1,25-dihydroxyvitamin D level supports the diagnosis.

Milk-Alkali Syndrome

The milk-alkali syndrome is characterized by the triad of hypercalcemia, metabolic alkalosis, and renal insufficiency. Originally described in patients ingesting significant amounts of dairy calcium along with absorbable antacids, the milk-alkali syndrome decreased in incidence over the years as physicians prescribed H_2-blockers and nonabsorbable antacids. However, it is seen more often now with the increased use of calcium carbonate in patients with osteoporosis. It should be a consideration in hypercalcemic patients who are ingesting >2 g of elemental calcium per day (>5 g of calcium carbonate).

Hyperthyroidism

Hyperthyroidism leads to a mild increase in the serum calcium concentration secondary to increased bone resorption. A level exceeding 11 mg/dL is unusual and should prompt a search for another etiology. A decreased serum TSH concentration in the setting of an increased free T_4 level establishes the diagnosis.

Thiazide Diuretic

Thiazide diuretics increase the reabsorption of calcium by the kidney. There may be a transient elevation in the serum calcium concentration in the patient who recently started thiazide diuretic therapy but the level returns to normal shortly thereafter. However, starting a thiazide diuretic agent in a patient with a high rate of bone turnover can lead to a sustained increase in the serum calcium concentration. Any patient who develops hypercalcemia while on thiazide diuretic therapy should have an evaluation for an additional underlying etiology, particularly primary hyperparathyroidism.

Vitamin D Intoxication

Vitamin D intoxication is usually iatrogenic. In rare instances, it may result from the surreptitious use of vitamin D. Typically, very large doses (50-100 times the physiologic requirement) are required in order to develop hypercalcemia. Since doses of this degree are only available by prescription, vitamin D intoxication is usually iatrogenic. Symptoms of intoxication include nausea, vomiting, altered mental status, and weakness. Because of fat storage of the vitamin, it may take a long period of time for the hypercalcemia to abate after cessation of vitamin D intake. An elevated 25-hydroxyvitamin D levels supports the diagnosis.

Immobilization

Increased bone resorption and hypercalcemia may occur when patients with high rates of bone turnover are subjected to prolonged bedrest. High rates of bone turnover are seen in children, adolescents, and young adults. High rates may also be appreciated with malignancy, Paget's disease, and hyperparathyroidism. One classic example is the young patient who has suffered a spinal cord injury.

Vitamin A Intoxication

Chronic ingestion of vitamin A (>50,000 units/day) is required for intoxication to occur. It is usually seen in intentional overdose, but more recently, it has been observed with greater frequency in patients taking cis-retinoic acid for the treatment of acne. In addition to the clinical manifestations of hypercalcemia, symptoms of intoxication may include itching, dry skin, bone pain, and headache due to pseudotumor cerebri. High levels of vitamin A confirm the diagnosis.

Familial Hypocalciuric Hypercalcemia

This is an autosomal dominant condition characterized by a gene mutation affecting the calcium-sensing receptor. As a result of the mutation, the parathyroid glands cannot recognize the actual extracellular calcium concentration, which then leads to hypercalcemia.

Patients with familial hypocalciuric hypercalcemia have mild to moderate hypercalcemia. Symptomatic hypercalcemia is not a feature of this condition and if symptoms are present, the clinician should search for another etiology. Serum PTH levels are typically normal but may be mildly elevated. Clues to the diagnosis are a family history of hypercalcemia, lack of symptoms, and low urinary calcium excretion (urinary calcium to creatinine clearance ratio <0.01). The clinician should realize that familial hypocalciuric hypercalcemia is not the only cause of hypercalcemia that presents with hypocalciuria. Two other considerations include thiazide diuretic use and the milk-alkali syndrome.

Miscellaneous Causes

Other causes of hypercalcemia include Addison's disease, pheochromocytoma, rhabdomyolysis, recovery phase of acute renal failure, Vipoma, hypophosphatasia, theophylline, tamoxifen (antiestrogens), dialysis using too high a calcium gradient, and parenteral nutrition.

References

Body JJ and Bouillon R, "Emergencies of Calcium Homeostasis," *Rev Endocr Metab Disord*, 2003, 4(2):167-75.

Bushinsky DA and Monk RD, "Calcium," *Lancet*, 1998, 352(9124):306-11.

Carroll MF and Schade DS, "A Practical Approach to Hypercalcemia," *Am Fam Physician*, 2003, 67(9):1959-66.

Deftos LJ, "Hypercalcemia in Malignant and Inflammatory Diseases," *Endocrinol Metab Clin North Am*, 2002, 31(1):141-58.

Esbrit P, "Hypercalcemia of Malignancy – New Insights Into an Old Syndrome," *Clin Lab*, 2001, 47(1-2):67-71.

Heys SD, Smith IC, and Eremin O, "Hypercalcaemia in Patients With Cancer: Aetiology and Treatment," *Eur J Surg Oncol*, 1998, 24(2):139-42.

Kinder BK and Stewart AF, "Hypercalcemia," *Curr Probl Surg*, 2002, 39(4):349-448.

Klee GG, "Maximizing Efficacy of Endocrine Tests: Importance of Decision-Focused Testing Strategies and Appropriate Patient Preparation," *Clin Chem*, 1999, 45(8 Pt 2):1323-30.

Krempl GA and Medina JE, "Current Issues in Hyperparathyroidism," *Otolaryngol Clin North Am*, 2003, 36(1):207-15.

Marx SJ, "Hyperparathyroid and Hypoparathyroid Disorders," *N Engl J Med*, 2000, 343(25):1863-75.

Sharma OP, "Hypercalcemia in Granulomatous Disorders: A Clinical Review," *Curr Opin Pulm Med*, 2000, 6(5):442-7.

Thirlwell C and Brock CS, "Emergencies in Oncology," *Clin Med*, 2003, 3(4):306-10.

Ziegler R, "Hypercalcemic Crisis," *J Am Soc Nephrol*, 2001, 12(Suppl 17):S3-9.

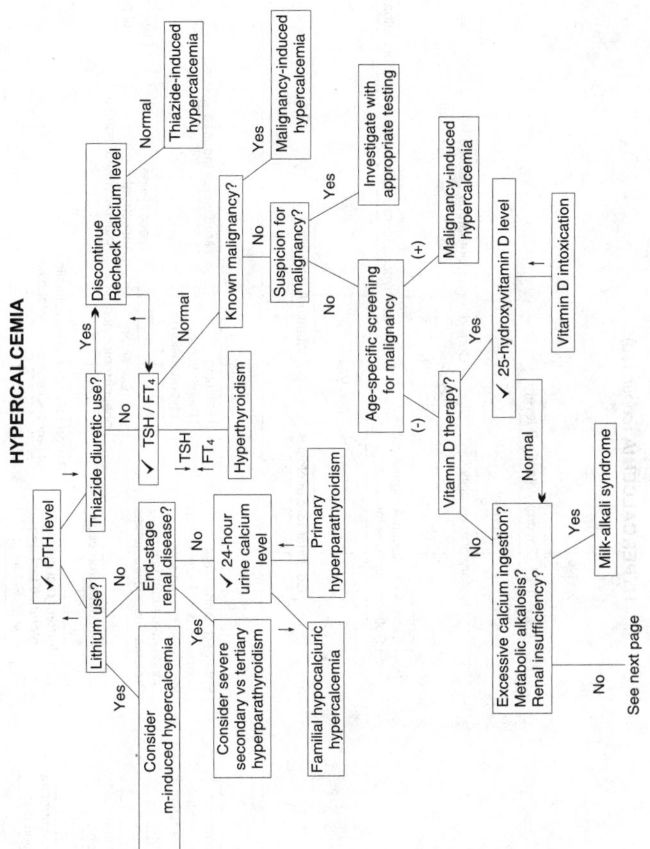
HYPERCALCEMIA
✓ PTH level
↑
Lithium use?
Yes
Consider
m-induced hypercalcemia
No
End-stage
renal disease?
Yes
Consider severe
secondary vs tertiary
hyperparathyroidism
No
✓ 24-hour
urine calcium
level
↓
Familial hypocalciuric
hypercalcemia
↑
Primary
hyperparathyroidism
↓
Thiazide diuretic use?
Yes
Discontinue
Recheck calcium level
↑
Normal
Thiazide-induced
hypercalcemia
No
✓ TSH / FT4
↓TSH
↑FT4
Hyperthyroidism
Normal
Known malignancy?
Yes
Malignancy-induced
hypercalcemia
No
Suspicion for
malignancy?
Yes
Investigate with
appropriate testing
No
Age-specific screening
for malignancy
(+)
Malignancy-induced
hypercalcemia
(-)
Vitamin D therapy?
Yes
✓ 25-hydroxyvitamin D level
↑
Vitamin D intoxication
Normal
No
Excessive calcium ingestion?
Metabolic alkalosis?
Renal insufficiency?
Yes
Milk-alkali syndrome
No
See next page

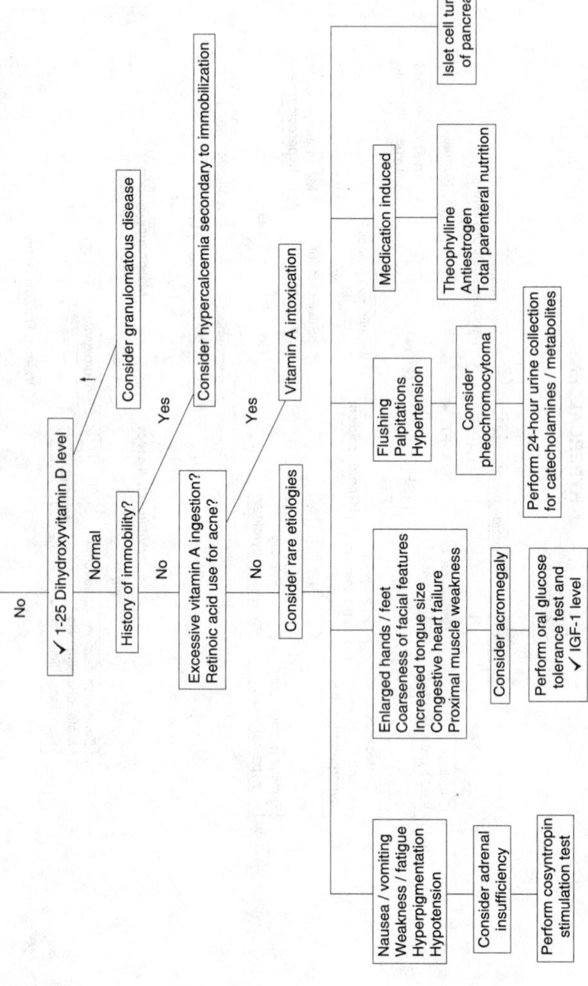
HYPERCALCEMIA (continued)
No
✓ 1-25 Dihydroxyvitamin D level
↑
Consider granulomatous disease
Normal
History of immobility?
Yes
Consider hypercalcemia secondary to immobilization
No
Excessive vitamin A ingestion?
Retinoic acid use for acne?
Yes
Vitamin A intoxication
No
Consider rare etiologies
Nausea / vomiting
Weakness / fatigue
Hyperpigmentation
Hypotension
Consider adrenal insufficiency
Perform cosyntropin stimulation test
Enlarged hands / feet
Coarseness of facial features
Increased tongue size
Congestive heart failure
Proximal muscle weakness
Consider acromegaly
Perform oral glucose tolerance test and ✓ IGF-1 level
Flushing
Palpitations
Hypertension
Consider pheochromocytoma
Perform 24-hour urine collection for catecholamines / metabolites
Medication induced
Theophylline
Antiestrogen
Total parenteral nutrition
Islet cell tumor of pancreas

ANION GAP

Calculating the Serum Anion Gap

In the extracellular fluid, the concentration of positive charges, or cations, always equals the concentration of negative charges, or anions. Most of the cationic charges are due to sodium. Potassium, calcium, magnesium, and other trace metals are also contributors, albeit to a much smaller extent.

Chloride and bicarbonate account for most of the anions in the extracellular fluid. Albumin is also a major contributor. Lactate, phosphate, and sulfate are also anions but are minor contributors to the total anionic charge.

With this in mind, the serum anion gap (AG) may be calculated using the following formula:

$$\mathbf{AG} = Na^{+} - (Cl^{-} + HCO_3^{-})$$

The serum anion gap is really a measure of the difference between the measured cations (serum sodium concentration) and the measured anions (chloride and bicarbonate). The other cations and anions are not present in the formula because sodium, chloride, and bicarbonate are the only charges that the lab routinely measures. Because some of the other anions and cations are not reflected in the formula, there is a disparity between the total positive and negative charges. Under normal circumstances, the negative charges (bicarbonate and chloride) are less than the positive charges (sodium). This difference is known as the serum anion gap.

Normal Serum Anion Gap

Traditionally, the reference range for the serum anion gap has been 12 mEq/L ± 4 mEq/L. This reference range, however, was established many years ago from electrolyte assays that have now been replaced by ion-selective electrode methodology.

This shift in methodology has resulted in a change in the reference range for a normal serum anion gap. The reference range is now considered to be 3-11 mEq/L. This new reference range should now be used in place of the old reference range of 12 mEq/L ±4 mEq/L only if ion-selective electrode techniques are used to measure serum electrolyte concentrations. Although most laboratories are using this newer method, it behooves the clinician to determine precisely what technique is being used at their particular institution. Many laboratories have established their own reference interval for the anion gap. If this is the case, the clinician should use this reference range in the interpretation of the patient's anion gap.

Causes of a High Serum Anion Gap

While a high serum anion gap is most often considered in patients with metabolic acidosis, there are other causes of an elevated serum anion gap, as shown in the following box.

CAUSES OF A HIGH SERUM ANION GAP

METABOLIC ACIDOSIS
- Uremia*
- Ketoacidosis (diabetic, alcoholic, starvation)
- Lactic acidosis†
- Intoxication
  - Salicylate
  - Ethylene glycol
  - Methanol‡

DEHYDRATION OR FLUID LOSS (relatively little unmeasured anions)

NONKETOTIC HYPEROSMOLAR COMA§

SALTS / ORGANIC ACIDS INFUSION (lactate, acetate, citrate, penicillin, carbenicillin)

REDUCED UNMEASURED CATIONS (magnesium, calcium, potassium)

ALKALEMIA¶

LABORATORY ERROR

*Patients with end-stage renal disease may have a normal anion gap metabolic acidosis, high anion gap metabolic acidosis, or a mixed type of metabolic acidosis. In one study of predialysis patients with end-stage renal disease, only 30% had a pure high anion gap metabolic acidosis. Twenty-four percent had a normal anion gap metabolic acidosis while 46% had a mixed pattern. With the institution of dialysis, a normal anion gap metabolic acidosis is more commonly encountered.

†Lactic acidosis is classically associated with a high anion gap metabolic acidosis. It is important to realize, however, that patients with mild to moderate lactic acidosis may present with a normal anion gap.

‡The metabolic acidosis of methanol intoxication is largely due to the metabolism of methanol to formic acid. This most often leads to the development of a high anion gap metabolic acidosis. Occasionally, patients present with both methanol and alcohol poisoning. In these patients, the alcohol ingestion may inhibit the metabolism of methanol. A high anion gap may not be noted in these patients (acidosis may be absent as well!). The absence of an elevated anion gap should not prompt the clinician to discard this diagnosis.

§A high anion gap may also be appreciated in patients with nonketotic hyperosmolar coma. In one study, the average serum anion gap was 34 mEq/L. This was not explained by concomitant lactic acidosis or ketoacidosis. Although, in some, the high anion gap was accompanied by metabolic acidosis, others had normal acid-base status.

¶A high anion gap is commonly encountered in patients with alkalosis. In one study, 47% of hospitalized patients with alkalosis were noted to have a high serum anion gap.

From the preceding box, it is quite obvious that there are many causes of an elevated serum anion gap. Therefore, the presence of a high serum anion gap is not synonymous with a diagnosis of metabolic acidosis. Studies of patients presenting with elevated serum anion gap have shown that metabolic acidosis is the explanation for only 50% of these cases. The other 50% have either a normal or alkalotic pH.

Furthermore, many of the causes of high anion gap metabolic acidosis may present with normal serum anion gap. The clinician should keep this consideration in mind when interpreting the serum anion gap in patients with metabolic acidosis.

Causes of a Low Serum Anion Gap

The causes of a low serum anion gap are listed in the following box.

CAUSES OF A LOW SERUM ANION GAP

INCREASED UNMEASURED CATIONS

NORMALLY PRESENT
- Potassium
- Calcium
- Magnesium

NOT NORMALLY PRESENT
- IgG multiple myeloma
- Polyclonal gammopathy
- Lithium
- Polymyxin B

DECREASED UNMEASURED ANIONS
- Hypoalbuminemia

SODIUM UNDERESTIMATION*
- Hyperviscosity
- Severe hypernatremia

CHLORIDE OVERESTIMATION
- Hypertriglyceridemia†
- Bromide‡
- Iodide

OTHER REPORTED CAUSES
- Renal transplantation
- Hyponatremia

*A low sodium underestimation is more likely to occur with the use of flame atomic emission spectrometry. Over the years, flame atomic emission spectrometry has largely been supplanted by ion-selective techniques. Sodium underestimation is less likely with these newer techniques.

†With the use of colorimetric assays.

‡Observed with all currently available laboratory methods.

Adapted from Jurado R, del Rio C, Nassar G, et al, "Low Anion Gap," *Southern Med J*, 1998, 91(7):626.

Significance of a Low Serum Anion Gap

The presence of a low serum anion gap should prompt the clinician to consider the causes of low serum anion gap listed in the preceding box. In these conditions, a low serum anion gap is a clue to the diagnosis, often occurring in patients who have signs or symptoms of the underlying disease. On occasion, however, the low serum anion gap may be the only manifestation of one of the above conditions (asymptomatic plasma cell dyscrasia).

The clinician should also realize that a low baseline serum anion gap may mask the identification of a condition that is normally associated with a high anion gap. For example, take the patient who has a baseline serum anion gap of 1 mEq/L. If this patient develops lactic acidosis, a common cause of high anion gap metabolic acidosis, the anion gap may rise to 9 mEq/L. This is a significant rise in the serum anion gap and had this patient had what we consider a normal anion gap, the increase of 8 mEq/L would have pushed this patient's serum anion gap above the normal range. Because the patient's baseline serum anion gap was low, however, the increase in the anion gap to 9 mEq/L may be interpreted as a normal anion gap metabolic acidosis. In such a patient, the clinician may erroneously discard the diagnosis of lactic acidosis.

To avoid missing a high anion gap metabolic acidosis in the patient with a low baseline serum anion gap, the clinician should compare the current anion gap with previous values. By doing so, the clinician will be able to recognize the presence of a low baseline serum anion gap, which will allow the clinician to correctly interpret the patient's current acid-base status.

Approach to the Patient With a Low Serum Anion Gap

The evaluation of the patient with low serum anion gap should begin with consideration of hyperkalemia, hypercalcemia, and hypermagnesemia. If hypercalcemia is present, it may be the sole cause of the reduced serum anion gap, as in patients with primary hyperparathyroidism, or may be a contributor, as in patients with multiple myeloma.

In patients treated with lithium, a reduced serum anion gap may be part of the presentation of acute lithium toxicity. An unexplained low serum anion gap warrants a serum protein electrophoresis to exclude the diagnosis of multiple myeloma, a common cause of a low serum anion gap.

Hypoalbuminemia is the most common cause of low serum anion gap in hospitalized patients.

Causes of a low serum anion gap include the following.

- Increased unmeasured cations

  Although serum potassium elevation could theoretically reduce the anion gap, the level at which it must be elevated (>10 mEq/L) is incompatible with life. Severe hypermagnesemia, presenting with a reduced serum anion gap, has been described.

  A reduced serum anion gap may also be noted in hypercalcemia. Interestingly, this is also related to the cause of the hypercalcemia. While primary hyperparathyroidism has been associated with a low serum anion gap, hypercalcemia of malignancy has not. A low serum anion gap may also be seen in patients with multiple myeloma. Hypercalcemia is thought to play a secondary role in the pathogenesis of the low serum anion gap in multiple myeloma patients.

- Not normally present cations

  When lithium is administered to maintain the serum lithium level in the therapeutic range (0.6-1.5 mEq/L), no reduction in the serum anion gap is noted. With an acute and massive overdose (serum lithium level >3.5 mEq/L), however, a low serum anion gap may be encountered.

  The serum anion gap is reduced in up to 27% of patients with multiple myeloma. Among the different types of multiple myeloma, IgG myelomas are most often associated with a reduction in the anion gap. Although hypercalcemia and hypoalbuminemia play a role in the development of a low serum anion gap, it is in large part due to the myeloma proteins behaving as cations.

  The parenteral administration of polymyxin B is also associated with a low serum anion gap. Because of its nephrotoxicity, this antibiotic is rarely used.

- Decreased unmeasured anions

  In hospitalized patients, hypoalbuminemia is the most common cause of a reduced serum anion gap. A useful relationship to remember is that for every 1 g/dL fall in the serum albumin below normal, the serum anion gap falls by 2.5 mEq/L.

- Serum sodium underestimation

  A falsely low serum sodium concentration may be reported in patients who have lipemic serum, particularly if flame atomic emission spectrometry is used for serum sodium measurement. The use of ion-selective electrodes has reduced the frequency of this problem but has not eliminated it.

In patients with severe hypernatremia (sodium concentration >170 mEq/L), laboratory techniques to measure the serum sodium level may underestimate the true sodium concentration, leading to a reduction in the serum anion gap.

Hyperviscosity may also be associated with a low serum anion gap, especially if flame atomic emission spectrometry is used. The major causes of hyperviscosity are multiple myeloma and Waldenström's macroglobulinemia.

- Serum chloride overestimation

  Hypertriglyceridemia leading to a reduction in the serum anion gap is only seen with the use of colorimetric assays. The high triglyceride levels interfere with the measurement of the serum chloride level, leading to an overestimation of the chloride concentration. Even modest degrees of hypertriglyceridemia (300 mg/dL) can reduce the serum anion gap.

  Bromide intoxication is another consideration in the differential diagnosis of a low serum anion gap. In the past, most cases were due to the use of over-the-counter sedatives containing bromides. Since these are no longer widely available, in recent years, most cases have been seen in myasthenia gravis patients treated with pyridostigmine bromide.

  Iodide intoxication has been reported to cause a low serum anion gap. Iodide is a component of many substances including medications, radiologic contrast, and expectorants. The ingestion of iodide in large quantities can result in iodinism, particularly in patients with renal insufficiency. These patients may certainly present with a low serum anion gap.

References

Gluck SL, "Acid-Base," *Lancet*, 1998, 352(9126):474-9.

Jurado RL, del Rio C, Nassar G, et al, "Low Anion Gap," *South Med J*, 1998, 91(7):624-9.

Laski ME and Kurtzman NA, "Acid-Base Disorders in Medicine," *Dis Mon*, 1996, 42(2):51-125.

Sirker AA, Rhodes A, Grounds RM, et al, "Acid-base Physiology: The Traditional and the Modern Approaches," *Anaesthesia*, 2002, 57(4):348-56.

Syabbolo N, "Measurement and Interpretation of Arterial Blood Gases," *Br J Clin Pract*, 1997, 51(3):173-6.

Williams AJ, "ABC of Oxygen: Assessing and Interpreting Arterial Blood Gases and Acid-Base Balance," *BMJ*, 1998, 317(7167):1213-6.

Williamson JC, "Acid-Base Disorders: Classification and Management Strategies," *Am Fam Physician*, 1995, 52(2):584-90.

APPROACH TO THE PATIENT WITH AN ACID-BASE DISORDER

STEP 1 – *What Is the pH*

The approach to the patient with an acid-base disorder begins with evaluation of the pH. A pH <7.37 is consistent with an acidemia whereas a pH >7.43 establishes the presence of alkalemia.

If the pH is <7.37, the patient has acidemia. ***Proceed to Step 2.***

If the pH is >7.43, the patient has alkalemia. ***Proceed to Step 3.***

If the pH is between 7.37 and 7.43, ***proceed to Step 4.***

STEP 2 – *What Is the $PaCO_2$?*

Patients with acidemia may have a respiratory or metabolic acidosis. These two types of acidosis can be distinguished from one another by consideration of the $PaCO_2$. A $PaCO_2$ <40 mm Hg is consistent with a metabolic acidosis whereas a $PaCO_2$ >40 mm Hg establishes the presence of a respiratory acidosis.

If the $PaCO_2$ is <40 mm Hg, the patient has a metabolic acidosis. ***Proceed to Step 5.***

If the $PaCO_2$ is >40 mm Hg, the patient has a respiratory acidosis. ***Proceed to Approach to the Patient With Respiratory Acidosis*** *on page 311.*

STEP 3 – *What Is the $PaCO_2$?*

Patients with alkalemia may have a respiratory or metabolic alkalosis. These two types of alkalosis can be distinguished from one another by consideration of the $PaCO_2$. A $PaCO_2$ <40 mm Hg is consistent with a respiratory alkalosis. Metabolic alkalosis is said to be present when the $PaCO_2$ exceeds 40 mm Hg.

If the $PaCO_2$ is <40 mm Hg, the patient has a respiratory alkalosis. ***Proceed to Approach to the Patient with Respiratory Alkalosis*** *on page 327.*

If the $PaCO_2$ is >40 mm Hg, the patient has a metabolic alkalosis. ***Proceed to Approach to the Patient With Metabolic Alkalosis*** *on page 317.*

STEP 4 – *Does a Normal pH Exclude the Presence of an Acid-Base Disorder?*

At first glance, a normal pH suggests the absence of an acid-base abnormality. While this is certainly the most common implication of a normal pH, the clinician should be aware of certain instances in which a normal pH may be misleading. To prevent this error from occurring, the clinician should always look at the $PaCO_2$ in the patient with a normal pH.

If the $PaCO_2$ is >40 mm Hg, then the patient has a mixed respiratory acidosis and metabolic alkalosis.

If the $PaCO_2$ is <40 mm Hg, then the patient has a mixed respiratory alkalosis and metabolic acidosis.

If the $PaCO_2$ is normal, then the patient may either have a combined metabolic acidosis and alkalosis or a normal acid-base balance. In these cases, the anion gap is helpful in the identification of the mixed metabolic disorder. The patient's clinical presentation and anion gap are helpful in differentiating between normal acid-base balance and a combined metabolic disorder.

End of Section.

STEP 5 – *What Is the Plasma Anion Gap (AG)?*

A metabolic acidosis is characterized by a serum bicarbonate that is below the lower limit of normal. When the presence of a metabolic acidosis is established, it is necessary to calculate the plasma anion gap. The plasma anion gap can be calculated as follows:

$$\textbf{Anion gap} = Na^{+} - (Cl^{-} + HCO_3^{-})$$

The normal plasma anion gap has traditionally been considered to be 12±4 mEq/L. This reference range for the normal plasma anion gap was established many years ago from electrolyte assays (flame photometry) that have largely been replaced by ion-selective electrode methodology. This shift in methodology has resulted in a change in the reference range for the normal plasma anion gap. The new reference range of 3-11 mEq/L should now be used in place of 12±4 mEq/L only if ion-selective electrode techniques are used for plasma electrolyte measurement. To avoid errors in patient diagnosis and management, it is wise to discuss these issues further with the laboratory. Many laboratories have established their own reference intervals for the plasma anion gap. If this is the case, the clinician should use this reference range in determining whether the patient has a high anion gap or normal anion gap metabolic acidosis.

Calculation of the anion gap is essential in categorizing the patient into one of the following two groups:

- High anion gap metabolic acidosis
- Normal anion gap (hyperchloremic) metabolic acidosis

If the calculated anion gap is elevated, the patient has a high anion gap metabolic acidosis. ***Proceed to Approach to the Patient With a High Anion Gap Metabolic Acidosis** on page 287.*

If the calculated anion gap is normal, the patient has a normal anion gap metabolic acidosis. ***Proceed to Approach to the Patient With a Normal Anion Gap Metabolic Acidosis** on page 299.*

References

Fall PJ, "A Stepwise Approach to Acid-Base Disorders. Practical Patient Evaluation for Metabolic Acidosis and Other Conditions," *Postgrad Med*, 2000, 107(3):249-50, 253-4, 257-8 passim.

Gluck SL, "Acid-Base," *Lancet*, 1998, 352(9126):474-9.

Kraut JA and Madias NE, "Approach to Patients With Acid-Base Disorders," *Respir Care*, 2001, 46(4):392-403.

Laski ME and Kurtzman NA, "Acid-Base Disorders in Medicine," *Dis Mon*, 1996, 42(2):51-125.

Syabbolo N, "Measurement and Interpretation of Arterial Blood Gases," *Br J Clin Pract*, 1997, 51(3):173-6.

Williams AJ, "ABC of Oxygen: Assessing and Interpreting Arterial Blood Gases and Acid-Base Balance," *BMJ*, 1998, 317(7167):1213-6.

Williamson JC, "Acid-Base Disorders: Classification and Management Strategies," *Am Fam Physician*, 1995, 52(2):584-90.

APPROACH TO THE PATIENT WITH AN ACID-BASE DISORDER

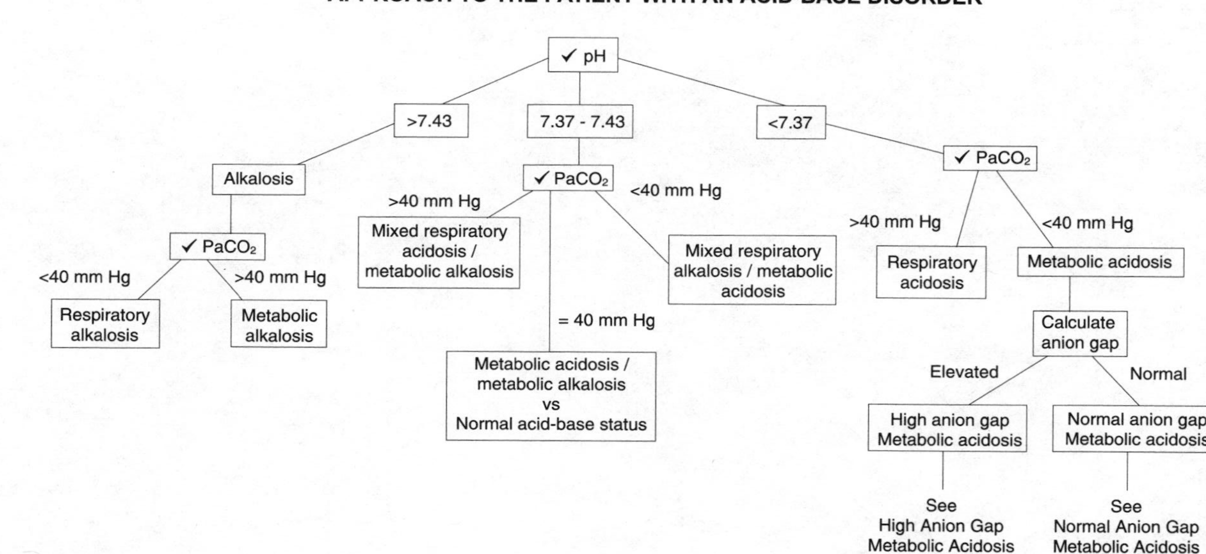

APPROACH TO THE PATIENT WITH A HIGH ANION GAP METABOLIC ACIDOSIS

STEP 1 – *Does the Patient Have a High Anion Gap Metabolic Acidosis?*

In this chapter, the evaluation of the patient with a high anion gap metabolic acidosis will be discussed. This chapter assumes that the presence of a high anion gap metabolic acidosis has been firmly established. For more information regarding how the diagnosis of high anion gap metabolic acidosis is established, please refer to the chapter, ***Approach to the Patient With an Acid-Base Disorder****on page 283.*

If the patient has a high anion gap metabolic acidosis, ***proceed to Step 2.***

STEP 2 – *Is Respiratory Compensation Adequate?*

Once it is determined that the patient has a high anion gap metabolic acidosis, it is then necessary to determine if a concomitant respiratory acid-base disorder is also present. This is evaluated by determining if the respiratory compensation is adequate for the degree of metabolic acidosis. The respiratory system will compensate for acidosis through hyperventilation. It is essential to always calculate the expected $PaCO_2$ in the patient with metabolic acidosis. By comparing the measured $PaCO_2$ with the expected $PaCO_2$, we can assess the degree of respiratory compensation as well as the presence of any concomitant respiratory acid-base disorder. The measured and calculated (expected) $PaCO_2$ should be about the same. If they differ, it is likely that another process exists. One can use the following formula to assess the adequacy of respiratory compensation:

$$\textbf{Expected } PaCO_2 = (1.5 \times HCO_3) + 8 \pm 2$$

Example: Let us consider the patient with a serum bicarbonate of 15 mEq/L. This patient should have a $PaCO_2$ between 28.5 and 32.5 mm Hg. If the $PaCO_2$ is outside this range, there exists a respiratory acid-base disorder as well.

If the measured $PaCO_2$ is greater than the expected $PaCO_2$, then a concomitant respiratory acidosis exists.

If the measured $PaCO_2$ is less than the expected $PaCO_2$, then a concomitant respiratory alkalosis is present.

One caveat to this formula is that it is based on the assumption that full compensation has occurred. In patients with metabolic acidosis, this usually requires 12-24 hours. Fortunately, most patients with a metabolic acidosis develop their acid-base abnormality relatively slowly allowing full compensation to take place prior to their presentation. An exception to this involves the patient who develops a metabolic acidosis fairly suddenly from a toxin, for example. In this instance, the formula may not be as useful.

The equation also has difficulty and may not be valid when the patient is markedly acidotic, particularly if the pH is <7.1.

Proceed to Step 3.

STEP 3 – *Are Any Other Metabolic Abnormalities Present?*

If a high anion gap metabolic acidosis exists, one must decide if there are any other metabolic disorders present as well. In the patient with a high anion gap metabolic acidosis, calculation of the gap:gap ratio can confirm the presence of a mixed metabolic disorder. The gap:gap ratio can be calculated as follows:

Gap:gap ratio = AG excess / HCO_3^- deficit

or

$$\textbf{Gap:gap ratio} = \frac{\text{calculated anion gap - normal anion gap}}{\text{normal bicarbonate - measured bicarbonate}}$$

where a normal AG = patient's baseline AG* and a normal bicarbonate = 24 mEq/L

*Baseline is best determined by looking at previous blood work (in the recent past).

If the ratio is >2.0, then the patient has a concomitant metabolic alkalosis (may also represent compensation for a respiratory acidosis).

If the ratio <1.0, then the patient has a concomitant normal anion gap metabolic acidosis (may also represent compensation for a respiratory alkalosis).

If the ratio is 1-2, then the patient has a pure high anion gap metabolic acidosis.

To determine the etiology of the high anion gap metabolic acidosis, ***proceed to Step 4.***

STEP 4 – *What Are the Causes of a High Anion Gap Metabolic Acidosis?*

Causes of a high anion gap metabolic acidosis are listed in the following box.

HIGH ANION GAP METABOLIC ACIDOSIS DIFFERENTIAL DIAGNOSIS	
METHANOL INTOXICATION	LACTIC ACIDOSIS
UREMIA	ETHYLENE GLYCOL POISONING
KETOACIDOSIS	SALICYLATE INTOXICATION
Diabetic, alcoholic, starvation	

Proceed to Step 5.

STEP 5 – *What Is the Osmolal Gap?*

Whenever a high anion gap metabolic acidosis exists, it is important to look for a significant osmolal gap. The osmolal gap is calculated by using the following formula.

Osmolal gap = measured serum osmolality - calculated serum osmolality

Where,

Calculated serum osmolality = $Na^+ \times 2$ + glucose / 18 + BUN / 2.8

Therefore...

CALCULATION OF OSMOLAL GAP
Osmolal gap = measured serum osmolality - $[2(Na^+) + (glucose / 18) + (BUN / 2.8)]$

The measured serum osmolality reflects all of the elements of the calculated serum osmolality but also includes any other osmotically active substances that may be present. A normal osmolal gap is usually <10-15 mOsm/kg. An elevated osmolal gap indicates the presence of osmotically active substances other than sodium, glucose, or urea. Examples include mannitol, radiocontrast media, ethanol, ethylene glycol, or methanol. Since methanol and ethylene glycol intoxication are major causes of a high anion gap metabolic acidosis, the osmolal gap should be calculated in every patient with this acid-base disorder.

One important point regarding the method used to measure the osmolality deserves mention here. There are two methods available to measure the osmolality: vapor pressure and freezing point depression. It is important to ensure that the laboratory performing these tests utilizes the freezing point depression method as this is the most reliable test.

If the osmolal gap is high (>10-15 mOsm/kg), ***proceed to Step 6.***

If the osmolal gap is normal (<10-15 mOsm/kg), ***proceed to Step 7.***

STEP 6 – *What Is the Differential Diagnosis of a High AG Metabolic Acidosis With an Increased Osmolal Gap?*

The differential diagnosis of an elevated osmolal gap in the setting of a high anion gap metabolic acidosis is listed in the following box.

CAUSES OF INCREASED OSMOLAL GAP IN THE PATIENT WITH A HIGH ANION GAP METABOLIC ACIDOSIS	
METHANOL INTOXICATION	ALCOHOLIC KETOACIDOSIS
ETHYLENE GLYCOL INTOXICATION	LACTIC ACIDOSIS
DIABETIC KETOACIDOSIS	CHRONIC RENAL FAILURE

Although methanol and ethylene glycol intoxication are the major considerations in the patient with elevated osmolal gap, other causes of a high anion gap metabolic acidosis, on occasion, may present with elevated osmolal gap as well. If the presentation is not consistent with ketoacidosis, lactic acidosis, and the patient does not have chronic renal failure, then the presence of increased osmolal gap strongly supports either methanol or ethylene glycol intoxication.

The serum ethanol level should always be determined at the same time the osmolal gap is calculated since many patients who ingest either methanol or ethylene glycol also abuse ethanol (most common cause of elevated osmolal gap). As ethanol is an osmotically active substance that affects the serum osmolality and therefore the osmolal gap, if ethanol is present, a correction must be made to the formula for serum osmolality.

If ethanol is present,

Osmolal gap = measured osmolality - $[2(Na^+) + BUN / 2.8 + glucose / 18 + ethanol (mg/dL) / 4.6]$

If the osmolal gap remains elevated after correction for ethanol, this suggests either methanol or ethylene glycol intoxication. Ethylene glycol and methanol intoxication are discussed in further detail in the remainder of this step.

Ethylene Glycol Intoxication

Ethylene glycol is a component of antifreeze and other solvents. It is metabolized into glycolic and oxalic acids by the action of alcohol dehydrogenase. These products are responsible for the metabolic acidosis that accompanies ethylene glycol intoxication. After ingestion, there are three clinical stages of varying severity. The first stage, which usually manifests in the first 12 hours, is characterized by neurologic abnormalities ranging from a drunken state to coma. Cardiopulmonary manifestations predominate the second stage (12-72 hours after ingestion), the severity of which may vary from tachypnea to pulmonary edema. Provided that the patient survives the first two stages, acute renal failure marks the third stage, occurring within 72 hours of ingestion.

The presence of these signs and symptoms in the setting of a high anion gap metabolic acidosis with an elevated osmolal gap provides strong evidence for the diagnosis. The presence of positively birefringent calcium oxalate crystals in the urine is pathognomonic for the diagnosis. However, the absence of oxalate crystals in the urine is not an infrequent finding even with severe intoxication. Additional laboratory clues include a urinalysis that reveals microscopic hematuria and proteinuria, fluorescence of the urine with Wood's lamp (fluorescein is present in many antifreezes), and hypocalcemia. Serum ethylene glycol levels should be obtained in all cases. Most laboratories are not equipped to perform the ethylene glycol assay. In most cases, the laboratory must send the specimen to an appropriate testing facility, in which case, several days may pass before the results are available. Herein lies the importance of starting treatment in patients suspected of having ethylene glycol intoxication even if a level is not available. Toxic levels are defined as a concentration >20 mg/dL.

Methanol Intoxication

Methanol (or wood alcohol) is present in shellac, varnish, as well as many other substances commonly found both in the workplace and home. Methanol is metabolized to formaldehyde by the action of alcohol dehydrogenase. Formaldehyde is then converted to formic acid. It is not unusual for the symptoms and high anion gap metabolic acidosis to be delayed up to 36 hours after ingestion because they are dependent on the accumulation of formic acid. The signs and symptoms of methanol intoxication include abdominal pain, blurred vision, vomiting, headache, cyanosis, respiratory depression, altered mental status, and cardiovascular collapse. Fundoscopic examination may reveal optic nerve swelling.

Comparison of Ethylene Glycol and Methanol

	↑ Osmolal Gap	High AG Metabolic Acidosis	Urine Oxalate Crystals	Fluorescence of Urine Under Wood's Lamp	ARF	Optic Nerve Swelling
Ethylene glycol	(+)	(+)	(+)	(+)	(+)	(-)
Methanol	(+)	(+)	(-)	(-)	(-)	(+)

End of Section.

STEP 7 – *What Is the Differential Diagnosis of a High AG Metabolic Acidosis With a Normal Osmolal Gap?*

The causes of a high anion gap metabolic acidosis in the setting of a normal osmolal gap are listed in the following box.

CAUSES OF NORMAL OSMOLAL GAP IN HIGH ANION GAP METABOLIC ACIDOSIS	
UREMIA	LACTIC ACIDOSIS
KETOACIDOSIS	SALICYLATE INTOXICATION
Diabetic, alcoholic, starvation	

While methanol and ethylene intoxication usually present with an elevated osmolal gap, they can present with a normal osmolal gap particularly if the patient presents early or late in the illness.

Proceed to Step 8.

STEP 8 – *Does the Patient Have Uremia?*

Once the clinician has excluded intoxication from either methanol or ethylene glycol, attention should focus on the renal function. As renal function deteriorates, the kidney's ability to excrete the daily acid load declines as well. It is the decrease in renal mass that leads to a decline in total ammonium ($NH4^+$) excretion. Early in the course of the renal insufficiency, the patient may have a normal anion gap metabolic acidosis but, as the renal function progressively worsens, a high anion gap metabolic acidosis will appear, particularly when the GFR falls to <15 mL/minute. It is, however, unusual for the serum bicarbonate to fall to <10 mEq/L in the patient with chronic renal failure. When such a bicarbonate level is encountered in the patient with chronic renal failure, the clinician should consider another process superimposed on the acidosis of chronic renal insufficiency.

If the metabolic acidosis is secondary to uremia, ***stop here***.

If the metabolic acidosis is not secondary to uremia, ***proceed to Step 9***.

STEP 9 – *Does the Patient Have Ketoacidosis?*

There are three forms of ketoacidosis:

- Diabetic ketoacidosis
- Alcoholic ketoacidosis
- Starvation ketoacidosis

To establish the diagnosis of ketoacidosis, it is necessary to demonstrate the presence of ketones in the blood or urine. The nitroprusside test (Acetest) can be used to detect ketonemia. When serum is diluted 1:1, a 4+ reaction provides strong support for the presence of ketoacidosis. Unfortunately, the situation is not so simple. The nitroprusside reaction detects the presence of two ketoacids, acetoacetate and acetone. It does not, however, react with β-hydroxybutyrate. This is important because the latter makes up between 66% and 75% of the ketoacids in diabetic ketoacidosis and up to 90% in alcoholic ketoacidosis. As a result, the nitroprusside test may underestimate the degree of ketonemia and ketonuria or even fail to recognize its presence. Since an assay for β-hydroxybutyrate is not available in most laboratories, a useful way of getting around this problem is to add a few drops of hydrogen peroxide to a specimen of urine. The addition of hydrogen peroxide results in the nonenzymatic conversion of β-hydroxybutyrate to acetoacetate. The acetoacetate can then be detected by the nitroprusside reaction as discussed above.

If the patient has ketoacidosis, ***proceed to Step 10***.

If the patient does not have ketoacidosis, ***proceed to Step 11***.

STEP 10 – *What Type of Ketoacidosis Is Present?*

The different types of ketoacidosis are discussed in further detail in the remainder of this step.

Diabetic Ketoacidosis

Diabetic ketoacidosis (DKA) typically develops in the insulin-dependent diabetic who is considerably hyperglycemic and manifests the symptoms of polyuria, polydipsia, and polyphagia. Other signs and symptoms include acetone breath, hyperventilation, and altered mental status. In many cases, an event may be identified that precipitated the DKA. The two leading causes are infection and noncompliance with insulin therapy. In 25% of patients, DKA may be the initial manifestation of diabetes. Other precipitants include alcohol abuse, myocardial infarction, pulmonary embolism, stroke, steroid treatment, and trauma. In a minority of cases, the precipitant is not known

Most experts agree that the diagnosis of DKA is fulfilled if the following criteria are met.

CRITERIA FOR DIAGNOSIS OF DKA	
GLUCOSE >250 mg/dL	pH <7.3
HCO_3^- <15 mEq/L	KETONEMIA / KETONURIA
HIGH ANION GAP METABOLIC ACIDOSIS	

Limitations of the above criteria include the following.

- Although most patients present with glucose levels exceeding 250 mg/dL, lower glucose levels have been described. While hyperglycemia is characteristic of DKA, other conditions causing a high anion gap metabolic acidosis may also present with hyperglycemia. Mild hyperglycemia (150-250 mg/dL) may be appreciated in alcoholic ketoacidosis and salicylate intoxication.
- The serum pH may be misleading in some DKA patients because other acid-base abnormalities may accompany the metabolic acidosis. For example, a respiratory alkalosis may be appreciated in the patient whose DKA was precipitated by pneumonia. Some patients including those with severe vomiting, diuretic therapy, or Cushing's syndrome may actually present with an alkalemic pH.
- Although 45% of DKA patients present with a pure high anion gap metabolic acidosis, almost an equivalent number present with a mixed anion gap metabolic acidosis. The remainder have a normal anion gap metabolic acidosis.
- As discussed above, ketonemia may be demonstrated by performing the nitroprusside test. The test, however, does not react with β-hydroxybutyrate which is the main metabolic product in DKA. As such, this test provides a poor reflection of the degree of ketonemia. In addition, the presence of a condition leading to tissue hypoxia may result in a negative or weakly positive nitroprusside reaction, because the serum ketones may be largely in the form of β-hydroxybutyrate.

Alcoholic Ketoacidosis

The typical case starts in the chronic alcoholic who has stopped alcohol use several days prior to admission because of abdominal pain and vomiting that may be due to gastritis or pancreatitis. These patients usually give a history of marked reduction of oral intake. Physical examination is often remarkable for hyperventilation, dehydration, and a tender abdomen.

While diabetic ketoacidosis is certainly more frequently encountered, the clinician should suspect alcoholic ketoacidosis in the patient who presents with a long-standing history of alcohol abuse in the setting of an unexplained high anion gap metabolic acidosis. The glucose level is usually normal but may be slightly elevated. The laboratory findings of alcoholic ketoacidosis are included in the following box.

ALCOHOLIC KETOACIDOSIS LABORATORY FINDINGS
KETONEMIA / KETONURIA* HIGH ANION GAP METABOLIC ACIDOSIS† DECREASED / UNDETECTABLE ETOH LEVEL‡ VARIABLE GLUCOSE LEVEL§

*Recall that the nitroprusside test may be negative or weakly reactive in the patient with alcoholic ketoacidosis because a high percentage of the circulating ketones are in the form of β-hydroxybutyrate.

†Because alcoholic patients may have other acid-base abnormalities, the clinician should not be dissuaded by a normal or even alkalemic pH. Careful inspection of the blood gas values will uncover the presence of an acidosis.

‡An ethanol level of zero is not uncommon in alcoholic ketoacidosis as most patients have stopped their alcohol intake because of vomiting.

§The glucose may be normal to slightly high but seldom exceeds 250 mg/dL. Rarely, hypoglycemia has been reported.

Not uncommonly, other acid-base disturbances are present in these patients such as metabolic alkalosis due to vomiting or respiratory alkalosis secondary to hyperventilation.

Starvation Ketoacidosis

Prolonged fasting can lead to ketoacidosis because of the cessation of carbohydrate intake. This leads to the same imbalance that is seen in patients with diabetic or alcoholic ketoacidosis. There is a relative decline in insulin activity along with an increase in glucagon secretion leading to the production of ketoacids. In contrast to the other two types, the ketoacidosis of starvation is not as severe. Rarely is the bicarbonate level <18 mEq/L.

End of Section.

STEP 11 – *Does the Patient Have Salicylate Intoxication?*

Aspirin is converted into salicylic acid. While it is not always easy to correlate symptoms with the serum salicylate concentration, the majority of patients manifest some signs and symptoms of salicylate intoxication when the level is >40 mg/dL. The therapeutic range is between 20 and 35 mg/dL.

The acid-base abnormalities of salicylate intoxication can be complex. Most patients have either a respiratory alkalosis or a combined respiratory alkalosis and metabolic acidosis. A pure metabolic acidosis is quite unusual. The respiratory alkalosis is due to salicylate induced stimulation of the respiratory center. Up to 33% of patients with salicylate intoxication abuse other drugs. Many of these drugs lead to respiratory depression. As a result, the patient with salicylate intoxication may have a concomitant respiratory acidosis.

There are two forms of salicylate intoxication, acute and chronic. The acid-base abnormalities described above are more typical of acute intoxication. Symptoms of the acute form include fever, seizures, stupor, and coma. Chronic salicylate intoxication is characterized by tinnitus, hearing loss, and vertigo.

The diagnosis is usually established by history. Soft laboratory findings supporting the diagnosis are hypouricemia and an elevated prothrombin time.

The clinician should realize that the urinary excretion of salicylate metabolites may result in false-positive test results for urine ketones and glucose.

To confirm the diagnosis, the clinician can add ferric chloride to the urine to check for salicylates (purple color will result if salicylates are present). Because a similar color change may occur if acetone and acetoacetate are present in the urine, the urine should be boiled prior to testing. The boiling will remove these volatile ketones.

A salicylate level may also be obtained. As mentioned above, the level does not always correlate with symptoms. In chronic intoxication, death has occurred at fairly low concentrations. In addition, the level must be interpreted with regards to the time elapsed since ingestion.

If salicylate intoxication is the cause of the high anion gap metabolic acidosis, ***stop here***.

If salicylate intoxication is not the cause of the high anion gap metabolic acidosis, ***proceed to Step 12***.

STEP 12 – *Does the Patient Have Lactic Acidosis?*

In the patient with a high anion gap metabolic acidosis, the diagnosis of lactic acidosis should be suspected if the patient has a clinical condition that may lead to lactic acidosis. An elevated serum lactate level >2 mmol/L confirms the diagnosis. The clinician should ensure that the blood specimen is placed on ice. Every effort should be made to transport the specimen immediately to the laboratory because a delay in testing will allow the lactate level in the specimen to climb because of continued production of lactate *in vitro*. This can lead to a falsely elevated lactate concentration.

As lactic acidosis may coexist with other causes of a metabolic acidosis, specifically ketoacidosis, it is important for the clinician to search for these other etiologies as well. In particular, the clinician should recall the limitation of the nitroprusside test in the diagnosis of alcoholic and diabetic ketoacidosis. These conditions may result in a negative or weakly positive test prompting the clinician to discard the diagnosis of ketoacidosis altogether.

Lactic acidosis may be divided into types A and B. Type A refers to those disorders that result in clinically evident tissue hypoxia while type B includes all other conditions. The causes of type A and B lactic acidosis are listed in the following box.

CAUSES OF LACTIC ACIDOSIS

TYPE A

SEIZURES

SEVERE EXERCISE

SHOCK / HYPOTENSION
- Cardiogenic
- Hypovolemic
- Sepsis
- Anaphylaxis
- Massive pulmonary embolism

SEVERE HYPOXEMIA
- Carbon monoxide poisoning
- Severe anemia
- Methemoglobinemia
- Acute respiratory failure

(continued)

(continued)

CAUSES OF LACTIC ACIDOSIS	
TYPE B	
DRUGS AND TOXINS	
Metformin	Salicylates
Acetaminophen	Cyanide
Niacin	Methanol
Lactulose	Isoniazid
Theophylline	Nitroprusside
Cocaine	Streptozotocin
Papaverine	Ethylene glycol
Sorbitol	Nalidixic acid
Ethanol	Others
MALIGNANCY	INFECTION
Leukemia	Malaria
Lymphoma	Cholera
Solid cancers	
INHERITED ENZYME DEFECTS	RENAL FAILURE
DIABETES MELLITUS	SEPSIS
LIVER FAILURE	D-LACTIC ACIDOSIS

Of note, the standard assay for lactic acid does not detect D-lactate. D-lactic acidosis should be suspected in patients who have a history of jejunoileal bypass or short bowel syndrome. In these patients, D-lactic acid is produced from the metabolism of starch and glucose in colon. To confirm the diagnosis, a special assay to detect the presence of D-lactic acid is required.

References

Chiasson JL, Aris-Jilwan N, Belanger R, et al, "Diagnosis and Treatment of Diabetic Ketoacidosis and the Hyperglycemia Hyperosmolar State," *CMAJ*, 2003, 168(7):859-66.

Fall PJ, "A Stepwise Approach to Acid-Base Disorders. Practical Patient Evaluation for Metabolic Acidosis and Other Conditions," *Postgrad Med*, 2000, 107(3):249-50, 253-4, 257-8.

Gauthier PM and Szerlip HM, "Metabolic Acidosis in the Intensive Care Unit," *Crit Care Clin*, 2002, 18(2):289-308, vi.

Ishihara K and Szerlip HM, "Anion Gap Acidosis," *Semin Nephrol*, 1998, 18(1):83-97.

Luft FC, "Lactic Acidosis Update for Critical Care Clinicians," *J Am Soc Nephrol*, 2001, 12(Suppl 17):S15-9.

Oster JR, Singer I, Contreras GN, et al, "Metabolic Acidosis With Extreme Elevation of Anion Gap: Case Report and Literature Review," *Am J Med Sci*, 1999, 317(1):38-49.

Piagnerelli M, Lejeune P, and Vanhaeverbeek M, "Diagnosis and Treatment of an Unusual Cause of Metabolic Acidosis: Ethylene Glycol Poisoning," *Acta Clin Belg*, 1999, 54(6):351-6.

Swenson ER, "Metabolic Acidosis," *Respir Care*, 2001, 46(4):342-53.

Williams GF, Hatch FJ, and Bradley MC, "Methanol Poisoning: A Review and Case Study of Four Patients From Central Australia," *Aust Crit Care*, 1997, 10(4):113-8.

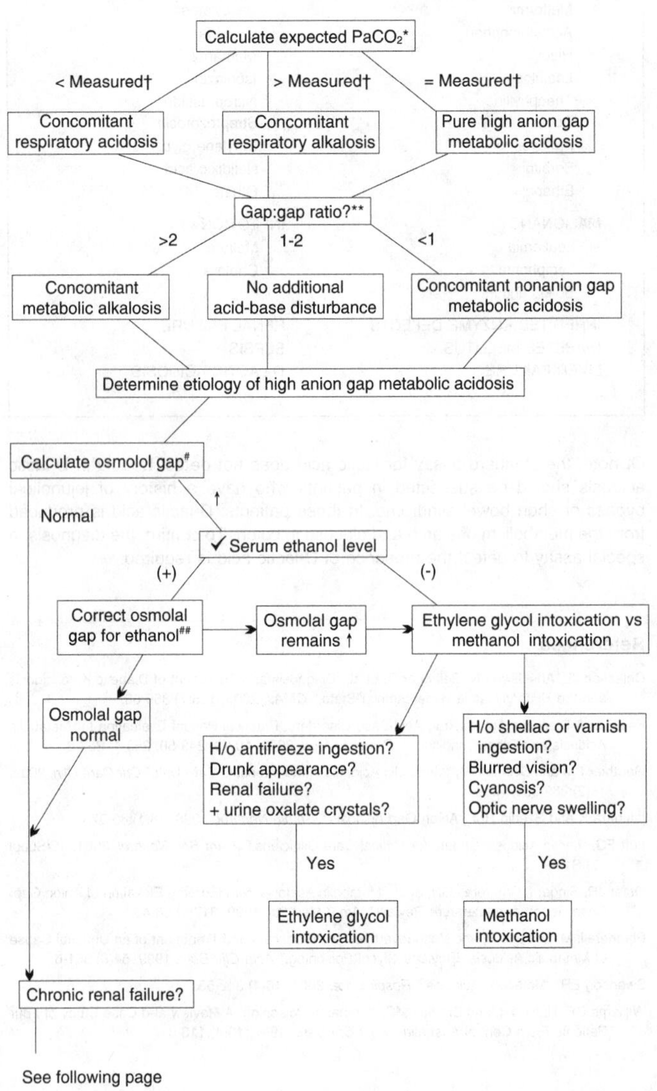

See following page

HIGH ANION GAP METABOLIC ACIDOSIS (*continued*)

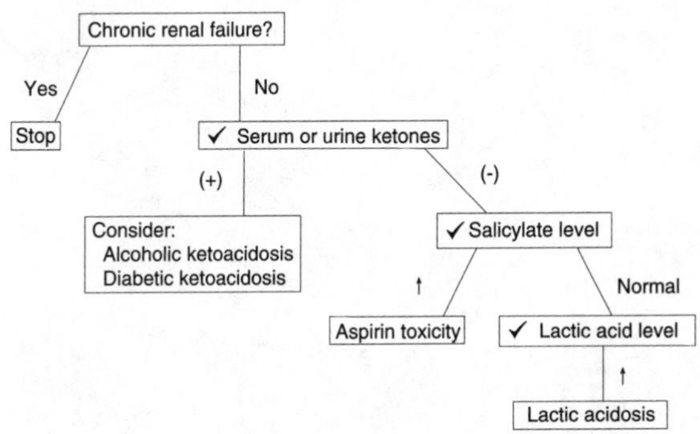

* Expected $PaCO_2 = [1.5 \times HCO_3^- + 8 \pm 2]$

† Measured $PaCO_2$ refers to the arterial blood gas value

** Gap:gap ratio $= \dfrac{\text{calculated AG - normal AG}}{\text{normal } HCO_3^- - \text{measured } HCO_3^-}$

Osmolal gap $=$ measured serum osmolality $- [2(Na^+) + \dfrac{\text{glucose}}{18} + \dfrac{\text{BUN}}{2.8}]$

Corrected osmolal gap for alcohol $=$ measured serum osmolality $- [2(Na^+) + \dfrac{\text{glucose}}{18} + \dfrac{\text{BUN}}{2.8} + \dfrac{\text{ETOH level (mg/dL)}}{4.6}]$

APPROACH TO THE PATIENT WITH A NORMAL ANION GAP METABOLIC ACIDOSIS

STEP 1 – *Does the Patient Have a Normal Anion Gap Metabolic Acidosis?*

In this chapter, the evaluation of the patient with a normal anion gap metabolic acidosis (hyperchloremic metabolic acidosis) will be discussed. This chapter assumes that the presence of a normal anion gap metabolic acidosis has been firmly established. For more information regarding how the diagnosis of normal anion gap metabolic acidosis is established, please refer to the chapter, ***Approach to the Patient With an Acid-Base Disorder*** *on page 283.*

If the patient has a normal anion gap metabolic acidosis, ***proceed to Step 2.***

STEP 2 – *Does the Patient Have Hypoalbuminemia?*

Before embarking on a workup of a normal anion gap metabolic acidosis, it is important to understand that hypoalbuminemia may lead to a decreased anion gap. There will be a 2.5 mEq/L decrease in the anion gap for every 1 g/dL decrease in the serum albumin because the serum albumin is the major component comprising the unmeasured anions. This is the most common cause of a decreased anion gap. In patients with hypoalbuminemia, the corrected anion gap may be calculated as follows:

CORRECTING THE ANION GAP IN HYPOALBUMINEMIA
Corrected AG = $AG_{measured}$ + 2.5 mEq (4 - albumin)

If the corrected anion gap is above the upper limit of normal, the patient has a high anion gap metabolic acidosis. Proceed to the chapter, ***Approach to the Patient With High Anion Gap Metabolic Acidosis*** *on page 287.*

If the corrected anion gap is normal, the patient has a normal anion gap metabolic acidosis. ***Proceed to Step 3.***

STEP 3 – *Is Respiratory Compensation Adequate?*

Once it is determined that the patient has a normal anion gap metabolic acidosis, it is then necessary to determine if a concomitant respiratory acid-base disorder is also present. This is evaluated by determining if the respiratory compensation is adequate for the degree of the metabolic acidosis.

The respiratory system will compensate for the acidosis through hyperventilation. It is essential to always calculate the expected $PaCO_2$ in the patient with a metabolic acidosis. By comparing the measured $PaCO_2$ with the expected $PaCO_2$, we can assess the degree of respiratory compensation as well as the presence of any concomitant respiratory acid-base disorder. The measured and calculated (expected) $PaCO_2$ should be about the same. If they differ, it is likely that another process exists. One can use the following formula to assess the adequacy of respiratory compensation.

$$\textbf{Expected } \mathbf{PaCO_2} = (1.5 \times HCO_3^-) + 8 \pm 2$$

Example:

Let us consider the patient with a serum bicarbonate of 15 mEq/L. This patient should have a $PaCO_2$ between 28.5 and 32.5 mm Hg. If the $PaCO_2$ is outside this range, there exists a respiratory acid-base disorder as well.

If the measured $PaCO_2$ is less than the expected $PaCO_2$, then a concomitant respiratory alkalosis is present.

If the measured $PaCO_2$ is greater than the expected $PaCO_2$, then a concomitant respiratory acidosis is present.

One caveat to this formula is that it is based on the assumption that full compensation has occurred. In patients with metabolic acidosis, this usually requires 12-24 hours. Fortunately, most patients with metabolic acidosis develop their acid-base abnormality relatively slowly allowing full compensation to take place prior to their presentation. An exception to this involves the patient who develops a metabolic acidosis fairly suddenly from a toxin, for example. In this instance, the formula may not be as useful.

The equation also may not be valid when the patient is markedly acidotic, particularly if the pH is <7.1.

To determine the etiology of the normal anion gap metabolic acidosis, ***proceed to Step 4.***

STEP 4 – *What Is the Differential Diagnosis of a Normal Anion Gap Metabolic Acidosis?*

The differential diagnosis of a normal anion gap metabolic acidosis is listed in the following box.

NORMAL ANION GAP METABOLIC ACIDOSIS DIFFERENTIAL DIAGNOSIS
RENAL TUBULAR ACIDOSIS
ASSOCIATED WITH HYPOKALEMIA
Distal or classical renal tubular acidosis (type I)
Proximal renal tubular acidosis (type II)
ASSOCIATED WITH HYPERKALEMIA
Type IV RTA
Medication-induced
Amiloride
Triamterene
Spironolactone
Trimethoprim
Pentamidine
ACE inhibitor
Angiotensin II receptor blocker
NSAIDs
Cyclosporine
ASSOCIATED WITH NORMOKALEMIA
Early renal failure
GASTROINTESTINAL LOSS OF ALKALI
DIARRHEA
PANCREATIC FISTULA
BILIARY FISTULA
ENTERIC FISTULA
PANCREATIC TRANSPLANTATION WITH DRAINAGE INTO URINARY BLADDER
URETEROSIGMOIDOSTOMY
JEJUNAL LOOP
MEDICATIONS
Calcium chloride
Magnesium sulfate
Cholestyramine
MISCELLANEOUS
RECOVERY FROM KETOACIDOSIS
POSTHYPOCAPNIA
EXPANSION ACIDOSIS
CATION EXCHANGE RESINS

Proceed to Step 5.

STEP 5 – *Does the Patient Have Diarrhea?*

Diarrhea is the most common cause of a normal anion gap metabolic acidosis. The resolution of the illness along with rehydration leads to correction of the metabolic acidosis.

If the normal anion gap metabolic acidosis is secondary to diarrhea, ***stop here***.

If the normal anion gap metabolic acidosis is not secondary to diarrhea, ***proceed to Step 6***.

STEP 6 – *Has the Patient Been Given HCl or a Chloride Salt?*

The administration of HCl or a chloride salt of NH_4^+, lysine, or arginine can lead to the development of a normal anion gap metabolic acidosis.

If the normal anion gap metabolic acidosis is secondary to the administration of HCl or a chloride salt, ***stop here***.

If the normal anion gap metabolic acidosis is not secondary to the administration of HCl or a chloride salt, ***proceed to Step 7***.

STEP 7 – *Is the Patient Recovering From Ketoacidosis?*

Recovery from diabetic, alcoholic, or starvation ketoacidosis is often associated with a normal anion gap metabolic acidosis.

If the normal anion gap metabolic acidosis is secondary to recovery from ketoacidosis, ***stop here***.

If the normal anion gap metabolic acidosis is not secondary to recovery from ketoacidosis, ***proceed to Step 8***.

STEP 8 – *Is the Patient Receiving an Anion Exchange Resin?*

The use of an anion exchange resin, such as cholestyramine, may lead to the development of a normal anion gap metabolic acidosis.

If the normal anion gap metabolic acidosis is secondary to an anion exchange resin, ***stop here***.

If the normal anion gap metabolic acidosis is not secondary to an anion exchange resin, ***proceed to Step 9***.

STEP 9 – *Has the Patient Had a Ureteral Division?*

A normal anion gap metabolic acidosis is not uncommon in the patient with a ureteral division (ureterosigmoidostomy, ileal conduit).

If the normal anion gap metabolic acidosis is secondary to a ureteral division, ***stop here***.

If the normal anion gap metabolic acidosis is not secondary to ureteral division, ***proceed to Step 10***.

STEP 10 – *What Is the Urine Anion Gap?*

The urine anion gap may be calculated using the following equation:

URINE ANION GAP
$\textbf{Urine}_{\textbf{anion gap}} = (U_{Na}^{+} + U_{K}^{+}) - U_{Cl}^{-}$

A negative urine anion gap in the patient with normal anion gap metabolic acidosis should prompt consideration of an extrarenal etiology. A positive urine anion gap should raise concern for the possibility of renal tubular acidosis.

If the urine anion gap is positive, ***proceed to Step 11.***

If the urine anion gap is negative, ***proceed to Step 14.***

STEP 11 – *What Is the Differential Diagnosis of a Positive Urine Anion Gap in the Patient With a Normal Anion Gap Metabolic Acidosis?*

The differential diagnosis of a positive urine anion gap in the patient with a normal anion gap metabolic acidosis is listed in the following box.

CAUSES OF POSITIVE URINE ANION GAP IN THE PATIENT WITH A NONANION GAP METABOLIC ACIDOSIS
Hypokalemic distal renal tubular acidosis (type I)
Hyperkalemic distal renal tubular acidosis (type IV)
Hypokalemic proximal renal tubular acidosis (type II)
Renal tubular acidosis of renal insufficiency

Determining the type of renal tubular acidosis that is present begins with consideration of the serum potassium concentration.

If the serum potassium is low, ***proceed to Step 12.***

If the serum potassium is high, ***proceed to Step 13.***

If the serum potassium is normal, ***proceed to Step 15.***

STEP 12 – *Does the Patient Have Type I or Type II RTA?*

Type I and II RTA are considerations in the hypokalemic patient who has a positive urine anion gap in the setting of a normal anion gap metabolic acidosis. These are discussed in further detail in the remainder of this step.

Proximal Renal Tubular Acidosis (Type II RTA)

Proximal renal tubular acidosis or type II RTA should be suspected in the patient who has the following findings at steady-state:

- Normal anion gap metabolic acidosis
- Hypokalemia
- Ability to acidify urine to pH <5.5
- Other findings of proximal tubular dysfunction may be present (glycosuria, hypophosphatemia, hypouricemia, and mild proteinuria)
- Positive urine anion gap

Proximal RTA may occur in isolation or in combination with other abnormalities of proximal tubular dysfunction (Fanconi syndrome). The causes of proximal RTA are listed in the following box.

CAUSES OF PROXIMAL (TYPE II) RTA
SELECTIVE (unassociated with Fanconi syndrome)
PRIMARY
Transient (infants)
Idiopathic or genetic
CARBONIC ANHYDRASE DEFICIENCY, INHIBITION, OR ALTERATION
Drugs: Acetazolamide, sulfanilamide
Carbonic anhydrase II deficiency with osteopetrosis
GENERALIZED (associated with Fanconi syndrome)
PRIMARY (without associated systemic disease)
Genetic
Sporadic
GENETICALLY TRANSMITTED SYSTEMIC DISEASE
Cystinosis
Wilson's disease
Lowe's syndrome
Tyrosinemia
Galactosemia
Hereditary fructose intolerance
Metachromatic leukodystrophy
Pyruvate carboxylase deficiency
Methylmalonic acidemia
DYSPROTEINEMIC STATES
Multiple myeloma
Monoclonal gammopathy
SECONDARY HYPERPARATHYROIDISM WITH CHRONIC HYPERCALCEMIA
Vitamin D deficiency or resistance
Vitamin D dependency
DRUGS OR TOXINS
Ifosfamide
Outdated tetracycline
Streptozotocin
Lead
Mercury
TUBULOINTERSTITIAL DISEASE
Sjögren's syndrome
Medullary cystic disease
Renal transplantation
MISCELLANEOUS
Nephrotic syndrome
Amyloidosis
Paroxysmal nocturnal hemoglobinuria

Adapted from *The Kidney*, Brenner BM and Rector FC, eds, Philadelphia, PA: WB Saunders Co, 2000, 952.

If type II RTA is suspected but the diagnosis is uncertain, the clinician may choose to perform a sodium bicarbonate infusion test. During this test, sodium bicarbonate is administered at a rate of 0.5-1.0 mEq/hour/kg body weight. The administration of sodium bicarbonate will cause the serum bicarbonate concentration to rise. As the serum bicarbonate concentration rises above the reabsorptive threshold, the pH of the urine will quickly climb to a value >7.5. In addition, the fractional excretion of bicarbonate will also increase to values >15%. The fractional excretion of bicarbonate may be calculated by sending a urine specimen for measurement of creatinine and bicarbonate. The equation to calculate the fractional excretion of bicarbonate is as follows:

FRACTIONAL EXCRETION OF BICARBONATE
$$FE_{HCO_3^-} (\%) = \frac{urine_{HCO_3^-} \times plasma_{Cr}}{plasma_{HCO_3^-} \times urine_{Cr}} \times 100$$
Normal $FE_{HCO_3^-}$ = 5%

Hypokalemic Distal Renal Tubular Acidosis (Type I RTA)

Hypokalemic distal renal tubular acidosis should be a consideration in patients who present with the following findings:

- Normal anion gap metabolic acidosis
- Hypokalemia
- Inability to lower urine pH maximally (urine pH >5.5 in setting of systemic acidosis)
- Positive urine anion gap

The causes of hypokalemic distal renal tubular acidosis are listed in the following box.

CAUSES OF HYPOKALEMIC DISTAL RENAL TUBULAR ACIDOSIS (TYPE I RTA)
PRIMARY
IDIOPATHIC
FAMILIAL
SECONDARY
AUTOIMMUNE DISORDERS
Hypergammaglobulinemia
Primary biliary cirrhosis
Systemic lupus erythematosus
Sjögren's syndrome
GENETIC DISEASES
Ehlers-Danlos syndrome
Marfan syndrome
Hereditary elliptocytosis
MEDICATION (amphotericin B)
TOXIN (toluene)
DISORDERS WITH NEPHROCALCINOSES
Hyperparathyroidism
Vitamin D intoxication
Idiopathic hypercalciuria
TUBULOINTERSTITIAL DISEASE
Obstructive uropathy
Renal transplantation

Adapted from *Comprehensive Clinical Nephrology*, Johnson R and Feehally J, eds, Harcourt Publishers Ltd, 2000, 3.12.8.

End of Section.

STEP 13 – *Does the Patient Have Hyperkalemic Distal Renal Tubular Acidosis (Type IV RTA)?*

Type IV RTA should be considered in the hyperkalemic patient who has a positive urine anion gap in the setting of a normal anion gap metabolic acidosis. Findings consistent with type IV RTA include the following:

- Normal anion gap metabolic acidosis
- Hyperkalemia
- Urine anion gap slightly positive
- Urine pH is variable (may be > or <5.5)

The causes of type IV RTA are listed in the following box.

CAUSES OF HYPERKALEMIC RENAL TUBULAR ACIDOSIS (TYPE IV RTA)

MINERALOCORTICOID RESISTANCE
- Pseudohypoaldosteronism (type I and II)
- Medications
  - Spironolactone
  - Triamterene
  - Amiloride
  - Trimethoprim
  - Pentamidine
- Chronic tubulointerstitial disease
  - Chronic urinary tract obstruction
  - Sickle cell nephropathy
  - Systemic lupus erythematosus

MINERALOCORTICOID DEFICIENCY
- Adrenal insufficiency
- Bilateral adrenalectomy
- Adrenal enzyme deficiency (congenital)
- Medications
  - ACE inhibitor
  - Angiotensin II receptor blocker
  - Heparin
  - Ketoconazole
- Hyporeninemic hypoaldosteronism

End of Section.

STEP 14 – *What Is the Differential Diagnosis of a Negative Urine Anion Gap in the Patient With a Normal Anion Gap Metabolic Acidosis?*

A negative urine anion gap in the patient with a normal anion gap metabolic acidosis may be secondary to the following:

- Diarrhea
- External loss of pancreatic or biliary secretions

In addition to diarrhea, there are other gastrointestinal conditions that may lead to the loss of alkali. Some of these include fistulas (biliary, pancreatic, enteric), ileus secondary to obstruction (large amounts of alkali may accumulate in the intestinal lumen), and some cases of villous adenoma, characterized by the elaboration of fluid high in bicarbonate. When no apparent gastrointestinal etiology is apparent in the patient with laboratory testing consistent with a gastrointestinal process, the clinician should entertain the possibility of laxative abuse.

End of Section.

STEP 15 – *Does the Patient Have Renal Tubular Acidosis of Renal Insufficiency?*

Patients with chronic renal insufficiency typically develop a normal anion gap metabolic acidosis as the glomerular filtration rate falls to <30 mL/minute. The serum potassium concentration typically remains in the normal range. With worsening renal function (glomerular filtration rate <10-15 mL/minute), the normal anion gap metabolic acidosis is replaced by a high anion gap metabolic acidosis.

References

Gregory MJ and Schwartz GJ, "Diagnosis and Treatment of Renal Tubular Disorders," *Semin Nephrol*, 1998, 18(3):317-29.

Kurtzman NA, "Renal Tubular Acidosis Syndromes," *South Med J*, 2000, 93(11):1042-52.

Penney MD and Oleesky DA, "Renal Tubular Acidosis," *Ann Clin Biochem*, 1999, 36 (Pt 4):408-22.

Rodriguez Soriano J, "Renal Tubular Acidosis: The Clinical Entity," *J Am Soc Nephrol*, 2002, 13(8):2160-70.

Smulders YM, Frissen PH, Slaats EH, et al, "Renal Tubular Acidosis. Pathophysiology and Diagnosis," *Arch Intern Med*, 1996, 156(15):1629-36.

Unwin RJ and Capasso G, "The Renal Tubular Acidoses," *J R Soc Med*, 2001, 94(5):221-5.

Unwin RJ, Shirley DG, and Capasso G, "Urinary Acidification and Distal Renal Tubular Acidosis," *J Nephrol*, 2002, 15(Suppl 5):S142-50.

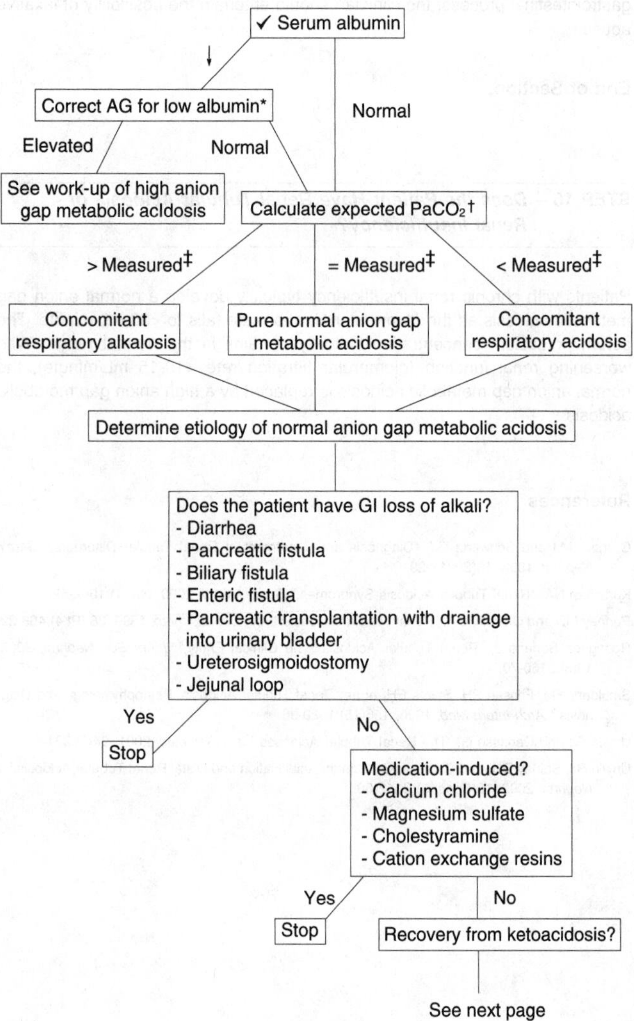
NORMAL ANION GAP METABOLIC ACIDOSIS
✓ Serum albumin
↓
Correct AG for low albumin*
Normal
Elevated
Normal
See work-up of high anion gap metabolic acidosis
Calculate expected PaCO2†
> Measured‡
= Measured‡
< Measured‡
Concomitant respiratory alkalosis
Pure normal anion gap metabolic acidosis
Concomitant respiratory acidosis
Determine etiology of normal anion gap metabolic acidosis
Does the patient have GI loss of alkali?
- Diarrhea
- Pancreatic fistula
- Biliary fistula
- Enteric fistula
- Pancreatic transplantation with drainage into urinary bladder
- Ureterosigmoidostomy
- Jejunal loop
Yes
Stop
No
Medication-induced?
- Calcium chloride
- Magnesium sulfate
- Cholestyramine
- Cation exchange resins
Yes
Stop
No
Recovery from ketoacidosis?
See next page

NORMAL ANION GAP METABOLIC ACIDOSIS *(continued)*

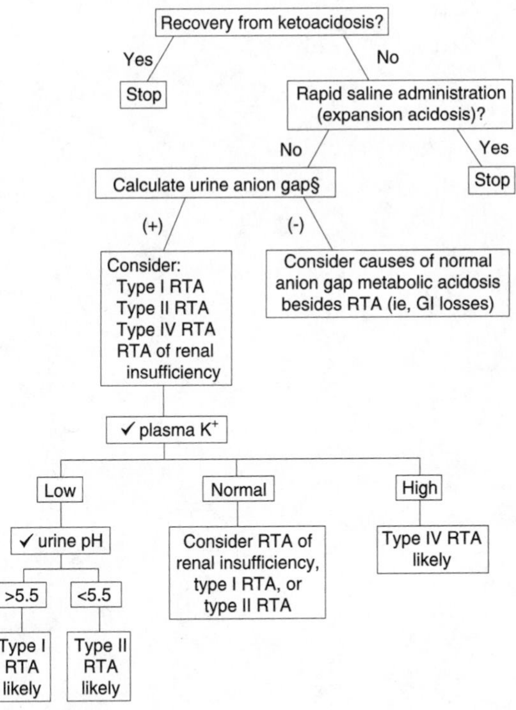

* Corrected AG = $AG_{measured} + 2.5\ (4\text{-albumin})$

† Expected $PaCO_2 = [(1.5 \times HCO_3^-) + 8 \pm 2]$

‡ Measured $PaCO_2$ refers to the arterial blood gas value

§ Urine AG = $U_{Na^+} + U_{K^+} - U_{Cl^-}$

APPROACH TO THE PATIENT WITH RESPIRATORY ACIDOSIS

STEP 1 – *Does the Patient Have Respiratory Acidosis?*

In this chapter, the evaluation of the patient with a respiratory acidosis will be discussed. This chapter assumes that the presence of a respiratory acidosis has been firmly established. For more information regarding how the diagnosis of respiratory acidosis is established, please refer to the chapter, ***Approach to the Patient With an Acid-Base Disorder*** *on page 283*

If the patient has a respiratory acidosis, ***proceed to Step 2***.

STEP 2 – *Is the Respiratory Acidosis Acute or Chronic?*

Once the presence of respiratory acidosis has been established, it is then necessary to determine if the process is acute or chronic. The body compensates for respiratory acidosis with the generation and reclamation of bicarbonate. When the respiratory acidosis is acute (less than 8 hours), there is a mild increase in bicarbonate. Since full compensation requires 12-24 hours to manifest, the clinician needs to be familiar with two equations. One equation is used in the evaluation of acute respiratory acidosis and the other with chronic respiratory acidosis. These equations are as follows.

In **acute** respiratory acidosis, there is a 0.08 fall in pH for every 10 mm Hg rise in $PaCO_2$ above normal (or 40 mm Hg).

In **chronic** respiratory acidosis, there is a 0.03 fall in pH for every 10 mm Hg rise in $PaCO_2$ above normal (or 40 mm Hg).

A pH that falls in between that which is expected for acute and chronic respiratory acidosis suggests a partially compensated disorder.

Proceed to Step 3.

STEP 3 – *Is There a Concomitant Metabolic Process That Accompanies the Respiratory Acidosis?*

In patients with respiratory acidosis, it is important to determine if a concomitant metabolic process accompanies the respiratory acidosis. The following points are helpful in this regard.

- If the pH is higher than the value that is calculated, then a concomitant metabolic alkalosis exists as well.
- If the pH is lower than the value that is calculated, then a concomitant metabolic acidosis exists as well.
- If the expected and measured pH are equal, then the patient has a pure respiratory acidosis.

To determine the etiology of the respiratory acidosis, ***proceed to Step 4***.

STEP 4 – *What Are the Causes of Acute and Chronic Respiratory Acidosis?*

The causes of acute respiratory acidosis are listed in the following box.

CAUSES OF ACUTE RESPIRATORY ACIDOSIS

UPPER AIRWAY OBSTRUCTION
- Coma-induced hypopharyngeal obstruction
- Aspiration of foreign body or vomitus
- Laryngospasm
- Angioedema
- Obstructive sleep apnea
- Inadequate laryngeal intubation
- Laryngeal obstruction postintubation

INCREASED VENTILATORY DEMAND
- High-carbohydrate diet
- High-carbohydrate dialysate (peritoneal dialysis)
- Sorbent-regenerative hemodialysis
- Pulmonary thromboembolism
- Fat, air pulmonary embolism
- Sepsis
- Hypovolemia

LOWER AIRWAY OBSTRUCTION
- Generalized bronchospasm
- Airways edema, secretions
- Severe episode of spasmodic asthma
- Bronchiolitis of infants and adults

LUNG STIFFNESS
- Severe bilateral pneumonia or bronchopneumonia
- Acute respiratory distress syndrome
- Severe pulmonary edema
- Atelectasis

CHEST WALL STIFFNESS
- Rib fractures with flail chest
- Pneumothorax
- Hemothorax
- Abdominal distention
- Ascites
- Peritoneal dialysis

MUSCLE DYSFUNCTION
- Fatigue
- Hyperkalemia
- Hypokalemia
- Hypoperfusion state
- Hypoxemia
- Malnutrition

DEPRESSED CENTRAL DRIVE
- General anesthesia
- Sedative overdose
- Head trauma
- CVA
- Central sleep apnea
- Cerebral edema
- Brain tumor
- Encephalitis
- Brainstem lesion

ABNORMAL NEUROMUSCULAR TRANSMISSION
- High spinal cord injury
- Guillain-Barré syndrome
- Status epilepticus
- Botulism; tetanus
- Crisis in myasthenia gravis
- Hypokalemic myopathy
- Familial periodic paralysis
- Drugs/toxic agents: Curare, succinylcholine, aminoglycosides, organophosphorus

Adapted from Johnson R and Feehally J, *Comprehensive Clinical Nephrology,* Harcourt Publishers Ltd, 2000, 3.14.2.

The causes of chronic respiratory acidosis are listed in the following box.

CAUSES OF CHRONIC RESPIRATORY ACIDOSIS

UPPER AIRWAY OBSTRUCTION
- Tonsillar and peritonsillar hypertrophy
- Paralysis of the vocal cords
- Tumor of the cords or larynx
- Airway stenosis postprolonged intubation
- Thymoma, aortic aneurysm

LOWER AIRWAY OBSTRUCTION
- Airway scarring
- Chronic obstructive lung disease
  - Bronchitis
  - Bronchiolitis
  - Bronchiectasis
  - Emphysema

LUNG STIFFNESS
- Severe chronic pneumonitis
- Diffuse infiltrative disease (eg, alveolar proteinosis)
- Interstitial fibrosis

CHEST WALL STIFFNESS
- Kyphoscoliosis, spinal arthritis
- Obesity
- Fibrothorax
- Hydrothorax
- Chest wall tumors

MUSCLE DYSFUNCTION (eg, polymyositis)

DEPRESSED CENTRAL DRIVE
- Sedative overdose
- Methadone / heroin addiction
- Sleep disordered breathing
- Brain tumor
- Bulbar poliomyelitis
- Hypothyroidism

ABNORMAL NEUROMUSCULAR TRANSMISSION
- Poliomyelitis
- Multiple sclerosis
- Muscular dystrophy
- Amyotrophic lateral sclerosis
- Diaphragmatic paralysis
- Myopathic disease (polymyositis)

Adapted from Johnson R and Feehally J, *Comprehensive Clinical Nephrology,* Harcourt Publishers Ltd, 2000, 3.14.2.

Proceed to Step 5.

STEP 5 – *What Laboratory Tests Should Be Obtained to Elucidate the Etiology of the Respiratory Acidosis?*

In most cases of respiratory acidosis, the etiology is readily apparent. Laboratory testing that may help elucidate the etiology of the respiratory acidosis include the following.

- Drug/toxicology screen

  Drug and toxicology screens may identify the recent use of barbiturates, benzodiazepines, and narcotics, all of which are associated with respiratory acidosis.

- Chest radiograph

  Pulmonary disease is a major cause of respiratory acidosis. The chest radiograph will often identify findings consistent with a particular type of pulmonary disease.

- CT scan of the chest

  CT scan of the chest is not necessary in all patients with respiratory acidosis. It should be considered, however, in patients who are thought to have a pulmonary disorder but have an unremarkable chest radiograph. It may also be obtained when the chest radiographic findings are inconclusive.

- CT scan of the brain

  When a central cause of respiratory acidosis is suspected, a CT scan of the brain should be obtained. CNS lesions such as strokes or tumors may be identified. The clinician should pay particular attention to the brainstem (pons, medulla).

- MRI of the brain

  A negative or inconclusive CT scan of the brain does not exclude a central cause of hypoventilation and respiratory acidosis. If a central cause is suspected but the CT scan is unrevealing, it is reasonable to proceed with a MRI of the brain, which may reveal findings not apparent on the CT scan.

- Fluoroscopy

  Not uncommonly, the chest radiograph in patients with diaphragmatic paralysis is unremarkable. In these cases, fluoroscopy can be performed to establish the diagnosis. During the fluoroscopic "sniff test", paradoxical elevation of the paralyzed diaphragm with inspiration is considered to be consistent with the diagnosis of diaphragmatic paralysis.

- Pulmonary function tests

  Pulmonary function tests are critical in not only establishing the diagnosis of obstructive lung disease but also in estimating the severity of the disease.

- EMG / NCV

  Respiratory acidosis may be due to respiratory muscle weakness. Respiratory muscle weakness may be a manifestation of a number of neuromuscular diseases. EMG / NCV are useful in the diagnosis of these diseases and may help differentiate a myopathic from neuropathic condition.

References

Epstein SK and Singh N, "Respiratory Acidosis," *Respir Care*, 2001, 46(4):366-83.

Gluck SL, "Acid-Base," *Lancet*, 1998, 352(9126):474-9.

Kraut JA and Madias NE, "Approach to Patients With Acid-Base Disorders," *Respir Care*, 2001, 46(4):392-403.

Laski ME and Kurtzman NA, "Acid-Base Disorders in Medicine," *Dis Mon*, 1996, 42(2):51-125.

Syabbolo N, "Measurement and Interpretation of Arterial Blood Gases," *Br J Clin Pract*, 1997, 51(3):173-6.

Williams AJ, "ABC of Oxygen: Assessing and Interpreting Arterial Blood Gases and Acid-Base Balance," *BMJ*, 1998, 317(7167):1213-6.

Williamson JC, "Acid-Base Disorders: Classification and Management Strategies," *Am Fam Physician*, 1995, 52(2):584-90.

APPROACH TO THE PATIENT WITH METABOLIC ALKALOSIS

STEP 1 – *Does the Patient Have Metabolic Alkalosis?*

In this chapter, the evaluation of the patient with metabolic alkalosis will be discussed. This chapter assumes that the presence of a metabolic alkalosis has been firmly established. For more information regarding how the diagnosis of metabolic alkalosis is established, please refer to the chapter, ***Approach to the Patient With an Acid-Base Disorder*** *on page 283.*

If the patient has metabolic alkalosis, ***proceed to Step 2.***

STEP 2 – *Is the Respiratory Compensation Adequate?*

Once the presence of metabolic alkalosis is established, it is then necessary to determine if respiratory compensation is adequate.

In a patient with a metabolic alkalosis, the following equation can be used to assess the adequacy of respiratory compensation:

$$\textbf{Expected PaCO}_2 = HCO_3^- + 15$$

Unfortunately, no derived equation predicting the respiratory compensation has been found to be completely reliable. However, the above equation is one of the best that is available to us. Some important points about the above equation in relation to patients with metabolic alkalosis include the following.

- If the measured $PaCO_2$ is greater than the expected $PaCO_2$, then a concomitant respiratory acidosis exists.
- If the measured $PaCO_2$ is less than the expected $PaCO_2$, then a concomitant respiratory alkalosis is present.
- If the measured $PaCO_2$ is equal to the expected $PaCO_2$, then the patient has a pure metabolic alkalosis.

It is important to recognize that this formula holds true only for patients who have had sufficient time for full compensation to take place, usually 12-24 hours. If the expected and measured $PaCO_2$ are not equal, there either exists a concomitant acid-base disorder as discussed above or sufficient time has not elapsed for full compensation to take place.

Remember also that this equation lacks reliability if the patient is markedly alkalemic, particularly if the pH is >7.6.

To determine the etiology of the metabolic alkalosis, ***proceed to Step 3.***

STEP 3 – *What Are the Causes of Metabolic Alkalosis?*

The differential diagnosis of metabolic alkalosis is listed in the following box.

CAUSES OF METABOLIC ALKALOSIS
EXOGENOUS ALKALI
Antacids
Citrate
Intravenous lactate
Massive blood transfusion
Plasmapheresis
NONABSORBABLE ANTACIDS WITH EXCHANGE RESIN
MILK-ALKALI SYNDROME
REFEEDING SYNDROME
HYPERCALCEMIA
CHLORIDE-RESPONSIVE METABOLIC ALKALOSIS
Vomiting or other gastric loss
Chloride losing diarrhea
Villous adenoma
Diuretic therapy (remote)
Poorly reabsorbable anions
Posthypercapnia
CHLORIDE-UNRESPONSIVE METABOLIC ALKALOSIS
Primary hyperaldosteronism
Renal artery stenosis
Renin-secreting tumor
Malignant hypertension
Cushing's syndrome
Exogenous mineralocorticoids
Adrenal enzyme deficiencies
Liddle's syndrome
Bartter's syndrome
Gitelman's syndrome
Magnesium deficiency
Potassium deficiency
Diuretic therapy

Proceed to Step 4.

STEP 4 – *Has the Patient Received Exogenous Alkali?*

The administration of exogenous alkali can lead to the development of metabolic alkalosis. Examples include:

- Ingestion of large amounts of medications containing sodium bicarbonate for gastritis or peptic ulcer disease
- Ingestion of large amounts of medications containing citrate or glutamate
- Intravenous administration of lactate or acetate in the setting of trauma or resuscitation of hypovolemia
- Massive blood transfusion
- Plasmapheresis
- Administration of large amounts of sodium bicarbonate in patients with metabolic acidosis may lead to rebound alkalosis after the acidosis resolves.

In all of these cases, the metabolic alkalosis is transient because the kidneys are able to excrete the excess bicarbonate.

If the metabolic alkalosis is secondary to exogenous alkali, ***stop here***.

If the metabolic alkalosis is not secondary to exogenous alkali, ***proceed to Step 5***.

STEP 5 – *Has the Patient Been Taking a Nonabsorbable Antacid in Conjunction With an Exchange Resin?*

Magnesium and aluminum hydroxide are known as nonabsorbable antacids. When these antacids are ingested along with a cation exchange resin, a transient metabolic alkalosis may result. Again, the kidneys are able to respond with the excretion of excess bicarbonate.

If the metabolic alkalosis is secondary to the ingestion of a nonabsorbable antacid in combination with an exchange resin, ***stop here***.

If the metabolic alkalosis is not secondary to the ingestion of a nonabsorbable antacid in combination with an exchange resin, ***proceed to Step 6***.

STEP 6 – *Does the Patient Have the Milk-Alkali Syndrome?*

This syndrome develops in the avid milk drinker who is also taking calcium-containing antacids.

MILK-ALKALI SYNDROME FEATURES	
CHRONIC RENAL FAILURE	NEPHROCALCINOSIS
HYPERCALCEMIA	METABOLIC ALKALOSIS

If the metabolic alkalosis is secondary to the milk-alkali syndrome, ***stop here***.

If the metabolic alkalosis is not secondary to the milk-alkali syndrome, ***proceed to Step 7***.

STEP 7 – *Does the Patient Have Refeeding Alkalosis?*

After fasting for several weeks, refeeding may result in a metabolic alkalosis, the etiology of which is unclear.

If the metabolic alkalosis is secondary to refeeding, ***stop here***.

If the metabolic alkalosis is not secondary to refeeding, ***proceed to Step 8***.

STEP 8 – *Does the Patient Have Hypercalcemia?*

A mild metabolic alkalosis has been reported in patients with hypercalcemia due to malignancy, sarcoidosis, or vitamin D intoxication. The etiology is unclear.

If the metabolic alkalosis is secondary to hypercalcemia, ***stop here***.

If the metabolic alkalosis is not secondary to hypercalcemia, ***proceed to Step 9***.

STEP 9 – *What Is the Urine Chloride Concentration?*

After exclusion of the above disorders, attention should focus on determination of the urine chloride concentration. Based on the urine chloride level, the metabolic alkalosis may be divided into one of the following:

- Chloride-responsive metabolic alkalosis (urine chloride <20 mEq/L)

- Chloride-unresponsive metabolic alkalosis (urine chloride >20 mEq/L)

In clinical practice, most patients have a chloride-responsive metabolic alkalosis. The most common causes include:

- Vomiting
- Gastric drainage
- Diuretic therapy

Less commonly, the patient is found to have a high urine chloride level, one that is >20 mEq/L. In these cases, the clinician should entertain the causes of chloride-unresponsive metabolic alkalosis. These are conditions in which there is excessive generation of bicarbonate by the kidneys.

Before delving any further, the clinician needs to be aware of some important exceptions.

- When metabolic alkalosis is due to diuretics, the urine chloride concentration may be high, particularly if the urine chloride determination is performed within the period of action of the diuretic.
- The urine chloride concentration may be low in patients with low chloride intake, who have excessive renal generation of bicarbonate.

If the urine chloride is <20 mEq/L, the patient has a chloride-responsive metabolic alkalosis. ***Proceed to Step 10.***

If the urine chloride is >20 mEq/L, the patient has a chloride-unresponsive metabolic alkalosis. ***Proceed to Step 16*** *on page 322.*

STEP 10 – *What Is the Differential Diagnosis of Chloride-Responsive Metabolic Alkalosis?*

The differential diagnosis of chloride-responsive metabolic alkalosis is listed in the following box.

CHLORIDE-RESPONSIVE METABOLIC ALKALOSIS DIFFERENTIAL DIAGNOSIS
VOMITING OR OTHER GASTRIC LOSS
CHLORIDE-LOSING DIARRHEA
VILLOUS ADENOMA
DIURETIC THERAPY (remote)
POORLY REABSORBABLE ANIONS
Ampicillin
Carbenicillin
POSTHYPERCAPNIA

Proceed to Step 11.

STEP 11 – *Is the Chloride-Responsive Metabolic Alkalosis Due to Gastric Losses?*

The most common type of metabolic alkalosis is that which is due to gastric losses, either vomiting or nasogastric suction. The diagnosis is usually apparent from the clinical history. The following laboratory findings support gastric losses as the etiology of the metabolic alkalosis.

GASTRIC LOSSES AS A CAUSE OF METABOLIC ALKALOSIS LABORATORY FEATURES	
DECREASED SERUM POTASSIUM	ACIDIC URINE
URINE POTASSIUM >20 mEq/L*	URINE CHLORIDE <20 mEq/L

*Vomiting is the only extrarenal cause of hypokalemia that presents with a high urine potassium level.

While gastric losses are usually evident, in the absence of a characteristic history, patients presenting with the above constellation of laboratory findings should be investigated for surreptitious vomiting. The following physical examination findings may provide clues to this possibility:

- Ulcers, calluses, and scarring on the dorsum of the hand
- Dental erosions due to chronic exposure to gastric secretions
- Puffy cheeks that result from salivary gland hypertrophy

If the metabolic alkalosis is secondary to gastric losses, ***stop here.***

If the metabolic alkalosis is not secondary to gastric losses, ***proceed to Step 12.***

STEP 12 – *Is Diuretic Therapy the Cause of the Chloride-Responsive Metabolic Alkalosis?*

Metabolic alkalosis can result from the administration of all diuretics except carbonic anhydrase inhibitors and potassium-sparing diuretics. Usually, the diagnosis is apparent from the history. Some patients, however, may surreptitiously abuse diuretics. These patients may be suspected of covert diuretic abuse based on the following laboratory findings.

DIURETIC USE AS A CAUSE OF METABOLIC ALKALOSIS LABORATORY FEATURES
DECREASED SERUM MAGNESIUM
URINE POTASSIUM >20 mEq/L
INCREASED URINE CHLORIDE (during diuretic's period of action) **or**
DECREASED URINE CHLORIDE (remote use)

If the metabolic alkalosis is secondary to diuretic use, ***stop here.***

If the metabolic alkalosis is not secondary to diuretic use, ***proceed to Step 13.***

STEP 13 – *Does the Patient Have Posthypercapnic Metabolic Alkalosis?*

This condition most commonly develops in the patient with COPD who has a chronic respiratory acidosis characterized by a high $PaCO_2$. In these patients, there is an increase in hydrogen ion secretion and therefore bicarbonate reabsorption. In essence, this is the kidney's compensatory response to the respiratory acidosis, in an attempt to return the pH back towards normal. When these patients require mechanical ventilation, posthypercapnic metabolic alkalosis may result with potentially catastrophic results. Metabolic alkalosis results when the $PaCO_2$ is rapidly decreased, because the bicarbonate concentration will remain elevated. The subsequent increase in pH can lead to serious neurologic abnormalities even death. As a result, the $PaCO_2$ should be lowered slowly in patients with chronic respiratory acidosis to prevent this complication.

If the metabolic alkalosis is secondary to the posthypercapnia, ***stop here.***

If the metabolic alkalosis is not secondary to the posthypercapnia, ***proceed to Step 14.***

STEP 14 – *Does the Patient Have Diarrhea?*

Recall that most patients with diarrhea have a normal anion gap metabolic acidosis. However, there are two fairly uncommon conditions that can present with metabolic alkalosis. These include the following.

- Congenital chloride diarrhea

  Most cases are diagnosed in infancy, but some have been identified in adults.
- Villous adenoma

  These are benign tumors typically affecting the rectosigmoid colon that can result in a metabolic alkalosis because of elaboration of large amounts of fluid with a high chloride concentration. These patients may also have significant hypokalemia.

If the metabolic alkalosis is secondary to diarrhea, ***stop here.***

If the metabolic alkalosis is not secondary to diarrhea, ***proceed to Step 15.***

STEP 15 – *Is the Patient Receiving Some Form of a Poorly Reabsorbable Anion?*

This is mainly seen in the setting of the intravenous administration of high doses of sodium carbenicillin or other derivative of penicillin, such as penicillin or ampicillin. As the sodium salt of the penicillin derivative is filtered through the kidney, the penicillin derivative acts as a poorly reabsorbable anion. At the level of the distal tubule, some sodium reabsorption occurs in exchange for the secretion of potassium and hydrogen ions. This leads to the development of metabolic alkalosis and hypokalemia in these patients.

End of Section.

STEP 16 – *What Is the Differential Diagnosis of Chloride-Unresponsive Metabolic Alkalosis?*

The differential diagnosis of chloride-unresponsive metabolic alkalosis is listed in the following box.

CHLORIDE-UNRESPONSIVE METABOLIC ALKALOSIS DIFFERENTIAL DIAGNOSIS	
PRIMARY HYPERALDOSTERONISM	LIDDLE'S SYNDROME
RENAL ARTERY STENOSIS	BARTTER'S SYNDROME
RENIN-SECRETING TUMOR	GITELMAN'S SYNDROME
MALIGNANT HYPERTENSION	MAGNESIUM DEFICIENCY
CUSHING'S SYNDROME	POTASSIUM DEFICIENCY (severe)
ADRENAL ENZYME DEFICIENCIES	DIURETIC THERAPY (early)
EXOGENOUS MINERALOCORTICOIDS	

Consideration of the patient's blood pressure helps the clinician to narrow the differential diagnosis.

If the patient has an elevated blood pressure, ***proceed to Step 17.***

If the patient has a normal blood pressure, ***proceed to step 18.***

STEP 17 – *What Is the Differential Diagnosis of Chloride-Unresponsive Metabolic Alkalosis In the Setting of Hypertension?*

The differential diagnosis of chloride-unresponsive metabolic alkalosis in the setting of hypertension is listed in the following box.

CAUSES OF CHLORIDE-UNRESPONSIVE METABOLIC ALKALOSIS IN THE HYPERTENSIVE PATIENT	
PRIMARY HYPERALDOSTERONISM	CUSHING'S SYNDROME
RENAL ARTERY STENOSIS	ADRENAL ENZYME DEFICIENCIES
RENIN-SECRETING TUMOR	LIDDLE'S SYNDROME
MALIGNANT HYPERTENSION	DIURETIC THERAPY (early)
EXOGENOUS MINERALOCORTICOIDS	

Measurement of plasma renin activity and aldosterone levels help to narrow the above differential diagnosis even further, as shown in the following table.

Using the Plasma Renin Activity and Aldosterone Level to Establish the Etiology of Metabolic Alkalosis and Hypertension

Test Results	Condition Suggested	Proceed to
Elevated plasma renin activity Elevated aldosterone	Renal artery stenosis Renin-secreting tumor Malignant hypertension Diuretic therapy	Step 15 of Hypokalemia chapter *on page 225*
Decreased plasma renin activity Elevated aldosterone	Primary hyperaldosteronism	Step 18 of Hypokalemia chapter *on page 228*
Decreased plasma renin activity Decreased aldosterone	Liddle's syndrome Exogenous mineralocorticoids Adrenal enzyme deficiencies	Step 16 of Hypokalemia chapter *on page 226*
Normal plasma renin activity Normal aldosterone	Cushing's syndrome	Step 17 of Hypokalemia chapter *on page 228*

End of Section.

STEP 18 – *What Is the Differential Diagnosis of Chloride-Unresponsive Metabolic Alkalosis in the Normotensive Patient?*

The differential diagnosis is listed in the following box.

CHLORIDE-UNRESPONSIVE METABOLIC ALKALOSIS IN THE NORMOTENSIVE PATIENT DIFFERENTIAL DIAGNOSIS	
BARTTER'S SYNDROME	POTASSIUM DEPLETION
GITELMAN'S SYNDROME	DIURETIC THERAPY
MAGNESIUM DEPLETION	

Patients with magnesium deficiency may develop a metabolic alkalosis. Many patients with hypomagnesemia have accompanying hypokalemia and it is thought that the hypokalemia predisposes to the development of the metabolic alkalosis in these patients. Hypokalemia, particularly when severe (K^+ <2 mEq/L), can lead to the development of a metabolic alkalosis.

Bartter's syndrome is a rare condition which is characterized by growth and mental retardation, muscle weakness, muscle cramps, polyuria, and polydipsia. Usually diagnosed during childhood, the characteristic features include hypokalemia, normomagnesemia (occasional hypomagnesemia), metabolic alkalosis, and high levels of renin and aldosterone. Urinary excretion of prostaglandin E_2 is also increased. The diagnosis of Bartter's syndrome requires excluding surreptitious vomiting, diuretic administration, and laxative abuse.

Gitelman's syndrome is a rare disorder that tends to be more benign than Bartter's syndrome. Forms of Gitelman's syndrome exhibiting both autosomal recessive and dominant inheritance have been described. Like Bartter's syndrome, it may be diagnosed in childhood but, in contrast to Bartter's syndrome, the diagnosis is often established later in childhood. Not uncommonly, the diagnosis is not made until adulthood. The syndrome presents with metabolic alkalosis and hypokalemia in the setting of a normal blood pressure. Plasma renin activity and aldosterone levels are elevated. Features favoring a diagnosis of Gitelman's syndrome over Bartter's syndrome include hypomagnesemia, low urine calcium excretion, and normal urinary prostaglandin excretion.

Comparison of Bartter's Syndrome and Gitelman's Syndrome

Bartter's Syndrome	Gitelman's Syndrome
Salt wasting	Salt wasting
Hypokalemia / alkalosis	Hypokalemia / alkalosis
Childhood	Adulthood
Hypercalciuria	Hypocalciuria
Increased PRA / aldosterone	Increased PRA / aldosterone
Na / K / Cl mutation	Na / Cl mutation

References

Galla JH, "Metabolic Alkalosis," *J Am Soc Nephrol*, 2000, 11(2):369-75.

Gluck SL, "Acid-Base," *Lancet*, 1998, 352(9126):474-9.

Khanna A and Kurtzman NA, "Metabolic Alkalosis," *Respir Care*, 2001, 46(4):354-65.

Kraut JA and Madias NE, "Approach to Patients With Acid-Base Disorders," *Respir Care*, 2001, 46(4):392-403.

Laski ME and Kurtzman NA, "Acid-Base Disorders in Medicine," *Dis Mon*, 1996, 42(2):51-125.

Palmer BF and Alpern RJ, "Metabolic Alkalosis," *J Am Soc Nephrol*, 1997, 8(9):1462-9.

Syabbolo N, "Measurement and Interpretation of Arterial Blood Gases," *Br J Clin Pract*, 1997, 51(3):173-6.

Webster NR and Kulkarni V, "Metabolic Alkalosis in the Critically Ill," *Crit Rev Clin Lab Sci*, 1999, 36(5):497-510.

Williams AJ, "ABC of Oxygen: Assessing and Interpreting Arterial Blood Gases and Acid-Base Balance," *BMJ*, 1998, 317(7167):1213-6.

Williamson JC, "Acid-Base Disorders: Classification and Management Strategies," *Am Fam Physician*, 1995, 52(2):584-90.

METABOLIC ALKALOSIS

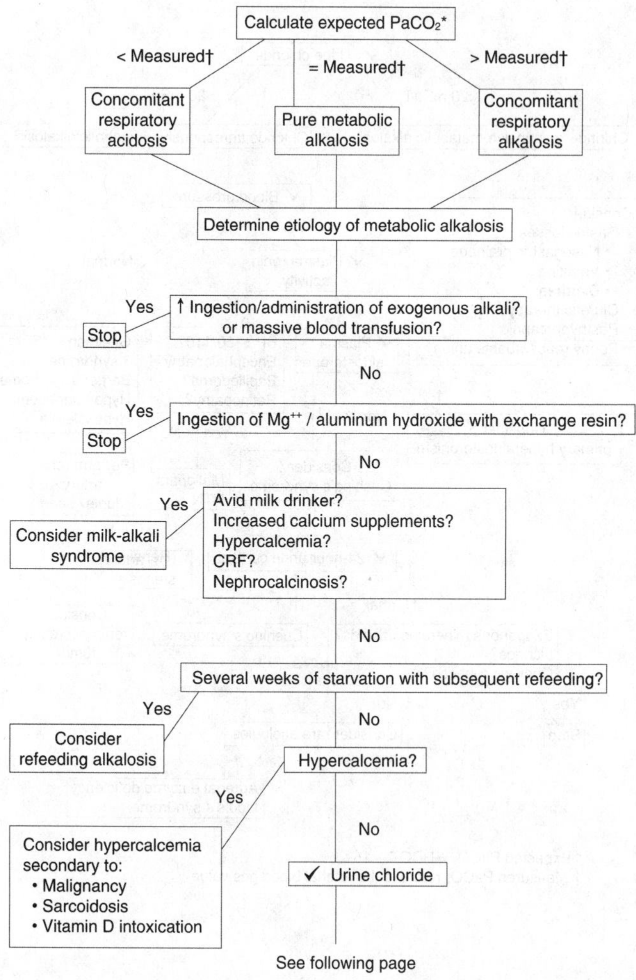

METABOLIC ALKALOSIS *(continued)*

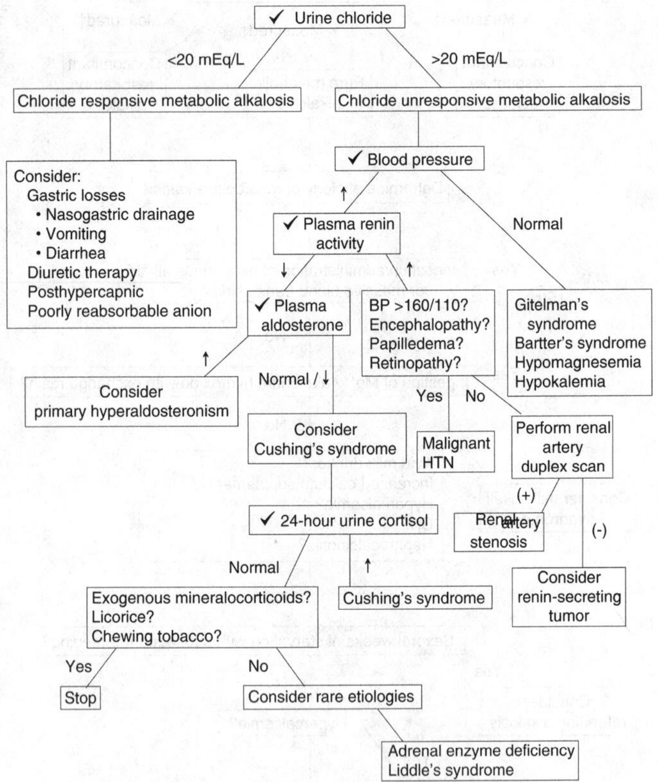

* Expected $PaCO_2 = HCO_3^- + 15$

† Measured $PaCO_2$ refers to the arterial blood gas value

APPROACH TO THE PATIENT WITH RESPIRATORY ALKALOSIS

STEP 1 – *Does the Patient Have a Respiratory Alkalosis?*

In this chapter, the evaluation of the patient with a respiratory alkalosis will be discussed. This chapter assumes that the presence of a respiratory alkalosis has been firmly established. For more information regarding how the diagnosis of respiratory alkalosis is established, please refer to the chapter, ***Approach to the Patient With an Acid-Base Disorder*** *on page 283.*

If the patient has a respiratory alkalosis, **proceed to Step 2.**

STEP 2 – *Is the Respiratory Alkalosis Acute or Chronic?*

Once it is determined that the patient has a respiratory alkalosis, it is then necessary to determine if the process is acute or chronic. The body compensates for a respiratory alkalosis by decreasing the generation and reclamation of bicarbonate. Acute respiratory alkalosis is characterized by a mild decrease in bicarbonate, whereas, in chronic respiratory alkalosis, there is a much more significant decrease after 12-24 hours as the full compensation takes place. The equations are divided into acute (<8 hours) or chronic (>24 hours). These equations are as follows.

In **acute** respiratory alkalosis, there is a 0.08 increase in the pH for every 10 mm Hg fall in the $PaCO_2$ below normal (or 40 mm Hg).
In **chronic** respiratory alkalosis, there is a 0.03 increase in the pH for every 10 mm Hg fall in the $PaCO_2$ below normal (or 40 mm Hg).

Proceed to Step 3.

STEP 3 – *Is There a Concomitant Metabolic Acid-Base Disturbance?*

In patients with a respiratory alkalosis, the following points are helpful in establishing whether a concomitant metabolic process exists.

- If the pH is higher than that expected, then the patient has a concomitant metabolic alkalosis.
- If the pH is lower than that expected, then the patient has a concomitant metabolic acidosis.
- If the measured and expected pH are equal, then the patient has a pure respiratory alkalosis.

A pH that falls in between that which is expected for acute and chronic respiratory alkalosis suggests a partially compensated disorder.

Proceed to Step 4.

STEP 4 – *What Are the Causes of Respiratory Alkalosis?*

The differential diagnosis of respiratory alkalosis is listed in the following box.

CAUSES OF RESPIRATORY ALKALOSIS

- CNS EVENT
  - CVA
  - Infection
    - Meningitis
    - Encephalitis
  - Tumor
  - Trauma
  - Fever
  - Psychosis
  - Pain
  - Anxiety
  - Hyperventilation syndrome
- DRUG USE
  - Salicylates
  - Progesterone
  - Nicotine
  - Methylxanthines
  - Catecholamines
- LUNG DISEASE
  - Interstitial lung disease
  - Pulmonary edema (cardiogenic or noncardiogenic)
  - Pneumonia
  - Pulmonary embolism
  - Asthma
  - Pneumothorax
  - Aspiration
  - Flail chest
- MISCELLANEOUS
  - Pregnancy
  - Sepsis
  - Liver cirrhosis or failure
  - Hemodialysis with acetate dialysis
  - Heat exposure
  - Severe anemia
  - Hyperthyroidism
  - High altitude
  - Right to left shunt
  - Aspiration
  - Laryngospasm

Proceed to Step 5.

STEP 5 – *What Laboratory Tests Should Be Obtained To Elucidate the Etiology of the Respiratory Alkalosis?*

In most cases of respiratory alkalosis, the etiology is readily apparent. Laboratory testing that may help elucidate the etiology of the respiratory alkalosis include the following.

- White blood cell count

  An elevated white blood cell count may be an indicator of sepsis, which is a common cause of respiratory alkalosis.

- Hemoglobin

  A low hemoglobin level should prompt consideration of severe anemia.

- Liver function tests

  Liver function test abnormalities should raise concern for the possibility of liver cirrhosis or hepatic failure as etiology of the respiratory alkalosis

- Cultures

  If the patient's clinical presentation is suggestive of sepsis, appropriate cultures should be obtained (ie, blood, urine, etc).

- Chest radiograph

  Pulmonary disease is a major cause of respiratory alkalosis. The chest radiograph will often reveal findings consistent with a particular pulmonary condition.

- CT scan of the chest

  CT scan of the chest is not necessary in all patients with respiratory alkalosis. It should be considered, however, in patients who have inconclusive chest radiographs. It may also be obtained if the chest radiograph was unremarkable but high suspicion for a pulmonary cause of respiratory alkalosis remains.

- CT scan of the brain

  When a central cause of respiratory alkalosis is suspected, the clinician should obtain a CT scan of the brain. CT scan of the brain may reveal findings consistent with CVA or tumor.

- Ventilation / perfusion scan

  Ventilation / perfusion scan of the lungs should be obtained if pulmonary embolism is a possibility.

- MRI of the brain

  MRI of the brain should be considered in patients suspected of having a central cause of respiratory alkalosis, particularly when the CT scan of the brain is inconclusive or unremarkable. The MRI may reveal abnormalities that are not apparent by CT scan.

- Lumbar puncture

  Lumbar puncture should be a consideration in patients who present with signs and symptoms of meningitis.

References

Foster GT, Vaziri ND, and Sassoon CS, "Respiratory Alkalosis," *Respir Care*, 2001, 46(4):384-91.

Gluck SL, "Acid-Base," *Lancet*, 1998, 352(9126):474-9.

Kraut JA and Madias NE, "Approach to Patients With Acid-Base Disorders," *Respir Care*, 2001, 46(4):392-403.

Laffey JG and Kavanagh BP, "Hypocapnia," *N Engl J Med*, 2002, 347(1):43-53.

Laski ME and Kurtzman NA, "Acid-Base Disorders in Medicine," *Dis Mon*, 1996, 42(2):51-125.

Syabbolo N, "Measurement and Interpretation of Arterial Blood Gases," *Br J Clin Pract*, 1997, 51(3):173-6.

Williams AJ, "ABC of Oxygen: Assessing and Interpreting Arterial Blood Gases and Acid-Base Balance," *BMJ*, 1998, 317(7167):1213-6.

Williamson JC, "Acid-Base Disorders: Classification and Management Strategies," *Am Fam Physician*, 1995, 52(2):584-90.

PART III:

ENDOCRINOLOGY

HYPOGLYCEMIA

STEP 1 – *Does the Patient Have Pseudohypoglycemia?*

Before embarking on an extensive workup for hypoglycemia, it is always wise to ensure that the patient does not have pseudohypoglycemia. Pseudohypoglycemia should be a consideration in hypoglycemic patients who have no signs or symptoms of hypoglycemia. This entity is classically seen in patients with chronic leukemias who have markedly elevated white blood cell counts. In these patients, there is an artifactual lowering of plasma glucose secondary to glycolysis *in vitro*. Pseudohypoglycemia may also be encountered in patients with hemolytic anemia or polycythemia. It can be definitively diagnosed by the finding of a normal glucose level in plasma that has been separated from the formed elements of the blood.

If the patient has pseudohypoglycemia, ***stop here***.
If the patient does not have pseudohypoglycemia, ***proceed to Step 2***.

STEP 2 – *Does the Patient Have Signs and Symptoms of Hypoglycemia?*

Symptoms and signs of hypoglycemia may be either adrenergic or neuroglycopenic in origin as demonstrated in the following table.

SIGNS AND SYMPTOMS OF HYPOGLYCEMIA	
ADRENERGIC SYMPTOMS	**NEUROGLYCOPENIC SYMPTOMS**
Diaphoresis	Warmth
Hunger	Weakness
Tingling sensation	Poor concentration / confusion
Shakiness / tremulousness	Fatigue
Palpitations ("pounding heart")	Drowsiness
Nervousness / anxiety	Lightheadedness
	Dizziness
	Difficulty with speech
	Blurred vision
	Focal neurologic deficits (rare)

Although the history is of major importance in identifying hypoglycemia, the signs and symptoms are nonspecific. Therefore, the diagnosis of hypoglycemia cannot be based on clinical presentation, nor solely on the basis of a plasma glucose level, unless it is markedly abnormal. The Third International Symposium on Hypoglycemia has defined hypoglycemia as an absolute plasma glucose level <50 mg/dL (2.8 mmol/L).

In usual clinical practice, the definition of hypoglycemia is based on Whipple's triad.

WHIPPLE'S TRIAD
1) Decreased plasma glucose
2) Symptoms consistent with hypoglycemia
3) Relief of symptoms by correction of hypoglycemia

In patients who have signs and symptoms suggestive of hypoglycemia but in whom a glucose level has not been obtained during a time when the patient is symptomatic, the plasma glucose level should be measured after an overnight fast in an attempt to document true hypoglycemia. The table below provides some guidance regarding the interpretation of the plasma glucose level after an overnight fast.

Interpreting Plasma Glucose Levels After an Overnight Fast

Plasma glucose level	Clinical significance
>70 mg/dL (3.9 mmol/L)	Normal response
50-70 mg/dL (2.8-3.9 mmol/L)	Suggestive of hypoglycemia
<50 mg/dL (2.8 mmol/L)	Postabsorptive hypoglycemia

Not all patients who have a history consistent with hypoglycemic episodes will experience hypoglycemia after an overnight fast. If the plasma glucose level is normal at least several times after an overnight fast, the decision to perform further evaluation for hypoglycemia should be based on the clinician's degree of suspicion. If the degree of suspicion for hypoglycemia is quite low, the clinician may choose not to pursue further evaluation. If the degree of suspicion is high, an extended fast should be performed. An extended fast of up to 48 hours may be done on an outpatient basis but fasts of 48-72 hours duration should be performed while the patient is hospitalized. An extended fast is also required when plasma glucose levels are suggestive of hypoglycemia following an overnight fast (50-70 mg/dL).

If the patient fulfills Whipple's triad for hypoglycemia, ***proceed to Step 3***.

If the patient has a normal glucose level during an episode of symptoms, no further evaluation is needed for hypoglycemia. ***Stop here.***

STEP 3 – *What Are the Causes of Hypoglycemia?*

The causes of hypoglycemia can be divided into postabsorptive (fasting) and postprandial (reactive) types.

SOME DEFINITIONS...

Postabsorptive hypoglycemia – fasting hypoglycemia
Postprandial hypoglycemia – hypoglycemia occurring exclusively after meals

The causes of hypoglycemia are listed in the following box.

CAUSES OF HYPOGLYCEMIA

FASTING

- Pancreatic disease
  - Insulinoma
- Liver disease
  - Cirrhosis
  - Hepatitis
  - Carcinomatosis
  - Ascending cholangitis
  - Circulatory failure
- Renal disease
- CNS disease
  - Hypothalamic disease
  - Brainstem disease
- Pituitary disease
  - Hypopituitarism
- Adrenal disease
  - Adrenal insufficiency
  - Congenital adrenal hyperplasia
- Nonpancreatic malignancy
- Medications
- Sepsis
- Miscellaneous
  - Prolonged strenuous exercise
  - Autoimmune hypoglycemia
  - Pregnancy
  - Lactation
  - Diarrheal states
  - Chronic starvation

REACTIVE

- Alimentary hypoglycemia
- Idiopathic postprandial (functional)

Hypoglycemia occurring in the fasting state is often due to serious disease. In contrast, reactive hypoglycemia rarely implies the presence of a serious abnormality. However, even with a history that is consistent with reactive hypoglycemia, the clinician must first rule out certain causes of fasting hypoglycemia (eg, insulinoma) since they may also present with reactive hypoglycemia.

If the patient has a history consistent with fasting hypoglycemia, ***proceed to Step 4.***

If the patient has a history consistent with reactive hypoglycemia, ***proceed to Step 9.***

STEP 4 – *How Are the Causes of Fasting Hypoglycemia Differentiated From One Another?*

The causes of fasting hypoglycemia are listed below.

PANCREATIC DISEASE	ADRENAL DISEASE
Insulinoma	Adrenal insufficiency
LIVER DISEASE	Congenital adrenal hyperplasia
Cirrhosis	NONPANCREATIC MALIGNANCY
Hepatitis	MEDICATIONS
Carcinomatosis	SEPSIS
Ascending cholangitis	MISCELLANEOUS
Circulatory failure	Prolonged / strenuous exercise
RENAL DISEASE	Autoimmune hypoglycemia
CNS DISEASE	Pregnancy
Hypothalamic disease	Lactation
Brainstem disease	Diarrheal states
PITUITARY DISEASE	Chronic starvation
Hypopituitarism	

Quite often, the cause of the fasting hypoglycemia can be determined after a thorough history, physical examination, and selected laboratory tests are obtained. Medications are a common cause of hypoglycemia. Insulin and sulfonylurea agents are most often involved. In fact, in IDDM patients receiving conventional insulin therapy, an average of one symptomatic hypoglycemic episode occurs per week. This average rises to two to three per week in patients treated intensively. Risk factors for the development of hypoglycemia in diabetic patients are listed in the following box.

RISK FACTORS FOR DEVELOPMENT OF HYPOGLYCEMIA IN DIABETIC PATIENTS	
EXCESSIVE INSULIN OR ORAL HYPOGLYCEMIC DOSE	ALCOHOL INTAKE
WRONG TYPE OF INSULIN	WORSENING RENAL FUNCTION
INCORRECT TIMING OF INSULIN ADMINISTRATION	ADVANCING AGE
MISSED MEAL / SNACK	POOR NUTRITION
EXERCISE	DRUG INTERACTION*
	HEPATIC DISEASE

*Commonly used drugs that can potentiate the effects of sulfonylureas include barbiturates, sulfonamides, thiazides, and salicylates.

Insulin and sulfonylurea use should be suspected even in nondiabetic patients presenting with hypoglycemia. This may be the result of surreptitious abuse or pharmacy error. The clinician should realize that nondiabetic medications may also cause hypoglycemia. Drugs that can cause hypoglycemia are listed in the following box.

MEDICATION-INDUCED HYPOGLYCEMIA	
INSULIN	AKEE NUT
SULFONYLUREAS	ANTIHISTAMINES
ALCOHOL	MONOAMINE OXIDASE INHIBITORS
PENTAMIDINE	PROPRANOLOL
QUININE	PHENYLBUTAZONE
SALICYLIC ACID (rare)	PHENTOLAMINE
SULFONAMIDES (rare)	ACE INHIBITORS
QUINIDINE	QUININE
DISOPYRAMIDE	CIBENZOLINE

Other causes of hypoglycemia that are often apparent from the patient's clinical presentation include hypoglycemia due to liver disease, renal disease, cardiac failure, sepsis, or inanition. Decreased plasma glucose levels may be seen in patients with severe liver disease. It is most commonly encountered in patients who have massive liver destruction of rapid onset. Cases of hypoglycemia have been reported in fulminant viral hepatitis, cholangitis, and fatty liver due to alcohol use. In most types of liver disease (hepatitis, cirrhosis), however, hypoglycemia is uncommon. Hypoglycemia has been noted in severe cardiac or circulatory failure but the pathophysiology remains unclear. The pathogenesis is also unclear in renal failure patients who develop hypoglycemia.

Patients with known pituitary or adrenal disease should be evaluated for adrenal insufficiency. Signs and symptoms of adrenal insufficiency are often nonspecific but may include weakness, fatigue, anorexia, weight loss, diarrhea, nausea, and ill-defined abdominal pain. Hyperpigmentation, hypotension, hyponatremia, and hyperkalemia are clues to the diagnosis. In patients who have a history of malignancy or a clinical presentation consistent with a non-beta cell tumor, the clinician should consider measuring IGF-II levels. Overproduction of IGF-II is the cause of hypoglycemia in these patients.

If the clinical presentation is not consistent with any of the above disorders, endogenous hyperinsulinism (insulinoma) and surreptitious sulfonylurea or insulin use should be considered.

If the cause of the fasting hypoglycemia is apparent, ***stop here.***

If the cause of the fasting hypoglycemia is not apparent, ***proceed to Step 5.***

STEP 5 – *What Are the Results of the 72-Hour Fast?*

If the patient does not have a medication-induced cause and no other etiology of fasting hypoglycemia can be easily identified, the clinician should consider having the patient perform a 48- to 72-hour fast. The purpose of the fast is to determine the role of insulin in the development of the patient's hypoglycemia. By differentiating insulin-mediated from noninsulin-mediated hypoglycemia, the differential diagnosis of fasting hypoglycemia can be narrowed considerably. The clinician should realize, however, that a prolonged fast may not be needed in some patients, especially those that develop symptomatic hypoglycemia after an overnight fast. These patients can be observed in the outpatient clinic and should symptomatic hypoglycemia occur, the tests listed below can then be obtained.

To perform a prolonged fast, the patient should be hospitalized. Blood specimens should be collected at 6-hour intervals for measurement of the following (some experts only measure the latter four tests if the plasma glucose <60 mg/dL):

- Plasma glucose level
- Plasma insulin concentration
- C-peptide level
- Proinsulin level
- Sulfonylurea screen

Once the plasma glucose level falls below 60 mg/dL (3.3 mmol/L), blood samples should be collected more frequently (every one to two hours). During the fast, when symptoms occur, a fingerstick blood glucose level should be obtained first to confirm the diagnosis of hypoglycemia, followed by a blood draw for the above tests.

The fast should be ended if one of the following criteria is met:

- Plasma glucose <45 mg/dL
- Signs or symptoms of hypoglycemia develop
- 72 hours have elapsed

Proceed to Step 6.

STEP 6 – *What Is the Insulin Level?*

To narrow the differential diagnosis of fasting hypoglycemia, the clinician should first consider the plasma insulin level when the patient has a plasma glucose <45 mg/dL.

If the insulin level is <6 μU/mL, ***proceed to Step 8.***

If the insulin level is >6 μU/mL, ***see below.***

The normal response to hypoglycemia is feedback inhibition of insulin secretion. Therefore, a plasma insulin concentration >6 μU/mL is an inappropriate response and suggests the presence of endogenous hyperinsulinism. The clinician should consider the following possibilities in the hypoglycemic patient with an elevated insulin level.

HYPERINSULINEMIA IN THE HYPOGLYCEMIC PATIENT DIFFERENTIAL DIAGNOSIS
INSULINOMA
FACTITIOUS INSULIN USE
SURREPTITIOUS SULFONYLUREA INGESTION

Of major concern is the possibility that the patient has an insulinoma.

Proceed to Step 7.

STEP 7 – *What Is the Plasma C-Peptide Level?*

The plasma C-peptide level is quite useful in differentiating among insulinoma, factitious insulin use, and surreptitious sulfonylurea ingestion. C-peptide is a fragment of endogenously produced proinsulin that is split from proinsulin as insulin is formed. As a result, the C-peptide level can only increase if endogenous insulin production is increased.

Low plasma C-peptide levels (<200 pmol/L) in the hypoglycemic patient (plasma glucose <45 mg/dL) with plasma insulin levels >6 μU/mL is consistent with factitious hypoglycemia due to insulin use. Factitial hypoglycemia occurs more often in women, usually in the third or fourth decades of life. Many of these women are employed in health-related occupations.

Plasma C-peptide levels ≥200 pmol/L in the hypoglycemic patient (plasma glucose <45 mg/dL) with plasma insulin levels >6 μU/mL should prompt consideration of insulinoma or surreptitious sulfonylurea ingestion. Sulfonylurea agents may produce hypoglycemia because they stimulate the pancreas to secrete insulin. As a result, the levels of the tests described will mimic the results seen in insulinoma patients. To distinguish between these two possibilities, it is useful to obtain a sulfonylurea screen of the blood or urine. If the screen is positive, the diagnosis is surreptitious sulfonylurea ingestion. A negative screen argues strongly for the presence of an insulinoma.

INTERPRETING THE RESULTS OF THE 72-HOUR FAST					
Condition	**Plasma Glucose Level**	**Plasma Insulin Level**	**Plasma C-Peptide Level**	**Plasma Proinsulin Level**	**Sulfonylurea Screen of Blood**
Insulinoma	<45 mg/dL	>6 μU/mL	≥200 pmol/L	≥5 pmol/L	Negative
Factitious hypoglycemia due to insulin use	<45 mg/dL	>6 μU/mL	<200 pmol/L	<5 pmol/L	Negative
Surreptitious sulfonylurea ingestion	<45 mg/dL	>6 μU/mL	≥200 pmol/L	≥5 pmol/L	Positive

If the results of the above tests are consistent with insulinoma, the clinician should focus on identifying the location of the tumor. The initial tests that are often ordered include CT and MRI of the abdomen. A negative result does not exclude the diagnosis as these tumors are often small. Other modalities used to localize the tumor include arteriography, octreotide scanning, endoscopic ultrasound, and intraoperative ultrasound.

End of Section

STEP 8 – *What Should Be Considered in the Patient With a Plasma Insulin Level <6 μU/mL?*

Plasma insulin levels <6 μU/mL in the hypoglycemic patient (plasma glucose <45 mg/dL) excludes the diagnosis of factitial hypoglycemia due to insulin use, surreptitious sulfonylurea ingestion, and insulinoma. The other causes of fasting hypoglycemia should be considered as shown in the box in step 4. Quite often, the etiology (eg, hepatic disease, renal disease, hypopituitarism, adrenal insufficiency, medications) can be determined after a thorough history, physical exam, and selected laboratory tests are performed. In rare cases, fasting hypoglycemia occurs secondary to overproduction of IGF-II by nonbeta cell tumors.

TUMORS ASSOCIATED WITH POSTABSORPTIVE HYPOGLYCEMIA	
FIBROSARCOMA	ADRENOCORTICAL TUMORS (rare)
MESOTHELIOMA	CARCINOID TUMORS (rare)
RHABDOMYOSARCOMA	RETICULUM CELL SARCOMA
LEIOMYOSARCOMA	BREAST CARCINOMA
LIPOSARCOMA	PHEOCHROMOCYTOMA
HEMANGIOPERICYTOMA	HEMATOLOGIC MALIGNANCY (leukemia, lymphoma, myeloma)
NEUROFIBROMA	CECAL CARCINOMA
LYMPHOSARCOMA	GASTRIC CARCINOMA
HEPATOCELLULAR CARCINOMA (rare)	CHOLANGIOCARCINOMA

End of Section.

STEP 9 – *Does the Patient Have Reactive Hypoglycemia?*

Reactive hypoglycemia is said to be present if hypoglycemia develops within five hours of food ingestion. The causes of reactive hypoglycemia are listed in the following box.

CAUSES OF REACTIVE HYPOGLYCEMIA	
IDIOPATHIC POSTPRANDIAL (functional)	CONGENITAL DEFICIENCIES OF ENZYMES INVOLVED IN CARBOHYDRATE METABOLISM
DIABETES MELLITUS Type 2 (early)	
RAPID GASTRIC EMPTYING (prior gastric surgery)	

Most cases of reactive hypoglycemia are idiopathic. Idiopathic reactive hypoglycemia is diagnosed if no other cause of reactive hypoglycemia is identified. In the past, the oral glucose tolerance test was used in the diagnosis of reactive hypoglycemia but it no longer plays a major role in the diagnosis. Even in patients with reactive hypoglycemia, a search is often undertaken for certain causes of fasting hypoglycemia, such as insulinoma, which can also present with reactive hypoglycemia.

References

Carroll MG, Burge MR, and Schade DS, "Severe Hypoglycemia in Adults," *Rev Endocr Metab Disord*, 2003, 4(2):149-57.

Cryer PE, Davis SN, and Shamoon H, "Hypoglycemia in Diabetes," *Diabetes Care*, 2003, 26(6):1902-12.

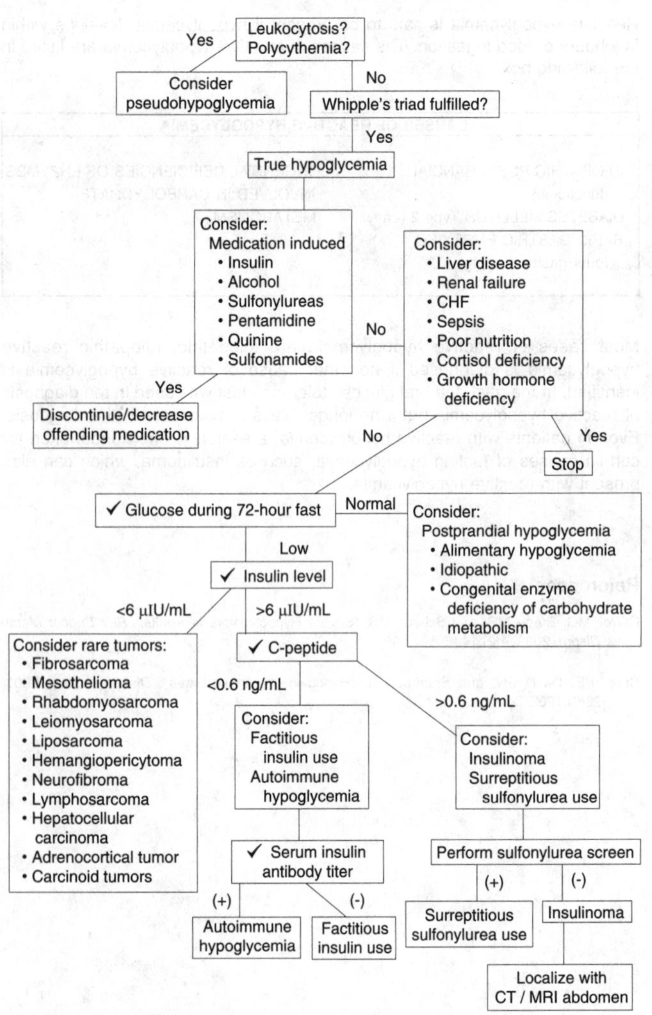
HYPOGLYCEMIA
Leukocytosis? Polycythemia?
Yes
Consider pseudohypoglycemia
No
Whipple's triad fulfilled?
Yes
True hypoglycemia
Consider: Medication induced
• Insulin
• Alcohol
• Sulfonylureas
• Pentamidine
• Quinine
• Sulfonamides
No
Consider:
• Liver disease
• Renal failure
• CHF
• Sepsis
• Poor nutrition
• Cortisol deficiency
• Growth hormone deficiency
Yes
Discontinue/decrease offending medication
No
Yes
Stop
✓ Glucose during 72-hour fast
Normal
Consider: Postprandial hypoglycemia
• Alimentary hypoglycemia
• Idiopathic
• Congenital enzyme deficiency of carbohydrate metabolism
Low
✓ Insulin level
<6 μIU/mL
>6 μIU/mL
Consider rare tumors:
• Fibrosarcoma
• Mesothelioma
• Rhabdomyosarcoma
• Leiomyosarcoma
• Liposarcoma
• Hemangiopericytoma
• Neurofibroma
• Lymphosarcoma
• Hepatocellular carcinoma
• Adrenocortical tumor
• Carcinoid tumors
✓ C-peptide
<0.6 ng/mL
>0.6 ng/mL
Consider: Factitious insulin use Autoimmune hypoglycemia
Consider: Insulinoma Surreptitious sulfonylurea use
✓ Serum insulin antibody titer
(+)
(-)
Autoimmune hypoglycemia
Factitious insulin use
Perform sulfonylurea screen
(+)
(-)
Surreptitious sulfonylurea use
Insulinoma
Localize with CT / MRI abdomen

HYPERGLYCEMIA

Hyperglycemia is the hallmark of diabetes mellitus, a disease characterized by a relative or absolute deficiency of insulin. Accompanying the insulin deficiency is relative or absolute excess of glucagon. Diabetes mellitus is a risk factor for myocardial infarction, stroke, and peripheral vascular disease. Other complications of diabetes mellitus include retinopathy, neuropathy, and nephropathy.

Causes of Hyperglycemia

Although the detection of hyperglycemia usually prompts concern for the possibility of diabetes mellitus, not all patients with hyperglycemia have diabetes mellitus. The causes of hyperglycemia are listed in the following box.

CAUSES OF HYPERGLYCEMIA	
DIABETES MELLITUS	STRESS HYPERGLYCEMIA
NONFASTING MEASUREMENT	CUSHING'S SYNDROME
RECENT I.V. INFUSION OF GLUCOSE	ACROMEGALY
CURRENT I.V. INFUSION OF GLUCOSE	PHEOCHROMOCYTOMA
MEDICATIONS	GLUCAGONOMA
Glucocorticoids	LIVER DISEASE
β-blockers	PANCREATITIS
Nicotinic acid	PANCREATECTOMY
Estrogens	CYSTIC FIBROSIS
Thiazide diuretics	HEMOCHROMATOSIS
Psychoactive agents	
Catecholamines	
Pentamidine	
Anti-HIV medications	

Hyperglycemia is commonly encountered in hospitalized patients. In some cases, the hyperglycemia is just a manifestation of previously diagnosed diabetes mellitus. Many patients, however, do not have a history of diabetes mellitus. In some of these patients, the detection of hyperglycemia while in the hospital may be the first indication of previously undiagnosed diabetes mellitus, especially if one considers the fact that over 5 million Americans have undiagnosed diabetes mellitus. It is difficult, however, to determine if hyperglycemia in a hospitalized patient reflects stress hyperglycemia (hyperglycemia occurring in acutely ill hospitalized patients due to elevations in counter-regulatory hormones such as glucagon, cortisol, epinephrine, and growth hormone) or true diabetes mellitus, especially since there are no criteria available to make the definitive diagnosis of diabetes mellitus in the hospital.

Screening Patients for Diabetes Mellitus

All patients >45 years of age should be screened for diabetes mellitus. Testing at an earlier age may be indicated if the patient is at high risk for developing diabetes. These risk factors are listed in the following box.

RISK FACTORS FOR DIABETES MELLITUS
AGE >45 YEARS*
OBESITY†
(+) FAMILY HISTORY‡
HIGH-RISK ETHNIC GROUP: African-American, Hispanic, Native American, Asian American, Pacific Islander
GESTATIONAL DIABETES / INFANT BIRTH WEIGHT >9 lb
HYPERTENSION
HDL CHOLESTEROL ≤35 mg/dL and/or TRIGLYCERIDES ≥250 mg/dL
HISTORY OF POLYCYSTIC OVARIAN SYNDROME
SEDENTARY
IMPAIRED GLUCOSE TOLERANCE OR IMPAIRED FASTING GLUCOSE ON PREVIOUS TESTING
HISTORY OF (+) OGTT OR INTERMEDIATE RESULT

*If normal, fasting glucose levels should be repeated at 3-year intervals.

†BMI ≥25 kg/m^2.

‡First degree relative with diabetes.

For screening purposes, the fasting plasma glucose is recommended over the oral glucose tolerance test (OGTT) because it is easier, faster, more convenient, more reproducible, and less expensive to perform.

Criteria for Diagnosis of Diabetes Mellitus

In order to make the diagnosis of diabetes mellitus, the criteria in the following box must be met.

CRITERIA FOR THE DIAGNOSIS OF DIABETES MELLITUS
1) Symptoms of diabetes plus casual plasma glucose ≥200 mg/dL* (11.1 mmol/L)
or
2) Fasting plasma glucose ≥126 mg/dL† (7 mmol/L)
or
3) Two-hour plasma glucose ≥200 mg/dL (11.1 mmol/L) during an observed glucose tolerance test (OGTT)‡

*Casual is defined as any time of the day without regard to time since a last meal. The classic symptoms of diabetes include polyuria, polydipsia, and unexplained weight loss.

†Fasting is defined as no caloric intake for at least 8 hours.

‡The test should be performed as described by WHO, using a glucose load containing the equivalent of 75 g of anhydrous glucose dissolved in water.

Obtained with permission from the Report of the Expert Committee on the Diagnosis and Classification of Diabetes Mellitus, *Diabetes Care*, 1997, 20(7):1183-97.

Note: In the absence of unequivocal hyperglycemia with acute metabolic decompensation, these criteria should be confirmed by repeat testing on a different day.

There exists a group of patients who do not meet the criteria for diabetes mellitus but have fasting glucose levels that exceed those found in normal individuals. This group, those with impaired fasting glucose (IFG), is characterized by a fasting plasma glucose ≥110 mg/dL (6.1 mmol/L) but <126 mg/dL (7 mmol/L). Impaired glucose tolerance (IGT) is said to be present if the 2-hour glucose value during a glucose tolerance test is ≥140 mg/dL (7.8 mmol/L) but <200 mg/dL (11.1 mmol/L).

Differentiating Normoglycemia, Impaired Fasting Glucose, Impaired Glucose Tolerance, and Diabetes From One Another*

Patient is normoglycemic if....	Patient has impaired fasting glucose if....	Patient has impaired glucose tolerance if....	Patient has diabetes if....
FPG <110 mg/dL 2-hour plasma glucose (OGTT) <140 mg/dL	FPG ≥110 mg/dL but <126 mg/dL	2-hour plasma glucose (OGTT) ≥140 but <200 mg/dL	FPG >126 mg/dL 2-hour plasma glucose (OGTT) ≥200 mg/dL Symptoms of diabetes + casual plasma glucose ≥200 mg/dL

FPG = fasting plasma glucose

OGTT = oral glucose tolerance test

*Abnormal results consistent with diabetes must be confirmed with repeat testing before the diagnosis can be firmly established.

It is important to realize that measurement of the Hb $A1_c$ is not part of the criteria for the diagnosis of diabetes mellitus. Although there has been considerable interest in the use of the Hb $A1_c$ in the diagnosis of diabetes mellitus, it has not been found to be an ideal screening test, partly due to the lack of standardization of the Hb $A1_c$ assays. In addition, patients with impaired glucose tolerance or mild diabetes mellitus may have Hb $A1_c$ levels within the normal range. An increased level supports the diagnosis but, in and of itself, cannot be used to establish the diagnosis.

Severe Hyperglycemia

The presence of severe hyperglycemia should always prompt consideration of diabetic ketoacidosis and nonketotic hyperosmolar syndrome, two complications of diabetes mellitus that have the potential to be life-threatening. In general, diabetic ketoacidosis is usually encountered in patients with type I diabetes mellitus whereas the nonketotic hyperosmolar syndrome is usually seen in patients with type II diabetes mellitus. The clinician should realize, however, that exceptions are not uncommon. For example, patients with type II diabetes mellitus may develop diabetic ketoacidosis. The clinical presentation of diabetic ketoacidosis and nonketotic hyperosmolar syndrome is compared in the following table.

Characteristic Clinical Findings in Diabetic Ketoacidosis and Nonketotic Hyperosmolar Syndrome

Finding	Diabetic Ketoacidosis	Nonketotic Hyperosmolar Syndrome
Age	Young (less commonly elderly)	Middle-aged to elderly
Type of diabetes	Type 1 (less often type 2)	Type 2
Onset	Acute or subacute	Insidious
Abdominal pain	Yes	No
Kussmaul's respiration	Yes	No
Acetone in breath	Yes	No
Temperature	Normothermic or hypothermic	Normothermic or hyperthermic
Volume depletion	Moderate	Severe
Blood pressure	Normotensive	Orthostatic hypotension
Change in mental status	Moderate	Severe (coma or seizures)

Adapted from Jabbour SA and Miller JL, "Uncontrolled Diabetes Mellitus," *Clin Lab Med*, 2001, 21(1):102.

Almost all patients with diabetic ketoacidosis and nonketotic hyperosmolar syndrome have plasma glucose levels >250 mg/dL. Plasma glucose levels are usually higher in nonketotic hyperosmolar syndrome with levels often >1000 mg/dL. In contrast, plasma glucose levels are typically <800 mg/dL in patients with diabetic ketoacidosis. The clinician should realize, however, that the degree of hyperglycemia alone cannot be used to differentiate between these two complications of diabetes mellitus.

Once the presence of severe hyperglycemia has been established, the clinician should measure serum and urine ketones. In addition, the clinician should consider performing an arterial blood gas to measure the pH. Measurement of the serum and urine ketones is important in establishing or excluding the diagnosis of diabetic ketoacidosis, which is characterized by the triad of hyperglycemia, ketosis, and acidosis.

Diabetic ketoacidosis should be strongly suspected when results of the ketone testing are strongly positive. In contrast to diabetic ketoacidosis, nonketotic hyperosmolar syndrome is typically not associated with the presence of ketones. On occasion, however, small amounts of ketones may be appreciated.

The clinician should beware of one limitation of ketone testing in differentiating diabetic ketoacidosis from nonketotic hyperosmolar syndrome. This limitation has to do with the fact that testing of the serum and urine for ketones is based upon the nitroprusside reaction. In diabetic ketoacidosis, three types of ketone bodies accumulate in the body: β-hydroxybutyrate, acetoacetate, and acetone. Seventy-five percent of the circulating ketones are in the form of β-hydroxybutyrate. A higher proportion of the ketones (up to 90%) may be in the form of β-hydroxybutyrate if the patient has recently consumed excessive amounts of alcohol or if lactic acidosis is also present. Because β-hydroxybutyrate is not detected by the nitroprusside reaction, when a high proportion of the ketones present are in the form of β-hydroxybutyrate, serum ketone testing may yield negative or weakly positive results. If diabetic ketoacidosis is suspected but ketone testing is unremarkable, it is wise to consider the possibility that the negative or weakly positive results of the ketone testing are due to the presence of ketones largely in the form of β-hydroxybutyrate. To make the diagnosis in these settings, several drops of hydrogen peroxide can be added to a urine specimen. The addition of hydrogen peroxide will result in conversion of β-hydroxybutyrate, if present, to acetoacetate, which can then be detected by the nitroprusside reaction. In recent years, direct measurement of β-hydroxybutrate has become available and can be used to diagnose patients with diabetic ketoacidosis.

The other cardinal feature of diabetic ketoacidosis is acidosis. In most patients, the pH is <7.30 whereas nonketotic hyperosmolar syndrome is associated with a pH >7.30. Mild cases of diabetic ketoacidosis are characterized by pH between 7.20 and 7.30. In severe cases, however, the pH may fall as low as 6.8. Most patients with diabetic ketoacidosis have a high anion gap metabolic acidosis. In some cases, a combined high anion gap and hyperchloremic metabolic acidosis is present. Rarely, patients with diabetic ketoacidosis have a hyperchloremic metabolic acidosis. On occasion, diabetic ketoacidosis may present with an alkalemic pH. In these cases, there is usually a combined metabolic acidosis and alkalosis. The alkalosis may be due to severe vomiting or diuretic therapy. In patients who present with an alkalemic pH, a markedly elevated anion gap is a clue to the presence of a concomitant metabolic acidosis.

It is important to calculate the effective plasma osmolality in patients with severe hyperglycemia. The effective plasma osmolality may be calculated using the following formula.

Effective plasma osmolality = [2 x (Na^+ + K^+)] + (plasma glucose / 18)

Normal plasma osmolality ranges between 285 and 295 mOsm/kg water. In nonketotic hyperosmolar syndrome, the plasma osmolality is often >330 mOsm/kg. Neurologic symptoms are uncommon until the effective plasma osmolality is >320-330 mOsm/kg. Values >350 mOsm/kg are considered to represent a severe hyperosmolar state. Patients with diabetic ketoacidosis typically have an effective plasma osmolality <320 mOsm/kg.

The characteristic laboratory test findings of diabetic ketoacidosis and nonketotic hyperosmolar syndrome are compared in the following table.

Laboratory Test Findings in Diabetic Ketoacidosis and Nonketotic Hyperosmolar Syndrome

Finding	Diabetic Ketoacidosis	Nonketotic Hyperosmolar Syndrome
Plasma glucose	>250 mg/dL	>600 mg/dL
Plasma osmolality	<330 mOsm/kg	>330 mOsm/kg
Ketones		
urine	>+3	- or small amounts
blood	+ at >1:2 dilution	- or small amounts
Serum bicarbonate	<15 mEq/L	>20 mEq/L
pH	<7.30	>7.30
BUN	<25 mg/dL	>30 mg/dL

Other laboratory test abnormalities that may be appreciated in patients presenting with diabetic ketoacidosis and nonketotic hyperosmolar state include the following.

- Hyponatremia / hypernatremia

  Hyponatremia is not uncommon in severe hyperglycemia. It is due to osmotic diuresis as well as a shift of water from the extracellular to intracellular fluid. A useful relationship to remember is that for every 100 mg/dL increase in the plasma glucose level >100 mg/dL, there is a fall in the serum sodium by 1.6 mmol/L. In contrast to diabetic ketoacidosis in which hyponatremia is more common, nonketotic hyperosmolar syndrome commonly presents with hypernatremia.

- Normal or high serum potassium (occasionally low)

  Patients with diabetic ketoacidosis and nonketotic hyperosmolar syndrome typically have a potassium deficit at the time of presentation. Despite the presence of potassium deficiency, the initial serum potassium level is either normal or elevated (33% of patients). In fact, the average serum potassium level at presentation is 5.3 mmol/L. Normal or high serum potassium levels in the setting of potassium deficiency are likely to be the result of hyperosmolality and insulin deficiency that accompany diabetic ketoacidosis and nonketotic hyperosmolar syndrome. With treatment, serum potassium levels will decrease.

- Prerenal azotemia

  Since marked hyperglycemia results in an osmotic diuresis, BUN levels may be elevated while the serum creatinine usually remains normal, resulting in a pattern consistent with prerenal azotemia due to volume depletion. If the laboratory measures the serum creatinine using alkaline picrate methodology, the serum creatinine may be falsely elevated due to the presence of high levels of acetoacetate. The increase in the serum creatinine may be as high as 3-4 mg/dL.

- Hyperamylasemia
- Normal / elevated / reduced serum magnesium or phosphorus levels
- Leukocytosis
- Hypertriglyceridemia

Glycosylated Hemoglobin

Glycosylated hemoglobin (Hb $A1_c$), also known as glycated hemoglobin or glycohemoglobin, is produced from the nonenzymatic reaction of protein and glucose. It is a component of hemoglobin which structurally is almost identical to hemoglobin A. The only difference is the presence of hexose residues covalently bound to certain parts of the hemoglobin. The formation of glycated hemoglobin depends on the blood glucose concentration; that is, the higher the serum glucose concentration over a period of time, the higher the percentage of glycated hemoglobin. The reference range for Hb $A1_c$ varies depending upon the methodology used, but a typical range is 4% to 6%. In some poorly controlled diabetic patients, the glycated hemoglobin may reach ≥15% of the total hemoglobin. Since the glycated hemoglobin is a measure of overall blood glucose control over a period of 60-120 days, its determination provides more information regarding glucose control than does an isolated blood glucose level.

In the past, the various techniques available for the measurement of the Hb $A1_c$ were not standardized. As a result, reference ranges varied depending upon the methodology used. Because this lack of standardization resulted in confusion with regard to the interpretation of test results, in recent years, there has a significant effort in developing standardized methods to measure the Hb $A1_c$. In the Diabetes Control and Complications Trial (DCCT), high-performance liquid chromatography (HPLC) was used to quantitate Hb $A1_c$. This technique is considered the reference method by which all other techniques are judged.

Hb $A1_c$ measurement is recommended in every patient with diabetes mellitus at the time of diagnosis. Thereafter, it should be obtained at 3-month intervals to ensure that the patient's glycemic control is within the recommended range. Some have advocated that testing can be done twice a year in diabetic patients who have levels consistently within the target range. The American Diabetes Association has recommended that clinicians strive for a level <7% in patients with diabetes mellitus. Therapy should be re-evaluated if the glycated hemoglobin levels are consistently >8%.

Although this test has been found to be very reliable, there are certain conditions other than diabetes mellitus that can affect the Hb $A1_c$ level. If not recognized, they may lead to errors in patient management. Depending on the assay used, Hb $A1_c$ levels may be decreased in hemolytic conditions and renal failure, states characterized by a reduction in the RBC lifespan. Levels may be artifactually increased in thalassemia patients. Again, depending on the assay used, there may be artifactual increases or decreases of the Hb $A1_c$ levels in patients with hemoglobinopathies. The clinician should consider the effects of these conditions on Hb $A1_c$ levels should these conditions exist. If the patient has a condition that significantly alters the half-life of red blood cells, fructosamine assays may be performed. Fructosamine is a measure of overall blood glucose over a period of 1-3 weeks.

Autoantibody Testing in Patients With Diabetes

Type I diabetes mellitus is an autoimmune disease characterized by the presence of autoantibodies directed against the pancreatic beta cells. The presence of autoantibodies places an individual at high risk for the development of diabetes mellitus type I. While autoantibodies have some predictive value, at the present time, routine testing for autoantibodies is not recommended for the following reasons.

- Cutoff values of some of the autoantibodies have not been well established.
- The appropriate course of action in the patient with a positive autoantibody test without clinical evidence of diabetes mellitus is unclear.

There are currently several studies focusing on the prevention of diabetes mellitus type I. In the event that investigators are able to find ways to prevent or delay the onset of diabetes, these autoantibody tests may become more widely used.

Autoantibody testing, however, may be useful in differentiating type I from type II diabetes mellitus when the clinical presentation does not allow the clinician to do so. In usual clinical practice, the patient's clinical presentation suffices in making the distinction between type I and type II diabetes mellitus.

Urine Glucose Testing

Paper strips impregnated with glucose-specific enzymes are available. The major limitation in the use of urine strips in the diagnosis and management of diabetes is that there is not always a good correlation between the plasma glucose and urine glucose concentrations. Normal tubular function allows reabsorption of glucose until a plasma glucose concentration of approximately 180 mg/dL is reached. This is known as the renal threshold. Unfortunately, this level is not absolute and there is significant individual variability. Some patients, for example, have a low renal threshold for glucose. In these patients, glucose may spill into the urine even when the blood glucose concentration is normal. In addition, because urine stays within the bladder for some time, urinary glucose concentration does not reflect current plasma glucose, but represents plasma glucose at the time urine left the kidney. The diagnosis of diabetes mellitus, therefore, cannot be based on urinary tests for glucose. While some use urinary glucose concentrations to guide diabetic therapy, self-monitored plasma glucose levels are superior in the management of diabetes.

Therapeutic Targets for Nonpregnant Diabetic Patients

Guidelines for glycemic control as well as control of other factors that increase the potential for diabetic complications are listed in the following table.

Therapeutic Targets for Nonpregnant Diabetic Patients

Parameter	Normal	Goal	Signals Possible Intervention*
Premeal glucose (mg/dL)	<110	80-120	<80 or >140
Bedtime glucose (mg/dL)	<120	100-140	<100 or >160
Hb $A1_c$ (%)†	<6	<7	>8
LDL cholesterol (mg/dL)	<130	<100	>100
HDL cholesterol (mg/dL)	>35	>35	<35
Fasting triglycerides (mg/dL)	<150	<150	>250-300
Blood pressure (mm Hg)	<140/90	<130/85	>130/85

*Targets may vary depending on assessment of risk:benefit ratio.

†Targets need to be adjusted for local laboratory differences in assay method and nondiabetic reference ranges.

Adapted from Goldman L and Bennett JC, eds, *Cecil's Textbook of Medicine*, Philadelphia, PA: WB Saunders Co, 2000, 1276.

References

Beisswenger PJ, Szwergold BS, and Yeo KT, "Glycated Proteins in Diabetes," *Clin Lab Med*, 2001, 21(1):53-78, vi.

Borg WP and Sherwin RS, "Classification of Diabetes Mellitus," *Adv Intern Med*, 2000, 45:279-95 (review).

Delaney MF, Zisman A, and Kettyle WM, "Diabetic Ketoacidosis and Hyperglycemic Hyperosmolar Nonketotic Syndrome," *Endocrinol Metab Clin North Am*, 2000, 29(4):683-705, v.

Jabbour SA and Miller JL, "Uncontrolled Diabetes Mellitus," *Clin Lab Med*, 2001, 21(1):99-110.

Kilpatrick ES, "Glycated Haemoglobin in the Year 2000," *J Clin Pathol*, 2000, 53(5):335-9.

McCowen KC, Malhotra A, and Bistrian BR, "Stress-Induced Hyperglycemia," *Crit Care Clin*, 2001, 17(1):107-24.

Montori VM, Bistrian BR, and McMahon MM, "Hyperglycemia in Acutely Ill Patients," *JAMA*, 2002, 288(17):2167-9.

APPROACH TO THE PATIENT WITH ELEVATED TSH

STEP 1 – *What Is the Differential Diagnosis of an Elevated TSH?*

The differential diagnosis of an increased TSH is listed in the following box.

ELEVATED TSH DIFFERENTIAL DIAGNOSIS
PRIMARY HYPOTHYROIDISM SUBCLINICAL HYPOTHYROIDISM RECOVERY PHASE OF NONTHYROIDAL ILLNESS INADEQUATE THYROID HORMONE REPLACEMENT MALABSORPTION OF THYROID HORMONE DRUG INHIBITION OF THYROID HORMONE SECRETION INTERMITTENT COMPLIANCE WITH THYROID HORMONE THERAPY ADRENAL INSUFFICIENCY TSH-PRODUCING PITUITARY TUMOR THYROID HORMONE RESISTANCE

Proceed to Step 2.

STEP 2 – *What Is the Free Thyroxine Index (FT_4I) or FT_4 Level?*

To determine the cause of TSH elevation, it is necessary to obtain a free thyroxine index or free T_4 level (FT_4).

If the FT_4I or free T_4 level is low, ***proceed to Step 3.***

If the FT_4I or free T_4 level is normal, ***proceed to Step 11** on page 353.*

If the FT_4I or free T_4 level is high, ***proceed to Step 16** on page 354.*

STEP 3 – *What Is the Differential Diagnosis of a Low FT_4 I or Free T_4 in the Patient Having an Elevated TSH?*

The differential diagnosis of a low FT_4I of free T_4 level in the patient who has an elevated TSH is listed in the following box.

ELEVATED TSH AND DECREASED FT_4 / FT_4I DIFFERENTIAL DIAGNOSIS
PRIMARY HYPOTHYROIDISM INADEQUATE THYROID HORMONE REPLACEMENT DRUG INHIBITION OF THYROID HORMONE SECRETION MALABSORPTION OF ORAL THYROID HORMONE RECOVERY FROM NONTHYROIDAL ILLNESS

If the patient is already taking thyroid hormone replacement, ***proceed to Step 8** on page 351.*

If the patient is not on thyroid hormone replacement, ***proceed to Step 4.***

STEP 4 – *Is the Patient Recovering From a Nonthyroidal Illness?*

Physical trauma, severe illness, or psychologic stress can lead to abnormal thyroid function tests. A decreased serum T_3 level is the most commonly encountered abnormality. In more seriously ill patients, however, the FT_4I or free T_4 level may be low as well. It is not uncommon for these patients to have a low TSH, but with recovery from the nonthyroidal illness, the TSH is often elevated in the setting of a decreased FT_4I or free T_4 level.

During the recovery phase, it is difficult to distinguish nonthyroidal illness from true hypothyroidism based on the thyroid function tests. A marked elevation in the TSH, however, supports hypothyroidism (>20 mU/L). Also suggestive of hypothyroidism in these patients is a low or low normal reverse T_3 (rT_3) level. In nonthyroidal illness, the rT_3 level should be increased. Resolution of the thyroid function test abnormalities over time establishes nonthyroidal illness as the etiology.

If the patient is in the recovery phase of nonthyroidal illness, repeat the thyroid function tests periodically to demonstrate normalization. ***Stop here***.

If the patient is not in the recovery phase of a nonthyroidal illness, ***proceed to Step 5***.

STEP 5 – *Does the Patient Have Primary Hypothyroidism?*

The most common cause of an elevated TSH is primary hypothyroidism. The term "primary" is used to describe hypothyroidism that results from disease of the thyroid gland. The clinical manifestations of primary hypothyroidism are listed in the following box.

SIGNS AND SYMPTOMS OF HYPOTHYROIDISM	
WEAKNESS	WEIGHT GAIN
DRY SKIN	LOSS OF HAIR
COARSE SKIN	PERIPHERAL EDEMA
LETHARGY	HOARSENESS
EDEMA OF EYELIDS	ANOREXIA
SENSATION OF COLD	NERVOUSNESS
COLD SKIN	MENORRHAGIA
COARSENESS OF HAIR	DIMINISHED SWEATING
MEMORY IMPAIRMENT	PARESTHESIA
CONSTIPATION	

Proceed to Step 6.

STEP 6 – *What Laboratory Features May Be Appreciated in Patients With Hypothyroidism?*

Laboratory test abnormalities found in patients with hypothyroidism are listed in the following box.

LABORATORY TEST ABNORMALITIES FOUND IN HYPOTHYROIDISM	
INCREASED CREATINE KINASE	INCREASED CHOLESTEROL / TRIGLYCERIDES
INCREASED AST	NORMOCYTIC OR MACROCYTIC ANEMIA
HYPONATREMIA	

Proceed to Step 7.

STEP 7 – *What Are the Causes of Primary Hypothyroidism?*

The causes of primary hypothyroidism are listed in the following box.

CAUSES OF PRIMARY HYPOTHYROIDISM
CHRONIC LYMPHOCYTIC THYROIDITIS (Hashimoto's disease)
SURGICAL THYROIDECTOMY
EXTERNAL RADIATION THERAPY (>2000 R)
RADIOIODINE THERAPY
INFILTRATIVE DISEASE
Amyloidosis
Lymphoma
Scleroderma
Hemochromatosis
Sarcoidosis
IODINE DEFICIENCY
CONGENITAL
DRUG-INDUCED
Thionamides
Iodine excess
Amiodarone
Lithium
Sertraline
Sulfonamides
Interleukins
Interferon alpha
DISRUPTIVE THYROIDITIS
Postpartum
Silent (painless)
Subacute (granulomatous)

Measurement of antithyroid antibodies can help elucidate the etiology of primary hypothyroidism. Chronic lymphocytic thyroiditis, also known as Hashimoto's disease, is associated with the presence of antithyroglobulin and antithyroid peroxidase antibodies. Sixty percent of patients with Hashimoto's disease are found to have antithyroglobulin antibodies while approximately 95% have circulating antithyroid peroxidase antibodies.

End of Section.

STEP 8 – *Is the Patient Taking a Medication That Is Interfering With the Absorption of Oral Thyroid Hormone?*

The medications which interfere with the absorption of oral thyroid hormone are listed in the following box.

MEDICATIONS INTERFERING WITH ORAL THYROID HORMONE ABSORPTION	
CHOLESTYRAMINE	FERROUS SULFATE
COLESTIPOL	CALCIUM CARBONATE
FIBER SUPPLEMENTS	ALUMINUM HYDROXIDE
SUCRALFATE	

The administration of these medications in a clinically euthyroid patient does not affect the TSH level. However, clinical deterioration has been reported in some hypothyroid patients taking these medications secondary to the inhibition of oral thyroid hormone absorption. Accompanying this deterioration is an increase in the TSH level. This problem can be avoided by having the patient take the above medications 4-8 hours after oral thyroid hormone dose.

If the patient is on a medication that inhibits absorption of oral thyroid hormone, ***stop here***.

If the patient is not on a medication that inhibits absorption of oral thyroid hormone, ***proceed to Step 9***.

STEP 9 – *Is the Patient Taking a Medication That Is Increasing the Metabolism of the Oral Thyroid Hormone?*

The medications which increase the metabolism of oral thyroid hormone are listed in the following box.

MEDICATIONS INCREASING METABOLISM OF ORAL THYROID HORMONE	
PHENYTOIN	CARBAMAZEPINE
PHENOBARBITAL	RIFAMPIN

These medications have no effect on the TSH level in clinically euthyroid individuals, but may precipitate hypothyroidism in patients taking oral thyroid hormone. Accompanying this is an increase in the TSH level.

If the patient is on a medication that is increasing metabolism of the oral thyroid hormone, ***stop here***.

If the patient is not on a medication that is increasing metabolism of the oral thyroid hormone, ***proceed to Step 10***.

STEP 10 – *Is the Patient Taking an Adequate Dose of Oral Thyroid Hormone?*

In the patient previously diagnosed with hypothyroidism, who is taking oral thyroid hormone replacement, a persistently elevated TSH level suggests an insufficient dose of medication. Approximately 6 weeks of adequate therapy is required before TSH normalizes. If the patient recently started on oral thyroid hormone, it is wise to wait 6 weeks before measuring the TSH level. Similarly, 6 weeks should pass before the TSH level is measured in a patient who receives an adjustment of oral thyroid hormone. If the TSH remains elevated after 6 weeks of therapy, then the diagnosis is likely to be inadequate hormone replacement.

End of Section.

STEP 11 – *What Is the Differential Diagnosis of a Normal FT_4I or Free T_4 Level in a Patient With an Elevated TSH?*

A normal FT_4I of free T_4 level in the patient with an elevated TSH should prompt consideration of the conditions listed in the following box.

NORMAL FT_4I / FT_4 AND ELEVATED TSH DIFFERENTIAL DIAGNOSIS
SUBCLINICAL HYPOTHYROIDISM RECOVERY PHASE OF NONTHYROIDAL ILLNESS POOR COMPLIANCE WITH ORAL THYROID HORMONE REPLACEMENT ADRENAL INSUFFICIENCY

If the patient is on oral thyroid hormone replacement, ***proceed to Step 12***.

If the patient is not on oral thyroid hormone replacement, ***proceed to Step 13***.

STEP 12 – *Is the Patient Poorly Compliant With Oral Thyroid Hormone Replacement?*

This is particularly a problem in the patient who intermittently takes oral thyroid hormone. An example is the patient who has missed multiple doses of oral thyroid hormone who decides to restart oral thyroid hormone several days before a visit to the physician's office. This may, in fact, normalize the T_4 level but the TSH will remain elevated. The clinician may erroneously conclude that the oral thyroid hormone dosage is inadequate. The importance of discussing compliance issues with the patient cannot be overemphasized.

End of Section.

STEP 13 – *Does the Patient Have Adrenal Insufficiency?*

In patients with adrenal insufficiency, corticosteroid deficiency may result in an increased TSH level. Adrenal insufficiency should be suspected in the patient presenting with the signs and symptoms listed in the following box.

ADRENAL INSUFFICIENCY SIGNS AND SYMPTOMS	
WEAKNESS	ABDOMINAL PAIN
ANOREXIA	WEIGHT LOSS
NAUSEA / VOMITING	ORTHOSTATIC HYPOTENSION / HYPOTENSION
DIARRHEA	HYPERPIGMENTATION

The cosyntropin stimulation test is required to establish the presence of adrenal insufficiency. Normalization of the TSH occurs with adequate corticosteroid replacement. The reader is referred to the Endocrine Section for further information regarding the diagnosis of adrenal insufficiency.

If the patient has adrenal insufficiency, ***stop here***.

If the patient does not have adrenal insufficiency, ***proceed to Step 14***.

STEP 14 – *Is the Patient Recovering From a Nonthyroidal Illness?*

Physical trauma, severe illness, or psychologic stress can lead to abnormal thyroid function tests. A decreased serum T_3 level is the most commonly encountered abnormality. In more seriously ill patients, however, the FT_4I or free T_4 level may be low as well. It is not uncommon for these patients to have a low TSH, but with recovery from the nonthyroidal illness, the TSH is often elevated in the setting of a decreased FT_4I or free T_4 level. As the FT_4I or free T_4 levels normalize, the TSH may remain elevated for some time.

If the patient is recovering from a nonthyroidal illness, repeat the thyroid function tests periodically to document normalization. ***Stop here.***

If the patient is not recovering from a nonthyroidal illness, ***proceed to Step 15***.

STEP 15 – *Does the Patient Have Subclinical Hypothyroidism?*

Some patients who appear clinically euthyroid have thyroid function tests (increased TSH, normal FT_4I or free T_4 level) consistent with early thyroid failure or subclinical hypothyroidism. In these patients, the TSH level is usually <20 mU/L.

If the thyroid function tests are consistent with subclinical hypothyroidism, the TSH level should be repeated. In some of these patients, the repeat TSH level may be normal. If the repeat TSH level is high and the FT_4I or free T_4 level remains normal, then the diagnosis of subclinical hypothyroidism is established.

Five percent to 18% of patients with subclinical hypothyroidism progress to overt hypothyroidism each year. Although it can difficult to predict those who will progress to overt hypothyroidism, it seems that progression is more likely if antithyroid antibodies are present. Patients with subclinical hypothyroidism who have a high TSH level, particularly one that is >20 mU/L, are also more likely to progress to overt hypothyroidism.

End of Section.

STEP 16 – *What is the Differential Diagnosis of an Elevated FT_4I or Free T_4 Level in the Patient Having an Increased TSH?*

The differential diagnosis of an elevated FT_4I or free T_4 in the setting of an elevated TSH is listed in the following box.

ELEVATED FT_4I / FREE T_4 AND ELEVATED TSH DIFFERENTIAL DIAGNOSIS
TSH-PRODUCING PITUITARY ADENOMA
THYROID HORMONE RESISTANCE

An increased TSH in the setting of an increased FT_4I of free T_4 level should prompt consideration of a TSH-producing pituitary adenoma. These tumors account for 0.5% to 3% of pituitary tumors. Not all patients present with CNS symptoms such as headache and visual field disturbance. In fact, headache and visual field disturbances are complaints in only 23% and 40% of patients, respectively.

While many patients with TSH-producing pituitary adenomas have increased TSH levels, 33% have levels <10 mU/L. A measurement of the α-subunit is helpful in supporting the diagnosis. An α-subunit:TSH ratio >1 is characteristic of a TSH-producing pituitary adenoma.

TSH-producing pituitary adenoma must be differentiated from thyroid hormone resistance. Both conditions may present with increased TSH levels. Features used to differentiate between TSH-producing pituitary adenoma and thyroid hormone resistance are listed in the following table.

Characteristics of TSH-Producing Pituitary Adenoma Versus Thyroid Hormone Resistance

Feature	TSH-Producing Pituitary Adenoma	Thyroid Hormone Resistance
TRH stimulation of TSH	8%	96%
T_3 suppression of TSH	12%	100%
Elevated sex hormone-binding globulin	94%	2%
Elevated alpha subunit/TSH ratio	81%	2%
Family history	0%	82%
MRI pituitary adenoma	98%	2%

Adapted from Beck-Peccoz P, Brucker-Davis F, Persani L, et al, "Thyrotropin-Secreting Pituitary Tumors," *Endocr Rev*, 1996, 17:610-38.

Cooper DS, *Medical Management of Thyroid Disease*, New York, MY: Marcel Dekker Inc, 2001.

End of Section.

References

Attia J, Margetts P, and Guyatt G, "Diagnosis of Thyroid Disease in Hospitalized Patients: A Systematic Review," *Arch Intern Med*, 1999, 159(7):658-65.

Camacho PM and Dwarkanathan AA, "Sick Euthyroid Syndrome. What to Do When Thyroid Function Tests Are Abnormal in Critically Ill Patients," *Postgrad Med*, 1999, 105(4):215-9.

Dayan CM, "Interpretation of Thyroid Function Tests," *Lancet*, 2001, 357(9256):619-24.

Fatourechi V, "Subclinical Thyroid Disease," *Mayo Clin Proc*, 2001, 76(4):413-6; quiz 416-7.

Kaplan MM, "Clinical Perspectives in the Diagnosis of Thyroid Disease," *Clin Chem*, 1999, 45(8 Pt 2):1377-83.

Langton JE and Brent GA, "Nonthyroidal Illness Syndrome: Evaluation of Thyroid Function in Sick Patients," *Endocrinol Metab Clin North Am*, 2002, 31(1):159-72.

O'Reilly DS, "Thyroid Function Tests-Time for a Reassessment," *BMJ*, 2000, 320(7245):1332-4.

Peery WH and Meek JC, "Interpretation of Thyroid Function Tests: An Update," *Compr Ther*, 1998, 24(11-12):567-73.

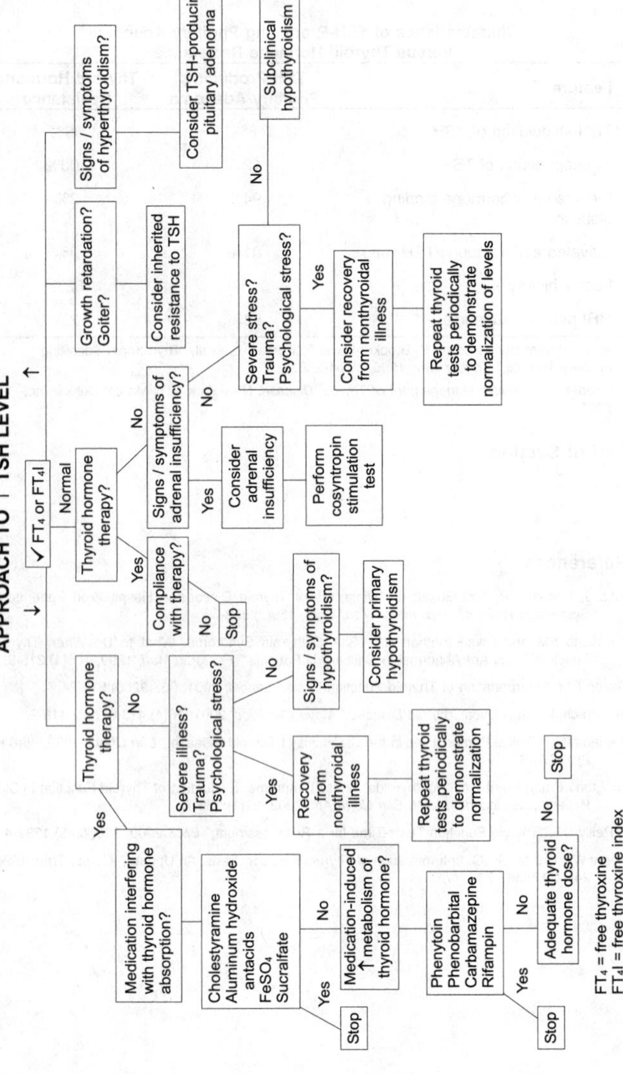
APPROACH TO ↑ TSH LEVEL
✓ FT_4 or FT_4I
↓
Normal
↑
Thyroid hormone therapy?
Yes
No
Medication interfering with thyroid hormone absorption?
Cholestyramine
Aluminum hydroxide antacids
$FeSO_4$
Sucralfate
Yes
Stop
No
Medication-induced ↑ metabolism of thyroid hormone?
Phenytoin
Phenobarbital
Carbamazepine
Rifampin
Yes
Stop
No
Adequate thyroid hormone dose?
No
Stop
Severe illness? Trauma? Psychological stress?
Yes
Recovery from nonthyroidal illness
Repeat thyroid tests periodically to demonstrate normalization
No
Signs / symptoms of hypothyroidism?
Consider primary hypothyroidism
Thyroid hormone therapy?
Yes
Compliance with therapy?
No
Stop
No
Signs / symptoms of adrenal insufficiency?
Yes
Consider adrenal insufficiency
Perform cosyntropin stimulation test
No
Severe stress? Trauma? Psychological stress?
Yes
Consider recovery from nonthyroidal illness
Repeat thyroid tests periodically to demonstrate normalization of levels
No
Subclinical hypothyroidism
Growth retardation? Goiter?
Consider inherited resistance to TSH
Signs / symptoms of hyperthyroidism?
Consider TSH-producing pituitary adenoma
FT_4 = free thyroxine
FT_4I = free thyroxine index

APPROACH TO THE PATIENT WITH DECREASED TSH

STEP 1 – *What Is the Differential Diagnosis of a Decreased TSH Level?*

The differential diagnosis of a decreased TSH level is listed in the following box.

DECREASED TSH DIFFERENTIAL DIAGNOSIS
HYPERTHYROIDISM SUBCLINICAL HYPERTHYROIDISM EXCESSIVE THYROID HORMONE REPLACEMENT ACUTE PSYCHIATRIC ILLNESS NONTHYROIDAL ILLNESS DRUG INHIBITION OF TSH RELEASE PITUITARY FAILURE T_3 THYROTOXICOSIS PREGNANCY

Proceed to Step 2.

STEP 2 – *What Is the Free Thyroxine Index (FT_4I) or FT_4 Level?*

The approach to the patient with a decreased TSH begins with the measurement of a FT_4I or free T_4 level (FT_4).

If the FT_4I or free T_4 level is increased, ***proceed to Step 3.***

If the FT_4I or free T_4 level is normal, ***proceed to Step 17** on page 363.*

If the FT_4I or free T_4 level is decreased, ***proceed to Step 18** on page 364.*

STEP 3 – *What Is the Differential Diagnosis of an Increased FT_4I or Free T_4 in the Patient Having a Decreased TSH Level?*

The differential diagnosis of an increased FT_4I of free T_4 level in the setting of a decreased TSH is listed in the following box.

ELEVATED FT_4I / FT_4 AND DECREASED TSH DIFFERENTIAL DIAGNOSIS
EXCESSIVE ORAL THYROID HORMONE REPLACEMENT ACUTE PSYCHIATRIC ILLNESS HYPERTHYROIDISM

Proceed to Step 4.

STEP 4 – *Is the Patient Taking Oral Thyroid Hormone Replacement?*

If the oral thyroid hormone dose is too high, hyperthyroidism may ensue. The hyperthyroidism may be subclinical or overt. In either instance, TSH will be decreased.

If the patient is on oral thyroid hormone, adjust the dose and repeat the thyroid function tests after 6 weeks. ***Stop here.***

If the patient is not on oral thyroid hormone replacement, ***proceed to Step 5***.

STEP 5 – *Does the Patient Have an Acute Psychiatric Illness?*

Patients with an acute psychiatric illness often have abnormal thyroid function tests. Early in the course of an acute psychiatric illness, a decreased TSH level may be appreciated. Since hyperthyroid patients often present with acute psychiatric problems, it may be difficult to distinguish hyperthyroid patients from those having acute psychiatric illness not due to hyperthyroidism. In both of these conditions, the T_4 levels may be elevated. In the absence of signs and symptoms strongly suggesting hyperthyroidism, it is reasonable to periodically follow these patients with serial thyroid function tests. In an acute psychiatric illness, the thyroid function abnormalities will normalize.

If the patient has an acute psychiatric illness, ***stop here***.

If the patient does not have an acute psychiatric illness, ***proceed to Step 6***.

STEP 6 – *Does the Patient Have Hyperthyroidism?*

The symptoms and signs of hyperthyroidism are listed in the following box.

SIGNS AND SYMPTOMS OF HYPERTHYROIDISM
NERVOUSNESS
EMOTIONAL LABILITY
TREMOR
INCREASED SWEATING
PALPITATIONS
FATIGUE
WEIGHT LOSS
TACHYCARDIA
ATRIAL FIBRILLATION
INCREASED DIFFERENCE BETWEEN SYSTOLIC / DIASTOLIC BLOOD PRESSURE
DIARRHEA
PROXIMAL MUSCLE WEAKNESS
WARM MOIST SMOOTH SKIN
HEAT INTOLERANCE
FINE HAIR
HAIR LOSS
WEAKNESS
INCREASED APPETITE

The presence of symptoms consistent with hyperthyroidism in the patient having a high FT_4I or free T_4 level in the setting of a decreased TSH establishes the diagnosis.

Proceed to Step 7.

STEP 7 – *What Laboratory Features May Be Appreciated in Patients With Hyperthyroidism?*

The laboratory test abnormalities that may be appreciated in the patient with hyperthyroidism are listed in the following box.

HYPERTHYROIDISM LABORATORY FEATURES
INCREASED CALCIUM INCREASED ALKALINE PHOSPHATASE ELEVATED TRANSAMINASES (mild) NORMOCYTIC NORMOCHROMIC ANEMIA LYMPHOCYTOSIS

Proceed to Step 8.

STEP 8 – *What Are the Causes of Hyperthyroidism?*

When a decreased TSH and elevated FT_4I or free T_4 level are found in a patient with signs and symptoms suggestive of hyperthyroidism, primary hyperthyroidism is said to be present. The term "primary" is used when the problem with thyroid function is a result of disease within the thyroid gland. The causes of primary hyperthyroidism are listed in the following box.

PRIMARY HYPERTHYROIDISM DIFFERENTIAL DIAGNOSIS

GRAVES' DISEASE
TOXIC MULTINODULAR GOITER
SOLITARY TOXIC ADENOMA
THYROIDITIS
    Subacute (granulomatous)
    Silent (painless)
    Postpartum
THYROTOXICOSIS FACTITIA
STRUMA OVARII (rare)
TROPHOBLASTIC DISEASE (rare)
FUNCTIONING THYROID FOLLICULAR CANCER (rare)
DRUG-INDUCED
    Iodine-induced*
    Amiodarone-induced
    Cytokine-induced†
    Lithium-associated

*A variety of iodine-containing substances, including medications, have been reported to cause hyperthyroidism. These substances include radiological contrast agents (oragraffin, telepaque, angio-conray, amipaque), topical agents (betadine, nu gauze, vioform, vytone), and medications (amiodarone, kelp, vitamins containing iodine). Patients with nodular goiter are particularly at risk for iodine-induced hyperthyroidism.

†2% of patients treated with alpha-interferon develop hyperthyroidism.

Proceed to Step 9.

STEP 9 – *What Clinical Clues Can Help Establish the Etiology of the Hyperthyroidism?*

Clinical clues that may help to establish the etiology of the hyperthyroidism are listed in the following table.

Clinical Clue	Disease Suggested
Infiltrative ophthalmopathy	Graves' disease
Infiltrative dermopathy	Graves' disease
Thyroid acropachy	Graves' disease
Symmetrical enlargement with bruits	Graves' disease
Large irregular gland with multiple nodules	Toxic multinodular goiter
Single, prominent thyroid nodule	Solitary toxic adenoma
Exquisitely tender gland	Subacute thyroiditis
Absence of goiter	Thyrotoxicosis factitia

Proceed to Step 10.

STEP 10 – *Does the Patient Have Graves' Disease?*

Graves' disease is a common cause of hyperthyroidism. While it may occur at any age, most patients present between the ages of 20 and 50 years. Classic physical exam findings that should prompt consideration of this disease include:

- Diffuse goiter with bruit
- Ophthalmopathy
- Pretibial myxedema

A clinical presentation classic for Graves' disease does not require further evaluation. If this is the case, ***stop here***.

The absence of these findings, however, does not exclude the diagnosis. If the patient does not have any of the above findings, ***proceed to Step 11***.

STEP 11 – *What Are the Results of the Radioactive Iodine Uptake Test (RAIU)?*

The radioactive iodine uptake test is useful in the evaluation of the hyperthyroid patient. The radioactive iodine uptake test may help separate high from low uptake causes of hyperthyroidism. Causes of a high RAIU test are listed in the following box.

DIFFERENTIAL DIAGNOSIS OF AN INCREASED RAIU TEST IN HYPERTHYROIDISM	
GRAVES' DISEASE	SOLITARY TOXIC ADENOMA
TOXIC MULTINODULAR GOITER	TROPHOBLASTIC DISEASE (rare)*

*Trophoblastic tumors include choriocarcinomas and hyatidiform moles. It is not uncommon for these tumors to elaborate hCG in high concentrations. The high levels of hCG stimulate the thyroid gland in the same way that TSH does. Although this is a rare cause of hyperthyroidism, it deserves consideration in the pregnant patient presenting with signs and symptoms of hyperthyroidism. The diagnosis may be established by demonstrating the presence of high hCG levels in the blood.

Causes of a low RAIU test are listed in the following box.

DIFFERENTIAL DIAGNOSIS OF A DECREASED RAIU TEST IN HYPERTHYROIDISM
THYROIDITIS Subacute (granulomatous) Silent (painless) Postpartum THYROTOXICOSIS FACTITIA STRUMA OVARII (rare)* THYROID CANCER†

*Struma ovarii refers to an ovarian tumor that is composed mainly of thyroid tissue. Although it accounts for up to 1% of all ovarian tumors, only 10% of these are complicated by the development of hyperthyroidism. It should be suspected in the hyperthyroid patient with a pelvic mass. The diagnosis may be established by demonstrating the accumulation of a radioiodine tracer in the pelvis.

†Thyroid cancer is an extremely rare cause of hyperthyroidism that usually presents after surgery has been performed for the cancer. Most cases have occurred in patients with follicular thyroid carcinoma that has spread to the bone. These functional metastases may be detected by whole body ^{131}I scanning.

If the RAIU test demonstrates high uptake, ***proceed to Step 12.***

If the RAIU test demonstrates low uptake, ***proceed to Step 13.***

STEP 12 – *What Are the Results of the Thyroid Scan?*

With the use of the thyroid scan, the remaining causes in the differential diagnosis of a high uptake RAIU test may be separated from one another, as shown in the following table.

Condition	Finding on Thyroid Scan
Graves' disease	Large hot gland with homogenous uptake
Toxic multinodular goiter	Localization of radioiodine in multiple nodules
Toxic solitary adenoma	Localization of radioiodine in a single nodule

End of Section.

STEP 13 – *Does the Patient Have Subacute Thyroiditis?*

The diagnosis of subacute thyroiditis, also known as granulomatous or de Quervain's thyroiditis, should be considered in the hyperthyroid patient with a low RAIU test. Subacute thyroiditis has a female predilection, with women outnumbering men in a ratio of 3 to 6:1. Not uncommonly, a history of recent upper respiratory tract infection is elicited.

Most patients describe the acute onset of fever, malaise, and anterior neck pain in the region of the thyroid gland. Radiation of the pain to the jaw, ears, or anterior chest is not uncommon. Precipitating and exacerbating factors include swallowing, head turning, and coughing. Some patients report that the pain is worse when wearing tight clothing. Nonspecific symptoms of malaise, myalgias, and anorexia are present in the majority of patients with subacute thyroiditis.

Physical examination typically reveals a tender and enlarged thyroid gland. Although the white blood cell count is often normal, in some patients, there is a moderate leukocytosis. The ESR is almost always elevated, often to a striking degree (as high as 100 mm/hour). When compared to Graves' disease, the T_4:T_3 ratio is usually higher.

If the patient has subacute thyroiditis, ***stop here***.

If the patient does not have subacute thyroiditis, ***proceed to Step 14***.

STEP 14 – *What Is the Serum Thyroglobulin Level?*

The clinician should also be aware of the possibility of thyrotoxicosis factitia. This refers to the deliberate and surreptitious intake of oral thyroid hormone. The classic patient is a medical professional who has a psychiatric condition. Thyrotoxicosis factitia has also been reported with inadvertent ingestion of thyroid hormone. Cases have been reported in individuals eating ground meat that was contaminated with thyroid tissue.

These patients can be differentiated from other patients with a low RAIU by measuring a serum thyroglobulin level. In true hyperthyroidism, the thyroglobulin level will be normal or elevated. In contrast, subnormal thyroglobulin levels argue for the diagnosis of thyrotoxicosis factitia.

If the thyroglobulin level is low, the patient has thyrotoxicosis factitia. ***Stop here***.

If the thyroglobulin level is normal or elevated, ***proceed to Step 15***.

STEP 15 – *Does the Patient Have Postpartum Thyroiditis?*

Postpartum thyroiditis occurs in about 5% of otherwise healthy women within 6 months of delivery. Approximately 25% of IDDM patients develop the disease. Postpartum thyroiditis seems to be a type of autoimmune thyroiditis, as most patients have circulating antithyroid antibodies.

If the patient has postpartum thyroiditis, ***stop here***.

If the patient does not have postpartum thyroiditis, ***proceed to Step 16***.

STEP 16 – *Does the Patient Have Silent Thyroiditis?*

Silent thyroiditis, also known as painless thyroiditis, also deserves consideration in the hyperthyroid patient with a low RAIU test. The following features can be used to differentiate silent thyroiditis from subacute thyroiditis.

Feature	Subacute Thyroiditis	Silent Thyroiditis
Preceding URI	(+)	(–)
Fever	(+)	(–)
Malaise	(+)	(–)
Headache	(+)	(–)
Myalgia	(+)	(–)
ESR	↑	Normal*
WBC	Normal / ↑	Normal
Anti-TPO antibodies	(–)	(+)†

*Over 50% of patients with silent thyroiditis will have a normal ESR. In the remainder, the ESR may be mildly elevated.

†Thyroid antibody levels are increased in up to 50% of patients with silent thyroiditis.

End of Section.

STEP 17 – *What Is the Differential Diagnosis of a Normal FT_4I or Free T_4 Level in the Patient With a Decreased TSH?*

The differential diagnosis of a normal FT_4I or free T_4 level in the setting of a decreased TSH is listed in the following box.

NORMAL FT_4I / FREE T_4 AND DECREASED TSH DIFFERENTIAL DIAGNOSIS
PREGNANCY
SUBCLINICAL HYPERTHYROIDISM
T_3 THYROTOXICOSIS
EXCESSIVE ORAL THYROID HORMONE REPLACEMENT
ACUTE PSYCHIATRIC ILLNESS
DRUG INHIBITION OF TSH RELEASE
Corticosteroid therapy
Dopamine therapy

These causes are considered in more detail in the remainder of this step.

Pregnancy

Human chorionic gonadotropin can stimulate the thyroid gland directly in pregnancy. This is the explanation for the decrease in TSH that is sometimes observed in normal pregnancy.

Acute Psychiatric Illness

Patients with an acute psychiatric illness often have abnormal thyroid function tests. Early in the course of an acute psychiatric illness, a decreased TSH level may be appreciated. Although the free T_4 level may be elevated, some patients have a normal free T_4 level. It is reasonable to periodically follow these patients with serial thyroid function tests. If the decreased TSH level is due to acute psychiatric illness, the TSH will normalize with time.

Excessive Oral Thyroid Hormone Replacement

A normal FT_4I or free T_4 level in the setting of a decreased TSH may be appreciated in the patient taking too much oral thyroid hormone. The appropriate dose of oral thyroid hormone is one that normalizes both the TSH and the FT_4I or free T_4 levels. If the patient is on oral thyroid hormone replacement, decrease the dose. Recheck the thyroid function tests in 6 weeks.

Subclinical Hyperthyroidism

Patients with subclinical hyperthyroidism are characteristically asymptomatic and have a normal FT_4I or free T_4 level despite a decreased TSH. Before labeling a patient with the diagnosis of subclinical hyperthyroidism, the clinician should consider other causes of a low TSH and normal FT_4I or free T_4 levels.

In patients thought to have subclinical hyperthyroidism, thyroid function tests (TSH, FT_4I or free T_4 level) should be repeated in several months. If repeat testing reveals normal or elevated TSH, the clinician should consider the possibility that the initially suppressed TSH was due to some other condition. If the repeat TSH is low and FT_4I or free T_4 level remains normal, then the diagnosis of subclinical hyperthyroidism is more secure.

T_3 Thyrotoxicosis

A small percentage of hyperthyroid patients have T_3 thyrotoxicosis. In this entity, levels of T_3 are high in the setting of a normal or even low FT_4I or free T_4 level. A similar biochemical profile may be obtained in the patient taking too much thyroid hormone in the form of T_3 (liothyronine). A T_3 level is required to establish the diagnosis.

Drug Inhibition of TSH Release

Corticosteroid and dopamine therapy may result in a depressed TSH but normal FT_4I or free T_4 levels.

End of Section.

STEP 18 – *What Is the Differential Diagnosis of a Decreased FT_4I or Free T_4 in the Patient Having a Decreased TSH Level?*

The differential diagnosis of a decreased FT_4I or free T_4 in the setting of a decreased TSH level is listed in the following box.

DECREASED FT_4I / FREE T_4 AND DECREASED TSH DIFFERENTIAL DIAGNOSIS
NONTHYROIDAL ILLNESS PITUITARY FAILURE

These causes will be discussed in more detail in the remainder of this step.

Pituitary Failure

In most patients with pituitary failure, there are signs and symptoms of other hormone deficiencies (ie, FSH, LH, ACTH, GH) in addition to the clinical manifestations of hypothyroidism.

Nonthyroidal Illness

Physical trauma, severe illness, or psychologic stress can lead to abnormalities of the thyroid function tests. A decreased serum T_3 level is the most commonly encountered abnormality. In more seriously ill patients, however, the FT_4I or free T_4 level may be low as well. It is not uncommon for these patients to have a low TSH.

End of Section.

References

Attia J, Margetts P, and Guyatt G, "Diagnosis of Thyroid Disease in Hospitalized Patients: A Systematic Review," *Arch Intern Med*, 1999, 159(7):658-65.

Camacho PM and Dwarkanathan AA, "Sick Euthyroid Syndrome. What to Do When Thyroid Function Tests Are Abnormal in Critically Ill Patients," *Postgrad Med*, 1999, 105(4):215-9.

Dayan CM, "Interpretation of Thyroid Function Tests," *Lancet*, 2001, 357(9256):619-24.

Fatourechi V, "Subclinical Thyroid Disease," *Mayo Clin Proc*, 2001, 76(4):413-6; quiz 416-7.

Kaplan MM, "Clinical Perspectives in the Diagnosis of Thyroid Disease," *Clin Chem*, 1999, 45(8 Pt 2):1377-83.

Langton JE and Brent GA, "Nonthyroidal Illness Syndrome: Evaluation of Thyroid Function in Sick Patients," *Endocrinol Metab Clin North Am*, 2002, 31(1):159-72.

O'Reilly DS, "Thyroid Function Tests-Time for a Reassessment," *BMJ*, 2000, 320(7245):1332-4.

Peery WH and Meek JC, "Interpretation of Thyroid Function Tests: An Update," *Compr Ther*, 1998, 24(11-12):567-73.

Toft AD, "Clinical Practice. Subclinical Hyperthyroidism," *N Engl J Med*, 2001, 24(11-12):567-73.

APPROACH TO ↓ TSH

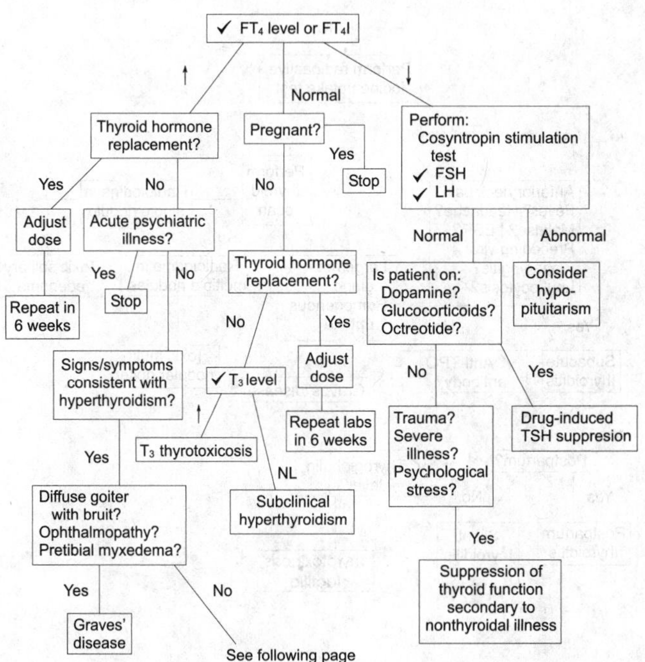

FT_4 = free thyroxine
FT_4I = free thyroxine index

APPROACH TO ↓ TSH (*continued*)

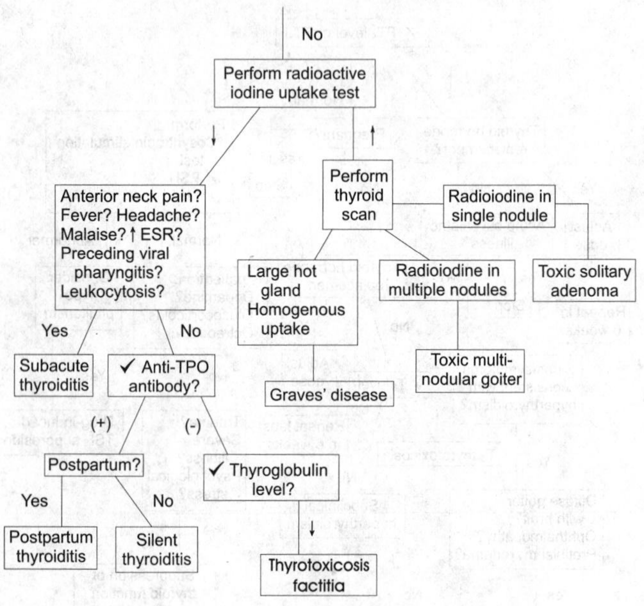

APPROACH TO THE PATIENT SUSPECTED OF HAVING HYPOTHYROIDISM

STEP 1 – *What Are the Clinical Manifestations of Hypothyroidism?*

The diagnosis of hypothyroidism should be considered when signs and symptoms of hypothyroidism are present, as shown in the following box.

HYPOTHYROIDISM SIGNS AND SYMPTOMS	
WEAKNESS	WEIGHT GAIN
DRY SKIN	LOSS OF HAIR
COARSE SKIN	PERIPHERAL EDEMA
LETHARGY	HOARSENESS
EDEMA OF EYELIDS	ANOREXIA
SENSATION OF COLD	NERVOUSNESS
COLD SKIN	MENORRHAGIA
COARSENESS OF HAIR	DIMINISHED SWEATING
MEMORY IMPAIRMENT	PARESTHESIAS
CONSTIPATION	

Proceed to Step 2.

STEP 2 – *What Laboratory Features May Be Appreciated in Patients With Hypothyroidism?*

Laboratory test abnormalities found in patients with hypothyroidism are listed in the following box.

LABORATORY TEST ABNORMALITIES FOUND IN HYPOTHYROIDISM
INCREASED CREATINE KINASE
INCREASED AST
HYPONATREMIA
INCREASED CHOLESTEROL / TRIGLYCERIDES
NORMOCYTIC OR MACROCYTIC ANEMIA
HYPERHOMOCYSTEINEMIA

Proceed to Step 3.

STEP 3 – *What Are the Results of the TSH and the Free T_4 Level?*

In the patient suspected of having hypothyroidism, confirmation of the diagnosis requires measurement of the serum TSH and free T_4 level.

If the patient has an increased TSH along with a decrease in the free T_4 level, then the diagnosis is primary hypothyroidism. ***Proceed to Step 4.***

If the patient has an increased TSH but a normal free T_4 level, this suggests the diagnosis of subclinical hypothyroidism. ***Proceed to Step 5.***

If the TSH is not increased in a patient who has a low free T_4 level, ***proceed to Step 6.***

If the TSH and free T_4 level are normal, then the patient does not have hypothyroidism.

STEP 4 – *What Are the Causes of Primary Hypothyroidism?*

An increased TSH along with a decreased free T_4 level is consistent with the diagnosis of primary hypothyroidism. The term "primary" is used when hypothyroidism results from disease of the thyroid gland. Primary hypothyroidism differs from secondary and tertiary hypothyroidism which reflect disease of the pituitary and hypothalamus, respectively.

The causes of primary hypothyroidism are listed in the following box. The two most common causes are chronic lymphocytic thyroiditis (Hashimoto's disease) and radioiodine-induced hypothyroidism.

CAUSES OF PRIMARY HYPOTHYROIDISM

- CHRONIC LYMPHOCYTIC THYROIDITIS (Hashimoto's disease)
- SURGICAL THYROIDECTOMY
- EXTERNAL RADIATION THERAPY (>2000 R)
- RADIOIODINE THERAPY
- INFILTRATIVE DISEASE
  - Amyloidosis
  - Lymphoma
  - Scleroderma
  - Hemochromatosis
  - Sarcoidosis
- IODINE DEFICIENCY
- CONGENITAL
- DRUG-INDUCED
  - Thionamides
  - Iodine excess
  - Amiodarone
  - Lithium
  - Sertraline
  - Sulfonamides
  - Interleukins
  - Interferon alpha
- DISRUPTIVE THYROIDITIS
  - Postpartum
  - Silent (painless)
  - Subacute (granulomatous)

Measurement of antithyroid antibodies can help elucidate the etiology of primary hypothyroidism. Chronic lymphocytic thyroiditis, also known as Hashimoto's disease, is associated with the presence of antithyroglobulin and antithyroid peroxidase antibodies. Sixty percent of patients with Hashimoto's disease are found to have antithyroglobulin antibodies while approximately 95% have circulating antithyroid peroxidase antibodies.

End of Section.

STEP 5 – *What Is Subclinical Hypothyroidism?*

Some patients who appear clinically euthyroid have thyroid function tests (increased TSH, normal free T_4 level) consistent with early thyroid failure or subclinical hypothyroidism. In these patients, the TSH level is usually <20 mU/L.

If the thyroid function tests are consistent with subclinical hypothyroidism, the TSH level should be repeated. In some of these patients, the repeat TSH level may be normal. If the repeat TSH level is high and the FT_4I or free T_4 level remains normal, then the diagnosis of subclinical hypothyroidism is established.

Five percent to 18% of patients with subclinical hypothyroidism progress to overt hypothyroidism each year. Although it can be difficult to predict those who will progress to overt hypothyroidism, it seems that progression is more likely if antithyroid antibodies are present. Patients with subclinical hypothyroidism who have a high TSH level, particularly one that is >20 mU/L, are also more likely to progress to overt hypothyroidism.

End of Section.

STEP 6 – *What Should Be Considered in the Patient Presenting With Signs and Symptoms of Hypothyroidism Who Has a Low Free T_4 Level but No Elevation in the TSH Level?*

When a patient suspected of having hypothyroidism has a low or normal TSH in the setting of a low free T_4 level, central hypothyroidism warrants consideration. Central hypothyroidism may be the result of a disease process in the pituitary gland or hypothalamus affecting the production or secretion of TSH and TRH, respectively. Since isolated deficiency of TSH or TRH is rare, these patients usually have signs and symptoms of other hormone deficiencies. Pituitary hormone deficiency is known as hypopituitarism. The reader is referred to the chapter, ***Hypopituitarism*** *on page 409* for more information regarding the evaluation of these patients.

References

Attia J, Margetts P, and Guyatt G, "Diagnosis of Thyroid Disease in Hospitalized Patients: A Systematic Review," *Arch Intern Med*, 1999, 159(7):658-65.

Camacho PM and Dwarkanathan AA, "Sick Euthyroid Syndrome. What to Do When Thyroid Function Tests Are Abnormal in Critically Ill Patients," *Postgrad Med*, 1999, 105(4):215-9.

Cooper DS, ed, "Clinical Practice. Subclinical Hypothyroidism," *N Engl J Med*, 2001, 345(4):260-5.

Dayan CM, "Interpretation of Thyroid Function Tests," *Lancet*, 2001, 357(9256):619-24.

Fatourechi V, "Subclinical Thyroid Disease," *Mayo Clin Proc*, 2001, 76(4):413-6; quiz 416-7.

Guha B, Krishnaswamy G, and Peiris A, "The Diagnosis and Management of Hypothyroidism," *South Med J*, 2002, 95(5):475-80.

Kaplan MM, "Clinical Perspectives in the Diagnosis of Thyroid Disease," *Clin Chem*, 1999, 45(8 Pt 2):1377-83.

O'Reilly DS, "Thyroid Function Tests-Time for a Reassessment," *BMJ*, 2000, 320(7245):1332-4.

Pearce EN, Farwell, AP, and Braverman LE, "Thyroiditis," *N Engl J Med*, 2003, 348(26):2646-55.

Peery WH and Meek JC, "Interpretation of Thyroid Function Tests: An Update," *Compr Ther*, 1998, 24(11-12):567-73.

APPROACH TO SUSPECTED HYPOTHYROIDISM

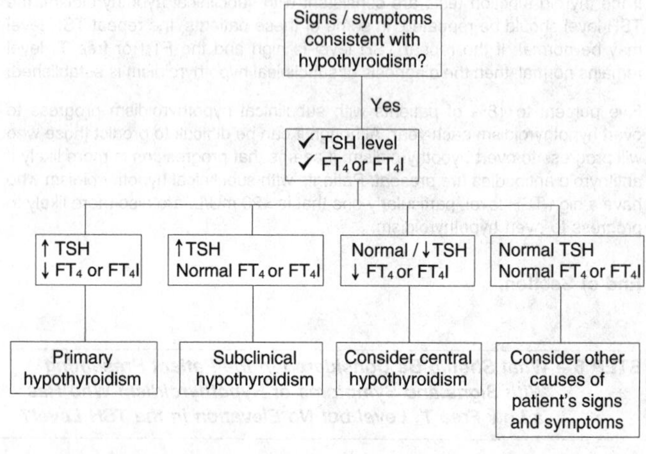

FT_4 = free thyroxine
FT_4I = free thyroxine index

APPROACH TO THE PATIENT SUSPECTED OF HAVING HYPERTHYROIDISM

STEP 1 – *What Are the Signs and Symptoms of Hyperthyroidism?*

Hyperthyroidism should be suspected when signs and symptoms of hyperthyroidism are present, as shown in the following box.

HYPERTHYROIDISM SIGNS AND SYMPTOMS	
NERVOUSNESS	DIARRHEA
EMOTIONAL LABILITY	PROXIMAL MUSCLE WEAKNESS
TREMOR	WARM MOIST SMOOTH SKIN
INCREASED SWEATING	HEAT INTOLERANCE
PALPITATIONS	FINE HAIR
FATIGUE	HAIR LOSS
WEIGHT LOSS	WEAKNESS
TACHYCARDIA	INCREASED APPETITE
ATRIAL FIBRILLATION	
INCREASED DIFFERENCE IN SYSTOLIC AND DIASTOLIC BLOOD PRESSURE	

Proceed to Step 2.

STEP 2 – *What Laboratory Features May Be Appreciated in Patients With Hyperthyroidism?*

The laboratory test abnormalities found in hyperthyroidism are listed in the following box.

HYPERTHYROIDISM LABORATORY FEATURES
INCREASED CALCIUM (mild)
INCREASED ALKALINE PHOSPHATASE
ELEVATED TRANSAMINASES (mild)
NORMOCYTIC NORMOCHROMIC ANEMIA
LYMPHOCYTOSIS
HYPOALBUMINEMIA
LEUKOPENIA (mild)
LOW TOTAL CHOLESTEROL
LOW HDL CHOLESTEROL
LOW TOTAL CHOLESTEROL / HDL CHOLESTEROL RATIO

Patients with Graves' disease may have laboratory test abnormalities related to other autoimmune diseases (eg, idiopathic thrombocytopenic purpura, pernicious anemia).

Proceed to Step 3.

STEP 3 – *What Are the Results of the Serum TSH and Free T_4 Level?*

In the patient suspected of having hyperthyroidism, a serum TSH and free T_4 level should be obtained.

A decreased TSH and elevated free T_4 establishes the diagnosis of primary hyperthyroidism. ***Proceed to Step 4.***

If the free T_4 is normal in the patient with decreased TSH, ***proceed to Step 13*** *on page 376.*

If the TSH is normal or increased with an increased free T_4 level, ***proceed to Step 15*** *on page 376.*

STEP 4 – *What Are the Causes of Primary Hyperthyroidism?*

When a decreased TSH and elevated free T_4 level are found in a patient with signs and symptoms suggestive of hyperthyroidism, primary hyperthyroidism is said to be present. The term "primary" is used when the problem with thyroid function is a result of disease within the thyroid gland. The causes of primary hyperthyroidism are listed in the following box.

PRIMARY HYPERTHYROIDISM DIFFERENTIAL DIAGNOSIS

- GRAVES' DISEASE
- TOXIC MULTINODULAR GOITER
- SOLITARY TOXIC ADENOMA
- THYROIDITIS
  - Subacute (granulomatous)
  - Silent (painless)
  - Postpartum
- THYROTOXICOSIS FACTITIA
- STRUMA OVARII (rare)
- TROPHOBLASTIC DISEASE (rare)
- FUNCTIONING THYROID FOLLICULAR CANCER (rare)
- DRUG-INDUCED
  - Iodine-induced*
  - Amiodarone-induced
  - Cytokine-induced†
  - Lithium-associated

*A variety of iodine-containing substances, including medications, have been reported to cause hyperthyroidism. These substances include radiological contrast agents (oragraffin, telepaque, angio-conray, amipaque), topical agents (betadine, nu gauze, vioform, vytone), and medications (amiodarone, kelp, vitamins containing iodine). Patients with nodular goiter are particularly at risk for iodine-induced hyperthyroidism.

†2% of patients treated with alpha-interferon develop hyperthyroidism.

The three most common causes of hyperthyroidism are Graves' disease, toxic multinodular goiter, and solitary toxic adenoma.

Proceed to Step 5.

STEP 5 – *What Clinical Clues Can Help Establish the Etiology of the Hyperthyroidism?*

Clinical clues that may help to establish the etiology of the hyperthyroidism are listed in the following table.

Clinical Clue	Disease Suggested
Infiltrative ophthalmopathy	Graves' disease
Infiltrative dermopathy	Graves' disease
Thyroid acropachy	Graves' disease
Symmetrical enlargement with bruits	Graves' disease
Large irregular gland with multiple nodules	Toxic multinodular goiter
Single, prominent thyroid nodule	Solitary toxic adenoma
Exquisitely tender gland	Subacute thyroiditis

Proceed to Step 6.

STEP 6 – *Does the Patient Have Graves' Disease?*

Graves' disease is a common cause of hyperthyroidism. While it may occur at any age, most patients present between the ages of 20 and 50 years. Classic physical exam findings that should prompt consideration of this disease include:

- Diffuse goiter with bruit
- Ophthalmopathy
- Pretibial myxedema

A clinical presentation classic for Graves' disease does not require further evaluation. If this is the case, ***stop here***.

The absence of these findings, however, does not exclude the diagnosis. If the patient does not have any of the above findings, ***proceed to Step 7***.

STEP 7 – *What Are the Results of the Radioactive Iodine Uptake Test (RAIU)?*

The radioactive iodine uptake test is useful in the evaluation of the hyperthyroid patient. The radioactive iodine uptake test may help separate high from low uptake causes of hyperthyroidism. Causes of a high RAIU test are listed in the following box.

DIFFERENTIAL DIAGNOSIS OF AN INCREASED RAIU TEST IN HYPERTHYROIDISM	
GRAVES' DISEASE	SOLITARY TOXIC ADENOMA
TOXIC MULTINODULAR GOITER	TROPHOBLASTIC DISEASE (rare)*

*Trophoblastic tumors include choriocarcinomas and hyatidiform moles. It is not uncommon for these tumors to elaborate hCG in high concentrations. The high levels of hCG stimulate the thyroid gland in the same way that TSH does. Although this is a rare cause of hyperthyroidism, it deserves consideration in the pregnant patient presenting with signs and symptoms of hyperthyroidism. The diagnosis may be established by demonstrating the presence of high hCG levels in the blood.

Causes of a low RAIU test are listed in the following box.

DIFFERENTIAL DIAGNOSIS OF A DECREASED RAIU TEST IN HYPERTHYROIDISM	
THYROIDITIS	THYROTOXICOSIS FACTITIA
Subacute (granulomatous)	STRUMA OVARII (rare)*
Silent (painless)	THYROID CANCER†
Postpartum	IODINE-INDUCED

*Struma ovarii refers to an ovarian tumor that is composed mainly of thyroid tissue. Although it accounts for up to 1% of all ovarian tumors, only 10% of these are complicated by the development of hyperthyroidism. It should be suspected in the hyperthyroid patient with a pelvic mass. The diagnosis may be established by demonstrating the accumulation of a radioiodine tracer in the pelvis.

†Thyroid cancer is an extremely rare cause of hyperthyroidism that usually presents after surgery has been performed for the cancer. Most cases have occurred in patients with follicular thyroid carcinoma that has spread to the bone. These functional metastases may be detected by whole body ^{131}I scanning.

If the RAIU test demonstrates high uptake, ***proceed to Step 8***.

If the RAIU test demonstrates low uptake, ***proceed to Step 9***.

STEP 8 – *What Are the Results of the Thyroid Scan?*

With the use of the thyroid scan, the remaining causes in the differential diagnosis of a high uptake RAIU test may be separated from one another, as shown in the following table.

Condition	Finding on Thyroid Scan
Graves' disease	Large hot gland with homogenous uptake
Toxic multinodular goiter	Localization of radioiodine in multiple nodules
Toxic solitary adenoma	Localization of radioiodine in a single nodule

End of Section.

STEP 9 – *Does the Patient Have Subacute Thyroiditis?*

The diagnosis of subacute thyroiditis, also known as granulomatous or de Quervain's thyroiditis, should be considered in the hyperthyroid patient with a low RAIU test. Subacute thyroiditis has a female predilection, with women outnumbering men in a ratio of 3 to 6:1. Not uncommonly, a history of recent upper respiratory tract infection is elicited.

Most patients describe the acute onset of fever, malaise, and anterior neck pain in the region of the thyroid gland. Radiation of the pain to the jaw, ears, or anterior chest is not uncommon. Precipitating and exacerbating factors include swallowing, head turning, and coughing. Some patients report that the pain is worse when wearing tight clothing. Nonspecific symptoms of malaise, myalgias, and anorexia are present in the majority of patients with subacute thyroiditis.

Physical examination typically reveals a tender and enlarged thyroid gland. Although the white blood cell count is often normal, in some patients, there is a moderate leukocytosis. The ESR is almost always elevated, often to a striking degree (as high as 100 mm/hour). When compared to Graves' disease, the T_4:T_3 ratio is usually higher. Thyroid-peroxidase (TPO) antibodies are often transiently present.

If the patient has subacute thyroiditis, ***stop here***.

If the patient does not have subacute thyroiditis, ***proceed to Step 10***.

STEP 10 – *What Is the Serum Thyroglobulin Level?*

The clinician should also be aware of the possibility of thyrotoxicosis factitia. This refers to the deliberate and surreptitious intake of oral thyroid hormone. The classic patient is a medical professional who has a psychiatric condition. Thyrotoxicosis factitia has also been reported with inadvertent ingestion of thyroid hormone. Cases have been reported in individuals eating ground meat that was contaminated with thyroid tissue.

These patients can be differentiated from other patients with a low RAIU by measuring a serum thyroglobulin level. In true hyperthyroidism, the thyroglobulin level will be normal or elevated. In contrast, subnormal thyroglobulin levels argue for the diagnosis of thyrotoxicosis factitia.

If the thyroglobulin level is low, the patient has thyrotoxicosis factitia. ***Stop here.***

If the thyroglobulin level is normal or elevated, ***proceed to Step 11.***

STEP 11 – *Does the Patient Have Postpartum Thyroiditis?*

Postpartum thyroiditis occurs in about 5% to 10% of otherwise healthy women between the third and ninth months after delivery. Approximately 25% of IDDM patients develop the disease, which is why this population should be screened periodically in the postpartum period. Postpartum thyroiditis seems to be a type of autoimmune thyroiditis, as most patients have circulating antithyroid antibodies. In contrast to subacute thyroiditis, TPO antibodies can be demonstrated before and after the episode of thyroiditis. In fact, higher TPO antibody titers confer greater susceptibility to the development of thyroiditis after delivery.

If the patient has postpartum thyroiditis, ***stop here.***

If the patient does not have postpartum thyroiditis, ***proceed to Step 12.***

STEP 12 – *Does the Patient Have Silent Thyroiditis?*

Silent thyroiditis, also known as painless thyroiditis, also deserves consideration in the hyperthyroid patient with a low RAIU test. Features that can be used to differentiate silent thyroiditis from subacute thyroiditis can be found in the following table

Feature	Subacute Thyroiditis	Silent Thyroiditis
Preceding URI	(+)	(–)
Fever	(+)	(–)
Malaise	(+)	(–)
Headache	(+)	(–)
Myalgia	(+)	(–)
ESR	↑	Normal*
WBC	Normal / ↑	Normal
Anti-TPO antibodies	(–)	(+)†

*Over 50% of patients with silent thyroiditis will have a normal ESR. In the remainder, the ESR may be mildly elevated.

†Thyroid antibody levels are increased in up to 50% of patients with silent thyroiditis.

End of Section.

STEP 13 – *What Is the Serum T_3 Level?*

If the free T_4 level is normal, then a serum T_3 level should be obtained. An elevated serum T_3 level suggests the diagnosis of T_3 thyrotoxicosis. T_3 thyrotoxicosis is most commonly encountered during early Graves' disease or during a relapse of Graves' disease.

If the patient has T_3 thyrotoxicosis, ***stop here.***

If the serum T_3 level is normal, ***proceed to Step 14.***

STEP 14 – *Does the Patient Have Subclinical Hyperthyroidism?*

In the patient not having signs and symptoms of hyperthyroidism, subclinical hyperthyroidism is the most likely diagnosis. These patients are characteristically asymptomatic and have a normal free T_4 level despite a decreased TSH. Before labeling a patient with the diagnosis of subclinical hyperthyroidism, the clinician should consider other causes of a low TSH and normal free T_4 levels. Other conditions to consider include nonthyroidal illness, transient thyroiditis, dopamine, corticosteroid, and amiodarone therapy.

In patients thought to have subclinical hyperthyroidism, thyroid function tests (TSH, free T_4 level) should be repeated in several months. If repeat testing reveals normal or elevated TSH, the clinician should consider the possibility that the initially suppressed TSH reflected nonthyroidal illness or transient thyroiditis. If the repeat TSH is low and free T_4 level remains normal, then the diagnosis of subclinical hyperthyroidism is more secure.

End of Section.

STEP 15 – *Does the Patient Have a TSH-Producing Pituitary Adenoma?*

A normal or increased TSH in the setting of an increased free T_4 level should prompt consideration of a TSH-producing pituitary adenoma. These tumors account for 0.5% to 3% of pituitary tumors. Not all patients present with CNS symptoms such as headache and visual field disturbance. In fact, headache and visual field disturbances are complaints in only 23% and 40% of patients, respectively.

While many patients with TSH-producing pituitary adenomas have increased TSH levels, 33% have levels <10 mU/L. A measurement of the α-subunit is helpful in supporting the diagnosis. An α-subunit:TSH ratio >1 is characteristic of a TSH-producing pituitary adenoma.

TSH-producing pituitary adenoma must be differentiated from thyroid hormone resistance. Both conditions are characterized by normal or increased TSH levels. Features used to differentiate between TSH-producing pituitary adenoma and thyroid hormone resistance are listed in the following table.

Characteristics of TSH-Producing Pituitary Adenoma Versus Thyroid Hormone Resistance

Feature	TSH-Producing Pituitary Adenoma	Thyroid Hormone Resistance
TRH stimulation of TSH	8%	96%
T_3 suppression of TSH	12%	100%
Elevated sex hormone-binding globulin	94%	2%
Elevated alpha subunit:TSH ratio	81%	2%
Family history	0%	82%
MRI pituitary adenoma	98%	2%

Adapted from Beck-Peccoz P, Brucker-Davis F, Persani L, et al, "Thyrotropin-Secreting Pituitary Tumors," *Endocr Rev*, 1996, 17:610-38.

Cooper DS, ed, *Medical Management of Thyroid Disease*, New York, NY: Marcel Dekker Inc, 2001.

End of Section.

References

Cooper DS, "Hyperthyroidism," *Lancet*, 2003, 362(9382):459-68.

Demura R, "Current Medical Approach to Thyroid Stimulating Hormone-Secreting Pituitary Adenomas," *Intern Med*, 1998, 37(12):999-1000.

Slatosky J, Shipton B, and Wahba H, "Thyroiditis: Differential Diagnosis and Management," *Am Fam Physician*, 2000, 61(4):1047-52, 1054.

Stagnaro-Green A, "Recognizing, Understanding, and Treating Postpartum Thyroiditis," *Endocrinol Metab Clin North Am*, 2000, 29(2):417-30, ix.

Summaria V, Salvatori M, Rufini V, et al, "Diagnostic Imaging in Thyrotoxicosis," *Rays*, 1999, 24(2):273-300.

Toft AD, "Clinical Practice. Subclinical Hyperthyroidism," *N Engl J Med*, 2001, 345(7):512-6.

Weetman AP, "Graves' Disease," *N Engl J Med*, 2000, 343(17):1236-48.

APPROACH TO SUSPECTED HYPERTHYROIDISM

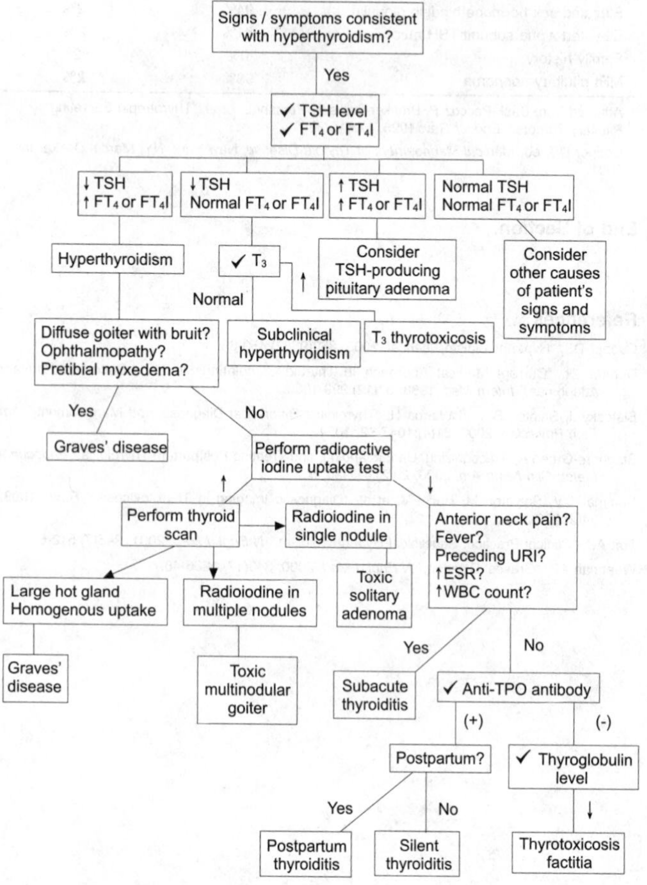

ADRENAL INSUFFICIENCY

STEP 1 – *What Are the Signs and Symptoms of Adrenal Insufficiency?*

The clinical presentation of adrenal insufficiency is variable. Quite often, the onset is insidious (chronic adrenal insufficiency). In chronic adrenal insufficiency, nonspecific signs and symptoms are typically present, as shown in the following box.

CHRONIC ADRENAL INSUFFICIENCY SIGNS AND SYMPTOMS

- WEAKNESS / FATIGUE
- ANOREXIA
- NAUSEA / VOMITING
- DIARRHEA
- CONSTIPATION
- ABDOMINAL PAIN
- DIZZINESS WHEN STANDING
- WEIGHT LOSS
- HYPOTENSION
- MYALGIAS
- ARTHRALGIAS
- SALT CRAVING
- PSYCHIATRIC SYMPTOMS
  - Depression
  - Apathy
  - Confusion
  - Paranoia
  - Psychosis
- AMENORRHEA
- HYPERPIGMENTATION

These nonspecific signs and symptoms may go undiagnosed until a stressful situation, such as infection, precipitates adrenal crisis. Patients with adrenal crisis or acute adrenal insufficiency often present with shock.

Proceed to Step 2.

STEP 2 – *What Are the Laboratory Findings in Patients With Adrenal Insufficiency?*

Before discussing laboratory findings in adrenal insufficiency, a distinction needs to be made between primary, secondary, and tertiary causes.

SOME DEFINITIONS...

Primary adrenal insufficiency: Failure of the adrenal gland to produce corticosteroids

Secondary adrenal insufficiency: Failure of the pituitary gland to produce adrenocorticotropin hormone (ACTH), resulting in corticosteroid deficiency

Tertiary adrenal insufficiency: Failure of the hypothalamus to produce corticotropin-releasing hormone (CRH), resulting in corticosteroid deficiency

Although the three forms of adrenal insufficiency have many laboratory abnormalities in common, there are some differences between primary adrenal insufficiency and the other two forms. Laboratory test abnormalities in primary adrenal insufficiency are listed in the following box.

PRIMARY ADRENAL INSUFFICIENCY LABORATORY FEATURES
INCREASED ACTH LEVELS
HYPONATREMIA
INCREASED THYROID STIMULATING HORMONE
HYPERPROLACTINEMIA (up to 50 ng/mL)
MILD HYPERCHLOREMIC METABOLIC ACIDOSIS
INCREASED BUN:CREATININE RATIO
HYPERCALCEMIA (occasional)
DECREASED / NORMAL GLUCOSE
INCREASED EOSINOPHILS
RELATIVE LYMPHOCYTOSIS
NORMOCYTIC, NORMOCHROMIC ANEMIA*
HYPERKALEMIA

*Anemia may be masked initially by volume depletion. Anemia may be macrocytic in patients with polyglandular autoimmune syndromes, particularly if pernicious anemia or hypothyroidism is present.

As discussed above, secondary and tertiary adrenal insufficiency have similar laboratory abnormalities to those found in primary adrenal insufficiency. However, there are several differences which are noted in the following table.

	Primary Adrenal Insufficiency	Secondary / Tertiary Adrenal Insufficiency
ACTH	↑	↓ / Low normal
K+	↑	Normal
Prerenal azotemia	More common	Less common
Hypoglycemia	More common	Less common
Hypercalcemia	More common	Less common

Proceed to Step 3.

STEP 3 – *What Is the AM Cortisol Level?*

AM cortisol levels are often obtained in the evaluation of patients suspected of having adrenal insufficiency. In the general population, the plasma cortisol level is elevated in the morning (before 8 AM). While low AM plasma cortisol levels (<3-5 μg/dL) argue strongly for the diagnosis of adrenal insufficiency, most experts recommend confirmation of the diagnosis with a more sensitive test (ACTH or cosyntropin stimulation test). Basal cortisol levels exceeding 15 μg/dL are highly predictive of a normally functioning hypothalamic-pituitary-adrenal axis. Intermediate cortisol levels are not diagnostic. There is no use in obtaining plasma cortisol levels in the afternoon or evening because they are normally low at this time.

If the morning plasma cortisol level is <3-5 μg/dL, the patient likely has adrenal insufficiency. ***Proceed to Step 4.***

If the basal plasma cortisol level is >15 μg/dL, adrenal insufficiency is very unlikely.

If the plasma cortisol level falls between 5 and 15 μg/dL, further testing needs to be performed to exclude or diagnose adrenal insufficiency. ***Proceed to Step 4.***

STEP 4 – *What Is the Result of the Cosyntropin Stimulation Test?*

In the standard ACTH (cosyntropin) stimulation test, plasma cortisol is measured before, and then 30 minutes after the intravenous or intramuscular administration of 250 μg of ACTH. It is preferable to perform the test at 9 AM since studies evaluating the usefulness of this test were often done at this time. If the peak plasma cortisol level exceeds 19 μg/dL, the patient is said to have normal adrenal function. It is wise, however, for the clinician to be familiar with the assay that is being used because the cutoff values may differ depending upon the assay. In the past, the difference between the peak and basal cortisol values was also used to assess patients for adrenal insufficiency but this has now fallen out of favor. The ACTH stimulation test can also be performed in patients who have already been started on corticosteroid therapy as long as they meet the following criteria:

- Corticosteroid replacement therapy has been of short duration
- Patient is not receiving hydrocortisone, which can interfere with the cortisol assay that is performed with the ACTH stimulation test

A subnormal response indicates the presence of adrenal insufficiency. There is one exception to this rule. This occurs in the patient who develops ACTH deficiency acutely, as found in the patient with recent hypophysectomy. Within the first few days after hypophysectomy, the adrenal glands retain the ability to respond to exogenously administered ACTH, but are unable to release ACTH in response to stress. Although the results of the cosyntropin stimulation test may be normal in these patients, the response to the insulin-induced hypoglycemia test will be abnormal. Alternatively, a metapyrone test may be performed to diagnose adrenal insufficiency in these patients.

Recently, there has been some focus on the use of a low-dose ACTH stimulation test (1 μg) for the diagnosis of adrenal insufficiency. Proponents maintain that the low-dose stimulation test may be more sensitive than the conventional dose but it remains to be seen whether studies will find this to be true.

If the cosyntropin stimulation test is consistent with adrenal insufficiency, ***proceed to Step 5***.

If the cosyntropin stimulation test is not consistent with adrenal insufficiency, ***stop here***.

STEP 5 – *What Is the Basal ACTH Level?*

The cosyntropin stimulation test only establishes the presence of adrenal insufficiency. It does not distinguish between primary, secondary, and tertiary forms of the disease. Once the presence of adrenal insufficiency has been established, attention should focus on determining whether the patient has primary, secondary, or tertiary adrenal insufficiency. This can be accomplished by the measurement of an ACTH level at 8 AM.

If the ACTH level is elevated, ***proceed to Step 6***.

If the ACTH level is low or low normal, ***proceed to Step 7***.

STEP 6 – *What Does an Elevated ACTH Level in the Patient With Adrenal Insufficiency Suggest?*

An elevated ACTH level indicates the presence of primary adrenal insufficiency. The many causes of primary adrenal insufficiency are listed in the following box.

CAUSES OF PRIMARY ADRENAL INSUFFICIENCY
AUTOIMMUNE
SEPSIS (WATERHOUSE-FRIDERICHSEN SYNDROME)
TUBERCULOSIS*
FUNGAL DISEASE†
Histoplasmosis
Paracoccidiodomycosis
Coccidioidomycosis
Blastomycosis
HEMOCHROMATOSIS
SARCOIDOSIS
AMYLOIDOSIS
MALIGNANCY
Lymphoma
Metastatic cancer (lung, melanoma, breast)
AIDS
Opportunistic infection
Cytomegalovirus
MAI
Cryptococcus
Malignancy
Kaposi's sarcoma
HEMORRHAGE‡
MEDICATIONS
Aminoglutethimide
Ketoconazole
Metapyrone
Rifampin
Suramin
BILATERAL ADRENALECTOMY
ADRENOLEUKODYSTROPHY / ADRENOMYELONEUROPATHY

*Tuberculosis was the most common cause of primary adrenal insufficiency in the past and, in some populations of the world, it remains the leading cause. Patients with adrenal insufficiency due to tuberculosis usually have evidence of active tuberculosis elsewhere. To help support this diagnosis, the clinician should obtain a chest x-ray, place a PPD, and obtain urine culture for mycobacteria.

†Fungal disease usually results in adrenal insufficiency when the disease is disseminated.

‡Adrenal insufficiency that develops in the anticoagulated patient should prompt the clinician to consider adrenal hemorrhage.

Of these conditions, autoimmune disease is the most common cause (in the developed world) of adrenal insufficiency, responsible for 70% to 90% of cases worldwide, tuberculosis is the most common etiology. It is not necessary to assay adrenal antibodies in the patient with primary adrenal insufficiency. Rather, the clinician should strive to exclude the other disorders that can cause primary adrenal insufficiency.

Not all patients with autoimmune adrenal insufficiency are found to have adrenal autoantibodies; however, 60% to 75% of these patients do have these antibodies. These antibodies are also occasionally found with other types of adrenal insufficiency, in the general population, and with other autoimmune endocrine disorders. In patients with autoimmune adrenal insufficiency, the clinician should consider screening the patient for other autoimmune diseases such as hypothyroidism and diabetes mellitus.

In patients with primary adrenal insufficiency, adrenal imaging is rarely helpful. Exceptions to this rule include patients suspected of having bilateral adrenal hemorrhage, infection, or malignancy, in which case CT scan of the adrenal glands may reveal suggestive or even conclusive findings. CT-guided biopsy may be needed if malignancy is suspected. A chest radiograph, PPD, and early morning urine samples should be obtained if tuberculosis is a consideration.

Infectious Agents and Clinical Manifestations at Time of Addison's Disease Diagnosis*

Infectious Agent	Possible Coexisting Skin Abnormalities	Potential CXR Findings	Adrenal Gland Appearance on CT Scan	DD*
TB	+PPD	Variable	Asymmetric adrenal enlargement and calcification	Yes
MAC	Rare; in setting of AIDS, may mimic Kaposi's sarcoma	Possible cavitary lesions or localized infiltrate	N/A	Yes
Meningococcus	Petechial rash	Pulmonary edema	Enlarged and poorly defined adrenal glands	Yes
CMV	Decreased skin turgor	Interstitial infiltrates	N/A	Yes
Pneumocystis carinii	None	Interstitial infiltrates	Bilateral adrenal enlargement	Yes
Histoplasma capsulatum	Indurated ulcers of mouth, tongue, and nose	Variable (granulomatous disease, discrete nodules, or miliary pattern, or CXR may be clear)	Nonenhancing (consistent with infarct or necrosis) bilaterally enlarged adrenals	Yes
Blastomyces dermatiditis	Wartlike lesions	Pulmonary infiltrates mimicking lobar pneumonia or mass lesion	Bilateral asymmetric enlargement	Yes
Paracoccidioides brasiliensis	Mucocutaneous lesions	Bilateral patchy infiltrates	Bilateral adrenal enlargement	Yes
Cryptococcus neoformans	Nodular lesions with ulceration	Variable (well-circumscribed, dense infiltrate or diffuse pneumonic infiltrate, or CXR may be clear)	Bilateral adrenal enlargement	Yes
Coccidioides immitis	Skin nodules	Reticulonodular infiltrate	Bilateral adrenal enlargement	Yes

*DD = Disseminated Disease

*CXR, chest x-ray; CT, computed tomographic; TB, tuberculosis; +PPD, positive for purified protein derivative; MAC, *Mycobacterium avium-intracellulare*; AIDS, acquired immunodeficiency syndrome; N/A, not available; CMV, cytomegalovirus.

Adapted from Alevritis EM, Sarubbi FA, Jordan RM, et al, "Infectious Causes of Adrenal Insufficiency," *Southern Med Assoc*, 2003, 96(9):888-90.

End of Section.

STEP 7 – *What Does a Low or Low-Normal ACTH Level in the Patient With Adrenal Insufficiency Suggest?*

A low or low normal ACTH level in the patient with adrenal insufficiency suggests a diagnosis of secondary or tertiary adrenal insufficiency. The most common cause of secondary/tertiary adrenal insufficiency is the administration of exogenous glucocorticoids or ACTH. If the patient has not been receiving exogenous glucocorticoids or ACTH, consideration should be given to the possibility of pituitary or hypothalamic disease resulting in ACTH deficiency. Evaluation of these patients begins with a CT or MRI scan to exclude tumor and other mass lesions. The causes of secondary and tertiary adrenal insufficiency, which are really the causes of panhypopituitarism, are listed in the following box.

CAUSES OF SECONDARY AND TERTIARY ADRENAL INSUFFICIENCY	
MALIGNANCY	INFILTRATION
Pituitary adenoma	Hemochromatosis
Hypothalamic tumors	Amyloidosis
Craniopharyngioma	VASCULAR EVENT
Germinoma	Sheehan's syndrome (postpartum pituitary necrosis)
Meningioma	Carotid aneurysm
Glioma	HEAD TRAUMA
Metastatic cancer	SURGERY
INFLAMMATORY DISEASE	RADIATION
Granulomatous disease	EXOGENOUS GLUCOCORTICOID THERAPY
Tuberculosis	
Sarcoidosis	
Syphilis	
Lymphocytic hypophysitis	
Histiocytosis X / eosinophilic granuloma	

In general, distinguishing between secondary and tertiary adrenal insufficiency is rarely important, because it does not impact on therapy. Nevertheless, the CRH test can differentiate between the two. In patients with secondary adrenal insufficiency, there is little or no ACTH secretion in response to CRH; whereas, in patients with tertiary adrenal insufficiency, CRH administration results in increased ACTH secretion.

References

Alevritis EM, Sarubbi FA, Jordan RM, et al, "Infectious Causes of Adrenal Insufficiency," *South Med J*, 2003, 96(9):888-90.

Don-Wauchope AC and Toft AD, "Diagnosis and Management of Addison's Disease," *Practitioner*, 2000, 244(1614):794-9.

Dorin RI, Qualls CR, and Crapo LM, "Diagnosis of Adrenal Insufficiency," *Ann Intern Med*, 2003, 139(3):194-204.

Hasinski S, "Assessment of Adrenal Glucocorticoid Function. Which Tests Are Appropriate for Screening?" *Postgrad Med*, 1998, 104(1):61-4, 69-72.

Marik PE and Zaloga GP, "Adrenal Insufficiency in the Critically Ill: A New Look at an Old Problem," *Chest*, 2002, 122(5):1784-96.

Shenker Y and Skatrud JB, "Adrenal Insufficiency in Critically Ill Patients," *Am J Respir Crit Care Med*, 2001, 163(7):1520-3.

ADRENAL INSUFFICIENCY

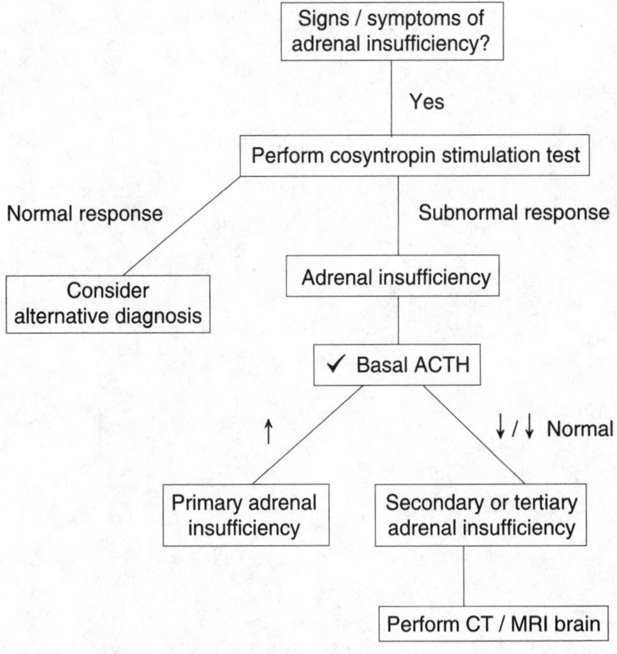

CUSHING'S SYNDROME

STEP 1 – *What Are the Signs and Symptoms of Cushing's Syndrome?*

Cushing's syndrome results from prolonged exposure to excessive amounts of endogenous or exogenous corticosteroids. The key to the diagnosis is recognizing that signs and symptoms of Cushing's syndrome are present. Signs and symptoms of Cushing's syndrome are listed in the following box.

CUSHING'S SYNDROME CLINICAL MANIFESTATIONS	
CENTRAL OBESITY	FACIAL PLETHORA
PROXIMAL MUSCLE WEAKNESS	ACNE
HYPERTENSION	HYPERPIGMENTATION
PSYCHIATRIC DISORDERS	HIRSUTISM
WIDE PURPLE STRIAE	HYPERGLYCEMIA
SPONTANEOUS ECCHYMOSES	HYPOKALEMIC METABOLIC ALKALOSIS

When a patient presents with some of these signs and symptoms, the diagnosis of Cushing's syndrome should be considered. Once suspected, screening tests can be performed to establish the presence of corticosteroid excess. Screening tests are indicated in all patients suspected of having Cushing's syndrome except for those taking exogenous glucocorticoids, in whom the diagnosis is usually apparent.

Proceed to Step 2.

STEP 2 – *What Are the Results of the 24-Hour Urine Collection for Cortisol?*

When Cushing's syndrome is suspected, the evaluation begins with screening tests to determine if the patient has hypercortisolism. Although a number of screening tests are available, the 24-hour urine collection for free cortisol is preferred by many investigators. Studies have shown that this test has a sensitivity and specificity that exceeds 95% and 98%, respectively.

The usefulness of this test is dependent upon the accuracy of the 24-hour urine collection. The 24-hour urine collection should begin after the patient wakes up in the morning and discards the first morning void. The patient should then collect all urine from this point on, terminating the collection after the next first morning void. To ensure adequacy of the 24-hour urine collection, urine creatinine should be measured as well. Recall that the following urine creatinine values confirm an adequate 24-hour collection.

NORMAL 24-HOUR URINE CREATININE
Male: 20-25 mg/kg creatinine
Female: 15-20 mg/kg creatinine

Ideally, at least three or four separate 24-hour urine collections for free cortisol are recommended. Multiple collections are recommended because about 10% of 24-hour urine collections for free cortisol are normal in patients with Cushing's syndrome. When all three values are in the normal range (typically 80-120 μg/day depending upon the assay used), Cushing's syndrome is very unlikely. If all three of the cortisol values exceed 3 times the upper limit of normal, Cushing's syndrome is likely and further evaluation is warranted. If the values are elevated but not to levels exceeding 3 times the upper limit of normal, repeat testing should be performed after several weeks or another type of screening test should be performed.

If the 24-hour urine free cortisol levels are > 3 times the upper limit of normal, the patient likely has Cushing's syndrome and further evaluation is necessary to determine the etiology of the Cushing's syndrome. ***Proceed to Step 4.***

If the 24-hour urine free cortisol levels are normal, the patient is unlikely to have Cushing's syndrome. ***Stop here.***

If the 24-hour urine free cortisol levels are elevated but not to levels exceeding 3 times the upper limit of normal, the clinician should either repeat the test after several weeks or perform another type of screening test. ***Proceed to Step 3.***

STEP 3 – *Does the Patient Have Cushing's Syndrome or a Pseudo-Cushing's State?*

When the results of the screening tests are intermediate, further evaluation is needed to differentiate Cushing's syndrome from other causes of hypercortisolism. These other causes of hypercortisolism can mimic the clinical presentation of Cushing's syndrome. These conditions can present with some of the same signs, symptoms, and laboratory test abnormalities seen in patients with Cushing's syndrome. These patients, who do not have Cushing's syndrome, are said to have a pseudo-Cushing's state.

In patients with the pseudo-Cushing's state, appropriate treatment or resolution of the underlying condition can lead to the disappearance of the signs, symptoms, and laboratory test abnormalities that are suggestive of Cushing's syndrome. It is important to make the distinction between Cushing's syndrome and pseudo-Cushing's state because misdiagnosis of the latter as Cushing's syndrome can lead to extensive testing that could potentially be harmful (eg, performance of invasive tests or even surgery in the patient with pseudo-Cushing's state who is misdiagnosed with Cushing's syndrome). Conditions associated with pseudo-Cushing's states are listed in the following box.

CONDITIONS ASSOCIATED WITH PSEUDO-CUSHING'S STATE
HIGH CORTISOL SECRETION RATE WITHOUT CONVINCING CLINICAL FEATURES OF CUSHING'S SYNDROME
STRESS
Surgery
Severe illness
Emotional
Caloric
Aerobic
ALCOHOLISM
Long-term active alcoholism
Ethanol withdrawal
PSYCHIATRIC DISORDERS
Depression (particularly melancholic depression)
Anorexia nervosa
Bulimia
Psychoses
Panic disorders
RENAL FAILURE
SEVERE OBESITY
PRIMARY GLUCOCORTICOID RECEPTOR RESISTANCE
EXCESSIVE FLUID INTAKE (psychogenic polydipsia or diabetes insipidus)
FACTITIOUS GLUCOCORTICOID INTAKE
UNCONTROLLED DIABETES
CONDITIONS ASSOCIATED WITH EUCORTISOLEMIA THAT MAY MIMIC CUSHING'S SYNDROME
OBESITY
METABOLIC SYNDROME
POLYCYSTIC OVARIAN SYNDROME
GROWTH HORMONE DEFICIENCY
HIV INFECTION
GLUCOCORTICOID HYPER-RESPONSIVITY
IMPAIRED CORTISOL CATABOLISM

To differentiate Cushing's syndrome from pseudo-Cushing's state, the clinician may wish to repeat the 24-hour urine collection for free cortisol after several weeks. If urine cortisol levels exceed 3 times the upper limit of normal, further evaluation for Cushing's syndrome is warranted (proceed to step 4). If the repeat urine cortisol level remains elevated but not to a level that exceeds 3 times the upper limit of normal, the clinician should consider performing another type of screening test. Other tests available to the clinician include the following:

- Overnight low-dose (1 mg) dexamethasone suppression test
- Late evening plasma cortisol level
- Late evening salivary cortisol level
- Dexamethasone-CRH test
- Naloxone test
- Insulin-induced hypoglycemia test

Of these tests, the first three, which are more widely used, are discussed in the remainder of this step.

Overnight Low-dose (1 mg) Dexamethasone Suppression Test

Traditionally, the 1 mg dexamethasone suppression test (DST) was considered to be the test of choice in screening patients suspected of having Cushing's syndrome. While the sensitivity of the dexamethasone suppression test exceeds 98%, it suffers from a relatively low specificity of 75%. As a result, the test has fallen out of favor, and has largely been replaced by measurement of the 24-hour urine free cortisol (see above). Nonetheless, this test continues to be performed as a screening test for the diagnosis of Cushing's syndrome.

The DST involves administration of 1 mg of dexamethasone at 11 PM, with a cortisol measurement obtained the following morning at 8 AM. The premise of this test is that all sources of steroid excess in Cushing's syndrome will not be inhibited by the administration of dexamethasone. As a result, the cortisol level will exceed 5 μg/dL. In the healthy patient, the administered dexamethasone will result in a decrease in ACTH secretion via negative feedback, resulting in a morning cortisol level <5 μg/dL.

The clinician should realize, however, that other causes of hypercortisolism besides Cushing's syndrome may present with morning cortisol levels >5 μg/dL. Examples include patients with alcoholic or psychiatric hypercortisolism. Estrogen therapy, liver disease, and administration of phenytoin, rifampin, or phenobarbital may also be associated with false-positive test results.

Because of its significant false-positivity rate, some experts prefer to perform a 48-hour low dose DST rather than the overnight test. This test can be performed in the outpatient setting (although traditionally performed in inpatients) but the patient must adhere carefully to the instructions. The patient is asked to take 0.5 mg of dexamethasone every 6 hours for 48 hours. The serum cortisol is measured at 9 AM before the start at the test and then again at this same time at 48 hours. In patients without Cushing's syndrome, serum cortisol levels will be <2 μg/dL (50 nmol/L). Values higher than this are supportive of Cushing's syndrome. While false-positive test results can occur, they are less common with this version of the DST.

Late Evening Plasma Cortisol Level

Normally, the nadir of ACTH secretion occurs at night. This can be assessed by measurement of a midnight plasma cortisol level, which will be low (<2 μg/dL in nonstressed patients) in healthy individuals. In patients with Cushing's syndrome, however, this nadir is lost. These patients have elevated nocturnal plasma cortisol levels.

To perform the test, an intravenous catheter is placed early on the first day of the test. A blood sample is drawn between 11 and 12 PM that evening and for the next 2 days, as well. Cortisol levels >7.5 μg/dL are consistent with the diagnosis of Cushing's syndrome. Cortisol levels <5 μg/dL strongly argue against the diagnosis. Repeat testing should be performed after several weeks in patients who have intermediate test results. One drawback to the performance of this test is the fact that results are easily influenced by acute stresses (false-positive test results may occur due to the stress of venipuncture, hospital admission, or intercurrent illness). For this reason, most clinicians perform several measurements to increase accuracy.

Late Evening Salivary Cortisol Level

The advantage of this test is that it can be performed by the patient at home. Studies have shown that the late-night (11 PM) salivary cortisol level is significantly higher in Cushing's syndrome when compared to normal individuals. Salivary cortisol levels that are repeatedly <1.3 ng/mL by radioimmunoassay or 1.5 ng/mL by competitive protein-binding assay exclude the diagnosis of Cushing's syndrome.

If the test results are consistent with Cushing's syndrome, ***proceed to Step 4***.

If the test results are consistent with a pseudo-Cushing's state, ***stop here***.

STEP 4 – *What Is the Plasma ACTH Level?*

Once the patient has been diagnosed as having a state of steroid excess, or Cushing's syndrome, the focus should center on tests to localize the source of the steroid excess. The causes of Cushing's syndrome along with their rate of occurrence are listed in the following table.

Sources of Hypercortisolism

Source	Rate of Occurrence
Exogenous (iatrogenic)*	Most common cause
Endogenous Pituitary adenoma (Cushing's disease) Adrenal adenoma carcinoma hyperplasia	 65% to 70% 20% to 25%
Ectopic (ACTH- or CRH-producing) nonpituitary tumors†	10% to 15%
Congenital	Rare
Other conditions (pseudo-Cushing's)‡	Transient

*Typically, prolonged administration of steroid therapy.

†Small cell cancer of the lung, pancreatic islet cell tumors, carcinoid, malignant thymoma, pheochromocytoma, medullary thyroid cancer.

‡Alcoholism, pregnancy, chronic renal failure, stress.

Adapted from Norton JA, Li M, Gillary J, at el, "Cushing Syndrome," *Curr Probl Surg*, 2001, 38:7(495).

The above causes of Cushing's syndrome can be divided into those that are ACTH-dependent and ACTH-independent, as shown in the following table.

Causes of Cushing's Syndrome

	Causes
ACTH dependent	ACTH-producing tumor (Cushing's disease) Ectopic secretion of ACTH by tumors
ACTH independent	Adrenal adenoma Adrenal carcinoma Adrenal micronodular or macronodular hyperplasia

Measurement of a plasma ACTH level is very useful in distinguishing between ACTH-dependent and ACTH-independent causes of Cushing's syndrome. It is recommended that ACTH levels be measured between midnight and 2 AM when levels are at their nadir. When measuring plasma ACTH levels, the clinician must exercise proper technique. For example, prechilled tubes on ice should be used to collect the sample. One cause of falsely low levels of plasma ACTH is platelet-associated protease degradation of ACTH. It is wise to discuss the procedure for plasma ACTH specimen collection with the laboratory prior to performing the test.

ACTH levels >10-15 pg/mL are consistent with an ACTH-dependent cause of Cushing's syndrome. In contrast, levels <5 pg/mL should prompt consideration of the ACTH-independent causes of Cushing's syndrome.

When the ACTH level is <5 pg/mL, the patient has an ACTH-independent cause of Cushing's syndrome. ***Proceed to Step 5***.

When the ACTH level is >10-15 pg/mL, the patient has an ACTH-dependent cause of Cushing's syndrome. ***Proceed to Step 6***.

STEP 5 – *What Type of Adrenal Problem Is the Cause of the Cushing's Syndrome?*

ACTH levels <5 pg/mL should prompt consideration of a primary adrenal cause of corticosteroid excess. Further evaluation begins with an abdominal CT scan to assess for the presence of an adrenal mass.

The presence of an adrenal mass should prompt consideration of an adrenal adenoma or carcinoma. The size of the mass can provide a clue to the diagnosis. An adrenal mass that is larger than 4-6 cm raises concern for the diagnosis of adrenal carcinoma. In recent years, many radiologists have recommended MRI in an effort to differentiate adrenal adenoma from carcinoma. On T2-weighted sequences, adrenal adenomas appear darker than the liver, whereas adrenal carcinoma typically looks much brighter than the liver. Additionally, measurement of dehydroepiandrosterone (DHEA) and a urinary 17-ketosteroid level can also be quite helpful. In patients with adrenal carcinoma, the levels are very high. In contrast, in patients with adrenal adenomas, DHEA and urinary 17-ketosteroid levels are low.

If the results of the imaging tests reveal no tumor or hyperplasia, the clinician should consider the possibility of primary pigmented nodular adrenocortical disease (PPNAD). To establish the diagnosis, radioisotope imaging of the adrenal glands with the use of labeled iodocholesterol is recommended.

End of Section.

STEP 6 – *Does the Patient Have Cushing's Disease or the Ectopic Production of ACTH by a Tumor?*

When ACTH levels exceed 10-15 pg/mL, the clinician should consider the causes of ACTH-dependent Cushing's syndrome. The major causes of ACTH-dependent Cushing's syndrome include pituitary adenoma (Cushing's disease) and ectopic production of ACTH by a tumor. To distinguish between these two possibilities, the clinician can perform one of the following tests.

- High-dose dexamethasone suppression test

  The high dose dexamethasone suppression test is useful in distinguishing Cushing's disease from the ectopic secretion of ACTH by a tumor, both of which are causes of ACTH-dependent Cushing's syndrome. The basis of the test is that high doses of dexamethasone will suppress ACTH secretion in patients with Cushing's disease, but will not have the same effect in patients having ectopic secretion of ACTH.

  In this test, 2 mg of dexamethasone are given every 6 hours for 2 days. Prior to the test, a baseline 24-hour urine free cortisol test is performed. A 24-hour urine collection is then repeated during the last 24 hours of dexamethasone administration.

  Most patients with Cushing's disease will have a considerable decline in the excretion of urine free cortisol and 17-hydroxycorticosteroids. Approximately 70% of patients have a decrease in urine free cortisol and 17-hydroxycorticosteroids exceeding 90% and 64%, respectively. Using these criteria, test sensitivity is 83% for Cushing's disease. While most patients with Cushing's disease suppress, it should be noted that there is a subset of patients who have higher secretion of ACTH that may be relatively resistant to suppression.

  The majority of patients with ectopic secretion of ACTH fail to suppress. However, about 5% of these patients, primarily those having bronchial carcinoid tumors, will have a decline in urine free cortisol and 17-hydroxycorticosteroids.

- Overnight 8 mg dexamethasone suppression test

  This test involves giving the patient 8 mg dexamethasone at 11 PM followed by measurement of an 8 AM cortisol level the next day. If the serum cortisol is suppressed to <50% of the baseline cortisol value, a pituitary adenoma is likely to be the cause of the Cushing's syndrome. The diagnostic accuracy of this test is about 70% to 80%.

- CRH test

  Corticotropin-releasing hormone (CRH) stimulates ACTH secretion in both normal individuals and in those who have Cushing's disease. This type of response is seldom seen in patients with the ectopic ACTH syndrome. The test involves measurement of plasma cortisol and ACTH every 15 minutes for two hours after the intravenous administration of 100 mcg of CRH. When 10 mcg of DDAVP is administered simultaneously (intravenously) with CRH, the test is even better at differentiating Cushing's disease from the ectopic ACTH disease. When both are administered, the test is consistent with Cushing's disease if the serum cortisol level increases by 37% or more.

If the test results are consistent with a pituitary adenoma (Cushing's disease), ***proceed to Step 7***.

If the test results are consistent with the ectopic secretion of ACTH by a tumor, ***proceed to Step 9***.

STEP 7 – *What Are the Results of the Imaging Studies?*

When the results of biochemical testing suggest the presence of Cushing's disease, the clinician should perform an imaging test of the sella to detect the pituitary tumor. Studies have shown that a CT scan of the sella detects a tumor in only 0% to 15% of patients. This low detection rate reflects the general inability of the CT scan to detect pituitary adenomas that are <5 mm in size. MRI with gadolinium provides greater resolution, resulting in a 40% detection rate. For this reason, MRI is preferred over CT when trying to locate the pituitary tumor. However, CT scan of the sella is often necessary to provide the neurosurgeon with information regarding the anatomy of the sella (complementary to the MRI).

If the MRI localizes a pituitary tumor, consult a surgeon for consideration of trans-sphenoidal surgery. ***Stop here***.

If the imaging study fails to reveal a pituitary tumor, the clinician should proceed to inferior petrosal vein sampling. ***Proceed to Step 8***.

STEP 8 – *What Are the Results of Inferior Petrosal Vein Sampling?*

The diagnosis of Cushing's disease should not be discarded if the imaging tests do not reveal the presence of a pituitary adenoma. In these cases, the pituitary adenoma may be too small to be detected by CT or MRI of the sella. In these cases, the clinician should proceed with inferior petrosal vein sampling.

Inferior petrosal vein sampling was developed because some pituitary microadenomas are not visualized by imaging studies. This test is usually recommended when results of biochemical testing are consistent with a pituitary tumor but the imaging tests do not reveal a pituitary mass. In this test, catheters are placed in the right and left inferior petrosal veins. A peripheral intravenous catheter is also inserted. Before CRH is injected peripherally, an ACTH level is obtained both peripherally and centrally. ACTH levels are again obtained at 2 and 5 minutes after injection.

A central:peripheral ACTH ratio >2 before CRH administration, and a ratio >3 after CRH administration, are diagnostic of Cushing's disease. The sensitivity and specificity of inferior petrosal vein sampling is 100% if both criteria are met.

If either value is exceeded, then the patient has a pituitary tumor not detected by imaging studies. ***Stop here.***

Ratios not diagnostic of Cushing's disease suggest the presence of the ectopic ACTH syndrome. Recall that a minority of patients with ectopic ACTH secretion will have biochemical test results suggestive of a pituitary adenoma. In these patients, the central:peripheral ratios are low. These patients should be further evaluated with imaging studies to localize the ectopic tumor. ***Proceed to Step 9.***

STEP 9 – *What Are the Results of the Imaging Studies?*

Most patients with ectopic secretion of ACTH have malignant tumors, of which 50% are small cell lung cancer. Tumors associated with ectopic secretion of ACTH are listed in the following table.

ECTOPIC ACTH-SECRETING TUMORS
SMALL CELL CARCINOMA (50%)
CARCINOID TUMORS
Bronchus
Thymus
Pancreas
MEDULLARY THYROID CANCER
PHEOCHROMOCYTOMA

If the patient is suspected of having ectopic secretion of ACTH by a tumor, evaluation begins with a CT or MRI scan of the chest, as ACTH-secreting tumors are most often found in this region of the body. If no lesion is discovered, then a CT of the abdomen, pelvis, and neck should be obtained. If any of the imaging tests suggests the presence of a tumor, immunoassay for ACTH can be performed on a biopsy specimen to confirm the diagnosis of ectopic ACTH secretion. Urinary catecholamines and plasma levels of calcitonin may be obtained if pheochromocytoma and medullary thyroid carcinoma, respectively, are considerations.

If CT or MRI scans reveal the tumor, ***stop here.***

If diagnostic tests are unrevealing, the clinician should proceed to octreotide scintigraphy. ***Proceed to Step 10.***

STEP 10 – *What Are the Results of the Octreotide Study?*

Octreotide scintigraphy is based on the fact that many neuroendocrine tumors have receptors for somatostatin. Since octreotide is an active fragment of somatostatin, radiolabeled octreotide can be used to localize these tumors. Unfortunately, the test is not very specific. Some non-neuroendocrine tumors can be detected as well. In addition, many inflammatory and granulomatous lesions can be identified using octreotide scintigraphy. In spite of these limitations, a single site of radiolabeled octreotide uptake can be considered as the source of ectopic ACTH secretion.

If an octreotide study demonstrates the tumor, ***stop here.***

If the results of octreotide scintigraphy are not helpful, the clinician should proceed to inferior petrosal sinus sampling (if the test has not been performed already) for ACTH, before and after CRH administration. ***Proceed to Step 11.***

STEP 11 – *What Is Inferior Petrosal Vein Sampling and How Does it Help Diagnostically?*

This test allows the clinician to determine whether steroid excess is a result of pituitary disease or ectopic ACTH syndrome. Recall that a minority of patients with Cushing's disease will have results of biochemical testing similar to that seen in patients who have ectopic secretion of ACTH by a tumor. When imaging tests do not identify a source of ectopic ACTH secretion, the clinician should reconsider the possibility that the patient has Cushing's disease. In these cases, inferior petrosal vein sampling will help make the distinction between Cushing's disease and the ectopic secretion of ACTH by a tumor.

In inferior petrosal vein sampling, catheters are placed in the left and right inferior petrosal veins. Another catheter is placed peripherally for the administration of CRH. ACTH levels are obtained peripherally and centrally prior to the test, 2 minutes after CRH injection peripherally, and then again at 5 minutes. The following are considered diagnostic of Cushing's disease:

- Central:peripheral ACTH ratio >2 before CRH administration
- Central:peripheral ACTH ratio >3 after CRH administration

Ratios lower than these suggest the presence of the ectopic ACTH syndrome.

End of Section.

References

Arnaldi G, Angeli A, Atkinson AB, et al, "Diagnosis and Complications of Cushing's Syndrome: A Concensus Statement," *J Clin Endocrinol Metab*, 2003, 88(12):5593-602.

Boscaro M, Barzon L, Fallo F, et al, "Cushing's Syndrome," *Lancet*, 2001, 357(9258):783-91.

Boscaro M, Barzon L, Fallo F, et al, "The Diagnosis of Cushing's Syndrome: Atypical Presentations and Laboratory Shortcomings," *Arch Intern Med*, 2000, 160(20):3045-53.

Katz J and Bouloux PM, "Cushing's: How to Make the Diagnosis," *Practitioner*, 1999, 243(1595):118-22, 124.

Kirk LF Jr, Hash RB, Katner HP, et al, "Cushing's Disease: Clinical Manifestations and Diagnostic Evaluation," *Am Fam Physician.*, 2000, 62(5):1119-27, 1133-4.

Klee GG, "Maximizing Efficacy of Endocrine Tests: Importance of Decision-Focused Testing Strategies and Appropriate Patient Preparation," *Clin Chem*, 1999, 45(8 Pt 2):1323-30.

Newell-Price J and Grossman AB, "The Differential Diagnosis of Cushing's Syndrome," *Ann Endocrinol (Paris)*, 2001, 62(2):173-9.

Norton JA, Li M, Gillary J, and Le HN, "Cushing's Syndrome," *Curr Probl Surg*, 200, 38(7):488-545.

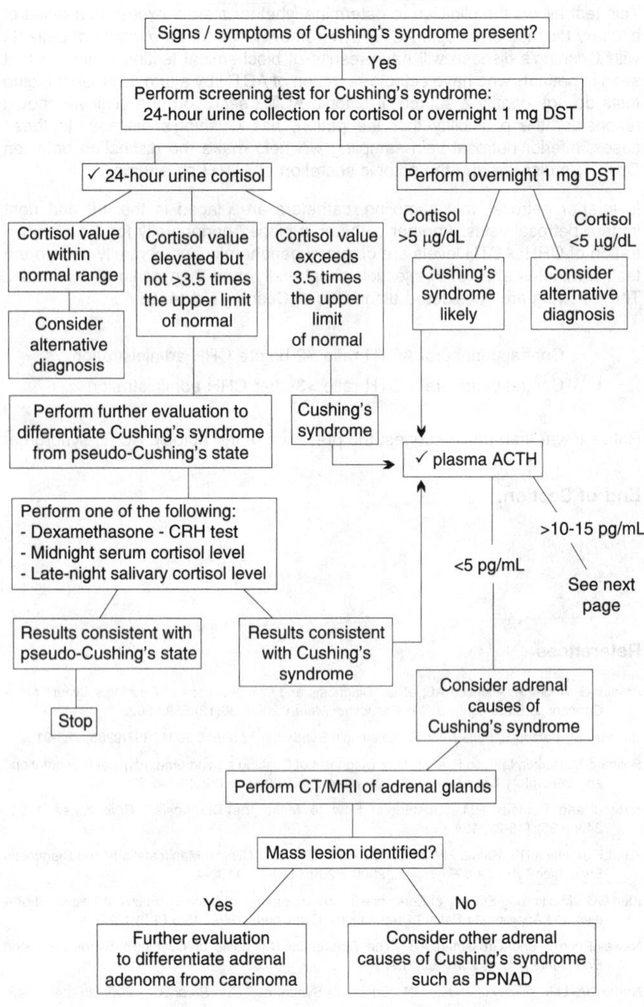

DST = dexamethasone suppression test

CUSHING'S SYNDROME *(continued)*

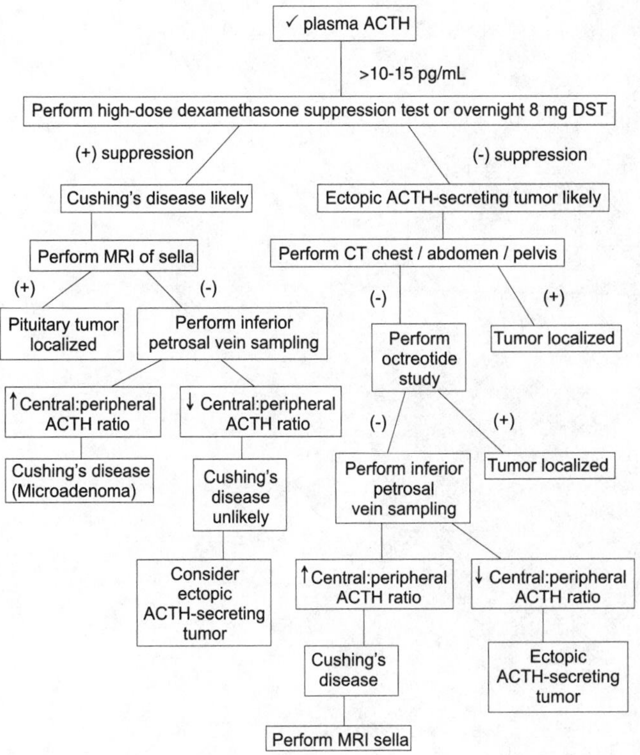

PRIMARY HYPERALDOSTERONISM

STEP 1 – *What Is Hyperaldosteronism?*

Hyperaldosteronism is a state of aldosterone excess, which may be divided into primary and secondary forms, as shown in the following box.

SOME DEFINITIONS...
Primary hyperaldosteronism: An inappropriate increase in aldosterone production **Secondary hyperaldosteronism**: Those conditions where aldosterone production is increased secondary to activation of the renin-angiotensin system

Although older studies indicated that primary hyperaldosteronism had a prevalence <1% in hypertensive patients, recent evidence suggests that primary hyperaldosteronism may occur in up to 15% of patients with hypertension. It is important to become familiar with the diagnosis of primary hyperaldosteronism because many of these patients can be cured of their disease with surgical treatment.

Proceed to Step 2.

STEP 2 – *When Should the Diagnosis of Primary Hyperaldosteronism Be Suspected?*

The key to the diagnosis of primary hyperaldosteronism is consideration of this disease as the cause of the patient's clinical presentation. Clinicians should suspect the diagnosis of primary hyperaldosteronism in patients who present with the following:

- Hypertensive patient with spontaneous or unprovoked hypokalemia
- Patients with refractory or severe (on three or more antihypertensive agents) hypertension
- Patients who develop severe and/or persistent hypokalemia with low doses of diuretic medications
- Diuretic-induced hypokalemia that is poorly responsive to potassium replacement
- Hypokalemia that persists in a hypertensive patient despite discontinuation of diuretic and replacement of potassium stores (repeat serum potassium measurement two weeks later)

It is important to realize that not all patients with primary hyperaldosteronism have hypokalemia. There is a subset of patients with primary hyperaldosteronism who present with normokalemia. In fact, some studies suggest that up to 38% of patients with primary hyperaldosteronism are normokalemic at the time of presentation. In this group of patients, the potassium level typically ranges between 3.5 and 4.0 mEq/L. Therefore, in patients who have refractory or severe hypertension but normal potassium levels, primary hyperaldosteronism remains a consideration, particularly when the potassium level is in the low-normal range.

Proceed to Step 3.

STEP 3 – *What Screening Tests Are Available in the Diagnosis of Primary Hyperaldosteronism?*

The evaluation of the patient suspected of having primary hyperaldosteronism often begins with the measurement of the plasma renin activity (PRA) and aldosterone level. In primary hyperaldosteronism, plasma aldosterone levels are elevated and PRA is suppressed. Low PRA levels argue against the diagnosis of secondary hyperaldosteronism, which occurs in conditions associated with decreased renal perfusion (congestive heart failure, intravascular volume loss, cirrhosis).

In recent years, the plasma aldosterone:PRA ratio has become popular as a screening test in the evaluation of patients suspected of having primary hyperaldosteronism. A ratio that exceeds 20 has a 95% sensitivity and 75% specificity for the diagnosis of primary hyperaldosteronism. This ratio is only valid if the aldosterone has been measured in ng/dL and the PRA in ng/mL/hour. A ratio >50 is almost diagnostic for this condition.

A number of medications can affect aldosterone and renin levels, and some must be discontinued prior to testing. It is recommended that β-blockers, diuretics, and ACE inhibitors be discontinued for at least 2-4 weeks. Spironolactone should be stopped at least 6-8 weeks before testing. Although many experts recommend holding all antihypertensives that can affect the renin system, in clinical practice, this is not always possible, especially in patients with severe hypertension. Calcium channel blockers and alpha blockers do not affect interpretation of this test.

In normal patients as well as those with essential hypertension, the mean value of the plasma aldosterone to PRA ratio is 4 to 10. This is in contrast to primary hyperaldosteronism patients in whom the ratio is typically >30-50.

If aldosterone and PRA are elevated, but the ratio of the two is <10, ***proceed to Step 4***.

If both the aldosterone and the PRA are low, ***proceed to Step 5***.

If the aldosterone:PRA ratio is >20, ***proceed to Step 6***.

STEP 4 – *What Is the Differential Diagnosis of an Elevated Aldosterone and PRA (Aldosterone to PRA Ratio <10 in the Hypertensive Patient?*

The differential diagnosis of an elevated aldosterone and PRA (aldosterone:PRA ratio <10) in the setting of hypertension is listed in the following box.

ELEVATED PRA AND ALDOSTERONE (Aldosterone:PRA Ratio <10) IN THE HYPERTENSIVE PATIENT DIFFERENTIAL DIAGNOSIS	
RENOVASCULAR HYPERTENSION	MALIGNANT HYPERTENSION
RENIN-SECRETING TUMOR	DIURETIC USE

Appropriate studies should be performed to determine the etiology.

End of Section.

STEP 5 – *What Is the Differential Diagnosis of a Decreased Aldosterone and PRA in the Hypertensive Patient?*

The differential diagnosis of a decreased aldosterone and PRA in the setting of hypertension is listed in the following box.

DECREASED PRA AND ALDOSTERONE IN THE HYPERTENSIVE PATIENT DIFFERENTIAL DIAGNOSIS
CUSHING'S SYNDROME*
EXOGENOUS MINERALOCORTICOID THERAPY
SYNDROME OF APPARENT MINERALOCORTICOID EXCESS
CONGENITAL ADRENAL HYPERPLASIA
LIDDLE'S SYNDROME
DEOXYCORTICOSTERONE-PRODUCING TUMOR
11-β-HYDROXYSTEROID DEHYDROGENASE DEFICIENCY

*PRA and aldosterone levels may be normal in patients with Cushing's syndrome.

Appropriate studies should be performed to determine the etiology.

End of Section.

STEP 6 – *What Confirmatory Tests Are Available in the Patient With Screening Test Results Consistent With Primary Hyperaldosteronism?*

When the results of the screening tests are consistent with the diagnosis of primary hyperaldosteronism, the clinician should perform further testing to confirm the diagnosis. Confirmatory tests that are available include the following:

- Intravenous salt loading test (saline infusion test)
- 24-hour urine aldosterone measurement after oral salt loading

These confirmatory tests are discussed in further detail below.

Intravenous Salt Loading Test (Saline Infusion Test)

During the intravenous salt loading test, 500 mL of normal saline is intravenously administered per hour for a total of 4 to 6 hours. The clinician should obtain serum aldosterone measurements at baseline and after the administration of saline. A normal test result is defined as suppression of the postsaline plasma aldosterone to levels to less than 10 ng/dL. Plasma aldosterone levels that exceed 10 ng/dL are consistent with the diagnosis of primary hyperaldosteronism. Recently, some have argued to lower the value from 10 ng/dL to 5-8 ng/dL but this has not yet been widely accepted.

24-Hour Urine Aldosterone Measurement After Oral Salt Loading

In this test, >200 mEq of sodium is given orally every day for 3 days. Because an increase in the dietary sodium stimulates kaliuresis and sometimes hypokalemia, potassium chloride may need to be administered. On the third day of oral salt loading, a 24-hour urine collection for aldosterone and sodium is performed. A 24-hour urine aldosterone level that exceeds 10-14 mcg/day is diagnostic of primary hyperaldosteronism as long as the sodium that is excreted in the urine collection exceeds 200 mEq/day. Creatinine should be measured in the urine collection to ensure that the urine collection was complete.

If the confirmatory test results are diagnostic of primary hyperaldosteronism, ***proceed to Step 7***.

If the confirmatory test results are not diagnostic of primary hyperaldosteronism, ***stop here***.

STEP 7 – *What Type of Primary Hyperaldosteronism Does the Patient Have?*

Once the diagnosis of primary hyperaldosteronism has been confirmed, the clinician should then focus efforts on determining the type of primary hyperaldosteronism present. The two major types of primary hyperaldosteronism include the following:

- Adrenal adenoma
- Bilateral adrenal hyperplasia

Adrenal adenoma is the most common cause of primary hyperaldosteronism, accounting for about 65% of primary hyperaldosteronism cases. Thirty to 40% of cases are due to bilateral adrenal hyperplasia.

To distinguish between these two types of primary hyperaldosteronism, a postural stimulation test is often performed. In this test, plasma aldosterone levels are measured in the morning after overnight recumbency. It is preferable to obtain this measurement while the patient is supine. After 2 to 4 hours of upright posture, the plasma aldosterone level should be measured again. In patients with bilateral adrenal hyperplasia, the plasma aldosterone level typically rises after the patient assumes an upright position. In contrast, patients with adrenal adenoma typically have a fall in the plasma aldosterone level. The sensitivity and specificity of the postural stimulation test in differentiating between adrenal adenoma and bilateral adrenal hyperplasia is about 80% to 85%. The clinician should realize that patients with glucocorticoid-remediable aldosteronism will also have a fall in the plasma aldosterone level after upright posture.

Another test that can help in differentiating between these two conditions is a measurement of the plasma 18-hydroxycorticosterone (18-OHC) level. Increased levels (>100 ng/dL) are typically found in patients with adenomas but are not characteristic of bilateral adrenal hyperplasia.

Some clinicians prefer to forego the diagnostic testing discussed in this step and proceed directly to adrenal CT or MRI. The basis behind their thinking is that if an imaging abnormality consistent with adenoma is noted, then the diagnosis of adrenal adenoma as the cause of the primary hyperaldosteronism has been established. Proceeding directly to imaging without biochemical confirmation (as discussed above in this step) can be problematic because there is a high incidence of nonfunctioning adrenal nodules, also known as adrenal incidentalomas. In other words, merely demonstrating the presence of an adrenal adenoma does not mean that the adenoma is the cause of the primary hyperaldosteronism.

If the postural stimulation test or plasma 18-hydroxycorticosterone level supports the diagnosis of an aldosterone-producing adenoma, ***proceed to Step 8***.

If the postural stimulation test or plasma 18-hydroxycorticosterone level supports the diagnosis of bilateral adrenal hyperplasia, ***stop here***.

STEP 8 – *What Are the Results of CT Imaging?*

Adrenal CT scanning with contrast is the radiologic test of choice for imaging the adrenal gland in patients who have biochemical evidence of aldosterone-producing adrenal adenoma (sensitivity of MRI is similar). CT scan has been shown to reliably detect adenomas that are at least 1-1.5 cm in diameter. The clinician should realize that the absence of a mass does not exclude the presence of an adenoma since small adenomas may be below the detection capability of CT imaging.

If the imaging test does not reveal findings consistent with adrenal adenoma or bilateral adrenal hyperplasia, the clinician may wish to perform iodocholesterol scanning of the adrenal glands with NP-59. Unilateral uptake is consistent with aldosteronoma while bilateral uptake is supportive of bilateral hyperplasia. The sensitivity of this test is about 88% if it is performed after dexamethasone suppression.

In cases where CT (and iodocholesterol scanning with NP-59, if available) is inconclusive, the clinician should proceed to adrenal venous sampling. When the ratio between the two adrenal vein aldosterone levels exceeds 10, an aldosterone-producing adenoma is very likely to be present. In patients with bilateral adrenal hyperplasia, simultaneously obtained adrenal vein aldosterone levels are roughly the same. The diagnostic accuracy of this test exceeds 95%.

References

Blumenfeld JD and Vaughan ED Jr, "Diagnosis and Treatment of Primary Aldosteronism," *World J Urol*, 1999, 17(1):15-21.

Brown CA, Bouldin MJ, Blackston JW, et al, "Hyperaldosteronism: The Internist's Hypertensive Disease," *Am J Med Sci*, 2002, 324(4):227-31.

Fardella CE and Mosso L, "Primary Aldosteronism," *Clin Lab*, 2002, 48(3-4):181-90.

Frey FJ, "The Hypertensive Patient With Hypokalaemia: The Search for Hyperaldosteronism," *Nephrol Dial Transplant*, 2001, 16(6):1112-6.

Ganguly A, "Primary Aldosteronism," *N Engl J Med*, 1998, 339(25):1828-34.

Stewart PM, "Mineralocorticoid Hypertension," *Lancet*, 1999, 353(9161):1341-7.

Thakkar RB and Oparil S, "Primary Aldosteronism: A Practical Approach to Diagnosis and Treatment," *J Clin Hypertens (Greenwich)*, 2001, 3(3):189-95.

Wheeler MH and Harris DA, "Diagnosis and Management of Primary Aldosteronism," *World J Surg*, 2003, 27(6):627-31.

Young WF Jr, "Minireview: Primary Hyperaldosteronism - Changing Concepts in Diagnosis and Treatment," *Endocrinology*, 2003, 144(6):2208-13.

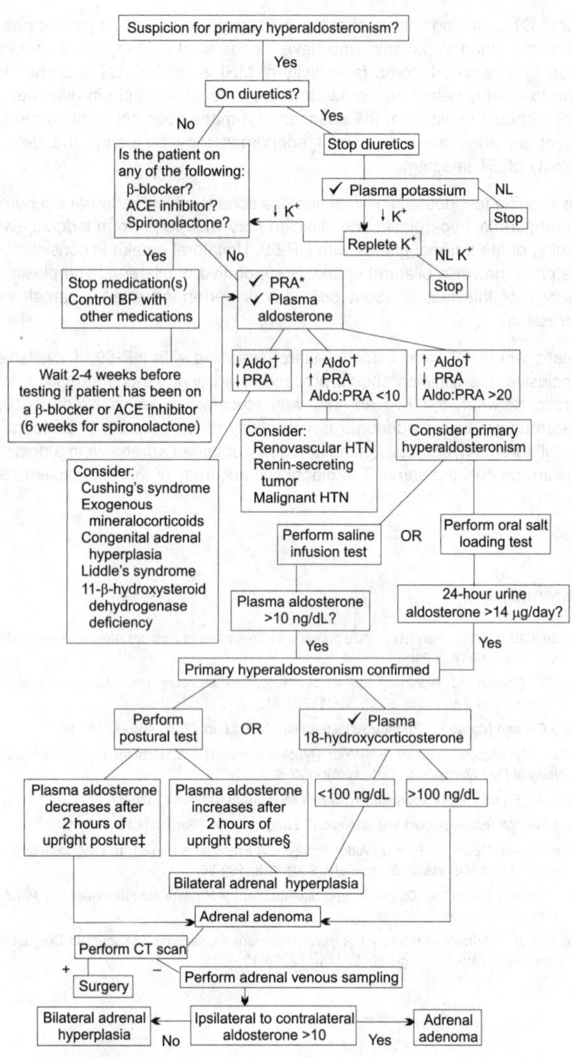

* PRA = plasma renin activity
† Aldo = aldosterone
‡ Plasma aldosterone level typically falls or does not rise to the extent seen in patients with bilateral adrenal hyperplasia
§ Plasma aldosterone level typically rises by at least 50% above baseline in patients with bilateral adrenal hyperplasia

HYPERPROLACTINEMIA

Prolactin plays a key role in the initiation and maintenance of lactation. It is produced in the anterior pituitary gland. Although the hypothalamic hormones that stimulate prolactin secretion are not known, prolactin release is inhibited by the hypothalamic secretion of dopamine.

Indications for Serum Prolactin Measurement

Serum prolactin levels should be obtained when signs or symptoms of hyperprolactinemia are present. In women, clinical features of hyperprolactinemia include amenorrhea, galactorrhea, and infertility. In men, diminished libido and impotence should prompt consideration of hyperprolactinemia.

Causes of Hyperprolactinemia

The causes of hyperprolactinemia are listed in the following box.

CAUSES OF HYPERPROLACTINEMIA

PHYSIOLOGIC

- NIPPLE STIMULATION
- PREGNANCY / LACTATION
- SLEEP
- STRENUOUS EXERCISE
- STRESS (physical or emotional)

PATHOLOGIC

HYPOTHALAMIC LESIONS
- Craniopharyngioma
- Metastatic neoplasms
- Germinoma
- Glioma
- Head trauma
- Encephalitis
- Radiation
- Surgical stalk resection
- Infiltrative disease
  - Histiocytosis X
  - Sarcoidosis
  - Tuberculosis

PITUITARY LESIONS
- Pituitary adenoma (secreting prolactin)
- Acromegaly
- Cushing's syndrome
- Empty sella syndrome

HYPOTHYROIDISM

CHRONIC RENAL FAILURE

IRRITATIVE LESIONS OF THE CHEST WALL
- Herpes zoster
- Tight-fitting garments
- Chest trauma
- Thoracotomy
- Mastectomy
- Reduction mammoplasty

SPINAL CORD LESIONS

MALIGNANCY
- Lung cancer
- Renal cell carcinoma
- Ovarian cystic teratoma
- Adrenal carcinoma

MEDICATIONS*

MACROPROLACTINEMIA

*A long list of medications is associated with hyperprolactinemia. Medication-induced hyperprolactinemia is one of the most common causes of serum prolactin elevation. With medication-induced hyperprolactinemia, rarely is the serum prolactin level >100 ng/mL. A potential offender should not be considered causative unless the clinician documents normalization of the prolactin level with discontinuation of the suspect medication. Common medicinal causes of hyperprolactinemia include methyldopa, reserpine, verapamil, chlorpromazine, cimetidine, domperidone, estrogens, fluphenazine, haloperidol, metoclopramide, opiates, perphenazine, promazine, tricyclic antidepressants, and sulpiride.

Degree of Hyperprolactinemia

With physiologic causes of hyperprolactinemia (except for pregnancy during which prolactin levels may rise to 200-300 ng/mL), prolactin elevation is typically mild, seldom rising to >50 ng/mL. Unfortunately, it is impossible to differentiate physiologic from pathologic elevation based on the degree of hyperprolactinemia. When the prolactin level is >200 ng/mL, the likelihood of a prolactinoma is very high, especially when imaging tests reveal the presence of a pituitary mass lesion.

It is important to realize, however, that prolactin levels may vary widely in patients with prolactinomas. In fact, prolactin levels <200 ng/mL are not uncommon. Therefore, in the patient with persistent hyperprolactinemia, an MRI of the sella should be performed.

Recently, hyperprolactinemia caused by macroprolactinemia has received considerable attention. In this condition, large prolactin polymers are formed. These polymers are unable to interact with the prolactin receptor but are recognized as prolactin by immunologically-based serum assays. It may be a relatively common cause of hyperprolactinemia, and, if suspected, specific testing to detect the presence of macroprolactinemia can be performed.

References

Biller BM, "Hyperprolactinemia," *Int J Fertil Womens Med*, 1999, 44(2):74-7.

Connor P and Fried G, "Hyperprolactinemia; Etiology, Diagnosis, and Treatment Alternatives," *Acta Obstet Gynecol Scand*, 1998, 77(3):249-62.

Molitch ME, "Diagnosis and Treatment of Prolactinomas," *Adv Intern Med*, 1999, 44:117-53.

Serri O, Chik CL, Ur E, et al, "Diagnosis and Management of Hyperprolactinemia," *CMAJ*, 2003, 169(6):575-81.

ACROMEGALY

The excessive secretion of growth hormone in adults is known as acromegaly. When excessive growth hormone secretion occurs in children, the term "gigantism" is used to describe the clinical syndrome that results.

Acromegaly is usually caused by a pituitary adenoma that secretes large amounts of growth hormone. Many years may pass from symptom onset to diagnosis of acromegaly. The delay in diagnosis is typically due to the clinician not suspecting the presence of the disease. Once suspected, laboratory confirmation of the diagnosis of acromegaly is usually not difficult. The tests used in the diagnosis of acromegaly are discussed in further detail below.

Growth Hormone Level

Because there is variation in growth hormone secretion throughout the day, random growth hormone measurements have no value in establishing the diagnosis of acromegaly. In fact, random growth hormone levels may be normal in patients with acromegaly. In no way should normal random growth hormone levels exclude the diagnosis.

Some patients with acromegaly have markedly elevated fasting growth hormone levels. Further testing is not needed in patients who have very high levels. In most patients with acromegaly, however, fasting growth hormone levels are only mildly elevated. In these patients, the measurement of growth hormone levels during an oral glucose tolerance test is recommended. This test is performed after an overnight fast. The morning after fasting, an intravenous catheter is placed. A growth hormone level should be measured approximately 1 hour after placement of the catheter (time 0). The patient should then be given 75-100 g oral glucose. Growth hormone levels are then obtained at 30, 60, 90, and 120 minutes after glucose ingestion.

The normal response is a decline in the growth hormone level to <2 g/L. In patients with acromegaly, serum growth hormone levels will not decrease to normal levels. These patients may have partial lowering of the growth hormone level, no change, or even a paradoxical increase in the growth hormone concentration.

Insulin-Like Growth Factor-1 (IGF-1)

The measurement of IGF-1, also known as somatomedin, is an excellent test for the diagnosis of acromegaly. An increased IGF-1 level is consistent with the diagnosis. Other causes of IGF-1 elevation include pregnancy, puberty, adolescence, and obesity.

Radiologic Imaging

Excessive secretion of GH is usually secondary to a benign pituitary tumor. Therefore, following biochemical confirmation of acromegaly, an MRI of the sella should be performed.

Other Laboratory Test Abnormalities in Acromegaly

Other laboratory test abnormalities that may be appreciated in patients with acromegaly include the following:

- Abnormal glucose tolerance / diabetes mellitus
- Elevated serum phosphate
- Hyperprolactinemia

  The prolactin level may be increased because of stalk compression. In other cases, the level may be elevated because of cosecretion with GH.
- Hypercalcemia

Because the growth hormone secreting pituitary adenoma may compress normal pituitary tissue, hypopituitarism may ensue. Testing for hypopituitarism includes assessment of adrenal, thyroid, and gonadal function. Evaluation for asymptomatic diabetes insipidus should also be considered. For further information regarding the evaluation of hypopituitarism, please refer to the chapter, ***Hypopituitarism*** *on page 409*.

While almost all cases of acromegaly are due to a pituitary tumor, more than 50 cases of growth hormone-releasing factor (GHRH) producing tumors have been reported. These tumors may occur in the lung, gastrointestinal tract, or adrenal glands. It is impossible to distinguish these tumors from a pituitary adenoma based upon clinical presentation alone.

References

Le Roith D, "Seminars in Medicine of the Beth Israel Deaconess Medical Center. Insulin-Like Growth Factors," *N Engl J Med,* 1997, 336(9):633-40.

Patel YC, Ezzat S, Chik CL, et al, "Guidelines for the Diagnosis and Treatment of Acromegaly: A Canadian Perspective," *Clin Invest Med,* 2000, 23(3):172-87.

Rosen CJ, "Serum Insulin-Like Growth Factors and Insulin-Like Growth Factor-Binding Proteins: Clinical Implications," *Clin Chem,* 1999, 45(8 Pt 2):1384-90.

HYPOPITUITARISM

The deficiency of one or more pituitary hormones is known as hypopituitarism. Recall that the pituitary gland is divided into anterior and posterior lobes.

Hormones Produced by the Anterior Pituitary

The hormones produced by the anterior pituitary gland are listed in the following box.

HORMONES PRODUCED BY THE ANTERIOR PITUITARY
GROWTH HORMONE LUTEINIZING HORMONE FOLLICLE STIMULATING HORMONE THYROID STIMULATING HORMONE ADRENOCORTICOTROPIN HORMONE PROLACTIN

These hormones are controlled by releasing hormones secreted by the hypothalamus, and by hormones produced by target organs in a feedback mechanism.

Causes of Hypopituitarism

The causes of hypopituitarism are listed in the following box.

CAUSES OF HYPOPITUITARISM

- MALIGNANCY
  - Pituitary adenoma
  - Hypothalamic tumors (craniopharyngioma, germinoma, meningioma, glioma)
  - Metastatic cancer
- INFLAMMATORY DISEASE
  - Granulomatous disease (tuberculosis, sarcoidosis, syphilis)
  - Lymphocytic hypophysitis
  - Histiocytosis X / eosinophilic granuloma
- INFILTRATION
  - Hemochromatosis
  - Amyloidosis
- VASCULAR EVENT
  - Sheehan's syndrome (postpartum pituitary necrosis)
  - Carotid aneurysm
- HEAD TRAUMA
- SURGERY
- RADIATION

HYPOPITUITARISM

Hypopituitarism may originate at the level of the pituitary gland (primary hypopituitarism) or at the level of the hypothalamus (secondary hypopituitarism). A clue to differentiating between the two is the presence of diabetes insipidus. Diabetes insipidus suggests that the origin is hypothalamic or high in the pituitary stalk.

Establishing the Diagnosis of Hormone Deficiency

Recommended screening tests for evaluation of the patient suspected of having hypopituitarism are listed in the following table.

Screening Test	Result
Morning cortisol	Normal* / ↓
Thyroid stimulating hormone	Normal† / ↓
Free thyroxine	↓
Luteinizing hormone	Normal / ↓
Follicle stimulating hormone	Normal / ↓
Testosterone (men only)	↓
Urine osmolality	↓‡

*A normal cortisol level should be further evaluated with a cosyntropin stimulation test. This test, however, may not diagnose all cases of adrenal insufficiency, particularly if the insufficiency is partial or of recent onset. In these cases, an insulin-induced hypoglycemia or metapyrone test will establish the diagnosis.

†In evaluating patients for thyrotropin deficiency, it is necessary to obtain both TSH and free thyroxine, because some patients have a normal TSH in the setting of a decreased free thyroxine level.

‡While the definitive diagnosis of diabetes insipidus requires a water deprivation test, the urine osmolality is a useful screening test.

Patients with hypopituitarism can have deficiencies of one or more hormones. As a result, in certain patients, some of the screening tests listed above may be normal. Diagnosis of individual hormone deficiencies is further detailed below.

ACTH Deficiency

Recall that ACTH is secreted from the anterior pituitary and subsequently stimulates the adrenal gland to produce corticosteroids, androgens, and has a permissive effect on mineralocorticoid production.

In cases of hypopituitarism, a morning plasma cortisol <3 μg/dL is diagnostic of adrenal insufficiency. Conversely, levels >18 μg/dL argues against adrenal insufficiency. Intermediate values require further testing with the cosyntropin stimulation test. In this test, a baseline cortisol is obtained, then 250 μg of cosyntropin (ACTH) is given, and cortisol levels are measured 30 minutes after. An abnormal result of this stimulation test establishes the diagnosis of adrenal insufficiency (either primary or secondary). Once adrenal insufficiency has been established, a morning ACTH is drawn. If it is low, a diagnosis of ACTH deficiency (or secondary adrenal insufficiency) is likely.

Of note, in patients with recent development of hypopituitarism, the cosyntropin stimulation test may be normal because adrenal atrophy from impaired ACTH production takes time to develop. In these cases, the adrenal glands may still have the ability to respond to exogenously administered ACTH. However, an insulin-induced hypoglycemia test will establish the diagnosis. Because this test is not without risk, the clinician may elect to perform a metapyrone test, which will provide the same information.

Gonadotropin (LH, FSH) Deficiency

Males

Under normal conditions, gonadotropins released from the anterior pituitary stimulate Leydig cells to produce testosterone, which in turn acts to inhibit LH and FSH secretion. A low testosterone level in males should thus prompt the measurement of gonadotropin levels in these patients. Failure to document high gonadotropin levels implies gonadotropin deficiency.

Females

In premenopausal women, an estrogen deficient state is suggested by any of the following:

- Amenorrhea
- Immature vaginal cytology
- Failure to bleed after administration of progesterone

In these conditions, FSH and LH levels should be measured. The appropriate feedback response to low estrogen levels is increased secretion of both hormones by the pituitary gland. Demonstration of low or normal FSH and LH levels supports the diagnosis of estrogen deficiency secondary to pituitary or hypothalamic disease.

In postmenopausal women, FSH and LH levels are normally high. Low or normal levels should prompt consideration of gonadotropin deficiency.

Since hyperprolactinemia also causes gonadotropin deficiency, it is essential to measure prolactin levels in patients with gonadotropin deficiency.

Thyrotropin (TSH) Deficiency

It is not uncommon for patients with pituitary or hypothalamic disease to have a normal TSH. Therefore, it is not possible to diagnose secondary hypothyroidism based on TSH alone. Establishing the presence of thyrotropin deficiency requires measurement of both TSH and free thyroxine levels. A low free thyroxine level, in the setting of a low or normal TSH, strongly suggests secondary hypothyroidism.

References

Freda PU and Wardlaw SL, "Clinical Review 110: Diagnosis and Treatment of Pituitary Tumors," *J Clin Endocrinol Metab*, 1999, 84(11):3859-66.

Lamberts SW, de Herder WW, and van der Lely AJ,"Pituitary Insufficiency," *Lancet*, 1998, 352(9122):127-34.

Schmidt DN and Wallace K, "How to Diagnose Hypopituitarism. Learning the Features of Secondary Hormonal Deficiencies," *Postgrad Med*, 1998, 104(1):77-8, 81-7.

Swallow CE and Osborn AG, "Imaging of Sella and Parasellar Disease," *Semin Ultrasound CT MR*, 1998, 19(3):257-71.

Vance ML, "Hypopituitarism," *N Engl J Med*, 1994, 330(23):1651-62.

Veznedaroglu E, Armonda RA, and Andrews DW, "Diagnosis and Therapy for Pituitary Tumors," *Curr Opin Oncol*, 1999, 11(1):27-31.

AMENORRHEA

STEP 1 – *What Is Amenorrhea?*

Amenorrhea can be divided into primary and secondary types. Primary amenorrhea refers to the situation where menses has not occurred by the age of 16. Secondary amenorrhea is said to exist when a previously menstruating woman has not had menstrual periods for more than 6 months. The reader is referred to other texts for the evaluation of primary amenorrhea. What follows is one approach to the patient with secondary amenorrhea.

Proceed to Step 2

STEP 2 – *Are There Any Clues in the Patient's History That Point to the Etiology of the Amenorrhea?*

Clues in the patient's history that point to the etiology of the amenorrhea are listed in the following table.

Clues in the Patient's History Pointing to the Etiology of Amenorrhea

Historical Clue	Condition Suggested
Acne Greasy or oily skin Hirsutism Obesity	Polycystic ovarian syndrome
History of chemotherapy	Ovarian failure
History of radiation therapy	Ovarian failure
History of diabetes mellitus, Addison's disease, or thyroid disease	Ovarian failure (autoimmune etiology)
Galactorrhea	Hyperprolactinemia
Weight loss	Functional amenorrhea
Excessive exercise	Functional amenorrhea
Psychological stress	Functional amenorrhea
Symptoms of early pregnancy	Pregnancy
Cessation of menstruation followed by hot flashes, vaginal dryness, or mood swings	Menopause
Rapid progression of hirsutism	Adrenal or ovarian androgen-secreting tumor
Bodybuilder	Exogenous androgen use
Medication history	Amenorrhea secondary to medication use (eg, danazol, deproprovera, LHRH agonists, oral contraceptives)
Severe dieting	Functional amenorrhea
Fatigue Nervousness Palpitations Sweating Weight loss	Hyperthyroidism

(continued)

Clues in the Patient's History Pointing to the Etiology of Amenorrhea *(continued)*

Historical Clue	Condition Suggested
Constipation Hoarseness Loss of hair Memory impairment Sensation of cold Weakness Weight gain	Hypothyroidism
Headache Neurological symptoms Visual field defect	CNS lesion (hypothalamic or pituitary)
History of pelvic inflammatory disease or endometriosis	Asherman's syndrome
History of cautery for cervical intraepithelial neoplasia or obstructive cervical malignancy	Cervical stenosis
Debilitating illness	Functional amenorrhea

Proceed to Step 3

STEP 3 – *Are There Any Clues in the Physical Examination That Point to the Etiology of the Amenorrhea?*

Clues in the patient's physical examination that point to the etiology of the amenorrhea are listed in the following table.

Clues in the Patient's Physical Examination Pointing to the Etiology of Amenorrhea

Physical Examination Finding	Condition Suggested
Tachycardia	Hyperthyroidism
Bradycardia	Hypothyroidism Physical or nutritional stress
Coarse skin Coarseness of hair Dry skin Edema of the eyelids Weight gain	Hypothyroidism
Exophthalmos Hyper-reflexia Lid lag or retraction Soft, moist skin Tremor	Hyperthyroidism
Galactorrhea	Hyperprolactinemia
Bradycardia Cold extremities Dry skin with lanugo hair Hypotension Hypothermia Minimum of body fat Orange discoloration of skin (hypercarotenemia)	Anorexia nervosa

Clues in the Patient's Physical Examination Pointing to the Etiology of Amenorrhea *(continued)*

Physical Examination Finding	Condition Suggested
Painless enlargement of parotid glands Ulcers or calluses on skin of dorsum of fingers or hands	Bulimia
Signs of virilization: Clitoromegaly Frontal balding Increased muscle bulk Severe hirsutism	Adrenal or ovarian androgen-secreting tumor
Centripetal obesity Hirsutism Hypertension Proximal muscle weakness Striae	Cushing's syndrome

If the history and physical examination provide clues to the etiology of the amenorrhea, the clinician should evaluate accordingly.

If the etiology of the amenorrhea is not clear after a thorough history and physical examination, ***proceed to Step 4.***

STEP 4 – *Is the Patient Pregnant?*

The most common cause of secondary amenorrhea is pregnancy. Pregnancy is usually suspected on the basis of the history and physical examination. Since the hCG that is secreted by the placenta enters the maternal circulation and is ultimately excreted in the urine, pregnancy can be diagnosed before symptoms and signs suggest it. It is now feasible to detect pregnancy 8-10 days after ovulation with determination of β-hCG in the urine.

Despite what the patient may say, every patient with secondary amenorrhea should have a pregnancy test. If the test is negative, then further evaluation is warranted.

If the pregnancy test is positive, ***stop here.***

If the pregnancy test is negative, ***proceed to Step 5.***

STEP 5 – *What Are the Results of the Thyroid Function Tests?*

Secondary amenorrhea may be an early manifestation of hypothyroidism. In fact, many patients with hypothyroidism may have no other signs or symptoms suggestive of hypothyroidism. Thyroid function tests will also exclude hyperthyroidism as the cause of amenorrhea.

If the results of the thyroid function tests indicate hypothyroidism, ***stop here***.

If the results of the thyroid function tests are not consistent with hypothyroidism, ***proceed to Step 6.***

STEP 6 – *What Is the Serum Prolactin Level?*

Once pregnancy has been excluded, a serum prolactin level should be obtained, particularly in the patient complaining of galactorrhea. The absence of galactorrhea should not dissuade the clinician from obtaining a serum prolactin level, since a fair number of patients with hyperprolactinemia do not have a history of galactorrhea.

Hyperprolactinemia is a common cause of secondary amenorrhea. Excessive secretion of prolactin may be the result of many different conditions. Before undertaking an extensive evaluation of hyperprolactinemia, it is wise to repeat the prolactin level, as nonspecific stimuli may cause an elevation. These include stress, sleep, and food intake.

If the patient has elevated prolactin levels, further evaluation is necessary to determine the etiology of the hyperprolactinemia.

If the patient does not have elevated prolactin levels, ***proceed to Step 7***.

STEP 7 – *What Is the Patient's Estrogen Status?*

Determining estrogen status can begin with assessment of the vaginal mucosa and cervical mucus. The following characteristics of the vaginal mucosa suggest adequate estrogen levels:

- Moist
- Rugated

The following characteristics of the cervical mucus suggest adequate estrogen levels:

- Mucus can be stretched
- Mucus ferns after drying

While these characteristics are helpful in providing information about estrogen status, more commonly, a progesterone challenge test is performed. In this test, either 10 mg of medroxyprogesterone acetate is taken orally once or twice a day or 100 mg of progesterone in oil is administered intramuscularly. In a woman with adequate estrogen levels and a normal outflow tract, withdrawal menstrual bleeding should be appreciated within 1 week of discontinuing the progesterone. The progesterone challenge test is superior to measurements of plasma estradiol, because estrogen levels fluctuate, and measuring estrogen levels is expensive.

If withdrawal bleeding occurs, then the patient has chronic anovulation with estrogen present. ***Proceed to Step 8***.

If withdrawal bleeding does not occur, ***proceed to Step 11***.

STEP 8 – *What Is the Differential Diagnosis in the Amenorrheic Patient Who Responds to the Progesterone Challenge With Uterine Bleeding?*

Withdrawal bleeding that occurs in response to the progesterone challenge test indicates adequate estrogen production. In these patients, the most common cause of amenorrhea is polycystic ovarian syndrome (Stein-Leventhal syndrome). In this syndrome, there is a mild to moderate excess in androgen levels. This results in the clinical manifestations listed in the following box.

STEIN-LEVENTHAL SYNDROME CLINICAL MANIFESTATIONS	
ACNE	MILD VIRILIZATION (severe cases only)
HIRSUTISM	OBESITY
INFERTILITY	OILY SKIN
IRREGULAR (absent) MENSES	

The diagnosis is supported by elevated LH levels with normal or low FSH levels. An LH:FSH ratio >2-3 argues for the diagnosis of polycystic ovarian syndrome.

Other causes of anovulation in the presence of estrogen include:

- Cushing's syndrome
- Late-onset congenital adrenal hyperplasia (21-hydroxylase or 11-β-hydroxylase deficiency)
- Ovarian tumors
- Adrenal tumors

Proceed to Step 9

STEP 9 – *Which Patients Should Have Further Evaluation?*

Not all patients with chronic anovulation with estrogen present require testing to differentiate between polycystic ovary syndrome (PCOS) and the other causes listed above. However, there are certain features that should prompt further evaluation. These include the sudden onset of hirsutism, virilization (clitoral enlargement, temporal hair loss, deepening of the voice), and signs and symptoms of Cushing's syndrome.

If the above features are not present, the diagnosis is polycystic ovarian syndrome. ***Stop here.***

If any of the above features are present, ***proceed to Step 10***.

STEP 10 – *What Tests Should Be Performed to Differentiate Between the Causes of Chronic Anovulation With Estrogen Present?*

These disorders may be differentiated from polycystic ovarian syndrome by measurement of serum testosterone and dehydroepiandrosterone sulfate (DHEA-S). Testosterone levels >2 ng/mL should prompt a search for an ovarian tumor.

DHEA-S levels >7 μg/mL should prompt a search for an adrenal source. In these patients, a CT scan should be performed to exclude the presence of an adrenal tumor. A normal CT scan should be followed by measurement of a basal 17-hydroxyprogesterone level. A level >9 nmol/L supports the diagnosis of late-onset adrenal hyperplasia.

In patients suspected of having Cushing's syndrome, evaluation should begin with a 24-hour urine collection for cortisol.

If the testosterone, DHEA-S, and 24-hour urine free cortisol levels are all normal, polycystic ovarian syndrome is the likely diagnosis.

End of Section.

STEP 11 – *What Is the FSH Level?*

In the amenorrheic patient with a failure to bleed after a progesterone challenge test, a plasma FSH level should be obtained.

If the FSH level is low or normal, ***proceed to Step 12***.

If the FSH level is >40 IU/L in a female <40 years of age, the diagnosis is premature ovarian failure. If the patient is <30 years of age, a karyotype should be ordered to exclude the presence of a Y chromosome.

Besides ovarian failure secondary to chromosomal abnormalities, other causes of ovarian failure include:

- Autoimmune disease
- Chemotherapy
- Radiation therapy
- 17-α-hydroxylase deficiency
- 17-, 20-lyase deficiency
- Resistant ovary syndrome
- Galactosemia

The most common cause of premature ovarian failure is autoimmune disease. While this may occur as an isolated condition, in some cases, autoimmune ovarian failure is accompanied by other endocrine disorders such as hypothyroidism, hypoparathyroidism, and adrenal insufficiency. Therefore, it is reasonable to assess the function of other endocrine organs with appropriate testing. The other causes listed above are rare and are usually suspected based on characteristic signs and symptoms.

End of Section.

STEP 12 – *What Is the Differential Diagnosis in the Amenorrheic Patient Who Fails to Bleed After Progesterone Challenge and Who Has a Low or Normal FSH?*

A low or normal FSH in the amenorrheic patient, who fails to bleed after the progesterone challenge test, is either due to a hypothalamic-pituitary disorder or anatomic defect of the outflow tract.

The diagnosis of an anatomic defect of the outflow tract is usually apparent from the history and physical examination. Scarring or stenosis of the cervix may occur following surgery, cryosurgery, electrocautery, or laser therapy. Destruction of the endometrium that ensues results in Asherman's syndrome.

If the history and physical examination does not establish the diagnosis of an outflow tract defect, then further testing can be done. To delineate between a hypothalamic-pituitary disorder and a defect of the outflow tract, cyclic estrogen and progesterone can be given. Specifically, 1.25 mg of orally conjugated estrogens are administered for 4 weeks, along with 10 mg of medroxyprogesterone acetate during the last 10 days.

If withdrawal bleeding does not occur in the patient with an intact uterus, the diagnosis is likely an anatomic defect of the outflow tract. Confirmation of the diagnosis requires either hysteroscopy or hysterosalpingography. ***Stop here.***

If withdrawal bleeding occurs, ***proceed to Step 13***.

STEP 13 – *What Are the Results of the MRI of the Sella?*

When withdrawal bleeding occurs in the amenorrheic patient with a low or normal FSH, a hypothalamic-pituitary disorder is present. These disorders can be divided into structural and functional causes. Structural causes are essentially the same as those that cause hypopituitarism. These causes are listed in the following box.

HYPOTHALAMIC – PITUITARY FAILURE STRUCTURAL CAUSES	
MALIGNANCY	INFILTRATION
Pituitary adenoma	Hemochromatosis
Hypothalamic tumors	Amyloidosis
Craniopharyngioma	VASCULAR EVENT
Germinoma	Sheehan's syndrome
Meningioma	(postpartum pituitary necrosis)
Glioma	Carotid aneurysm
Metastatic cancer	
INFLAMMATORY DISEASES	
Granulomatous disease	
Tuberculosis	
Sarcoidosis	
Syphilis	
Lymphocytic hypophysitis	
Histiocytosis X / eosinophilic granuloma	

Functional etiologies of amenorrhea are listed in the following box.

HYPOTHALAMIC – PITUITARY FAILURE NONSTRUCTURAL CAUSES	
ANOREXIA NERVOSA / BULIMIA	DRUG-RELATED
CHRONIC DEBILITATING ILLNESS	EXERCISE
AIDS	MALNUTRITION
Malabsorption	STRESS
Malignancy	WEIGHT LOSS
Uremia	

The clinician should obtain an MRI scan to differentiate between structural and functional etiologies.

End of Section.

References

Aloi JA, "Evaluation of Amenorrhea," *Compr Ther*, 1995, 21(10):575-8.

Baird DT, "Amenorrhoea," *Lancet*, 1997, 350(9073):275-9.

Crosignani PG and Vegetti W, "A Practical Guide to the Diagnosis and Management of Amenorrhoea," *Drugs*, 1996, 52(5):671-81.

Kiningham RB, Apgar BS, and Schwenk TL, "Evaluation of Amenorrhea," *Am Fam Phys*, 1996, 53(4):1185-94 (review).

McIver B, Romanski SA, and Nippoldt TB, "Evaluation and Management of Amenorrhea," *Mayo Clin Proc*, 1997, 72(12):1161-9.

SECONDARY AMENORRHEA / OLIGOMENORRHEA

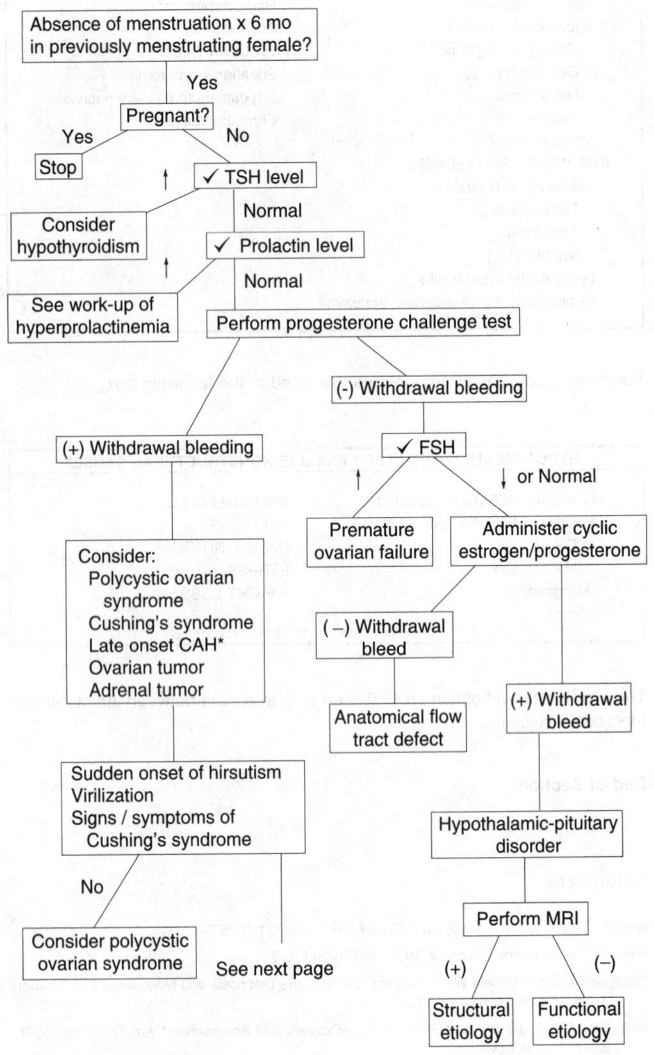
Absence of menstruation x 6 mo in previously menstruating female?
Yes
Pregnant?
Yes
No
Stop
↑
✓ TSH level
Consider hypothyroidism
Normal
✓ Prolactin level
↑
See work-up of hyperprolactinemia
Normal
Perform progesterone challenge test
(-) Withdrawal bleeding
(+) Withdrawal bleeding
✓ FSH
↑
↓ or Normal
Premature ovarian failure
Administer cyclic estrogen/progesterone
Consider:
Polycystic ovarian syndrome
Cushing's syndrome
Late onset CAH*
Ovarian tumor
Adrenal tumor
(–) Withdrawal bleed
Anatomical flow tract defect
(+) Withdrawal bleed
Sudden onset of hirsutism
Virilization
Signs / symptoms of Cushing's syndrome
Hypothalamic-pituitary disorder
No
Perform MRI
Consider polycystic ovarian syndrome
See next page
(+)
(–)
Structural etiology
Functional etiology

*CAH = congenital adrenal hyperplasia

SECONDARY AMENORRHEA / OLIGOMENORRHEA (*continued*)

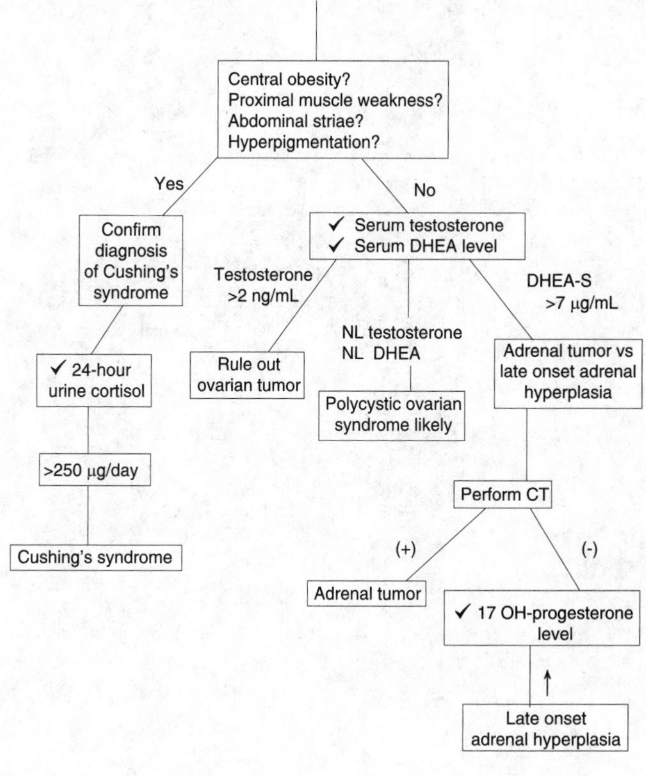

PART IV:

PULMONARY

PLEURAL FLUID ANALYSIS

The approximate annual incidence of various types of pleural effusions in the United States is listed in the following table.

Approximate Annual Incidence of Various Types of Pleural Effusions in the United States

Type of Effusion	Number of Patients
Congestive heart failure	500,000
Pneumonia (bacterial)	300,000
Malignancy	200,000
Lung	60,000
Breast	50,000
Lymphoma	40,000
Other	50,000
Pulmonary embolism	150,000
Pneumonia (viral)	100,000
Cirrhosis with ascites	50,000
Gastrointestinal disease	25,000
Collagen vascular disease	6000
Tuberculosis	2500
Asbestos exposure	2000
Mesothelioma	1500

Adapted from Light, *Pleural Diseases*, 3rd ed, Philadelphia, PA: Lea and Febiger, 1995, 76.

Differentiating among the above causes of pleural effusion requires consideration of the patient's clinical presentation along with analysis of the pleural fluid.

Tests to Order on Pleural Fluid

Of key importance in elucidating the etiology of a pleural effusion is differentiating a transudative from exudative pleural effusion. To do so, the following tests must be obtained:

- Serum protein level
- Pleural fluid protein level
- Serum LDH
- Pleural fluid LDH

These tests from the basis of Light's criteria which are used to separate transudative from exudative pleural effusions. Light's criteria will be discussed shortly.

There are, of course, many other tests of the pleural fluid. Too often, a laundry list of tests is obtained without consideration of the patient's clinical presentation. This often leads to extensive testing which is not cost-effective. Therefore, after the above tests are obtained, further testing of the pleural fluid should be individualized. For example, when the clinician suspects that a pleural effusion is transudative, only protein and LDH levels of the pleural fluid and serum should be obtained.

In those who have an exudative pleural effusion, the following tests of the pleural fluid are routinely indicated:

- Protein
- LDH
- Glucose
- Amylase
- Differential cell count
- Microbiologic studies
- Cytologic studies

Other tests of the pleural fluid, such as pH, ANA, complement levels, lipid analysis, and rheumatoid factor, should not be obtained in every patient with an exudative pleural effusion. The clinician should order these tests if the patient's clinical presentation is suggestive of a condition in which the performance of one or more of these tests would be useful.

Gross Appearance / Odor

Even before pleural fluid is sent to the laboratory for analysis, some important information can be gleaned at the bedside. At times, gross inspection of pleural fluid may provide some clues as to the underlying etiology of the effusion.

Straw color is characteristic of transudative effusions. In the absence of trauma, thoracentesis revealing bloody fluid should raise concern about the possibility of malignancy, pulmonary infarct, benign asbestos-related pleural effusion, tuberculosis, or postcardiac injury syndrome. If the pleural fluid is bloody, a pleural fluid hematocrit should be obtained. A ratio of the pleural fluid hematocrit to the blood hematocrit exceeding 50% satisfies the definition of a hemothorax. Such a finding should prompt the clinician to consider chest tube placement.

Pleural fluid turbidity usually reflects the presence of increased cells or lipids. Centrifugation can be used to distinguish between the two. Turbidity that does not clear with centrifugation indicates increased lipids as the etiology. Increased cellularity is likely if the supernatant clears with centrifugation.

Aspiration of milky fluid is consistent with either chylothorax or chyliform effusion. A pleural aspirate that is of anchovy paste consistency suggests a possible amebic pleural effusion. Obtaining an aspirate that is the same color as enteral feeding fluid indicates that a feeding tube has been inserted into the pleural space. A highly viscous effusion may be the result of a malignant mesothelioma. The odor of the aspirate may be revealing as well. A putrid odor is consistent with an empyema secondary to anaerobic infection. An ammonia odor suggests a urinothorax.

Gross Inspection of Pleural Fluid and Differential Diagnosis

Characteristic of Fluid	Etiology
Straw colored	Transudative
Bloody	Trauma Malignancy Pulmonary infarct Postcardiac injury syndrome Tuberculosis Asbestos-related
Milky	Chylothorax Chyliform
Anchovy paste consistency	Amebic infection
Color of enteral feed	Misplacement of feeding tube in pleural space
Color of central venous catheter infusate	Extravascular catheter migration
Putrid odor	Empyema from anaerobic infection
Ammonia-like odor	Urinothorax
Black	Aspergillus infection
Dark green	Biliothorax
Viscous	Mesothelioma

PLEURAL EFFUSIONS

Evaluating the Appearance

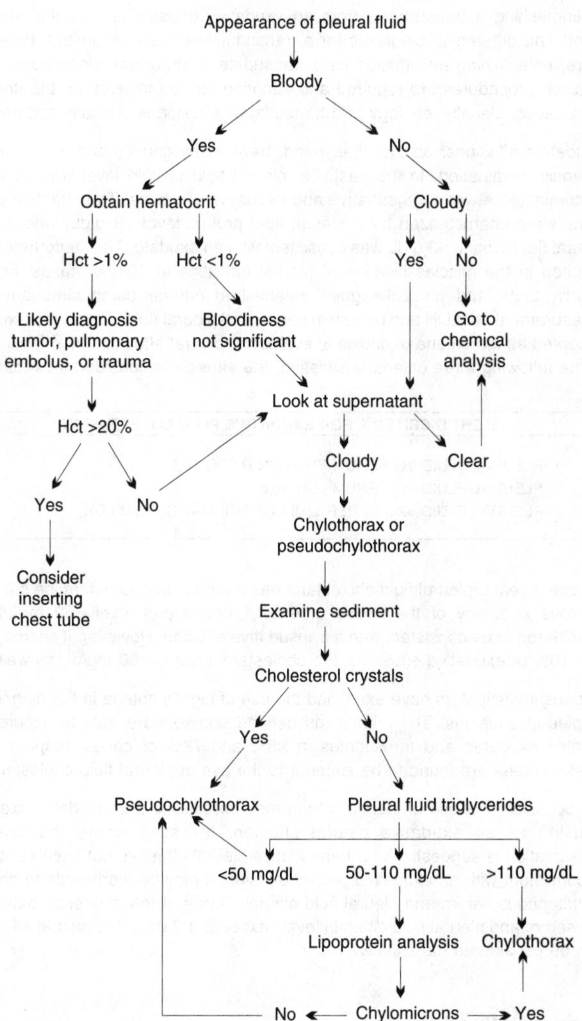

Adapted from Light R, *Pleural Diseases*, 4th ed, Philadelphia, PA: Lippincott Williams & Wilkins, 2001, 90.

Differentiating Transudative From Exudative Pleural Effusion

After gross inspection, pleural fluid should be sent to the laboratory for analysis. Distinguishing a transudative from an exudative effusion is essential at this point. The differential diagnosis for a transudative effusion is limited. Furthermore, establishing an effusion as a transudate is important, since no further invasive procedures are required and attention can be focused on the underlying cause. Usually, etiology of a transudative effusion is clinically apparent.

Exudative effusions, on the other hand, have many causes and may require extensive evaluation. In the past, the pleural fluid protein level was used to discriminate between transudative and exudative effusions. Transudative effusions were characterized by a pleural fluid protein level <3 g/dL, whereas a pleural fluid protein >3 g/dL was consistent with an exudate. This, unfortunately, resulted in the misclassification of pleural effusions in 10% of cases. Fortunately, Light and his colleagues established criteria using simultaneous measurements of LDH and protein in serum and pleural fluid. This is now widely accepted as the criteria of choice in evaluating pleural effusions. If at least one of the following three criteria is satisfied, the effusion is considered exudative.

LIGHT'S CRITERIA FOR EXUDATIVE PLEURAL EFFUSION
• PLEURAL FLUID TO SERUM PROTEIN RATIO >0.5 • PLEURAL FLUID TO SERUM LDH >0.6 • PLEURAL FLUID >2/3 UPPER LIMIT OF NORMAL SERUM LDH

In recent years, pleural fluid cholesterol has been studied to determine if it can improve accuracy of the above criteria. A cholesterol level <60 mg/dL is considered to be consistent with a transudative effusion. However, it seems that in ~10% of exudative effusions, the cholesterol level is <60 mg/dL as well.

Various investigators have examined the use of Light's criteria in the diagnosis of pleural effusions. The criteria, as defined above, were able to accurately identify exudates and transudates in 98% and 77% of cases, respectively. These criteria are found to be superior to the use of pleural fluid cholesterol.

On occasion, the use of Light's criteria may misclassify a transudative pleural effusion as an exudative pleural effusion. In cases where the clinical presentation is suggestive of a transudative pleural effusion, but Light's criteria is consistent with an exudative pleural effusion, it may be worthwhile to obtain simultaneous serum and pleural fluid albumin levels. If the difference between the serum and pleural fluid albumin levels exceeds 1.2 g/dL, the pleural effusion can be considered transudative.

Transudative Effusion

Pleural fluid that is transudative is typically straw colored and odorless. In approximately 80% of cases, the white blood cell count is <1000/μL. It is relatively unusual to observe a white blood cell count >10,000/μL in a transudative effusion. In about 85% of patients, the red blood cell count is <10,000/μL. There is characteristically a mononuclear cell predominance with lymphocytes, mesothelial cells, macrophages, and monocytes commonly found. Transudative effusions do not typically have low pleural fluid glucose. The pH is alkaline. The amylase level is always lower in the pleural fluid than in the serum.

TRANSUDATIVE EFFUSION CHARACTERISTICS	
STRAW COLORED	pH ALKALINE
ODORLESS	GLUCOSE NORMAL
WBC USUALLY <1000/μL*	RBC <10,000/μL
MONONUCLEAR CELL PREDOMINANCE	
PLEURAL FLUID AMYLASE < SERUM AMYLASE	

*Almost never >10,000/μL.

Causes of a Transudative Pleural Effusion

The causes of a transudative pleural effusion are listed in the following box.

TRANSUDATIVE EFFUSION DIFFERENTIAL DIAGNOSIS	
CONGESTIVE HEART FAILURE	MYXEDEMA
CIRRHOSIS	PULMONARY EMBOLISM
NEPHROTIC SYNDROME	URINOTHORAX
SUPERIOR VENA CAVA OBSTRUCTION	PERITONEAL DIALYSIS
TRAPPED LUNG	ATELECTASIS
PERICARDIAL DISEASE	FONTAN'S PROCEDURE
SARCOIDOSIS	

Causes of transudative pleural effusions are discussed in more detail in the chapter, ***Transudative Pleural Effusions*** *on page 439*.

Exudative Effusion

The causes of an exudative pleural effusion are listed in the following box.

CAUSES OF EXUDATIVE PLEURAL EFFUSION	
MALIGNANCY	INFECTION
Metastatic pleural disease	Bacterial pneumonia
Mesothelioma	Tuberculous pleuritis
Body cavity lymphoma	Viral
PULMONARY EMBOLISM	*Mycoplasma*
GASTROINTESTINAL DISEASE	Actinomycosis
Acute pancreatitis	Nocardiosis
Chronic pancreatitis	Fungal disease
Intra-abdominal abscess	Histoplasmosis
Bilious pleural effusion	Coccidioidomycosis
Diaphragmatic hernia	Aspergillosis
Liver transplantation	Blastomycosis
Postabdominal surgery	Cryptococcosis
Endoscopic variceal sclerotherapy	Parasitic disease
POSTCARDIAC INJURY SYNDROME	Paragonimiasis
HEMOTHORAX	Amebiasis
CHYLOTHORAX	Echinococcosis
	Pneumocystis carinii

(continued)

CAUSES OF EXUDATIVE PLEURAL EFFUSION *(continued)*	
DRUG-INDUCED PLEURAL DISEASE	MISCELLANEOUS
Nitrofurantoin	Uremia
Dantrolene	Lung transplantation
Methysergide	Bone marrow transplantation
Bromocriptine	Asbestos exposure
Procarbazine	Sarcoidosis
Amiodarone	Therapeutic radiation exposure
Ergot alkaloids	Yellow-nail syndrome
Interleukin-2	Extramedullary hematopoiesis
Methotrexate	Urinary tract obstruction
Clozapine	Meig's syndrome
CONNECTIVE TISSUE DISEASE	Endometriosis
Pleural effusion of rheumatoid arthritis	Ovarian hyperstimulation syndrome
Lupus arthritis	Iatrogenic
Churg-Strauss syndrome	Misplaced percutaneously placed catheter
Wegener's granulomatosis	
Immunoblastic lymphadenopathy	Misplaced nasogastric tube
Sjögren's syndrome	Translumbar aortographic examination
Familial Mediterranean fever	Trapped lung

Adapted from Light R, *Pleural Diseases*, 4th ed, Philadelphia, PA: Lippincott Williams and Wilkins, 2001, 88.

For further discussion regarding the clinical and laboratory features of many of the causes listed above, please refer to the chapter, ***Exudative Pleural Effusions*** *on page 443.*

Establishing the Etiology of an Exudative Pleural Effusion

The following tests may be helpful in establishing the etiology of an exudative pleural effusion.

Red Blood Cell Count

Approximately 15% of transudative and 40% of exudative effusions are blood tinged. If thoracentesis reveals grossly bloody pleural fluid, it is essential to obtain a pleural fluid hematocrit. A pleural fluid hematocrit that is >50% of the blood hematocrit defines the existence of a hemothorax and consideration should be given to insertion of a chest tube.

Three common causes of a hemothorax include malignancy, trauma, and pulmonary embolism.

Sometimes it is difficult to tell whether a bloody aspirate is the result of a traumatic thoracentesis or whether the blood was present prior to aspiration. In general, bloody pleural fluid that results from a traumatic thoracentesis should not be uniformly bloody during the entire aspiration.

White Blood Cell Count and Differential

A white blood cell count alone is seldom diagnostically helpful. Most transudative effusions are characterized by white blood cell counts <1000/μL while most exudative effusions exceed this value. A white blood cell count exceeding >50,000/μL can be seen in complicated parapneumonic effusion or empyema, but is unusual with other causes of exudative pleural effusion.

The differential white blood cell count is often more revealing than the absolute white blood cell count. When reporting the differential, laboratories, in general, report the percentage of polymorphonuclear and mononuclear cells. It is helpful, however, to subdivide even further. Polymorphonuclear cells include neutrophils, eosinophils, and basophils. Mononuclear cells include lymphocytes, mesothelial cells, macrophages, and plasma cells. Malignant cells may be noted as well.

WBC Differential and Etiology of Exudative Effusion

Cell Type	Etiology
Neutrophilia	Inflammation
	Pneumonia
	Pulmonary embolism
	Subphrenic abscess
	Pancreatitis
	Early tuberculosis
Eosinophilia	Air*
	Blood*
	Parasitic infection
	Paragonimiasis
	Hydatid disease
	Amebiasis
	Ascariasis
	Fungal infection
	Coccidioidomycosis
	Histoplasmosis
	Cryptococcal infection
	Medication reaction
	Dantrolene
	Nitrofurantoin
	Bromocriptine
	Malignancy (carcinoma, lymphoma)
	Churg-Strauss syndrome
	Pulmonary infarction
	Asbestos-related pleural effusion
Lymphocytosis†	Malignancy
	Tuberculosis
	Sarcoidosis
	Chronic rheumatoid pleurisy
	Chylothorax
	Yellow nail syndrome

(continued)

WBC Differential and Etiology of Exudative Effusion *(continued)*

Cell Type	Etiology
Mesothelial cells‡	↑ # argues against tuberculosis
Macrophage	No clinical significance
Plasma cells§	Multiple myeloma

*Pleural fluid eosinophilia is defined as a pleural fluid eosinophil count >10% of the total white blood cell count. Air and blood in the pleural space are the most common causes of eosinophilia in pleural fluid. Unusual causes of pleural fluid eosinophilia should be considered if the cause is not evident. Unusual causes of pleural fluid eosinophilia include benign asbestos pleural effusion, drug reaction, paragonimiasis, and Churg-Strauss syndrome. Pulmonary embolism, one cause of blood in the pleural space, deserves consideration in unexplained effusions characterized by eosinophilia.

One should realize that the cause of pleural fluid eosinophilia is not always established. Indeed, up to 25% of eosinophilic pleural effusions remain undiagnosed. If no diagnosis is apparent after routine studies of the pleural fluid, further evaluation should be nonaggressive since spontaneous resolution occurs in the majority of cases.

†A lymphocytic percentage that exceeds 50% suggests either malignancy or tuberculous infection. If the clinical setting is concerning for either of these two diseases, the finding of lymphocytic predominance indicates the need for a pleural biopsy. If the clinical presentation is suggestive of chronic lymphocytic leukemia or lymphoma, it may be worthwhile to differentiate between T and B lymphocytes in the pleural fluid. With CLL or lymphoma, all the pleural fluid lymphocytes will be of the same type.

‡Mesothelial cells are cells that line the pleural cavity. Mesothelial cells are found in normal pleural fluid because of exfoliation. The absence of mesothelial cells is helpful when one is considering a diagnosis of tuberculosis. Tuberculous pleural effusions are usually characterized by a paucity of mesothelial cells. It is important to realize that mesothelial cells may be mistaken for malignant cells. Therefore, it is necessary to have the pleural fluid examined by a skilled pathologist to make this distinction. In one study of 65 patients with tuberculous pleurisy, only one patient had >1 mesothelial cell per 1000 cells. In general, tuberculosis is not likely to be the cause of the effusion if there are >5% mesothelial cells. It is important to realize, however, that a lack of mesothelial cells is not specific for tuberculous pleurisy as such a finding has been described in other causes of an exudative pleural effusion.

§The presence of a significant number of plasma cells should raise concern about the possibility of multiple myeloma.

Protein

Earlier in this section, recall that protein was one of the criteria used in separating transudative from exudative pleural effusion. However, a protein level does not help in further determining the cause of an exudative effusion. A protein level >4.0 g/dL should, however, prompt the clinician to consider the possibility of tuberculous pleurisy. Higher protein levels (7-8 g/dL) should prompt consideration of multiple myeloma or Waldenström's macroglobulinemia.

Glucose

Unlike cerebrospinal fluid, a concomitant serum glucose level does not need to be obtained for interpretation of the pleural fluid glucose level. The causes of a low pleural fluid glucose level (<60 mg/dL) are listed in the following box.

DIFFERENTIAL DIAGNOSIS OF GLUCOSE <60 mg/dL IN EXUDATIVE EFFUSION	
MALIGNANCY*	HEMOTHORAX
TUBERCULOSIS	CHURG-STRAUSS SYNDROME
RHEUMATOID ARTHRITIS	PARAGONIMIASIS
COMPLICATED PARAPNEUMONIC EFFUSION† / EMPYEMA	ESOPHAGEAL RUPTURE
LUPUS PLEURITIS	

*Approximately 15% of malignant pleural effusions have a pleural fluid glucose level <60 mg/dL. As a general rule, as the tumor mass increases the pleural fluid glucose level decreases. Successful treatment of a malignant pleural effusion with chemical pleurodesis is less likely when the pleural fluid glucose is <60 mg/dL. These patients are more likely to have a positive pleural biopsy or cytology. Their life expectancy seems to be reduced as well, with a mean survival of less than 2 months.

†The finding of a low pleural fluid glucose in a parapneumonic effusion suggests the possibility of a complicated parapneumonic effusion. In fact, a glucose level <40 mg/dL argues for chest tube thoracostomy.

Amylase

Pleural fluid amylase levels are said to be elevated if the level exceeds the upper limit of normal for serum amylase or if the pleural fluid to serum amylase ratio is >1.0. Causes of an exudative pleural effusion which are characterized by increased pleural fluid amylase levels are listed in the following box.

CAUSES OF ELEVATED PLEURAL FLUID AMYLASE
MALIGNANCY
ESOPHAGEAL RUPTURE
PANCREATIC DISEASE
Acute pancreatitis
Chronic pancreatitis

Up to 50% of patients with acute pancreatitis have an associated pleural effusion. In most cases, the signs and symptoms of acute pancreatitis dominate the clinical picture. On occasion, however, the predominant symptoms may be related to the pleural effusion (shortness of breath and pleuritic chest pain). In these cases, acute pancreatitis as the etiology of the pleural effusion may not be considered. An increased pleural fluid amylase level is a clue to the diagnosis.

Patients with chronic pancreatic disease may also present with an associated pleural effusion. In chronic pancreatic disease, the pleural fluid accumulates via a sinus tract from a pancreatic pseudocyst. The diagnosis of pleural effusion secondary to chronic pancreatic disease can be difficult to establish. Many of these patients deny abdominal complaints suggestive of pancreatic disease. They appear chronically ill which often prompts the clinician to consider malignancy as the cause of the effusion. If a pleural fluid amylase level is not obtained, the pleural effusion may go undiagnosed. If obtained, the pleural fluid amylase often exceeds 4000 IU/mL.

Patients with malignancy may have an elevation of pleural fluid amylase. The degree of elevation tends to be less than in patients with either esophageal rupture or pancreatitis. In malignancy-related effusions, the amylase isozyme is of salivary origin. This can be helpful, then, in distinguishing the pleural fluid of malignancy from that of acute or chronic pancreatic disease.

Esophageal rupture also presents with an increase in salivary amylase. It is important for the clinician to make this diagnosis quickly because mortality rises considerably if the mediastinum is not explored within 24 hours of the onset of the esophageal perforation.

LDH

Recall that LDH, along with protein, forms the basis of Light's criteria used in distinguishing an exudative from a transudative effusion. Once a pleural effusion has been established as exudative, the LDH is usually only of limited value. In pleural effusions due to *Pneumocystis carinii*, pleural fluid analysis characteristically reveals a pleural fluid to serum LDH ratio exceeding 1.0. In these cases, the pleural fluid to serum protein ratio is typically <0.5. Pleural fluid LDH levels >1000 IU/L may be seen in empyema, malignancy, rheumatoid pleurisy, and paragonimiasis.

The LDH level does correspond directly with the extent of pleural inflammation. If repeat thoracentesis demonstrates a serial increase in the pleural fluid LDH level, the clinician should be more aggressive in pursuing the etiology of the pleural effusion as this finding is indicative of increasing inflammation in the pleural space.

pH

Causes of pleural effusion characterized by a pH <7.20 are listed in the following box.

PLEURAL FLUID pH <7.20 DIFFERENTIAL DIAGNOSIS
URINOTHORAX*
PARAGONIMIASIS
COMPLICATED PARAPNEUMONIC EFFUSION / EMPYEMA
ESOPHAGEAL RUPTURE†
TUBERCULOUS PLEURAL EFFUSION
HEMOTHORAX
MALIGNANT PLEURAL EFFUSION
SYSTEMIC ACIDOSIS
SLE-ASSOCIATED PLEURAL EFFUSION
RHEUMATOID ARTHRITIS-ASSOCIATED PLEURAL EFFUSION

*This is the only cause of a transudative pleural effusion with a low pH in the absence of systemic acidosis.

†A pH that falls below 6.0 is consistent with esophageal rupture. Other conditions, however, can rarely lead to this acidic of a pH.

Measurement of the pleural fluid pH is not indicated in every patient with an exudative pleural effusion. It is, however, recommended in all patients with parapneumonic effusions. In these cases, measurement of the pH is useful in determining the need for chest tube placement.

When obtaining a specimen for pH measurement, the clinician should exercise proper technique in specimen collection. Pleural fluid should be anaerobically collected in a heparinized syringe and sent to the laboratory on ice. The pH will be spuriously elevated if the specimen is exposed to air. Measurement of the pH should be performed using a blood gas machine.

In patients with a malignant pleural effusion, a low pH, similar to a low glucose, indicates that chemical pleurodesis is less likely to be successful. It also portends a reduced life expectancy. The diagnostic yield of cytology is higher in patients with malignant effusion who have a low pH.

A low pH accompanied by pleural fluid eosinophilia is seen in only two conditions. These include Churg-Strauss disease and paragonimiasis.

Cytology

Cytology can establish the diagnosis of malignant pleural effusions in >50% of patients. Cytologists use many characteristics to distinguish malignant cells from other cells.

CHARACTERISTICS OF MALIGNANT CELLS
LARGER CELLS LARGE NUCLEI LARGER NUCLEOLI HIGH NUCLEUS:CYTOPLASM RATIO TENDENCY TO AGGREGATE INTO CLUMPS

In various studies, accuracy of cytologic analysis in diagnosis of malignancy varies from 40% to 87%. Some reasons for this broad range include the following.

- Type of tumor

  As is the case with ascitic fluid, obtaining a positive result on cytology is contingent upon the type of tumor. In patients with lymphoma, for example, studies indicate that positive cytology is appreciated in approximately 75% of patients with the diffuse histiocytic subtype as compared to 25% in patients with Hodgkin's disease.

- Cell preparation

  Preparation of the cytologic examination is important as well. The efficacy of cytologic examination is greater if cell blocks and smears are used.

- Relation of malignancy and pleural effusion

  If the effusion is not related to a malignancy invading the pleura, then cytology is not likely to be positive. There may be other reasons why a patient with malignancy develops a pleural effusion, such as a pulmonary embolism. Malignancy resulting in obstruction of the lymphatic system, for example, is not likely to have a positive cytology.

- Number of specimens obtained

  The percentage of positive cytologic studies will increase if multiple pleural fluid specimens are sent for analysis. Cytology will be positive in 90% of patients if three separate specimens are obtained and analyzed.

- Cytologist

  The expertise of the cytologist cannot be undervalued.

Other tests that may be useful in establishing the diagnosis of malignant pleural effusion include electron microscopy, histochemical studies, immunohistochemical tests, and flow cytometry.

Adenosine Deaminase (ADA)

ADA levels are increased in almost all patients with tuberculous pleural effusions (HIV patients may have normal levels). There are other conditions (parapneumonic effusion, empyema, lymphoma, leukemia, lung cancer, rheumatoid pleurisy, mesothelioma) that can increase pleural ADA levels. Differentiating tuberculosis pleurisy from other causes of an elevated pleural fluid ADA level is usually not difficult if one carefully considers the clinical presentation.

A number of studies have been done to evaluate the usefulness of pleural fluid ADA levels for the diagnosis of tuberculous pleural effusion. Some of these studies have shown excellent sensitivity and specificity. For example, in a 1999 study, the sensitivity and specificity of the test was found to be 95% and 96%, respectively, if the cutoff value of 60 units/L is used. It is important to realize that these studies have used different ADA cutoff values. Using a lower cutoff value will increase sensitivity but at the cost of reduced specificity. The specificity of an elevated pleural fluid ADA level is increased if pleural fluid lymphocytosis is noted.

At the current time, pleural fluid ADA levels should not be relied on alone for the diagnosis of tuberculous pleural effusion. It is particularly useful, however, when tuberculous pleural effusion remains a consideration despite negative histology and mycobacterial cultures.

Pleural fluid interferon gamma levels are increased in patients with tuberculous pleural effusion. One study demonstrated that 99% of patients with tuberculous effusion had interferon gamma levels above 3.7 units/mL. Some studies have suggested that elevated pleural fluid interferon gamma levels are more specific than increased ADA levels for the diagnosis. Another advantage interferon gamma levels have over ADA levels is that the former seems to be increased consistently in HIV patients with tuberculous effusion.

Rheumatoid Factor

Five percent of patients with rheumatoid arthritis develop a pleural effusion at some point in the course of their disease. In most cases, the pleural effusion develops after the diagnosis of rheumatoid arthritis has been established. On occasion, a pleural effusion may be the initial manifestation of rheumatoid arthritis. In these cases, the exudative effusion may go undiagnosed if the clinician does not consider the possibility that the pleural effusion is secondary to rheumatoid arthritis.

To diagnose the pleural effusion of rheumatoid arthritis, it is necessary to obtain a pleural fluid rheumatoid factor titer. The pleural fluid rheumatoid factor is typically high (>1:320). The titer is usually equal to or greater than the serum rheumatoid factor titer.

ANA

Fifty percent of patients with SLE develop a pleural effusion at some point in the course of the disease. While diagnosis of SLE has often been made by the time a pleural effusion is noted, on occasion, the pleural effusion may be the initial manifestation of SLE. Traditionally, measurement of the pleural fluid ANA level has been considered the best test in the diagnosis of lupus pleuritis. Recent studies, however, suggest that the pleural fluid ANA level offers no advantage over the serum ANA titer in establishing the diagnosis of lupus pleuritis. Of note, a positive pleural fluid ANA is not entirely specific for lupus pleuritis as it has been found in up to 30% of patients with non-SLE pleural effusions.

Lipid Studies

On occasion, milky or turbid fluid may be obtained at the time of thoracentesis. In these cases, the cloudiness of the fluid may be explained by either increased cellularity or high lipid content in the pleural fluid. Centrifugation of the specimen can help differentiate between these possibilities. When centrifugation results in a clear supernatant, the likely etiology is increased cellularity. When the cloudiness persists after centrifugation, the pleural fluid is likely to have high lipid content. The following are two situations in which the pleural fluid may have a high lipid content:

- Chylothorax (chylous pleural effusion)
- Pseudochylothorax (chyliform pleural effusion)

To confirm the presence of high lipid content in the pleural fluid, lipid studies (ie, triglyceride level) of the pleural fluid may be obtained. Chylothorax and pseudochylothorax will be discussed in more detail in the chapter, ***Exudative Pleural Effusions*** *on page 443*.

Microbiology

In patients with an unexplained pleural effusion that is exudative, pleural fluid should be sent for bacterial, fungal, and mycobacterial cultures. For bacteria, aerobic and anaerobic cultures at the bedside are recommended.

Gram stain of the pleural fluid should be sent as well in patients with an undiagnosed exudative pleural effusion.

AFB smears are of low yield in determining the etiology of an exudative pleural effusion. An exception to this is in the case of a tuberculous empyema.

Counterimmunoelectrophoresis (CIE) can be done on pleural fluid in the hope of establishing the presence of a particular bacterial organism within hours, rather than days, as required with routine bacterial culture. This test detects bacterial antigens. It may also be helpful when antibiotic therapy has been instituted prior to thoracentesis and pleural fluid analysis, as it remains positive even in the face of several days of antibiotic treatment. Unfortunately, pleural effusions secondary to anaerobic bacterial infections may be missed because CIE does not test for these antigens.

References

Ansari T and Idell S, "Management of Undiagnosed Persistent Pleural Effusions," *Clin Chest Med*, 1998, 19(2):407-17.

Azoulay E, "Pleural Effusions in the Intensive Care Unit," *Curr Opin Pulm Med*, 2003, 9(4):291-7.

Heffner JE, "Evaluating Diagnostic Tests in the Pleural Space. Differentiating Transudates From Exudates as a Model," *Clin Chest Med*, 1998, 19(2):277-93.

Kalomenidis I and Light RW, "Eosinophilic Pleural Effusions," *Curr Opin Pulm Med*, 2003, 9(4):254-60.

Light RW, "Useful Tests on the Pleural Fluid in the Management of Patients With Pleural Effusions," *Curr Opin Pulm Med*, 1999, 5(4):245-9.

Morelock SY and Sahn SA, "Drugs and the Pleura," *Chest*, 1999, 116(1):212-21.

Parfrey H and Chilvers ER, "Pleural Disease – Diagnosis and Management" *Practitioner*, 1999, 243(1598):412, 415-21.

Perez-Rodriguez E and Jimenez Castro D, "The Use of Adenosine Deaminase and Adenosine Deaminase Isoenzymes in the Diagnosis of Tuberculous Pleuritis," *Curr Opin Pulm Med*, 2000, 6(4):259-66.

Rubins JB and Colice GL, "Evaluating Pleural Effusions. How Should You Go About Finding the Cause?" *Postgrad Med*, 1999, 105(5):39-42, 45-8.

Tam AC and Lapworth R, "Biochemical Analysis of Pleural Fluid: What Should We Measure?" *Ann Clin Biochem*, 2001, 38(Pt 4):311-22.

Wich MR, Moran CA, Mills SE, et al, "Immunohistochemical Differential Diagnosis of Pleural Effusions, With Emphasis on Malignant Mesothelioma," *Curr Opin Pulm Med*, 2001, 7(4):187-92.

PLEURAL EFFUSIONS

Distinguishing Transudative From Exudative

Patient with abnormal chest radiograph

↓

Suspect pleural disease

↓

Blunting of costrophrenic angle?

↓

Yes

↓

Lateral decubitus chest radiographs, chest CT or ultrasound

↓

Fluid thickness >10 mm

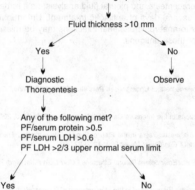

Yes → Diagnostic Thoracentesis

No → Observe

Diagnostic Thoracentesis ↓

Any of the following met?
PF/serum protein >0.5
PF/serum LDH >0.6
PF LDH >2/3 upper normal serum limit

Yes → Probable exudate

No → Transudate → Treat CHF, cirrhosis, or nephrosis

Probable exudate ↓

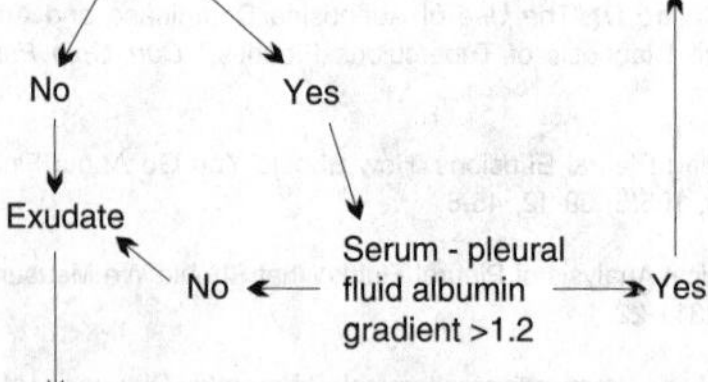

Patient has CHF or cirrhosis?

No → Exudate

Yes → Serum - pleural fluid albumin gradient >1.2

Serum - pleural fluid albumin gradient >1.2: No → Exudate; Yes → Treat CHF, cirrhosis, or nephrosis

Exudate ↓

Appearance of pleural fluid
Glucose of pleural fluid
Cytology and differential cell count of pleural fluid
Pleural fluid marker for TB

Adapted from Light R, *Pleural Diseases*, 4th ed, Philadelphia, PA: Lippincott Williams & Wilkins, 2001, 89.

TRANSUDATIVE PLEURAL EFFUSIONS

Causes of Transudative Pleural Effusion

The causes of transudative pleural effusion are listed in the following box.

CAUSES OF TRANSUDATIVE PLEURAL EFFUSION	
CONGESTIVE HEART FAILURE	MYXEDEMA¶
HEPATIC HYDROTHORAX	FONTAN'S PROCEDURE§
NEPHROTIC SYNDROME	SARCOIDOSIS
PULMONARY EMBOLISM*	SVC OBSTRUCTION
PERICARDIAL DISEASE†	ATELECTASIS
PERITONEAL DIALYSIS‡	TRAPPED LUNG

*Twenty-five percent of patients with pulmonary embolism who present with a pleural effusion are found to have a transudate. Further information regarding pulmonary embolism as a cause of pleural effusions can be found in the chapter, Exudative Pleural Effusions.

†There is a high incidence of pleural effusion in patients with pericardial disease. In one study of patients with constrictive pericarditis, 60% were found to have pleural effusions. Most commonly, the pleural effusion of pericardial disease is left-sided. Bilateral pleural effusions may also be noted. Less commonly, a right-sided pleural effusion may be seen in patients with pericardial disease. To summarize, pericardial disease should be considered in every patient with transudative pleural effusion, particularly if the effusion is left-sided. These effusions may be small to massive.

‡Peritoneal dialysis is an uncommon cause of transudative pleural effusion. 50% of cases are encountered in the first 30 days after the start of dialysis. In nearly 20% of cases, the pleural effusion develops at least 1 year after the initiation of dialysis.

¶Patients with myxedema may also present with pleural effusion. In most cases, a pericardial effusion is also present. When both are present together, pleural fluid analysis is usually consistent with a transudate. In myxedema patients who have an isolated pleural effusion, the effusion may be transudative or exudative.

§Fontan's procedure refers to a surgical anastomosis that is created between the superior vena cava, right atrium, or inferior vena cava and the pulmonary artery. This procedure may be performed to bypass the right ventricle in patients with congenital heart disease, especially in patients with tricuspid atresia or univentricular heart.

The laboratory tests needed to establish a diagnosis of transudative pleural effusion have already been discussed in the chapter, ***Pleural Fluid Analysis** on page 425*. In this chapter, we will discuss the clinical and laboratory features of the above causes of transudative pleural effusion in more detail.

Congestive Heart Failure

Congestive heart failure is the most common cause of transudative pleural effusions in the United States. In patients with congestive heart failure, the incidence of pleural effusion is quite high. In one study of 114 patients with congestive heart failure, 58% were found to have a pleural effusion on chest radiograph.

In most cases, patients present with signs and symptoms of congestive heart failure. These may include dyspnea, orthopnea, paroxysmal nocturnal dyspnea, peripheral edema, nocturia, distended jugular veins, crackles, and S3. Studies have shown that pleural effusions are much more common in left ventricular rather than right ventricular dysfunction. In fact, the presence of a pleural effusion in the patient with right ventricular dysfunction should prompt the clinician to consider other causes of pleural effusion, including undiagnosed left ventricular dysfunction.

Besides demonstrating the presence of a pleural effusion, chest radiography usually reveals cardiomegaly. The absence of cardiomegaly should prompt the clinician to consider other causes of the pleural effusion. In one study of 78 patients who had bilateral pleural effusions but a normal sized heart, congestive heart failure was the ultimate diagnosis in only 4% of patients. Other radiographic features of congestive heart failure may also be present, including perihilar congestion, cephalization, and Kerley's B lines.

Most often, bilateral pleural effusions are present. In fact, congestive heart failure is the most common cause of bilateral pleural effusions. However, unilateral pleural effusions are also commonly seen. When unilateral, there seems to be a predilection for the right side, although some studies have shown an equal frequency of right- and left-sided pleural effusions in patients with congestive heart failure.

Not all patients with congestive heart failure who have a pleural effusion require diagnostic thoracentesis to ensure that the effusion is secondary to congestive heart failure. To determine whether thoracentesis is needed in the patient with congestive heart failure, the clinician should decide if the patient has any of the following clinical features:

- Unilateral pleural effusion
- Bilateral pleural effusion but effusions are not comparable in size
- Fever
- Pleuritic chest pain
- No cardiomegaly

If one or more of the above features are present in the patient with congestive heart failure who has a pleural effusion, a diagnostic thoracentesis is warranted. In the absence of any of the above clinical features, it is appropriate to optimize treatment for congestive heart failure. In these cases, thoracentesis should be considered if the pleural effusion fails to resolve with appropriate treatment of the heart failure.

The pleural effusion of congestive heart failure is usually transudative by Light's criteria. In cases where congestive heart failure is the likely etiology of the pleural effusion, the most cost-effective use of pleural fluid laboratory tests is to only obtain protein and LDH levels of the pleural fluid and serum. A pleural effusion due to congestive heart failure is supported if Light's criteria is consistent with a transudate. Of note, congestive heart failure patients are at increased risk for the development of pulmonary embolism. Twenty-five percent of pleural effusions due to pulmonary embolism are transudative. Therefore, pulmonary embolism should be a consideration in all congestive heart failure patients with transudative pleural effusion.

Should pleural fluid analysis reveal the presence of an exudative pleural effusion, further tests to elucidate the etiology of the exudative pleural effusion may then be obtained. It is important to realize, however, that in 20% of congestive heart failure patients, the effusion may be exudative. This is more likely to be the case after a period of diuresis.

With several days of diuresis, there may be a rise in protein and LDH concentrations which result in an elevation of the ratios that form the basis of Light's criteria. In some cases, the ratios may enter the exudative range. How does one differentiate an exudative effusion due to diuresis in a congestive heart failure patient from another cause of exudative pleural effusion? First of all, although the protein and LDH ratios may move into the exudative range with diuresis, the values are usually just above the exudative range. If the clinical presentation is very suggestive of congestive heart failure but evaluation of the pleural fluid reveals an exudate by Light's criteria, it is also useful to obtain pleural fluid and serum albumin levels. If the difference between the pleural fluid and serum albumin exceeds 1.2 g/dL, the pleural effusion can be considered to be secondary to congestive heart failure so long as the clinical presentation is not suggestive of another cause of an exudative effusion.

Hepatic Hydrothorax

Hepatic hydrothorax should be a consideration in every cirrhotic patient who presents with a pleural effusion. The clinician should realize, however, that other causes of pleural effusion are common in the patient with cirrhosis. In one study, hepatic hydrothorax was not the etiology of the pleural effusion in nearly 20% of cirrhotic patients presenting with pleural effusion.

The incidence of hepatic hydrothorax is increased in cirrhotic patients who have ascites. Although ascites is commonly present, the absence of ascites does not exclude the diagnosis. In most cases, the signs and symptoms of cirrhosis and ascites overshadow the pleural effusion. Not uncommonly, hepatic hydrothorax may present with a large effusion, in which case, shortness of breath may dominate the clinical picture. In some cases, the effusion may occupy the entire hemithorax. It is has a predilection for the right side but, on occasion, may be bilateral or even left-sided. When hepatic hydrothorax is a possibility, both paracentesis and thoracentesis should be performed to confirm that the ascitic fluid and pleural fluid are both transudative.

The clinical and laboratory features of hepatic hydrothorax are listed in the following box.

USUAL CLINICAL AND LABORATORY FEATURES OF HEPATIC HYDROTHORAX
CLINICAL FEATURES
Right-sided (85%)
Left-sided (13%)
Bilateral (2%)
LABORATORY FEATURES
Cell count <1000 cells/mm^3
Total protein concentration <2.5 g/dL
Total protein pleural fluid to serum ratio <0.5
LDH pleural fluid to serum ratio <2:3
Serum to pleural fluid albumin gradient >1.1 g/dL
Pleural fluid amylase concentration < serum amylase concentration
pH 7.40-7.55

From Lazaridis KN, Frank JW, Krowka MJ, et al, "Hepatic Hydrothorax: Pathogenesis, Diagnosis, and Management," *Am J Med*, 1999, 107(3):262-7.

One complication of hepatic hydrothorax that the clinician should be aware of is spontaneous bacterial pleuritis. It should certainly be a consideration in patients with hepatic hydrothorax who present with fever. Spontaneous bacterial pleuritis is defined as an infection within a pre-existing hepatic hydrothorax (pneumonia and parapneumonic effusion must not be present). Spontaneous bacterial pleuritis is synonymous with spontaneous bacterial empyema. The latter term is to be avoided since these patients do not require chest tube placement for resolution of the infection. Of importance, not all patients with spontaneous bacterial pleuritis have spontaneous bacterial peritonitis.

To establish the diagnosis of spontaneous bacterial pleuritis, it is necessary to obtain the following tests:

- Pleural fluid culture
- Pleural fluid neutrophil count

A pleural fluid neutrophil count >250 cells/µL is supportive of the diagnosis. A positive pleural fluid culture corroborates the diagnosis of spontaneous bacterial pleuritis. Culture-negative spontaneous bacterial pleuritis is diagnosed if the pleural fluid neutrophil count is >500 cells/µL but the culture is negative.

Nephrotic Syndrome

The incidence of pleural effusion in patients with nephrotic syndrome is high. In one study of 52 patients with nephrotic syndrome, 21% of these patients were found to have pleural effusions. A diagnostic thoracentesis is warranted in all patients with nephrotic syndrome who present with a pleural effusion to demonstrate that the effusion is indeed a transudate.

The clinician should realize, however, that the nephrotic syndrome may be complicated by pulmonary embolism. The pleural effusion of pulmonary embolism may also be transudative. For this reason, many authorities recommend ventilation/perfusion lung scan or spiral CT in all patients with nephrotic syndrome who have a transudative pleural effusion to differentiate between nephrotic syndrome and nephrotic syndrome complicated by pulmonary embolism.

References

Johnson JL, "Pleural Effusions in Cardiovascular Disease. Pearls for Correlating the Evidence With the Cause," *Postgrad Med*, 2000, 107(4):95-101, quiz 257.

Kinasewitz GT, "Transudative Effusions," *Eur Respir J*, 1997, 10(3):714-8.

Kinasewitz GT and Keddissi JI, "Hepatic Hydrothorax," *Curr Opin Pulm Med*, 2003, 9(4):261-5.

Lazaridis KN, Frank JW, Krowka MJ, et al, "Hepatic Hydrothorax: Pathogenesis, Diagnosis, and Management," *Am J Med*, 1999, 107(3):262-7.

Light RW, "Pleural Effusions Due to Pulmonary Emboli," *Curr Opin Pulm Med*, 2001, 7(4):198-201.

Light RW, "Useful Tests on the Pleural Fluid in the Management of Patients With Pleural Effusions," *Curr Opin Pulm Med*, 1999, 5(4):245-9.

Tam AC and Lapworth R, "Biochemical Analysis of Pleural Fluid: What Should We Measure?" *Ann Clin Biochem*, 2001, 38(Pt 4):311-22.

EXUDATIVE PLEURAL EFFUSIONS

Causes of Exudative Pleural Effusions

The causes of exudative pleural effusion are listed in the following box.

CAUSES OF EXUDATIVE PLEURAL EFFUSION	
MALIGNANCY	INFECTION
Metastatic pleural disease	Bacterial pneumonia
Mesothelioma	Tuberculous pleuritis
Body cavity lymphoma	Viral
PULMONARY EMBOLISM	*Mycoplasma*
GASTROINTESTINAL DISEASE	Actinomycosis
Acute pancreatitis	Nocardiosis
Chronic pancreatitis	Fungal disease
Intra-abdominal abscess	Histoplasmosis
Bilious pleural effusion	Coccidioidomycosis
Diaphragmatic hernia	Aspergillosis
Liver transplantation	Blastomycosis
Postabdominal surgery	Cryptococcosis
Endoscopic variceal sclerotherapy	Parasitic disease
POSTCARDIAC INJURY SYNDROME	Paragonimiasis
HEMOTHORAX	Amebiasis
CHYLOTHORAX	Echinococcosis
DRUG-INDUCED PLEURAL DISEASE	*Pneumocystis carinii*
Nitrofurantoin	MISCELLANEOUS
Dantrolene	Uremia
Methysergide	Lung transplantation
Bromocriptine	Bone marrow transplantation
Procarbazine	Asbestos exposure
Amiodarone	Sarcoidosis
Ergot alkaloids	Therapeutic radiation exposure
Interleukin-2	Yellow-nail syndrome
Methotrexate	Extramedullary hematopoiesis
Clozapine	Urinary tract obstruction
CONNECTIVE TISSUE DISEASE	Meig's syndrome
Pleural effusion of rheumatoid arthritis	Endometriosis
Lupus arthritis	Ovarian hyperstimulation syndrome
Churg-Strauss syndrome	Iatrogenic
Wegener's granulomatosis	Misplaced percutaneously placed catheter
Immunoblastic lymphadenopathy	Misplaced nasogastric tube
Sjögren's syndrome	Translumbar aortographic examination
Familial Mediterranean fever	Trapped lung

Adapted from Light R, *Pleural Diseases*, 4th ed, Philadelphia, PA: Lippincott Williams and Wilkins, 2001, 88.

The clinical and laboratory features of some of the more common causes of exudative pleural effusion will be discussed in further detail in the remainder of this chapter. For more information regarding the various tests available to elucidate the etiology of an exudative effusion, please refer to the chapter, ***Pleural Fluid Analysis*** *on page 425*.

Parapneumonic Effusion / Empyema

Parapneumonic effusion is defined as any pleural effusion that is associated with bacterial pneumonia or lung abscess. It is the most common cause of exudative pleural effusion in the United States. Bacterial pneumonia is commonly accompanied by pleural effusion, occurring in 40% to 60% of cases. In many of these cases, the effusion is clinically insignificant, not requiring thoracentesis, and resolving with appropriate treatment of the bacterial pneumonia. The clinician, however, must be able to differentiate these patients with uncomplicated parapneumonic effusion from patients with complicated parapneumonic effusion or empyema. The term "complicated" is used to describe parapneumonic effusions that do not resolve without chest tube placement. Empyema is defined as the presence of gross pus within the pleural space.

Failure to make the distinction between uncomplicated parapneumonic effusion and complicated parapneumonic effusion or empyema can have grave consequences for the patient. Although the possibility of complicated parapneumonic effusion and empyema should be considered in every patient presenting with bacterial pneumonia and pleural effusion, not all patients with bacterial pneumonia and pleural effusion require thoracentesis. To decide whether or not the patient requires thoracentesis, it is useful to determine the amount of free pleural fluid present on a lateral decubitus chest radiograph. The amount of free pleural fluid can be determined by measuring the distance between the inside chest wall and outside the lung. If this distance is <10 mm, the effusion can be considered clinically insignificant and therefore does not require thoracentesis. If the distance is >10 mm, however, it is possible that a complicated parapneumonic effusion or empyema is present. These patients require thoracentesis to establish or exclude complicated parapneumonic effusion or empyema.

Analysis of pleural fluid in patients with bacterial pneumonia will allow the clinician to determine whether or not the patient has a complicated parapneumonic effusion or empyema, which would require placement of a chest tube for resolution of the infection. If the decision is made to perform thoracentesis in the patient with bacterial pneumonia, the following studies of the pleural fluid should be obtained:

- Protein level
- LDH concentration
- Glucose level
- pH
- Amylase level
- Cell count and differential
- Gram stain
- Aerobic and anaerobic bacterial cultures

If gross pus is obtained during pleural fluid analysis, the patient is said to have an empyema. Patients with empyema require chest tube placement. If gross pus is not obtained, the clinician still needs to differentiate a complicated from uncomplicated pleural effusion. In the following box, pleural fluid parameters that can help the clinician make this distinction are listed.

BAD PROGNOSTIC SIGNS FOR PARAPNEUMONIC EFFUSIONS AND EMPYEMA*
PUS PRESENT IN PLEURAL SPACE
GRAM STAIN OF PLEURAL FLUID POSITIVE
PLEURAL FLUID GLUCOSE <40 mg/dL
PLEURAL FLUID CULTURE POSITIVE
PLEURAL FLUID pH <7.0
PLEURAL FLUID LDH >3x UPPER LIMIT OF NORMAL FOR SERUM
PLEURAL FLUID LOCULATED

*Listed in order of decreasing importance.

Adapted from Light R, *Pleural Diseases*, 4th ed, Philadelphia, PA: Lippincott Williams and Wilkins, 2001.

The results of these pleural fluid tests can be categorized to provide the clinician with guidance regarding the most appropriate treatment for the parapneumonic effusion, as shown in the following table.

Class	Pleural Fluid Characteristics	Recommended Management
Class 1: Nonsignificant pleural effusion	Small (<10 mm thick on decubitus x-ray study)	No thoracentesis indicated
Class 2: Typical parapneumonic pleural effusion	More than 10 mm thick; glucose >40 mg/dL; pH >7.2; LDH <3x upper limit of normal for serum; Gram stain negative; culture negative	Antibiotics alone
Class 3: Borderline complicated pleural effusion	7.0 < pH < 7.20 and/or LDH >3x upper limit of normal and glucose >40 mg/day; Gram stain negative; culture negative	Antibiotics plus serial thoracentesis
Class 4: Simple complicated pleural effusion	pH <7.0 or glucose <40 mg/dL or Gram stain or culture positive; not loculated, not frank pus	Tube thoracostomy plus antibiotics
Class 5: Complex complicated pleural effusion	pH <7.0 and/or glucose <40 mg/dL or Gram stain or culture positive; multiloculated	Tube thoracostomy plus fibrinolytics (rarely require thoracoscopy or decortication)
Class 6: Simple empyema	Frank pus present; single locule or free flowing	Tube thoracostomy ± decortication
Class 7: Complex empyema	Frank pus present; multiple locules	Tube thoracostomy ± fibrinolytics

Adapted from Light R, *Pleural Diseases*, 4th ed, Philadelphia, PA: Lippincott Williams and Wilkins, 2001, 163.

Malignant Pleural Effusion

Among the causes of an exudative pleural effusion, malignancy is second only to infection. Although almost every type of malignancy has been associated with the development of a pleural effusion, three neoplasms account for 75% of malignant pleural effusions. These include lung cancer (30%), breast cancer (25%), and lymphoma (20%). Metastatic ovarian cancer and sarcoma are responsible for 6% and 3% of malignant pleural effusions, respectively. Of note, in about 6% of patients, the primary tumor is never identified.

While 20% of patients with malignant pleural effusion are asymptomatic at the time of diagnosis, more often, these patients present with symptoms such as dyspnea (>50%) or chest pain (25%). Contrary to popular belief, the chest pain of malignant pleural effusion is more commonly dull and aching rather than pleuritic in nature. Quite often, constitutional symptoms such as anorexia, fatigue, malaise, and weight loss are present. Signs and symptoms of the underlying malignancy may also be present.

The pleural effusion of malignancy may vary from small to massive in size. In these latter cases, the effusion may occupy the entire hemithorax. When the pleural effusion is this large, a shift in the mediastinum to the contralateral side is usually noted. If the mediastinum is not shifted to the contralateral side, the clinician should give consideration to the presence of one of the following possibilities:

- Bronchogenic carcinoma causing obstruction of main-stem bronchus
- Malignant mesothelioma
- Fixed mediastinum due to tumor involvement

The chest radiograph may also be helpful in elucidating the etiology of the malignant pleural effusion. A parenchymal abnormality is usually present in patients with bronchogenic carcinoma. However, it may not be apparent in patients with massive pleural effusion until a therapeutic thoracentesis has been performed. The presence of a parenchymal abnormality in no way clinches the diagnosis of bronchogenic carcinoma as other cancers may present with metastases to the lung parenchyma.

In cases of malignant pleural effusion due to lung cancer, the pleural effusion usually develops on the same side as the cancer but, on occasion, it may be bilateral. In patients with breast cancer complicated by malignant pleural effusion, the effusion is on the same side as the breast cancer in approximately 60% of patients. It may be contralateral to the breast cancer in 25% and bilateral in about 15% of patients.

The third most common cause of malignant pleural effusion is lymphoma. Both non-Hodgkin's and Hodgkin's lymphoma may be complicated by the development of malignant pleural effusion. In fact, about 15% of patients with non-Hodgkin's or Hodgkin's lymphoma have pleural effusion at some point in their disease course. In most cases, the pleural effusion is present at the time of diagnosis. In these cases, there is almost always evidence of lymphoma elsewhere. In Hodgkin's lymphoma, 90% of patients with malignant pleural effusion will have associated mediastinal lymphadenopathy. Up to 70% of patients with non-Hodgkin's lymphoma with malignant pleural effusion will have mediastinal involvement.

Examination of the pleural fluid is consistent with an exudative pleural effusion. The clinician should seriously consider malignancy when only the absolute LDH concentration (but not the protein or LDH ratio) meets exudative criteria. The pleural fluid laboratory features of malignant pleural effusion are listed in the following box.

PLEURAL FLUID LABORATORY TEST ABNORMALITIES SUPPORTIVE OF MALIGNANT PLEURAL EFFUSION
EXUDATIVE BY LIGHT'S CRITERIA
GROSS APPEARANCE* – Bloody or nonbloody
CELL COUNT – Normal or elevated
DIFFERENTIAL
Lymphocytic predominance most common (45%)
Less commonly other mononuclear cells (40%) or neutrophils (15%) predominate
Eosinophilia may also be noted
GLUCOSE† – Normal or low
pH‡ – Normal or low
AMYLASE# – Normal or high

*It has classically been taught that bloody effusions are the rule in patients with malignant pleural effusion. While malignancy is likely to be the most common cause of grossly bloody pleural effusion, approximately 50% of cases are not characterized by the presence of bloody pleural fluid.

†Glucose levels <60 mg/dL have been described in approximately 20% of patients.

‡Low pleural fluid pH has also been described in malignant pleural effusions (33% of patients have pH <7.30). In general, low pleural fluid pH is usually accompanied by low pleural fluid glucose levels. These pleural fluid findings are usually indicative of large tumor burden within the pleural space and portend a poor prognosis, with a mean survival of 1-2 months.

#Amylase levels are increased in about 10% of patients with malignant pleural effusions. An elevated amylase level in a patient with malignant pleural effusion can be due to pancreatic or nonpancreatic cancer.

The above laboratory tests may support the diagnosis of malignant pleural effusion but the definitive diagnosis rests upon the demonstration of malignant cells in the pleural fluid or in the pleura itself. In most cases, the diagnosis is established by pleural fluid cytology. Pleural fluid cytology has been found to be positive in 40% to 87% of patients. This, of course, depends upon the following factors.

- Type of malignancy

  Pleural fluid cytology will be positive in most cases of metastatic adenocarcinoma but are unlikely to be diagnostic in patients with squamous cell carcinoma. In patients with Hodgkin's disease, pleural fluid cytology is positive in approximately 25% of patients. The yield is higher in patients with non-Hodgkin's lymphoma (50% to 60%). It is important to note that the cytologic exam only establishes the presence of malignant pleural effusion; in most cases, it cannot identify the primary site of the tumor.

- Skill of cytologist

- Mechanism of malignant pleural effusion

  The yield of cytology is also dependent upon the mechanism of the malignant pleural effusion. Mechanisms by which cancer leads to the development of pleural effusion are listed in the following box.

MECHANISMS BY WHICH MALIGNANT DISEASE LEADS TO PLEURAL EFFUSION
DIRECT RESULT
Pleural metastases with increased permeability
Pleural metastases with obstruction of pleural lymphatic vessels
Mediastinal lymph node involvement with decreased pleural lymphatic drainage
Thoracic duct interruption (chylothorax)
Bronchial obstruction (decreased pleural pressures
Pericardial involvement
INDIRECT RESULT
Hypoproteinemia
Postobstructive pneumonitis
Pulmonary embolism
Postradiation therapy

Adapted from Light R, *Pleural Diseases*, 4th ed, Philadelphia, PA: Lippincott Williams and Wilkins, 2001, 110.

As shown in the above box, there are many mechanisms of pleural effusion in patients with malignancy. Pleural fluid cytology will be of lower yield in patients who do not have direct pleural metastases.

- Number of pleural fluid specimens submitted

  Eighty percent of patients with malignant pleural effusion will be diagnosed if three separate pleural fluid specimens are submitted for cytologic analysis.

- Extent of tumor

  Those who have a higher tumor burden in the pleural space are more likely to have positive cytologic studies.

Pleural fluid cytology is superior to needle biopsy of the pleura (40% to 87% vs 39% to 75%) in the diagnosis of malignant pleural effusion. Studies have shown that needle biopsy of the pleura is diagnostic of malignant pleural effusion in only 20% of patients with malignant pleural effusion who have negative cytology. In recent years, needle biopsy of the pleura has been supplanted by thoracoscopy so much so that needle biopsy is only recommended if thoracoscopy is unavailable. Thoracoscopy will allow the clinician to establish the diagnosis of malignancy in about 90% of patients with malignancy.

Should all patients with an undiagnosed exudative effusion and negative pleural fluid cytology be referred for thoracoscopy? Prior to considering thoracoscopy in these patients, many experts recommend obtaining a spiral CT scan of the chest. The spiral CT scan of the chest may reveal one of the following:

- Pulmonary emboli (establishes diagnosis of pulmonary embolism)
- Parenchymal lesions
- Findings consistent with mesothelioma

If parenchymal lesions are noted, the clinician should refer the patient for bronchoscopy. If the CT scan findings are suggestive of mesothelioma, thoracoscopy is indicated to establish the diagnosis. If the CT scan is unrevealing (no other findings except pleural effusion), the decision to proceed with thoracoscopy should be based upon the patient's clinical presentation. The clinician should perform thoracoscopy if any of the following criteria are met:

- Patient's symptoms are worsening
- Clinical presentation is consistent with malignancy

If thoracoscopy is indicated but not available, the clinician may wish to proceed with needle biopsy of the pleura or thoracotomy with open pleural biopsy. The clinician may forego thoracoscopy if the patient's symptoms are improving and there is no evidence to support malignancy in the patient's clinical presentation.

In most cases, the diagnosis of malignant pleural effusion is made in a patient with known history of malignancy. On occasion, however, a malignant pleural effusion may be the initial manifestation of malignancy. If the patient has symptoms or signs suggestive of malignancy, an appropriate investigation should be pursued. When the primary site of the tumor is unknown, the clinician should obtain a CT scan of the chest, abdomen, and pelvis. Mammography and pelvic exam should be performed in women. If the site of the primary tumor remains unclear after this workup, no further investigation is recommended.

Tuberculous Pleuritis

Although tuberculous pleuritis can present as a chronic illness, most patients have acute disease characterized by nonproductive cough (70%) and chest pain (75%), which is frequently pleuritic. Fever is commonly present but a normal temperature should not exclude the diagnosis.

The chest radiograph usually reveals a unilateral effusion of varying size. Coexisting parenchymal lung disease is only present in approximately 20% of patients. When present, the radiographic lesions are usually on the same side as the effusion.

It is important to realize that a negative PPD does not exclude the diagnosis of tuberculous pleuritis. If the initial PPD is negative, the clinician may choose to repeat the test at least 8 weeks after symptom onset. A negative repeat PPD at this time argues against the diagnosis unless the patient has HIV or is severely malnourished.

Examination of pleural fluid is essential in establishing the diagnosis of tuberculous pleuritis. Pleural fluid laboratory findings are listed in the following box.

PLEURAL FLUID LABORATORY FINDINGS IN TUBERCULOUS PLEURITIS
EXUDATIVE EFFUSION
TOTAL PROTEIN CONCENTRATION >5 g/dL
DIFFERENTIAL CELL COUNT
>50% with lymphocytic predominance
Possible PMN predominance if symptoms present <2 weeks
Eosinophils >10% argue strongly against diagnosis
Mesothelial cells >5% argue strongly against diagnosis

Although the above pleural fluid findings are supportive of the diagnosis of tuberculous pleuritis, establishing the diagnosis definitively requires the performance of one or more of the following tests.

- Pleural fluid ADA level

  In one study, all patients with tuberculous pleuritis had pleural fluid ADA levels >70 units/L. A pleural fluid level <40 units/L argues strongly against the diagnosis of tuberculous pleuritis. Other causes of pleural effusion that may be associated with increased pleural fluid ADA levels include rheumatoid arthritis, malignancy, and empyema.

  The specificity of an increased pleural fluid ADA level for the diagnosis of tuberculous pleuritis can be increased if this finding is combined with a pleural fluid lymphocyte:neutrophil ratio >0.75. If both are present, most experts feel that the diagnosis of tuberculous pleuritis is established. A presumptive diagnosis of tuberculous pleuritis can be established if the pleural fluid ADA level is between 40 and 70 units/L and the lymphocyte:neutrophil ratio >0.75. In this group of patients, the clinician should consider needle biopsy or thoracoscopy of the pleura if the clinical presentation is not consistent with tuberculous pleuritis.

Tuberculous pleuritis is highly unlikely if the pleural fluid ADA level is <40 units/L. This finding should prompt the clinician to consider other causes of exudative pleural effusion. Even in these patients, the clinician may wish to consider needle biopsy or thoracoscopy of the pleura if the clinical presentation is suggestive of tuberculous pleuritis.

- Pleural fluid interferon-gamma level

  In one study, 33 of 35 patients with tuberculous pleuritis had interferon-gamma levels >140 pg/mL. Testing of pleural fluid for interferon-gamma is more expensive than pleural fluid ADA testing, but may be more readily available.

- PCR

  In recent years, there has been much interest in PCR testing of pleural fluid for the diagnosis of tuberculous pleuritis. Currently, PCR testing is not superior to ADA or interferon-gamma levels.

- Acid-fast smear of pleural fluid

  The yield of acid-fast smears of the pleural fluid is low in immunocompetent patients with tuberculous pleuritis unless tuberculous empyema is present. In HIV patients with tuberculous pleuritis, acid-fast smears may be positive in approximately 20%.

- Pleural fluid culture for mycobacteria

  A pleural fluid culture is indicated in all patients suspected of having tuberculous pleuritis. Cultures of both sputum and pleural fluid should be obtained. Pleural fluid culture is positive for *M. tuberculosis* in <40% of patients.

- Pleural biopsy

  For years, needle biopsy of the pleura has been the test of choice for establishing the diagnosis of tuberculous pleuritis. When granulomas are seen on histologic examination of tissue obtained by pleural biopsy, one can make a strong argument for the diagnosis. While it is true that there are other causes of granulomatous pleuritis (fungal disease, sarcoidosis, tularemia, rheumatoid arthritis), >95% of patients found to have granulomas have tuberculous pleuritis. If granulomas are not demonstrated, the clinician should perform an acid-fast smear on the specimen because, on occasion, the acid-fast smear may reveal the tuberculous organisms when granulomas are not identified. Culture of the biopsy specimen is positive in about 55% of patients. Recently, needle biopsy of the pleura has been supplanted, to some extent, by sensitive tests such as pleural fluid ADA. One advantage of pleural biopsy over ADA levels is that biopsy will provide specimen for culture. This allows the clinician to determine sensitivity of the organisms to the various antituberculous agents.

Pulmonary Embolism

In most studies, pulmonary embolism has been noted to account for <5% of cases of pleural effusion. This figure is likely to be a gross underestimate, however. Autopsy studies have shown that many cases of pulmonary embolism are not diagnosed until the time of autopsy. It is likely that many cases of undiagnosed pleural effusion are due to pulmonary embolism.

In the PIOPED study, 56% of patients with pulmonary embolism presenting with pleuritic chest pain or hemoptysis had a pleural effusion. Fewer patients with pulmonary embolism presenting with dyspnea alone had a pleural effusion (26%). Parenchymal abnormalities may or may not be present on the chest radiograph in patients with pulmonary embolism who present with pleural effusion. When present, parenchymal abnormalities usually have the following characteristics:

- Lower lobe location
- Pleural based
- Convex towards the hilum

Pleural effusions seen in pulmonary embolism tend to be small and usually unilateral. Pleural fluid analysis in patients with pleural effusion secondary to pulmonary embolism does not allow the clinician to establish the diagnosis. This is because the pleural fluid findings can vary widely. Both transudative and exudative pleural effusions have been described in patients with pulmonary embolism. The pleural red and white blood cell counts are not helpful in differentiating pulmonary embolism from other causes of pleural effusion. The differential white blood cell count may reveal a predominance of PMNs or lymphocytes. Despite the fact that pleural fluid analysis is not diagnostic of pulmonary embolism, a thoracentesis should be done to exclude other causes of pleural effusion.

When the etiology of a transudative or exudative pleural effusion remains unclear, an evaluation for pulmonary embolism is warranted. Even when a transudative pleural effusion is present in the patient with congestive heart failure, the clinician should consider the possibility of pulmonary embolism. Remember that congestive heart failure is a risk factor for pulmonary embolism. Pulmonary embolism should especially be a consideration in congestive heart failure patients who present with a unilateral effusion. It should also be a consideration in those with bilateral effusions, particularly when there is a disparity in size between the two effusions.

The ventilation/perfusion scan is difficult to interpret in patients with pulmonary embolism who present with a pleural effusion. In these cases, the utility of the ventilation/perfusion scan in the diagnosis of pulmonary embolism is improved if a therapeutic thoracentesis is performed prior to the scan. Because of the difficulty of interpreting ventilation/perfusion scans in patients with pulmonary embolism who have pleural effusions, clinicians are now turning to spiral CT scans in order to make the diagnosis. Since most pulmonary emboli originate in the deep venous system of the legs, the clinician may also choose to perform studies of the leg veins (ultrasound, impedance plethysmography, venography). When the results of these studies are unrevealing or equivocal, pulmonary angiography should be considered.

Chylothorax

Chylothorax should be considered whenever milky or turbid fluid is obtained during a thoracentesis. When such a specimen is obtained, the clinician should have the laboratory centrifuge the specimen. If the supernatant clears, the cause of the cloudiness is probably increased cellularity. Persistence of cloudiness after centrifugation is indicative of high lipid content within the pleural fluid. There are two situations in which the pleural fluid may contain high amounts of lipid.

1. Chylothorax or chylous effusion

   Chylothorax develops when there is a disruption of the thoracic duct. This disruption leads to the accumulation of chyle in the pleural space.

2. Pseudochylothorax or chyliform effusion

   Pseudochylothorax typically develops in the setting of a long-standing pleural effusion. The milky appearance of the pleural fluid is due to the presence of lecithin-globulin complexes.

It is usually not difficult to distinguish chylothorax from pseudochylothorax based on the patient's clinical presentation. Pseudochylothorax usually develops in the setting of a long-standing pleural effusion (>5 years). It is also characterized by the presence of markedly thickened or calcified pleura which is not usually seen in patients with chylothorax. Examination of the pleural fluid may reveal cholesterol crystals, consistent with the diagnosis of pseudochylothorax. Not all patients, however, will be demonstrated to have cholesterol crystals; therefore, the absence of these crystals does not exclude the diagnosis.

When difficulty remains in differentiating chylothorax from pseudochylothorax, the clinician can obtain triglyceride and cholesterol levels in both the serum and pleural fluid. Chylothorax is the probable diagnosis if the following criteria are met:

- Pleural fluid triglyceride level >110 mg/dL
- Ratio of pleural fluid to serum triglyceride level >1.0
- Ratio of pleural fluid to serum cholesterol level <1.0

If uncertainty remains, the clinician may wish to perform a lipoprotein analysis of the pleural fluid. A lipoprotein analysis that reveals the presence of chyle in the pleural fluid establishes the diagnosis of chylothorax. Once the presence of a chylothorax has been established, the clinician should search for the etiology. The causes of chylothorax are listed in the following box.

CAUSES OF CHYLOTHORAX

MALIGNANCY*	MISCELLANEOUS
TRAUMA	High translumbar aortography
Penetrating	Esophagoscopy
Nonpenetrating	Stellate ganglion blockade
SURGERY†	Weight lifting
Cardiovascular	Straining
Thoracic	Severe coughing or vomiting
Esophageal resection	Childbirth
Thoracic sympathectomy	Vigorous stretching while yawning
Cervical node dissection	Intestinal lymphangiectasia
Pneumonectomy	SVC thrombosis
Spinal surgery	Subclavian thrombosis
CHYLOUS ASCITES	Filariasis
(movement of fluid through diaphragm)	Mediastinal tuberculosis
PULMONARY LYMPHANGIOMYOMATOSIS	Lymphangitis of thoracic duct
IDIOPATHIC	Lymph node enlargement
	Tuberous sclerosis
	Amyloidosis
	Gorham's syndrome

*Malignancy is the most common cause of chylothorax, accounting for >50% of cases. The majority of these cases are secondary to lymphoma.

†Surgery is also a common cause of chylothorax. There is a 0.5% incidence of chylothorax development following cardiovascular surgery. In particular, surgery that involves mobilization of the left subclavian artery is more likely to be complicated by chylothorax.

Of major importance is an evaluation for malignancy, particularly lymphoma, since this is the most common cause of chylothorax. In women, the possibility of pulmonary lymphangiomyomatosis should always be considered. In general, CT scan of the mediastinum and abdomen is recommended in all patients with nontraumatic chylothorax (in the absence of a clear etiology). The clinician may also consider lymphangiography in the evaluation of these patients.

Pseudochylothorax

Pseudochylothorax, also known as a chyliform effusion, is less common than chylothorax. It should be considered whenever pleural fluid aspiration reveals a turbid or milky pleural fluid. In these cases, the clinician should centrifuge the specimen. When the cloudiness clears, the likely diagnosis of the cloudiness is increased cellularity. Persistence of the cloudiness after centrifugation warrants consideration of chylothorax or pseudochylothorax. The features used to distinguish these two causes of an exudative pleural effusion have already been discussed above under chylothorax. Although some patients with pseudochylothorax have cholesterol crystals that can be seen with microscopic analysis of the pleural fluid, the absence of these crystals does not exclude the diagnosis. A pleural fluid cholesterol level >250 mg/dL supports the diagnosis of pseudochylothorax.

Hemothorax

Hemothorax is defined as a pleural fluid hematocrit that is at least 50% of the peripheral blood hematocrit. A pleural fluid hematocrit should be obtained in every patient who is found to have bloody fluid during a thoracentesis. It is important to establish the diagnosis of hemothorax since chest tube placement is indicated in many cases.

Once the presence of hemothorax has been established, the clinician should consider the causes of hemothorax. These causes are listed in the following box.

CAUSES OF HEMOTHORAX
TRAUMA
Penetrating
Nonpenetrating
IATROGENIC
Thoracic surgery
Perforation of central vein or artery secondary to percutaneously inserted catheter
Leaking from aorta after translumbar aortographic study
Thoracentesis
Endoscopic esophageal variceal therapy
Pleural biopsy
NONTRAUMATIC
Metastatic pleural disease
Anticoagulation (in patients with or without pulmonary embolism)
Aortic aneurysm rupture
Rupture of pulmonary artery aneurysm
Patent ductus arteriosus
Aortic coarctation
Bleeding disorder - hemophilia, thrombocytopenia
Spontaneous pneumothorax
Thoracic endometriosis
Bronchopulmonary sequestration
Chickenpox pneumonia
Intrathoracic extramedullary hematopoiesis
Rupture of splenic artery aneurysm (through diaphragm)
IDIOPATHIC

Esophageal Perforation

Esophageal perforation deserves consideration in every patient with an exudative pleural effusion. This is because a delay in the diagnosis and treatment of esophageal perforation can have grave consequences for the patient. Sixty percent of patients with esophageal perforation have an accompanying pleural effusion. Although most are left-sided, patients may also have bilateral or right-sided effusions.

Patients are acutely ill with symptoms of chest pain, epigastric pain, or shortness of breath. Over 50% of patients report small amounts of hematemesis. Physical exam may reveal subcutaneous emphysema of the suprasternal notch. While this finding is very suggestive of esophageal perforation, the absence of this finding in no way excludes the diagnosis. In one study, subcutaneous emphysema was present in <10% of patients within the first 4 hours after symptom onset. Cases of esophageal perforation that follow esophagoscopy often are not realized by the endoscopist during the procedure. Several hours may pass before symptoms of chest or epigastric pain begin.

The pleural fluid amylase is the best test to obtain in patients suspected of having esophageal perforation because almost all patients will have an elevation in the amylase level. The pH of the pleural fluid is usually <7.00. The diagnosis can be established by contrast studies of the esophagus.

Acute Pancreatitis

The development of a pleural effusion is quite common in acute pancreatitis, occurring in up to 60% of patients. The pleural effusion may be bilateral (77%), left-sided (15%), or right-sided (8%). Interestingly, acute pancreatitis patients who do develop a pleural effusion are likely to have more severe disease. Many of these patients go on to form pancreatic pseudocysts.

The abdominal complaints of acute pancreatitis usually overshadow the pleural effusion. On occasion, however, patients may develop symptoms related to the pleural effusion, such as pleuritic chest pain and shortness of breath, that dominate the clinical picture. For precisely this reason, all acutely ill patients with an exudative pleural effusion should have measurement of the pleural fluid amylase level. An increased amylase level is supportive of the diagnosis so long as esophageal perforation has been excluded. The differential cell count often reveals a neutrophilic predominance.

The pleural effusion of pancreatitis usually resolves with treatment of the acute pancreatitis. Pancreatic abscess or pseudocyst should be considered if the effusion persists for longer than 2 weeks.

Chronic Pancreatitis

Chronic pancreatic disease as the etiology of pleural effusion is not as well recognized as acute pancreatitis. Most patients with chronic pancreatic disease who develop pleural effusion have a pancreatic pseudocyst. Unlike the patient with acute pancreatitis, most of these patients have symptoms related to the pleural effusion, including shortness of breath, cough, and chest pain. The majority do not have abdominal complaints. The lack of abdominal symptoms plays a large role in the delay in diagnosis in patients with pleural effusion secondary to chronic pancreatic disease.

In contrast to acute pancreatitis, the effusion of chronic pancreatitis is often massive. It is usually left-sided but may be right-sided or even bilateral. Establishing the diagnosis requires measuring the pleural fluid amylase level. Of course, an elevation in the amylase level is not entirely specific for pancreatic disease. The main consideration in the differential diagnosis is malignancy. However, patients with increased pleural fluid amylase levels due to malignancy usually have a less impressive elevation in the pleural fluid amylase level when compared to chronic pancreatic disease. If diagnostic confusion remains, the clinician may wish to obtain amylase isoenzymes. In malignancy, the increase in the pleural fluid amylase is due to the salivary isoenzyme. Further evaluation in patients with pleural effusion secondary to chronic pancreatitis may include ultrasound or CT scan of the abdomen to identify the pseudocyst.

Intra-abdominal Abscess

Pleural effusion is quite common in patients with intra-abdominal abscess. Of the different types of intra-abdominal abscess, subphrenic abscess is most commonly associated with the development of pleural effusion. Studies have shown that up to 80% of patients with subphrenic abscess have an accompanying pleural effusion. The approximate incidence of pleural effusion in different types of intra-abdominal abscess is listed in the following table.

Approximate Incidence of Pleural Effusion in Patients With Intra-abdominal Abscess

Type of Intra-Abdominal Abscess	Approximate Incidence of Pleural Effusion
Subphrenic abscess	80%
Pancreatic	40%
Splenic	30%
Intrahepatic	20%

Subphrenic abscess should be suspected in patients who present with fever and abdominal pain 1-3 weeks after surgery. In 10% of patients, however, a history of surgery cannot be elicited. In these patients, the etiology of the subphrenic abscess may be due to perforation of the stomach, duodenum, colon, diverticula, or appendix. In other cases, the abscess may result from acute cholecystitis, pancreatitis, or diverticulitis. Leukocytosis is common.

Fever and abdominal pain, particularly right upper quadrant, are quite common in patients with intrahepatic abscess. Physical exam may reveal a tender, enlarged liver. Leukocytosis, normocytic anemia, and an elevated alkaline phosphatase level are all supportive of the diagnosis.

Pancreatic abscess should be considered in any patient with acute pancreatitis who fails to improve with appropriate therapy. It also deserves consideration if fever, abdominal pain, or leukocytosis develop within 1 month of an episode of acute pancreatitis.

Splenic abscess is rare. The most common cause of splenic abscess is bacterial endocarditis.

In patients with intra-abdominal abscess, the pleural fluid is exudative with a neutrophilic predominance. On occasion, very high white blood cell counts may be appreciated, with counts even >50,000/µL. The pH and glucose are usually >7.20 and 60 mg/dL, respectively.

Bilious Pleural Effusion

Another uncommon cause of exudative pleural effusion is bilious pleural effusion. This type of effusion results from the development of a fistula from the biliary tree to the pleural space. Risk factors for the development of bilious pleural effusion include trauma, surgery, and biliary tract infection. The gross appearance of pleural fluid is often bilious. A ratio of pleural fluid to serum bilirubin >1.0 is consistent with bilious pleural effusion. Of note, there is high incidence of empyema (50%) in patients with bilious pleural effusion.

Rheumatoid Arthritis

Five percent of patients with rheumatoid arthritis develop pleural effusion at some point during their disease course. Pleural effusion tends to have a predilection for male patients. In addition, most patients are older than 35 years of age. Eighty percent of rheumatoid arthritis patients who develop a pleural effusion have subcutaneous nodules on physical exam. Most cases of pleural effusion develop after the diagnosis of rheumatoid arthritis has been established. On occasion, however, the pleural effusion may precede the diagnosis.

Patients may be symptomatic with complaints of shortness of breath, fever, or pleuritic chest pain. The effusion is typically small to moderate in size. In 25% of cases, bilateral effusions are present. In up to 33% of patients, the pleural effusion is accompanied by other pulmonary manifestations of rheumatoid arthritis.

The development of a pleural effusion in a patient with rheumatoid arthritis should always prompt consideration of the diagnosis. Characteristic features of the pleural fluid that support the diagnosis include the following:

- Glucose level <30 mg/dL
- LDH >700 IU/L
- pH <7.20
- Rheumatoid factor >1:320

The major consideration in the differential diagnosis of pleural effusion with the above pleural fluid lab findings is bacterial pneumonia with parapneumonic effusion. For this reason, every patient with rheumatoid arthritis with pleural effusion should have a Gram stain and bacterial culture of the pleural fluid to exclude parapneumonic effusion.

Lupus Pleuritis

Pleural effusions develop in 40% of SLE patients at some point in the disease course. Most of these patients provide a history of arthritis or arthralgia prior to their presentation with pleural effusion. On occasion, the pleural effusion precedes the other manifestation of SLE. Although not all patients are symptomatic, those that are complain of pleuritic chest pain and fever. In many cases, the symptoms of lupus pleuritis occur in conjunction with other symptoms suggestive of lupus exacerbation.

The pleural effusion of lupus pleuritis is usually small. Bilateral pleural effusions are noted in 50% of cases. The diagnosis should be entertained in every patient with an undiagnosed exudative pleural effusion. Differential cell count reveals a predominance of neutrophils or mononuclear cells, depending upon when the thoracentesis is performed. Traditionally, an increased pleural fluid ANA titer has been said to be very supportive of the diagnosis. Recently, however, it has been realized that the ANA is not sensitive or specific for the diagnosis of lupus pleuritis. Therefore, the diagnosis is now based on compatible clinical presentation and supported by serum ANA testing.

References

Ferrer-Sancho J, "Pleural Tuberculosis: Incidence, Pathogenesis, Diagnosis, and Treatment," *Curr Opin Pulm Med*, 1996, 2(4):327-34.

Garcia-Zamalloa A, Ruiz-Irastorza G, Aguayo FJ, et al, "Pseudochylothorax. Report of 2 Cases and Review of the Literature," *Medicine (Baltimore)*, 1999, 78(3):200-7.

Heffner JE, "Infection of the Pleural Space," *Clin Chest Med*, 1999, 20(3):607-22.

Light RW, "Pleural Effusion Due to Pulmonary Emboli," *Curr Opin Pulm Med*, 2001, 7(4):198-201.

Light RW, "The Management of Parapneumonic Effusions and Empyema," *Curr Opin Pulm Med*, 1998, 4(4):227-9.

Perez-Rodriguez E and Jimenez Castro D, "Always Remember Chylothorax," *South Med J*, 1999, 92(8):833-5.

Perez-Rodriguez E and Jimenez Castro D, "The Use of Adenosine Deaminase and Adenosine Deaminase Isoenzymes in the Diagnosis of Tuberculous Pleuritis," *Curr Opin Pulm Med*, 2000, 6(4):259-66.

Putnam JB Jr, "Malignant Pleural Effusions," *Surg Clin North Am*, 2002, 82(4):867-83.

Sasse SA, "Parapneumonic Effusions and Empyema," *Curr Opin Pulm Med*, 1996, 2(4):320-6.

Wang DY, "Diagnosis and Management of Lupus Pleuritis," *Curr Opin Pulm Med*, 2002, 8(4):312-6.

PART V:

NEUROLOGY

CEREBROSPINAL FLUID ANALYSIS

CSF Pressure

Normal CSF opening pressure varies with age and body weight. In general, values <250 mm H20 are considered normal in adults. In young children, 100 mm H20 is often considered to be the upper limit of normal. When measuring the opening pressure, patients should be instructed not to strain or hyperventilate because the opening pressure may be increased and decreased, respectively.

CSF opening pressures less than 60 mm H20 is considered to be low. Such a value satisfies the definition of intracranial hypotension. Previous lumbar puncture and CSF leak due to previous trauma are the major considerations in patients with low CSF opening pressures.

When the CSF opening pressure exceeds 250 mm H20, the patient is said to have intracranial hypertension. Intracranial hypertension is not a diagnosis in and of itself but rather a manifestation of another illness. There are many causes of increased intracranial pressure some of which include malignancy, hemorrhage, and meningitis.

Gross Appearance

CSF is normally clear and colorless. It may become turbid or discolored in pathologic states. Turbidity may reflect the presence of cells, bacteria, or fungi.

CSF may also be discolored by the presence of breakdown products of red blood cells, by increased levels of protein, bilirubin, or other pigments.

In the patient with a subarachnoid hemorrhage, lysis of red blood cells entering the CSF manifests as a yellowish discoloration, or xanthochromia.

CSF Supernatant Colors and Associated Conditions or Causes

Color or Supernatant	Condition or Causes
Yellow	Blood breakdown products (hyperbilirubinemia) CSF protein >150 mg/dL (>1.5 g/L) >100,000 red blood cells/mm^3
Orange	Blood breakdown products High carotenoid ingestion
Pink	Blood breakdown products
Green	Hyperbilirubinemia Purulent CSF
Brown	Meningeal melanomatosis

Adapted from Seehusen DA, *Am Fam Physician*, 2003, 68(6):1103-8.

WBC Count and Differential

While the number of white blood cells varies with age, a count >5 WBCs/mm^3 is clearly abnormal after the age of 10 weeks. The white blood cells normally found in CSF are mononuclear cells (lymphocytes and monocytes). An occasional neutrophil, however, may be appreciated. It is abnormal, however, to have more than 3 neutrophils/mm^3 in adults.

A traumatic tap may cause difficulty in the interpretation of the white blood cell count. In these cases, it may be difficult to distinguish true CSF pleocytosis from white blood cells introduced into the CSF from the peripheral blood by the spinal tap. One option available to the clinician is to repeat the lumbar puncture through another lumbar interspace after a few hours have passed. Since this requires the patient to have a repeat procedure, it is not often done. Another way of making the distinction between true CSF pleocytosis and the introduction of white blood cells into the CSF from a traumatic tap is to obtain a red blood cell count on tubes 1 and 4. A traumatic tap is very likely if the number of red blood cells decreases from tube 1 to tube 4.

A more precise method entails the use of a correction factor. The true number of white blood cells in the CSF may be estimated by taking into account the number of red blood cells present. For every 1000 RBCs/mm^3 counted, one WBC/mm^3 is subtracted from the total CSF white blood cell count. This relationship holds true as long as the peripheral white blood cell and red blood cell counts are normal. If anemia or leukocytosis exists, the formula in the following box should be used.

TRUE WHITE BLOOD CELL COUNT IN CSF PRIOR TO LUMBAR PUNCTURE

$$W = WBC_{CSF} - \frac{WBC_{blood} \times RBC_{CSF}}{RBC_{blood}}$$

Where:
W = Corrected CSF white blood cell count
WBC_{CSF} = WBC count in the CSF as reported by the lab

The cell count may be spuriously low if the count is measured 30-60 minutes after the lumbar puncture is performed. Therefore, it is important for the clinician to transport the specimen to the laboratory as quickly as possible and for the laboratory to analyze the specimen expeditiously.

Whenever the white blood cell count in the CSF is >5 cells/mm^3, pleocytosis is said to exist. The causes of CSF pleocytosis are listed in the following box.

CSF PLEOCYTOSIS DIFFERENTIAL DIAGNOSIS

- INFECTION
  - Bacterial
  - Viral
  - Tuberculous
  - Fungal
  - Protozoal
- INTRACRANIAL LESION NEAR THE SUBARACHNOID SPACE
  - Malignancy
  - Abscess
  - Demyelination
  - Infarct
  - Hemorrhage
  - Vasculitis
- RECENT SEIZURE
- RADIATION THERAPY
- INJECTION OF DRUG INTO THE INTRATHECAL SPACE

While there are both noninfectious and infectious causes of pleocytosis, infection is always a major concern.

When evaluating the patient with a suspected CNS infection, the differential count may provide important information. A preponderance of neutrophils suggests the presence of bacterial meningitis. In fact, adults with bacterial meningitis, on average, have >80% neutrophils. Contrast this with a 30% neutrophil average in patients with aseptic meningitis. The cell count differential alone cannot be used to differentiate bacterial meningitis from other causes of infectious meningitis. While viral, fungal, and tuberculous meningitis usually present with a preponderance of lymphocytes, PMN predominance may be noted early in the course of these infections. Although bacterial meningitis is usually characterized by PMN predominance, a lymphocytic preponderance has been described in as many as 10% of cases, especially early in the course of the infection and when the total white blood cell count is less than 1000 WBC/mm^3.

Normally, CSF does not contain plasma cells. Plasma cells may be appreciated in both infectious and noninfectious conditions. Their presence suggests inflammation, but has little diagnostic significance otherwise.

Normally, CSF does not contain eosinophils. When the CSF contains more than 10 eosinophils/mm^3 or the total CSF white blood cell count consists of more than 10% eosinophils, the patient is said to have eosinophilic meningitis. CSF eosinophilia should raise suspicion for a parasitic infection. However, CSF eosinophils have been demonstrated in noninfectious conditions as well. The causes of CSF eosinophilia are listed in the following box.

CSF EOSINOPHILIA
DIFFERENTIAL DIAGNOSIS

PARASITIC INFECTION
- *Taenia solium*
- *Angiostrongylus cantonensis*
- *Gnathostoma spinigerum*
- *Trichinella spiralis*
- *Toxoplasma gondii*
- *Toxocara cati*
- *Toxocara canis*
- *Ascaris lumbricoides*

OTHER INFECTION
- *Mycobacterium tuberculosis*
- Fungal meningitis
- *Treponema pallidum*
- Rocky Mountain spotted fever
- Lymphocytic choriomeningitis virus
- Subacute sclerosing panencephalitis
- *Mycoplasma pneumoniae*

MALIGNANCY
- Malignant lymphoma
- Leukemia
- Hodgkin's disease

MULTIPLE SCLEROSIS

SUBARACHNOID HEMORRHAGE

OBSTRUCTIVE HYDROCEPHALUS WITH SHUNT

GRANULOMATOUS MENINGITIS

IDIOPATHIC EOSINOPHILIC MENINGITIS

RBC Count

An occasional red blood cell is normal when cerebrospinal fluid is analyzed following a lumbar puncture. If the red blood cell count exceeds 5/mm^3, the patient is said to have an abnormal number of CSF red blood cells.

When a significant number of red blood cells are found in the CSF, considerations such as traumatic tap and subarachnoid hemorrhage come to mind. A number of factors may help the clinician make the distinction between these two causes of increased CSF red blood cell counts:

1. Assessment of fluid color throughout spinal tap

   A traumatic tap is likely if grossly bloody CSF clears as the CSF is being collected.

2. Comparison of red cell number between first and last tubes collected

   If clearing is not evident, the number of red blood cells in tubes 1 and 4 should be compared. A decrease in the number of red blood cells in tube 4, as compared to tube 1, strongly suggests that the tap was traumatic.

3. Presence / absence of xanthochromia

   The presence of xanthochromia (yellowish discoloration) in a specimen centrifuged immediately after collection strongly supports the diagnosis of a subarachnoid hemorrhage. A traumatic lumbar puncture will give rise to a colorless supernatant. If, however, the specimen is allowed to stand for some time before analysis, lysis of red blood cells will occur causing xanthochromia even in a traumatic tap specimen. The causes of CSF xanthochromia are listed in the following box.

CAUSES OF XANTHOCHROMIA

SUBARACHNOID HEMORRHAGE
TRAUMATIC LUMBAR PUNCTURE
DELAYED PROCESSING OF SAMPLE
JAUNDICE (especially bilirubin >4 mg/dL)
CSF PROTEIN >150 mg/dL
PRESENCE OF CAROTENE PIGMENT

   It is important to note that the supernatant usually remains clear for at least 2-4 hours (even up to 12 hours) after the onset of a subarachnoid hemorrhage.

4. Quantity of white blood cells / differential

   Blood that enters the CSF either during a subarachnoid hemorrhage or traumatic tap will contain white blood cells. The number of white blood cells present in the CSF can provide useful information in distinguishing between these two conditions. After a traumatic lumbar puncture, the number of white blood cells, in relation to the number of red blood cells, should mimic that found in peripheral blood. The differential count should be similar as well. In contrast, patients with a subarachnoid hemorrhage often have an increased white blood cell count in the CSF. In addition, the differential usually shows a preponderance of lymphocytes.

Summary: Traumatic Tap vs Subarachnoid Hemorrhage

	Traumatic Tap	Subarachnoid Hemorrhage
Xanthochromia	Absent	Present
Reduction in RBC number from tube 1 to tube 4	Present	Absent
CSF pressure	Normal	Elevated
Spontaneous coagulation	Present	Absent
WBC:RBC ratio	Similar to peripheral blood	Ratio exceeds that of peripheral blood
CSF protein level	Corrected protein level is normal	Corrected protein level remains elevated

Glucose

The normal glucose concentration in the CSF is less than that of the serum. Glucose concentration in the CSF is dependent on the serum glucose level. Because of this, a serum glucose level should always be obtained at the time of a spinal tap. If this is done, then a CSF to serum glucose ratio may be calculated. Since the normal ratio is approximately 0.6, a ratio below this signifies the presence of low CSF glucose.

It is better to rely on this ratio rather than the absolute CSF glucose level. Hyperglycemia, for example, will artificially elevate CSF glucose, and may lull the clinician into believing the CSF glucose concentration is normal, when in fact it is low. The ratio may not be as useful, however, in patients with marked hyperglycemia because CSF glucose levels rarely exceed 300 mg/dL, even in patients with dramatically elevated blood glucose levels. If a serum glucose concentration is not available, then the lower limit of normal of CSF glucose (45 mg/dL) can be used.

When determination of CSF glucose is important, it is best to measure CSF and blood glucose simultaneously, with patients in a fasting state (at least 4 hours without food).

The presence of decreased glucose levels in the CSF is known as hypoglycorrhachia. The differential diagnosis of hypoglycorrhachia is listed in the following box.

HYPOGLYCORRHACHIA DIFFERENTIAL DIAGNOSIS
BACTERIAL MENINGITIS
TUBERCULOUS MENINGITIS
FUNGAL MENINGITIS
CARCINOMATOUS MENINGITIS
SARCOIDOSIS
HYPOGLYCEMIA
SUBARACHNOID HEMORRHAGE
CYSTICERCOSIS
TRICHINELLA MENINGITIS
SYPHILIS (acute)
VIRAL MENINGOENCEPHALITIS*

*While infectious meningitis is a major concern in the patient with hypoglycorrhachia, it is important to recognize that viral infections are usually not characterized by a decrease in the CSF glucose level. There are exceptions to this, however, as low glucose concentrations may be appreciated in patients with meningoencephalitis secondary to mumps, enterovirus, lymphocytic choriomeningitis, herpes simplex, and herpes zoster.

While any of the conditions in the above box may present with hypoglycorrhachia, CSF glucose levels <18 mg/dL are very suggestive of bacterial meningitis.

As patients recover from infectious meningitis, the glucose level tends to return towards normal earlier than the other elements of the CSF including the cell count and protein level. As a result, the glucose concentration is a useful parameter to follow to gauge the response of the patient to therapy.

A normal glucose level does not exclude bacterial meningitis as this finding is noted in up to 50% of cases.

Protein

The upper limit of normal for the CSF protein concentration is usually 40-50 mg/dL. An increased protein concentration is a nonspecific finding, appreciated in many conditions. It can occur in any patient who has a condition that increases permeability of the blood brain barrier, or with a condition that leads to the increased production of local protein. An elevation in the protein concentration >150 mg/dL may result in xanthochromia.

Protein concentration may be spuriously elevated in any condition that causes deterioration of red blood cells. Examples include the introduction of red blood cells in a subarachnoid hemorrhage or after a traumatic tap. A correction factor should be used in these cases. For every 1000 RBCs/mm^3 in the CSF, the protein level will increase by approximately 1 mg/dL. For this to hold true, a normal hemoglobin and serum protein concentration are required. In addition, it is important that the RBC count and CSF protein level be determined on the same tube.

An elevated CSF protein level can occur in both infectious and noninfectious conditions. When CNS infection is suspected, an elevation in the protein concentration has little discriminatory value. In fact, it can even be normal in bacterial meningitis. Some suggest, however, that a viral etiology is very unlikely when the protein level is >220 mg/dL. In fact, most patients with viral meningitis have levels <100 mg/dL. Unlike the CSF glucose levels, the protein concentration may remain elevated during recovery from meningitis. In fact, persistent elevation, lasting weeks or months, has been described in some patients. As a result, the CSF protein concentration has limited usefulness in assessing the patient's response to therapy.

Protein levels >500 mg/dL are infrequent. Such elevations occur mainly in meningitis, spinal block, arachnoiditis, or subarachnoid hemorrhage. A protein concentration >1000 mg/dL suggests the presence of loculation of the CSF, also known as CSF block. The clinician may note very yellow CSF fluid. In addition, it may easily clot because of the presence of fibrinogen. These characteristics satisfy the definition for Froin's syndrome.

Low protein levels may be appreciated in conditions listed in the following box.

LOW PROTEIN LEVELS IN THE CSF DIFFERENTIAL DIAGNOSIS
AGE <2 YEARS
PRESENCE OF CSF EXTRADURAL LEAK
BENIGN INTRACRANIAL HYPERTENSION
HYPERTHYROIDISM
ACUTE WATER INTOXICATION ASSOCIATED WITH INCREASED INTRACRANIAL PRESSURE

References

Blaney SM and Poplack DG, "Neoplastic Meningitis: Diagnosis and Treatment Considerations," *Med Oncol*, 2000, 17(3):151-62.

Coyle PK, "Overview of Acute and Chronic Meningitis," *Neurol Clin*, 1999, 17(4):691-710.

Garcia-Monco JC, "Central Nervous System Tuberculosis," *Neurol Clin*, 1999, 17(4):737-59.

Grossman SA and Krabak MJ, "Leptomeningeal Carcinomatosis," *Cancer Treat Rev*, 1999, 25(2):103-19.

Jerrard DA, Hanna JR, and Schindelheim GL, "Cerebrospinal Fluid," *J Emerg Med*, 2001, 21(2):171-8.

Lo Re V 3rd and Gluckman SJ, "Eosinophilic Meningitis," *Am J Med*, 2003, 114(3):217-23.

Roos KL, "Encephalitis," *Neurol Clin*, 1999, 17(4):813-33.

Roos KL, "Lumbar Puncture," *Semin Neurol*, 2003, 23(1):105-14.

Weber T, "Cerebrospinal Fluid Analysis for the Diagnosis of Human Immunodeficiency Virus-Related Neurologic Diseases," *Semin Neurol*, 1999, 19(2):223-33.

Weisberg LA, "Neurologic Abnormalities in Human Immunodeficiency Virus Infection," *South Med J*, 2001, 94(3):266-75.

Zunt JR and Marra CM, "Cerebrospinal Fluid Testing for the Diagnosis of Central Nervous System Infection," *Neurol Clin*, 1999, 17(4):675-89.

ACUTE BACTERIAL MENINGITIS

In acute bacterial meningitis, bacterial infection causes inflammation of the leptomeninges. To make the diagnosis, the clinician must not only be able to recognize the manifestations of the illness but also be comfortable confirming the diagnosis with CSF analysis. This will ensure that this potentially deadly infection will not go untreated.

Clinical Manifestations

Fever, headache, and neck stiffness are the major symptoms of acute bacterial meningitis. Other symptoms such as nausea, vomiting, and confusion are also often present. Physical exam may reveal meningismus and the presence of meningeal signs (Kernig's and/or Brudzinski).

Laboratory Testing

CBC

Not uncommonly, patients with acute bacterial meningitis will present with a leukocytosis. Examination of the differential count will typically reveal a neutrophilic predominance, often with a shift toward immature cells (left shift). Although the platelet count is often normal, thrombocytopenia may be present. If present, the clinician should consider the possibility of disseminated intravascular coagulation, which can complicate the course of acute bacterial meningitis.

BLOOD CULTURES

Blood cultures should routinely be obtained in patients suspected of having acute bacterial meningitis. Culture results are often positive (50% of cases) and are particularly useful in patients in whom antibiotic therapy was started before lumbar puncture was performed. Of course, cultures are of lower yield if they are obtained after the start of antibiotic therapy.

CSF FINDINGS

Ultimately, the diagnosis of acute bacterial meningitis rests on the examination of the CSF. Before performing lumbar puncture, the clinician should assess the patient for any contraindications to the procedure. Prior to lumbar puncture, CNS imaging tests should be obtained in patients who have papilledema, coma, or focal neurologic findings.

Regardless of the causative bacterial agent, CSF findings are quite similar and are useful in differentiating acute bacterial meningitis from viral meningitis, which is the main consideration in the differential diagnosis. CSF tests that should be obtained include cell count, cell count differential, protein, glucose, Gram stain, and culture. CSF findings include the following:

1. Increased CSF opening pressure

   CSF opening pressure is elevated in almost all patients with acute bacterial meningitis. CSF pressure that exceeds 600 mm H_2O should prompt consideration of cerebral edema, intracranial suppurative foci, or communicating hydrocephalus.

2. Increased CSF white blood cell count

   The CSF white blood cell count in bacterial meningitis typically ranges between 1000-10,000 cells/mm^3, with a median white blood cell count of 1200 cells/mm^3. In contrast, viral meningitis is characterized by a median cell count of 100 cells/mm^3. Investigators have determined that a total WBC >2000 cells/mm^3 is highly predictive of bacterial meningitis.

Lower counts lack diagnostic specificity because of the overlap between bacterial and viral meningitis at these levels. Up to 4% of patients with acute bacterial meningitis may not have CSF pleocytosis. Groups that may not present with pleocytosis include infants, alcoholics, the elderly, and the immunocompromised. Thus, a Gram stain and culture should be performed in all patients suspected of having bacterial meningitis regardless of the cell count.

A cell count <20 cells/mm^3 is associated with a poor prognosis. It is also important to note that the white blood cell count often increases 18-36 hours after the start of antibiotic therapy. This does not imply that the patient is not responding to therapy.

3. Neutrophilic pleocytosis

   In most cases of bacterial meningitis, there is a neutrophilic predominance with neutrophils exceeding 90% to 95% of the total white blood cell count. However, 10% of patients with acute bacterial meningitis present with a lymphocytic predominance. This is more commonly observed with gram-negative organisms, especially in newborns, and *L. monocytogenes.* With *L. monocytogenes,* up to 30% of infections may be characterized by a preponderance of lymphocytes. A lymphocytic predominance is also more likely when the total WBC count is <1000 cells/mm^3. In these cases, the differential may not be as useful in separating bacterial from viral causes of meningitis.

4. Elevated protein level

   The protein concentration is usually elevated in patients with acute bacterial meningitis. In most cases, the protein concentration ranges from 100-500 mg/dL. However, it is not uncommon for the protein concentration to approach 1000 mg/dL. Levels exceeding this value should prompt the clinician to consider the possibility of spinal block. The mean protein level in bacterial meningitis is about 175 mg/dL. Contrast this with a mean of 45 mg/dL in patients with viral meningitis. Investigators maintain that a level >220 mg/dL provides strong evidence for the diagnosis of bacterial meningitis. It should be noted, however, that a normal protein level does not exclude the diagnosis.

5. Decreased glucose level

   It is important to determine the CSF glucose level promptly after lumbar puncture because the level will decrease the longer the specimen sits at room temperature, with potentially misleading results. In patients with acute bacterial meningitis, the glucose level is often decreased. A level <40 mg/dL is noted in 60% of patients.

   Investigators have determined that the CSF:blood glucose ratio is a more reliable measure than the CSF glucose level alone in evaluating patients with acute bacterial meningitis. A ratio <0.31 is found in 70% of cases. The clinician must realize that normal glucose levels do not exclude the diagnosis of bacterial meningitis.

   Note that a minority of patients with viral meningitis will also have low CSF glucose levels. Therefore, a low glucose level does not conclusively differentiate bacterial from viral meningitis.

   The return of the CSF glucose level to normal tends to parallel the improvement in the patient's clinical condition. On occasion, however, the glucose may remain low for up to 10 days.

6. Gram stain / culture

   Whenever acute bacterial meningitis is suspected, a Gram stain should be obtained. Gram stain is useful in directing therapy, providing information well before the results of culture testing become available. The sensitivity of the Gram stain ranges from 60% to 90%, while the specificity approaches 100%. Sensitivity varies depending on the particular organism, as outlined in the following table.

Organism	Sensitivity of Gram Stain
Streptococcus pneumoniae	90%
Staphylococcus aureus	90%
Haemophilus influenzae	85%
Neisseria meningitidis	75%
Gram-negative organisms	>50%
Listeria monocytogenes	<50%
Anaerobic organisms	<50%

Note that acute bacterial meningitis due to *L. monocytogenes* infection often presents with a negative Gram stain. When *Listeria* infection presents with both a negative Gram stain and CSF pleocytosis with lymphocytic predominance (up to 25% to 30% of cases), the clinician may mistakenly make the presumptive diagnosis of viral meningitis. In patients who have risk factors for Listeria infection (ie, elderly, immunocompromised, chronically ill), however, it is best to treat for this infection while waiting for culture results.

If possible, Gram stain should be obtained before instituting antimicrobial therapy. When antimicrobial therapy is started before Gram stain is obtained, it can decrease the diagnostic yield of the study. The clinician should realize, however, that the test may still be positive, even in patients who have received therapy for a few days. In fact, in partially treated cases, Gram stain is positive in 40% to 60% of cases.

Culture is also necessary in all patients suspected of having bacterial meningitis. It is important to realize that up to 10% of patients may have negative CSF cultures despite having a positive Gram stain. As with the Gram stain, the diagnostic yield of the culture is lower when the culture is obtained after the start of antimicrobial therapy. It should still be obtained, however, since it may be positive even in partially treated cases.

7. Lactic acid level

   Many investigators advocate the use of a lactic acid level in differentiating bacterial from nonbacterial meningitis. In one study of patients with acute bacterial meningitis following neurosurgery, the mean CSF lactate levels were higher in cases of proven bacterial meningitis (versus nonbacterial meningitis). Despite data such as this, CSF lactate levels are not often obtained in the evaluation of acute bacterial meningitis, mainly because the information provided by the test results is not perceived to have additional value over the results of standard CSF testing.

8. Counterimmunoelectrophoresis

   Counterimmunoelectrophoresis (CIE) is a rapid diagnostic test that detects bacterial antigens. It has the capability of detecting antigens of the following organisms:

   - *N. meningitidis* (A, C, Y, W135)
   - *H. influenzae* type b
   - *S. pneumoniae*
   - Group B *Streptococcus*
   - *Escherichia coli* K1

Sensitivity of the test ranges from 50% to 95%. The test has fallen out of favor with the development of more sensitive rapid diagnostic tests, such as latex agglutination.

9. Latex agglutination

   Latex agglutination is a more sensitive and rapid test in the diagnosis of acute bacterial meningitis when compared to CIE, and it has the capability of detecting the same organisms detected by CIE. Unfortunately, both CIE and latex agglutination are hindered by the fact that not all bacterial organisms can be detected, limiting their role in the evaluation of the patient with bacterial meningitis. Latex agglutination does play a unique role in the patient with suspected bacterial meningitis who has a negative Gram stain, particularly if lumbar puncture is performed after the institution of antimicrobial therapy. It must be stressed that a negative result does not exclude bacterial meningitis. The sensitivity and specificity of latex agglutination varies with the etiologic organism, as shown in the following table.

Sensitivity and Specificity of Latex Agglutination

	Sensitivity	Specificity
S. pneumoniae	69% to 100%	96%
H. influenzae	78% to 86%	100%
N. meningitidis	33% to 70%	100%

Effect of Antibiotic Treatment on the CSF Parameters in Bacterial Meningitis

CSF findings can certainly be altered in patients with acute bacterial meningitis when antimicrobial therapy is started before performing lumbar puncture. This may cause a considerable amount of diagnostic confusion. Even as little as several doses of antibiotics may seriously impact the yield of the Gram stain and culture. If the etiologic organism is sensitive to the antibiotic, then the Gram stain and culture is often unrevealing 24 hours after the start of antibiotic therapy. During the first 2-3 days, however, antibiotic therapy does not affect the cell count, differential, protein, and glucose levels. These parameters may help the clinician make the diagnosis.

With more prolonged antibiotic therapy, the cell count may decrease and neutrophilic predominance may give way to lymphocytic pleocytosis. In these patients, particularly if the glucose is low, the clinician may be misled into thinking that fungal and tuberculous meningitis are strong possibilities.

The CSF abnormalities that characterize bacterial meningitis return to normal as the patient's clinical condition improves. After 24 hours of antibiotic treatment, CSF cultures are usually negative. The total WBC count often increases during the first day of antibiotic treatment. This should not cause alarm. By day 3 of therapy, most patients have lymphocytic predominance. The parameter that usually returns to normal first is the CSF glucose. However, some patients have depressed glucose levels for more than 10 days despite clinical improvement and normalization of other CSF parameters. A persistently low glucose level in a patient who is improving clinically should not cause concern.

Repeat CSF Analysis in Patients With Bacterial Meningitis

Repeat CSF analysis during or after a course of antibiotic therapy is usually not required. Exceptions to this rule include:

- Infants and children - repeat lumbar puncture is often performed 24-36 hours after starting therapy
- Poor response to therapy
- Signs and symptoms of relapse
- Cases of bacterial meningitis due to resistant organisms
- 48-72 hours after starting therapy in patients with bacterial meningitis due to Gram negative rod infection

References

Thomson RB Jr and Bertram H, "Laboratory Diagnosis of Central Nervous System Infections," *Infect Dis Clin North Am*, 2001, 15(4):1047-71.

ACUTE VIRAL MENINGITIS

Acute viral meningitis is often used synonymously with acute aseptic meningitis. However, it is important to realize that the former is just one type of acute aseptic meningitis. The term "acute aseptic meningitis" refers to the presence of acute meningeal irritation with a sterile CSF. Most cases of acute viral meningitis are benign and self-limiting. Patients typically make a complete recovery.

Causes of Acute Viral Meningitis

Major causes of acute viral meningitis are listed in the following box.

MAJOR CAUSES OF ACUTE VIRAL MENINGITIS
Enterovirus (coxsackievirus, echovirus) Herpes simplex virus type 1 and 2 Mumps Varicella-zoster Lymphocytic choriomeningitis HIV

Clinical Manifestations

The clinical manifestations of acute viral meningitis are similar to that of acute bacterial meningitis. Although the illness is often described as less severe and shorter in duration, these features are not discriminating enough to be helpful in the differentiation of these two major causes of meningitis.

CSF Findings

Ultimately, the distinction between acute bacterial meningitis and acute viral meningitis depends upon analysis of the CSF. Although many viruses can cause meningitis, CSF findings are similar, regardless of the etiologic agent. Typical CSF findings in acute viral meningitis are described in the following box.

TYPICAL CSF FINDINGS IN ACUTE VIRAL MENINGITIS

Normal or mildly elevated opening pressure
CSF pleocytosis
  Usually up to 1000 WBC/mm^3
  Typically lymphocytic predominance
  Neutrophilic predominance may be noted early in the course of the infection
Mildly elevated protein concentration
Normal glucose level (decreased levels may be seen, especially in infection due to mumps or lymphocytic choriomeningitis viruses)
Negative Gram stain
Negative bacterial culture

The CSF findings of acute viral meningitis described above can also be seen in patients with early bacterial meningitis, partially treated bacterial meningitis, fungal meningitis, and parasitic meningitis. To help differentiate early viral meningitis (which can present with neutrophilic pleocytosis) from acute bacterial meningitis, it is often useful to repeat the lumbar puncture 12-24 hours later. If lymphocytosis is found, a bacterial etiology becomes less likely (*L. monocytogenes* should still be considered, however).

Other Testing

Although serologic testing of the blood (acute and convalescent titers) can be performed to identify the specific viral etiology, it is not often done since acute viral meningitis is typically a self-limiting and benign illness. Viral antigen, IgM antibody testing, and PCR techniques of the CSF are also available but once again, testing is not often performed since establishing the precise etiologic agent seldom changes management with the illness resolving several days to a few weeks later.

References

Redington JJ and Tyler KL, "Viral Infections of the Nervous System, 2002: Update on Diagnosis and Treatment," *Arch Neurol*, 2002, 59(5):712-8.

Rotbart HA, "Viral Meningitis," *Semin Neurol*, 2000, 20(3):277-92.

Thomson RB Jr and Bertram H, "Laboratory Diagnosis of Central Nervous System Infections," *Infect Dis Clin North Am*, 2001, 15(4):1047-71.

TUBERCULOUS MENINGITIS

The incidence of tuberculous meningitis has been increasing, especially in developing countries, where the prevalence of HIV infection is high.

Clinical Manifestations

Unlike acute bacterial meningitis, tuberculous meningitis typically presents with a subacute to chronic course. Symptoms and signs of the illness include headache, fever, neck stiffness, lethargy, confusion, meningeal signs, and cranial nerve palsies.

Laboratory Testing

Test	Clinical Significance
CBC	Findings may be consistent with subacute/chronic infection (ie, anemia of chronic disease, etc)
Electrolytes	Hyponatremia may be present due to SIADH or concomitant tuberculous infection of the adrenal glands
PPD	Positive test indicates previous or recent exposure to *M. tuberculosis* Positive test does not establish diagnosis of active tuberculosis Test may be negative in patients early in the course of the illness, with overwhelming infection, and in immunocompromised patients
Sputum acid-fast smear/culture	Quite often, pulmonary involvement is present in patients with tuberculous meningitis
Chest radiograph	To assess for pulmonary tuberculosis
Urinalysis	Genitourinary tuberculosis may be present in the patient with tuberculous meningitis

Although abnormalities of the above test results may be supportive of the diagnosis, confirmation of the tuberculous meningitis diagnosis requires examination of the CSF. The typical CSF profile in tuberculous meningitis is described in the following box.

TYPICAL CSF PROFILE IN TUBERCULOUS MENINGITIS

GROSS APPEARANCE
- Typically clear but may be slightly turbid
- Pellicle may form in tube if it is left standing for some time

ELEVATED CSF OPENING PRESSURE

CELL COUNT
- Usually between 50 and 500/mm^3 but higher counts not unusual
- Mean WBC count 223/mm^3
- Acellular CSF described in HIV and elderly

CELL COUNT DIFFERENTIAL
- Typically lymphocytic*
- Early in the course of the illness, neutrophilic predominance may be noted

ELEVATED PROTEIN CONCENTRATION
- Mean level 224 mg/dL
- 6% of adults have normal levels

DECREASED GLUCOSE LEVEL
- 72% have levels <45 mg/dL

POSITIVE ACID-FAST SMEAR
- Present in 10% to 20%

(continued)

(continued)

TYPICAL CSF PROFILE IN TUBERCULOUS MENINGITIS
POSITIVE CULTURE
Requires weeks for results to return
Positive in 50% to 80% of cases

*Interestingly, the initial lymphocytic predominance may give way to neutrophilic pleocytosis in patients treated with antituberculous medications. This is known as the therapeutic paradox.

Quite often, antituberculous therapy is started when the clinical presentation and CSF findings are consistent with the diagnosis, even if microbiologic confirmation is lacking. This is because the results of culture are not quickly available. Should the culture results return negative in a patient who is not responding to therapy, other causes of subacute to chronic meningitis such as fungal meningitis should be considered.

References

Roos KL, "Laboratory Diagnosis of Central Nervous System Infections," *Infect Dis Clin North Am*, 2001, 15(4):1047-71.

Thomson RB Jr and Bertram H, "*Mycobacterium* Tuberculosis Meningitis and Other Etiologies of the Aseptic Meningitis Syndrome," *Semin Neurol*, 2000, 20(3):329-35.

NEOPLASTIC MENINGITIS

The diagnosis of meningeal carcinomatosis requires the demonstration of neoplastic cells in the CSF. The yield of the CSF analysis is improved with repeated lumbar punctures.

	First Lumbar Puncture	Repeated Lumbar Punctures
Elevated CSF pressure*	50%	71%
Cell count >5 cells/mm^3†	57%	72%
Protein >50 mg/dL	81%	89%
Glucose level <40 mg/dL	31%	41%
Positive cytology	54%	91%

*A normal CSF pressure is not uncommon early in the course of meningeal carcinomatosis. With disease progression, the CSF pressure rises.

†The cell count typically does not exceed 500 cell/mm^3. The differential cell count may reveal low or high proportion of neutrophils.

Adapted from Wasserstrom WR, Glass JP, and Posner JB, "Diagnosis and Treatment of Leptomeningeal Metastases From Solid Tumors: Experience With 90 Patients," *Cancer*, 1982, 49:759-72.

The classic CSF profile of neoplastic meningitis includes the following:

- High opening pressure
- High protein concentration
- Low glucose level
- Lymphocytic pleocytosis

Many patients, however, do not have all elements of this classic profile. Although a completely normal CSF analysis can occur in neoplastic meningitis, it is uncommon, occurring in <10% of cases.

Even in patients who have all elements of the classic profile listed above, this combination of findings is nonspecific. This is one of the reasons why a firm diagnosis of neoplastic meningitis rests on the identification of malignant cells within the CSF. CSF cytology has excellent specificity. This is true as long as testing is performed by experienced personnel.

Although false-positive test results are rare, false-negative test results are not uncommon. Measures to decrease the false-negativity rate include the removal of large amounts of CSF for cytology, expeditious processing of the specimen, and repeating lumbar puncture if cytologic analysis of the initial specimen is unrevealing in the patient suspected of having neoplastic meningitis (see table above).

Despite these measures, some patients with neoplastic meningitis will have negative cytologic test results. In these patients, the clinical presentation or imaging test results may be consistent with the diagnosis.

In recent years, considerable attention has focused on testing the CSF for the presence of biological markers. Assays for tumor antigens and biochemical markers are available but because of their poor sensitivity and specificity, they have not been adopted for widespread use. These markers may have some utility, however, in assessing the response to therapy.

If lymphomatous meningitis is suspected, several other tests should be considered. In these patients, CSF flow cytometry and immunoglobulin gene rearrangement testing are often superior to cytologic analysis.

The malignancies that most often spread to the meninges in decreasing order of incidence are listed in the following box.

MENINGEAL CARCINOMATOSIS ASSOCIATED MALIGNANCIES
BREAST LYMPHOMA LUNG ADENOCARCINOMA OF THE PANCREAS BRAIN GLIOMA

Occasionally, viscous CSF is obtained in patients with meningeal carcinomatosis. When present, if often implies the presence of a mucin-producing adenocarcinoma usually from the gastrointestinal tract.

References

Blaney SM and Poplack DG, "Neoplastic Meningitis: Diagnosis and Treatment Considerations," *Med Oncol*, 2000, 17(3):151-62.

Chamberlain MC, "Neoplastic Meningitis: A Guide to Diagnosis and Treatment," *Curr Opin Neurol*, 2000, 13(6):641-8.

Kim L and Glantz MJ, "Neoplastic Meningitis," *Curr Treat Options Oncol*, 2001, 2(6):517-27.

SUBARACHNOID HEMORRHAGE

Patients with subarachnoid hemorrhage classically present with abrupt onset of a severe headache. Many patients describe the headache to be the "worst headache" of their lives. Physical exam findings may include alteration in mental status, nuchal rigidity, other meningeal signs, and focal neurologic findings. The laboratory test findings in patients with subarachnoid hemorrhage are discussed below.

Laboratory Testing

Lumbar puncture is not indicated in all patients suspected of having subarachnoid hemorrhage. When the clinical presentation is consistent with the diagnosis of subarachnoid hemorrhage, a CT scan of the brain should be obtained to confirm the diagnosis. In 95% to 97% of cases, CT evidence of subarachnoid hemorrhage will be demonstrated by imaging.

In 3% to 5% of cases, however, the CT may not reveal findings consistent with subarachnoid hemorrhage. It is in these patients that lumbar puncture is necessary. In other words, when a patient presents with signs and symptoms of subarachnoid hemorrhage but has an unremarkable CT, the clinician should not discard the diagnosis because 3% to 5% of patients present this way. In these patients, lumbar puncture is warranted. CSF findings of subarachnoid hemorrhage are described in the following box.

CSF ANALYSIS IN PATIENTS WITH SUBARACHNOID HEMORRHAGE

- If onset of sudden headache was <3 days before
  - Wait until at least 12 hours have elapsed since symptom onset before performing lumbar puncture*
  - If CSF is not only clear/colorless but also acellular (no more than a few RBC/mm^3), a ruptured aneurysm has been excluded and there is no need for further evaluation
  - If CSF is blood stained:

    A. Spin down CSF immediately. If it contains RBC from trauma and it is allowed to stand, oxyhemoglobin will form *in vitro*. Bilirubin will not but the absence of bilirubin in the CSF cannot exclude the diagnosis of subarachnoid hemorrhage.

    B. Perform spectrophotometric analysis† of supernatant unless yellow color (xanthochromia) is evident to the naked eye. If analysis has to be deferred for practical reasons, store CSF wrapped in tin foil because daylight may induce breakdown of bilirubin.

- If onset of sudden headache was >3 days before
  - Do lumbar puncture immediately (after brain CT)
  - If CSF is unequivocally xanthochromic (with or without RBCs), no further CSF tests are necessary.
  - If the CSF is clear, colorless, and acellular, spectrophotometric analysis must still be performed (the red blood cells may have lysed and the presence of pigment may not be visible to the naked eye).
  - If the time interval is more than two weeks from headache onset, xanthochromia may still be detectable (up until 4 weeks) but normal results of spectrophotometric testing cannot exclude the diagnosis of subarachnoid hemorrhage.

*In patients who are suspected of having subarachnoid hemorrhage despite negative CT findings, lumbar puncture should certainly be performed. It is important, however, not to perform the procedure until 12 hours have passed since the onset of the headache. If the lumbar puncture is performed before this amount of time has elapsed, the clinician will not be able to reliably distinguish between subarachnoid hemorrhage and traumatic tap. The reason for this is that it typically takes 12 hours for red blood cells to lyse. With the lysis of red blood cells, hemoglobin will be broken down into oxyhemoglobin and bilirubin. When these products have formed, centrifugation of CSF will result in a yellowish color of the supernatant. This is known as xanthochromia, the hallmark CSF finding of subarachnoid hemorrhage. Testing for xanthochromia is the most reliable way to make the distinction between subarachnoid hemorrhage and traumatic tap.

†The presence of oxyhemoglobin and bilirubin, which are the main breakdown products of hemoglobin, in the CSF can be detected by spectrophotometry.

Modified from *Stroke A Practical Guide To Management*, 2nd ed, Warlow CP, et al (eds), 2001, Blackwell Science, 206.

References

Edlow JA, "Diagnosis of Subarachnoid Hemorrhage in the Emergency Department," *Emerg Med Clin North Am*, 2003, 21(1):73-87.

Edlow JA and Caplan LR, "Avoiding Pitfalls in the Diagnosis of Subarachnoid Hemorrhage," *N Engl J Med*, 2000, 342(1):29-36.

Shah KH and Edlow JA, "Distinguishing Traumatic Lumbar Puncture From True Subarachnoid Hemorrhage," *J Emerg Med*, 2002, 23(1):67-74.

TRANSIENT ISCHEMIC ATTACKS (TIA) / STROKE

Both transient ischemic attacks (TIA) and stroke are characterized by the loss of focal brain (or monocular) function. Classically, the symptoms are maximal at the onset of the illness. The difference between these two conditions is the duration of time the symptoms are present. In TIA, symptoms last no longer than 24 hours. In contrast, stroke patients have symptoms of at least 24 hours duration. In this chapter, we will discuss laboratory testing that is performed in TIA / stroke patients.

Laboratory Testing

The time window for the use of thrombolytic agents in the treatment of acute stroke is short (inclusion threshold of three hours) and patients who are eligible for these agents must be identified quickly. For these reasons, the evaluation of suspected TIA/stroke must be emergent. In addition to the history and physical examination, neuroimaging is a standard part of the evaluation. Routine blood tests should also be obtained. Essential laboratory testing in patients with transient ischemic attack or stroke are listed in the following box.

ESSENTIAL LABORATORY TESTING IN PATIENTS WITH TIA OR STROKE
HEMOGLOBIN / HEMATOCRIT PLATELET COUNT WHITE BLOOD CELL COUNT ERYTHROCYTE SEDIMENTATION RATE (ESR) URINALYSIS PLASMA GLUCOSE PLASMA CHOLESTEROL ELECTROLYTES BUN CREATININE LIVER FUNCTION TESTS PT PTT EKG NEUROIMAGING

The clinical significance of the above testing is described in the following table.

Essential Laboratory Testing in TIA / Stroke and What it May Reveal

Test(s)	Indicated in All Patients?	Why?
Hemoglobin / hematocrit	Yes	In anemic patients, focal cerebral ischemia can occur in the setting of severe arterial disease TIA/stroke can occur in patients with polycythemia vera
Platelet count	Yes	TIA/stroke can occur in essential thrombocythemia Manifestations of TIA/stroke can occur in certain patients with thrombocytopenia (eg, thrombotic thrombocytopenic purpura or heparin-induced thrombocytopenia) Severe thrombocytopenia, itself, can result in intracerebral hemorrhage, one form of stroke
White blood cell count	Yes	TIA/stroke can occur in leukemic patients because of increased whole blood viscosity
Urinalysis	Yes	May show evidence of renal disease, infective endocarditis, vasculitis, or diabetes mellitus
ESR	Yes	Elevated ESR may be supportive of vasculitis, infective endocarditis, or atrial myxoma Elevated ESR may also be noted in malignancy and other chronic diseases, both of which may be associated with a hypercoagulable state
Plasma cholesterol/ lipid profile	Yes	Hypercholesterolemia (risk factor for atherothromboembolism)
Plasma glucose	Yes	Hypoglycemia can present with symptoms similar to that of TIA or stroke Presence of hyperglycemia may indicate previously undiagnosed diabetes mellitus, a risk factor for cerebrovascular disease Marked hyperglycemia (ie, nonketotic hyperglycemia) can present with manifestations seen in stroke patients
Electrolytes	Yes	Hyponatremia can present with focal neurologic symptoms/signs
Liver function tests	Yes	Hepatic encephalopathy is in the differential diagnosis of TIA/stroke
PT PTT	Yes	In intracerebral hemorrhage patients, elevated PT and/or PTT may be due to underlying coagulopathy or anticoagulant use Elevated PTT may be a manifestation of the lupus anticoagulant

Essential Laboratory Testing in TIA / Stroke and What it May Reveal *(continued)*

Test(s)	Indicated in All Patients?	Why?
BUN Creatinine	Yes	Uremia is in the differential diagnosis of TIA/stroke Certain causes of TIA/stroke (ie, TTP) are often characterized by the presence of renal failure BUN and creatinine are indices of dehydration
EKG	Yes	May detect previously undiagnosed atrial fibrillation Absence of atrial fibrillation does not rule out diagnosis since the arrhythmia is often intermittent Necessary to exclude silent myocardial infarction Useful to assess for left ventricular hypertrophy

Other Testing / Investigation

Many other tests may be obtained in the evaluation of TIA/stroke patient. These tests should be performed if indicated based on the patient's clinical presentation.

Other Tests Available for the Evaluation of the TIA / Stroke (If Indicated)

Test	Obtain if....
Hemoglobin AIC	Patient has elevated fasting plasma glucose
VDRL/RPR FTA-ABS	Meningovascular syphilis is suspected
ANA	Vasculitis is a possibility
Blood cultures	Endocarditis is a concern
Creatine kinase (with fractionation)	Myocardial infarction is suspected
Thyroid function tests	Patient has atrial fibrillation
Toxicology screen/blood alcohol level	Drug overdose is suspected since its manifestations can mimic that of stroke or drug-induced stroke is a concern (certain recreational drugs like cocaine or amphetamine can cause stroke)
Serum protein electrophoresis Immunoelectrophoresis Serum viscosity	Hyperviscosity syndrome secondary to a paraproteinemia is suspected
Blood for type and crossmatch	There is a need to reverse coagulopathy
Lumbar puncture	Neurosyphilis, vasculitis, or multiple sclerosis are suspected

(continued)

Other Tests Available for the Evaluation of the TIA / Stroke (If Indicated) *(continued)*

Test	Obtain if....
Hypercoagulability evaluation (antithrombin III, protein C, protein S, lupus anticoagulant, anticardiolipin antibodies)	TIA occurs in patient who is or has: <50 years Personal or family history of premature arterial or venous thrombosis Thrombocytopenia History of recurrent miscarriages Positive VDRL/RPR
Temporal artery biopsy	Temporal arteritis is suspected

Tests such as Holtor monitoring, echocardiography (transthoracic, transesophageal), carotid artery ultrasound, and other imaging tests may also be indicated depending on the patient's clinical presentation. Discussion of these tests and their role in the evaluation of TIA/stroke are beyond the scope of this chapter.

References

Demaerschalk BM, "Diagnosis and Management of Stroke (Brain Attack)," *Semin Neurol*, 2003, 23(3):241-52.

Thurman RJ and Jauch EC, "Acute Ischemic Stroke: Emergent Evaluation and Management," *Emerg Med Clin North Am*, 2002, 20(3):609-30, vi.

Warlow C, Sudlow C, Dennis M, et al, "Stroke," *Lancet*, 2003, 362(9391):1211-24.

Wityk RJ and Beauchamp NJ Jr, "Diagnostic Evaluation of Stroke," *Neurol Clin*, 2000, 18(2):357-78.

SEIZURE / STATUS EPILEPTICUS

A seizure is the result of excessive aberrant synchronous firing of cortical neurons. Status epilepticus is a medical emergency defined as continuous seizure activity lasting 30 minutes or more. Two or more discrete seizures occurring in a patient who does not regain consciousness between the seizures also satisfies the definition of status epilepticus (>30 minutes).

Diagnosis of Seizure

The evaluation of the patient suspected of having a seizure (especially if the event is not witnessed by the physician) begins with an evaluation to exclude other causes of an event that mimics or resembles seizure. Considerations include syncope, transient ischemic attacks, migraine, hyperventilation, and psychogenic seizure. A careful history and physical exam often allows the clinician to make the distinction between seizure and these other possibilities.

Laboratory testing has a very limited role in this regard. An exception to this rule is in the patient who may be having psychogenic seizures. Psychogenic seizures, also known as pseudoseizures, may resemble seizures but are not due to excessive aberrant electrical discharge from cortical neurons. Clinically, it can be quite challenging to make the distinction between them. Although continuous video monitoring combined with EEG telemetry is the best test to distinguish seizure from pseudoseizure, measurement of the serum prolactin level may also be of some benefit. Serum prolactin levels rise after an epileptic seizure. Normal levels should prompt consideration of pseudoseizures or other causes (ie, syncope). Because serum prolactin levels decline to baseline 60 minutes or so after seizure activity, it is important to measure the level within the first 30 minutes. Since elevated levels have been described in syncope patients and some patients with seizure have normal serum prolactin levels, this test is far from perfect.

Laboratory Testing for First Seizure

In the patient who has had seizure for the first time, an evaluation should be performed to identify the cause of the seizure. In addition to a thorough history and physical exam, laboratory testing should also be performed. The laboratory test evaluation should include CBC, electrolytes, BUN, creatinine, calcium level, magnesium level, liver function tests, and a toxicology screen. This battery of tests may identify the cause (hypoglycemia, hyponatremia, hypocalcemia, hypomagnesemia, substance abuse, uremia, etc) or a precipitant (a factor that lowered the seizure threshold in a patient with epilepsy). Neuroimaging should be obtained, especially if the patient has focal neurologic findings, altered consciousness, or evidence of head trauma. Even in the absence of these findings, however, neuroimaging is often a standard part of the evaluation. If the patient is febrile or has other manifestations of CNS inflammation/infection, a lumbar puncture is warranted. An EEG is useful for the diagnosis and classification of the type of seizure.

Causes of Status Epilepticus

Causes of status epilepticus are listed in the following box.

ANTIEPILEPTIC DRUG THERAPY
- Noncompliance
- Recent cessation
- Recent decrease in dose

STROKE

FEVER

INFECTION (systemic infection occurring in a patient with chronic seizure disorder)

CNS INFECTION
- Meningoencephalitis
- Brain abscess

CNS MALIGNANCY (primary or metastatic)

BRAIN TRAUMA

DRUG WITHDRAWAL
- Alcohol
- Barbiturates
- Benzodiazepines
- Opiates

DRUG OVERDOSE
- Phenothiazines
- Theophylline
- Tricyclic antidepressants
- Cocaine
- Amphetamines
- PCP
- Chemotherapy medications
- Isoniazid

TOXINS

METABOLIC DISORDERS
- Hyponatremia
- Uremia
- Hepatic encephalopathy
- Hyponatremia
- Hypocalcemia
- Hypomagnesemia
- Hypoglycemia

HYPOXIC ENCEPHALOPATHY

Laboratory Testing in Patients With Status Epilepticus

Laboratory and diagnostic testing that are often obtained in patients with status epilepticus are listed in the following box. Many of the tests are obtained to identify the etiology of the status epilepticus.

LABORATORY / DIAGNOSTIC TESTS THAT ARE OFTEN OBTAINED IN PATIENTS WITH STATUS EPILEPTICUS

COMPLETE BLOOD COUNT*
ESR†
BUN
CREATININE
ELECTROLYTES
PLASMA GLUCOSE‡
CALCIUM
MAGNESIUM
PHOSPHATE
TOXICOLOGY SCREEN
LIVER FUNCTION TESTS
ARTERIAL BLOOD GAS ANALYSIS§
ANTIEPILEPTIC DRUG LEVEL¶
LUMBAR PUNCTURE#
CT BRAIN
EEG

*Leukocytosis may be a manifestation of systemic (systemic infection can lower seizure threshold in patient with seizure disorder or other predisposition to seizure development) or CNS infection (meningitis, encephalitis, cerebral abscess).

†An elevated ESR may be a clue to the presence of a vasculitis. The clinician should realize, however, that seizure alone would be a rare manifestation of vasculitis. If suspected, further testing may be indicated (anti-double stranded DNA antibodies, complement levels, rheumatoid factor, urinalysis to identify renal disease due to vasculitis, etc).

‡Always obtain fingerstick glucose because the results are quickly available (blood glucose should also be obtained but it takes longer for results to become available)

§Analysis will typically reveal the presence of a metabolic acidosis but may uncover other acid-base disturbances. It is also useful in assessing oxygenation and ventilation.

¶Since subtherapeutic anticonvulsant drug levels are a common cause of seizure recurrence in patients with chronic seizure disorder, levels are certainly indicated in the evaluation of these patients.

#If CNS infection suspected, lumbar puncture should be obtained (as long as there are no contraindications). In patients with idiopathic seizure disorder, examination of the CSF may reveal the presence of a few lymphocytes/mm^3 (in the absence of infection). The clinician should, however, suspect infection or another condition if the CSF has more than 5-10 lymphocytes/mm^3. Of note, abnormalities of the protein or glucose concentration should not be attributed to seizure activity.

DEMENTIA

Although dementia is a clinical diagnosis, laboratory testing is an essential part of the evaluation. The two most common causes of dementia are Alzheimer's disease and vascular dementia, both of which are diagnosed mainly by careful consideration of the patient's clinical presentation. Laboratory testing is most often performed to exclude other (less common but potentially reversible) causes of dementia.

REVERSIBLE CAUSES OF DEMENTIA		
Alcoholism (chronic)	Infection	Neurosyphilis
Connective tissue diseases	AIDS	Normal pressure hydrocephalus
Systemic lupus erythematosus	Chronic meningitis	Nutritional
Temporal arteritis	Tuberculosis	Vitamin B_{12} deficiency
Rheumatoid vasculitis	Fungal	Thiamine deficiency
Sarcoidosis	Parasitic	Pellagra
TTP	Lyme neuroborelliosis	Whipple's disease
Granulomatous angiitis	Mass lesions	Miscellaneous
Endocrine disorders	Tumor	Obstructive sleep apnea
Adrenal insufficiency	Subdural hematoma	Chronic obstructive pulmonary disease
Hyperparathyroidism	Medications	Congestive heart failure
Hyperthyroidism	Metabolic disorders	Radiation-induced dementia
Hypothyroidism	Electrolyte abnormalities	Dialysis dementia
	Hepatic encephalopathy	
	Hypoxemia	
	Renal failure	

Adapted from Arnold SE and Kumar A, "Reversible Dementias," *Med Clin N Am*, 1994, 77(1):215-30.

Laboratory Testing

The American Academy of Neurology recommends routinely performing the tests in the following box in the evaluation of every patient with dementia.

ROUTINE LABORATORY TESTS INDICATED IN EVERY PATIENT WITH DEMENTIA
BUN
CREATININE
CBC
ELECTROLYTES
CALCIUM
GLUCOSE
LIVER FUNCTION TESTS
SERUM VITAMIN B_{12} LEVEL
SYPHILIS SEROLOGY (RPR or VDRL)
THYROID FUNCTION TESTS (TSH)

Tests that are not considered routine but that may be indicated in certain situations are listed in the following box.

LABORATORY TESTS THAT MAY BE INDICATED IN THE EVALUATION OF DEMENTIA
CHEST RADIOGRAPH
ESR
ANTINUCLEAR ANTIBODIES*
RHEUMATOID FACTOR*
ANTINEUTROPHILIC CYTOPLASMIC ANTIBODY OR ANCA*
SERUM / URINE PROTEIN ELECTROPHORESIS†
HIV‡
24-HOUR URINE FOR HEAVY METALS
TOXICOLOGY SCREEN (SERUM / URINE)
URINALYSIS

*If vasculitis is suspected

†If paraproteinemia is suspected

‡Of note, testing for HIV should be performed in any patient with risk factors for HIV. Up to 20% of patients with HIV develop dementia. However, most patients with HIV dementia are known to have HIV prior to the diagnosis. Dementia as the initial presentation of HIV would be particularly unusual.

Lumbar puncture should not be a routine part of the dementia evaluation. The indications for lumbar puncture are listed in the following box.

INDICATIONS FOR LUMBAR PUNCTURE IN PATIENTS WITH DEMENTIA
ACUTE OR SUBACUTE ONSET
FEVER
HISTORY OF METASTATIC CANCER
IMMUNOSUPPRESSION
MENINGEAL ENHANCEMENT ON IMAGING
MENINGEAL SIGNS
SUSPICION FOR PRIORI DEMENTIA
PRESENTATION CONSISTENT WITH NORMAL PRESSURE HYDROCEPHALUS
RAPIDLY PROGRESSIVE DEMENTIA
REACTIVE SYPHILIS SEROLOGY
SUSPECTED CNS VASCULITIS
YOUNGER PATIENT (<55 years of age)

Prior to performing lumbar puncture, it is important to ensure that there are no contraindications to the procedure. Neuroimaging is often obtained in the evaluation of the dementia patient but details regarding such testing are beyond the scope of this chapter.

MULTIPLE SCLEROSIS

Multiple sclerosis is a demyelinating disease of the central nervous system, which primarily affects women. The diagnosis of this disease is mainly a clinical one. However, laboratory testing (particularly CSF analysis) may provide support for the diagnosis.

CSF Analysis

Examination of the CSF provides important information in the diagnosis of multiple sclerosis. The CSF is abnormal in close to 90% of patients with multiple sclerosis. CSF findings in multiple sclerosis include the following.

1. Mononuclear pleocytosis

   Studies have revealed that 66% of patients with multiple sclerosis have a normal cell count. In the remaining 33%, a mild degree of pleocytosis is noted. When present, a lymphocytic predominance is typical. Approximately 95% of multiple sclerosis patients have a white blood cell count <16 cells/mm^3. It is unusual to appreciate a WBC count >50 cells/mm^3. Such a level should prompt the clinician to consider other causes. Many investigators feel that there is a greater likelihood of noting pleocytosis during exacerbation, compared to times when the disease is quiescent. There is little data to support this, however, as diagnostic lumbar punctures are usually only done during times of exacerbation.

2. Mildly increased / normal protein concentration

   Sixty-six percent of patients with multiple sclerosis have a normal protein concentration. The remaining 33% have a mildly increased protein level. A protein concentration >70 mg/dL is unusual in patients with multiple sclerosis. In fact, levels >100 mg/dL should prompt the clinician to question the diagnosis of multiple sclerosis or, alternatively, search for another disease process superimposed on multiple sclerosis.

3. Increased immunoglobulin level

   A healthy individual has a significantly lower immunoglobulin concentration in the CSF as compared to the serum. In patients with multiple sclerosis, however, the CSF immunoglobulin concentration is increased. This reflects the increased production of immunoglobulin in the central nervous system. Although the IgG fraction is predominantly increased, both IgM and IgA levels may be elevated as well.

   There is, however, no correlation between the degree of immunoglobulin elevation and the activity of multiple sclerosis. In fact, patients with severe multiple sclerosis may have normal immunoglobulin levels while others with milder disease may have a considerable increase in the immunoglobulin concentration.

4. Oligoclonal bands

   The persistent demonstration of oligoclonal bands in the CSF is also useful in the diagnosis of multiple sclerosis. In approximately 90% of patients with multiple sclerosis, oligoclonal bands are appreciated on the agarose gel. In general, the presence of oligoclonal bands correlates well with an increase in the CSF immunoglobulin level. Abnormal results of both tests support the diagnosis in a patient with a clinical presentation consistent with multiple sclerosis. Their presence alone is not diagnostic of this illness.

   The treatment of multiple sclerosis with immunosuppressive therapy may decrease CSF immunoglobulin, but has no affect on the oligoclonal band pattern. False-positive test results do occur, which should serve as a reminder that these tests are not specific to multiple sclerosis, but reflect the presence of an immune-mediated process in the nervous system. For example, oligoclonal bands have been reported with chronic CNS infection. As such, abnormalities are most helpful when used in conjunction with the patient's clinical presentation.

References

Lublin FD, "The Diagnosis of Multiple Sclerosis," *Curr Opin Neurol*, 2002, 15(3):253-6.

Poser CM and Brinar VV, "Diagnostic Criteria for Multiple Sclerosis," *Clin Neurol Neurosurg*, 2001, 103(1):1-11.

PART VI:

NEPHROLOGY

RENAL FUNCTION TESTING

Before embarking on the evaluation of abnormal renal function, it is important to understand the terms that are often used and have some understanding about the tools used to assess renal function.

Glomerular Filtration Rate

The GFR, which is an index of renal function, is defined in the following box.

DEFINITIONS...

GFR: The rate at which plasma is filtered through glomeruli

Normal range:

Male: 115-125 mL/minute

Female: 90-100 mL/minute

The serial measurement of GFR enables the clinician to monitor the course of renal disease. Knowing the GFR also allows the clinician to make medication dose adjustments based on renal excretion. GFR cannot be measured directly. In clinical practice, an estimation of GFR is possible based on serum creatinine or creatinine clearance.

Serum Creatinine

Serum creatinine is defined in the following box.

DEFINITION...

Creatinine: A substance that is formed from creatine phosphate, which is primarily stored in muscle. Creatine is formed at a fairly constant rate and, therefore, creatinine production is related directly to muscle mass.

Normal serum creatinine varies between 0.8 and 1.2 mg/dL (slightly lower in women). Since serum creatinine and GFR are inversely related, an increase in serum creatinine usually reflects renal disease. For every 50% reduction in the GFR, there is a doubling of the serum creatinine. A creatinine level that doubles from 1-2 mg/dL indicates a 50% loss of renal function. A further increase in serum creatinine to 4 mg/dL indicates that only 25% of normal renal function remains.

One can make use of the reciprocal of serum creatinine (or 1/serum creatinine) to follow the progression of renal disease. A plot can be made of 1/serum creatinine versus time. This can be used to predict the progression of the patient's renal disease, including the time it will take for the patient to reach end-stage renal disease. It is important to realize that in some patients, worsening renal function is not linear.

Creatinine Clearance

Creatinine clearance is a measure of the GFR. Its value can be calculated using the results of a 24-hour urine collection for creatinine and a concomitant serum creatinine.

GLOMERULAR FILTRATION RATE (GFR)
GFR $= Cr_{cl}^{*} = \dfrac{urine_{Cr\ (mg/dL)} \times urine_{volume\ (mL)}}{plasma_{Cr\ (mg/dL)}}$ where Cr_{cl} = creatinine clearance

*Using the above equation, the calculated creatinine clearance will be in mL/day. This value needs to be divided by 1440 (# of minutes in one day) to yield a value expressed in mL/minute.

It is important to ensure that the 24-hour urine collection is complete. The adequacy of the collection can be determined by recognizing the following expected values.

NORMAL VALUES 24-HOUR CREATININE EXCRETION
Male: 20-25 mg/kg creatinine/day   **Female:** 15-20 mg/kg creatinine/day

If the total creatinine in the 24-hour urine specimen falls below the normal range, the collection may have been incomplete. An incomplete collection may give spurious results.

Limitations of the Serum Creatinine for GFR Estimation

Creatinine clearance is a more accurate measurement of the GFR than serum creatinine. Both, however, have their limitations. In general, serum creatinine is more often used to approximate the GFR, mainly because of the difficulty in obtaining an adequate 24-hour urine collection needed to calculate creatinine clearance. There are limitations to the accuracy of the serum creatinine test that the clinician must be aware of. These include the following.

1. A large decline in the GFR is required before creatinine will increase. As a result, in early renal insufficiency, serum creatinine may be within the normal range.
2. With advancing renal disease, tubular secretion of creatinine increases. This makes the serum creatinine an unreliable approximation of the GFR as renal disease worsens.
3. Certain groups of patients have a lower baseline serum creatinine.

   Therefore, serum creatinine may remain in the normal range despite a decrease in the GFR. In such cases, the clinician may erroneously conclude that renal function is normal. These patient groups include:

   - Women
   - Children
   - Malnourished individuals
   - Elderly
   - Poor meat eaters

4. Some drugs interfere with renal handling of creatinine by decreasing tubular secretion or by interfering directly with the creatinine assay.

   The following drugs interfere with tubular secretion of creatinine.

MEDICATIONS INTERFERING WITH THE TUBULAR SECRETION OF CREATININE*
SALICYLATES
CIMETIDINE
TRIMETHOPRIM
TRIAMTERENE
SPIRONOLACTONE
AMILORIDE

*In these instances, the GFR has not changed but the creatinine clearance may be falsely low. It can be difficult to discern whether a rise in serum creatinine reflects worsening renal insufficiency or is the result of an alteration in the renal handling of creatinine in a patient taking one of the above medications.

Depending on the assay used, causes of false-positive elevations in the serum creatinine include glucose, fructose, uric acid, ketonemia (acetoacetate), ascorbic acid, cephalosporin antibiotics, guanidine, bilirubin, hemolysis, lipemia, and 5-flucytosine.

Limitations of the Creatinine Clearance for GFR Estimation

The limitations of creatinine clearance include:

- Difficulty in obtaining an adequate 24-hour urine collection. Inadequate collection yields spurious results.
- Difficulty in obtaining the serum creatinine during a steady state of creatinine balance. When serum creatinine levels are increasing or decreasing, as in the development and resolution of acute renal failure, respectively, the creatinine clearance is not an accurate approximation of the GFR.
- Overestimation in patients with renal disease

The use of creatinine clearance as an adequate marker of GFR is based on the assumption that creatinine is an ideal substance for such an approximation. While creatinine is freely filtered at the glomerulus, some degree of tubular secretion takes place as well. As a result, creatinine clearance will always overestimate the GFR. While this overestimation is not an important issue in individuals with normal renal function, it becomes relevant in patients with renal disease and decreased GFR. In these cases, overestimation of the GFR is disproportionately greater, and may inaccurately lull the clinician into believing that creatinine clearance is higher than it truly is.

A modification of the creatinine clearance determination involves the administration of oral cimetidine (1200 mg) two hours before starting the 24-hour urine collection. Because cimetidine blocks the tubular secretion of creatinine, its use increases the accuracy of the creatinine clearance measurement, even in patients with advanced renal disease.

Cockcroft-Gault Equation

Recognizing that there are difficulties with the 24-hour urine collection, Cockcroft and Gault devised a formula that can be used to estimate creatinine clearance using serum creatinine.

COCKROFT-GAULT EQUATION

$$\textbf{Creatinine clearance} = \frac{[(140 - \text{age}) \times \text{wt (kg)}]}{(72 \times \text{serum creatinine [mg/dL]})}$$

Note: In females, it is necessary to multiply the value obtained from the equation by 0.85.

Urea (BUN)

Urea is defined in the following box.

DEFINITION...
Urea: A crystallizable substance found in urine, blood, lymph, and all body fluids that is formed by the metabolism of protein and nucleic acids. The kidneys filter and reabsorb urea, with reabsorption governed mainly by the urinary flow rate.

Because urea production is dependent on many factors, including protein ingestion, catabolism, and GI protein loss, the blood urea nitrogen (BUN) is not a good measure of glomerular filtration.

Causes of Increased BUN

The causes of an elevated BUN are listed in the following box.

CAUSES OF ELEVATED BUN
DECREASED FLOW TO KIDNEY
Prerenal causes
Postrenal causes
CORTICOSTEROID USE
TETRACYCLINE
ABSORPTION OF BLOOD FROM GASTROINTESTINAL TRACT
CATABOLIC STATES
Fever
Sepsis
Tissue necrosis
Trauma
INCREASED PROTEIN INTAKE

Causes of Decreased BUN

The causes of a decreased BUN are listed in the following box.

CAUSES OF DECREASED BUN
DECREASED PROTEIN DIET
HEMODIALYSIS*
LIVER DISEASE (severe)
OVERHYDRATION
COMPULSIVE WATER DRINKING
SIADH
PREGNANCY

*This occurs because urea is better dialyzed than creatinine.

References

Bennett JC and Plum F, eds, *Cecil Textbook of Medicine*, 20th ed, Philadelphia, PA: WB Saunders Company, 1996.

Brenner BB, ed, *Brenner and Rector's The Kidney*, 5th ed, Philadelphia, PA: WB Saunders Company, 1996.

Fauci AS, Braunwald E, Isselbacher KJ, et al, eds, *Harrison's Principles of Internal Medicine*, 14th ed, New York, NY: McGraw-Hill, 1998.

Greenberg A, Cheung AK, et al, eds, *Primer on Kidney Diseases*, 2nd ed, San Diego, CA: Academic Press, 1998.

Kallenberg CG, Brouwer E, Weening JJ, et al, "Anti-neutrophil Cytoplasmic Antibodies: Current Diagnostic and Pathophysiological Potential," *Kidney Int*, 1994, 46(1):1-15.

Schrier RW and Guttschalk CW, eds, *Diseases of the Kidney*, 6th ed, Boston, MA: Little, Brown and Company, 1997.

APPROACH TO THE PATIENT WITH ACUTE RENAL FAILURE

STEP 1 – *Is the Renal Failure Acute or Chronic?*

The occurrence of acute renal failure (ARF) in hospitalized patients is increasing. At the current time, approximately 5% of hospitalized patients develop acute renal failure. In the intensive care unit setting, however, acute renal failure is more common, occurring in up to 20% to 30% of the patients. Although a consensus definition for acute renal failure is lacking, it is characterized by worsening renal function, occurring over hours to days. The decline in renal function leads to the accumulation of nitrogenous waste products, which is reflected as an increase in the serum BUN and creatinine. Note that oliguria (urine volume <400 mL/day or <20 mL/hour) is not part of the definition because acute renal failure patients can be oliguric or nonoliguric.

Before embarking on a search for the etiology of acute renal failure, it is wise to first establish if the renal failure is an acute process. Acute renal failure must be differentiated from chronic renal failure, which is defined as a decline in kidney function over an extended period of time. Not uncommonly, however, patients with chronic renal failure develop worsening renal function, beyond that expected from the natural history of their kidney disease. These patients are said to have acute on chronic renal failure. Patients with acute on chronic renal failure deserve the same evaluation as those with acute renal failure.

There are a number of ways to differentiate acute from chronic renal failure. The best proof of chronicity is serial BUN and creatinine levels that have been elevated for a prolonged period of time (at least 3-6 months). However, these levels are not always available. Other ways to differentiate acute from chronic renal failure (CRF) are listed in the following table.

ARF vs CRF

	History	Kidney Size	Bone X-ray	Hemoglobin	Broad Casts
ARF	Normal renal function	Normal*	Normal	Normal‡	Absent
CRF	↑ BUN and Cr	Small bilaterally†	Renal osteodystrophy	↓‡	Present

*The kidneys may be enlarged in ARF secondary to obstructive uropathy.

†Chronic renal failure secondary to multiple myeloma, autosomal dominant polycystic kidney disease, diabetic nephropathy, or amyloidosis may be associated with normal or enlarged kidneys.

‡Acute renal failure due to a thrombotic microangiopathy (TTP, HUS) typically presents with anemia (microangiopathic hemolytic anemia). In addition, remember that anemia can complicate acute renal failure after a sufficient period of time, irrespective of the cause of the acute renal failure. It is also important to realize that anemia may not be a feature of certain chronic renal diseases, such as polycystic kidney disease.

Ultrasound is useful in differentiating acute from chronic renal failure. In adults, the normal kidney size ranges from 9-12 cm in length. In contrast to acute renal failure, most cases of chronic renal failure are characterized by a reduction in kidney size. Other features of a chronic process include reduction of cortical thickness, increased echo density and scarring.

The presence of normocytic, normochromic anemia is common in patients with chronic renal failure. Although it is uncommon in acute renal failure, it can be seen, especially if the acute renal failure is prolonged or is a feature of a systemic illness.

Although radiologic findings consistent with renal osteodystrophy are indicative of chronic renal failure, these findings are usually a manifestation of severe chronic renal failure. Therefore, milder degrees of chronic renal failure may not present with these radiologic changes (ie, erosion of lateral end of clavicle or radial edge of 2nd phalanx).

In most cases, the degree of BUN and creatinine elevation does not allow the clinician to differentiate acute from chronic renal failure. On occasion, patients appear well despite marked increases in BUN (>300 mg/dL) and creatinine (>13.5 mg/dL). In these patients, chronic renal failure is more likely to be present. Patients with acute renal failure who present with BUN and creatinine elevations to this extent usually do not appear well because they have not had time to adapt to the renal failure.

If the patient has chronic renal failure and does not have an accompanying acute process, ***proceed to the section on Chronic Renal Failure*** *on page 535.*

If the patient has acute renal failure or acute on chronic renal failure, ***proceed to Step 2.***

STEP 2 – *How Is Acute Renal Failure Classified?*

Acute renal failure can be divided into three categories, as shown in the following box.

CLASSIFICATION OF ACUTE RENAL FAILURE
Prerenal azotemia (55% of cases)
Renal azotemia (40% of cases)
Postrenal azotemia (5% of cases)

The three types of acute renal failure are defined in the following box.

SOME DEFINITIONS...

Prerenal azotemia: Increased BUN and/or creatinine secondary to a decrease in renal perfusion

Postrenal azotemia: Acute renal failure resulting from a structural or functional impediment of urine flow, affecting any portion of the urinary tract from the tubules to the urethra

Renal azotemia: Acute renal failure resulting from disease affecting the renal vasculature, glomeruli, tubules, or interstitium

The initial evaluation of the patient with acute renal failure focuses on determining whether the patient has prerenal azotemia, renal azotemia, or postrenal azotemia.

Proceed to Step 3.

STEP 3 – *Does the Patient Have Postrenal Azotemia?*

Although postrenal azotemia accounts for only 5% of acute renal failure cases, most cases are easily treatable. For this reason, every effort should be made to exclude this type of acute renal failure. Postrenal azotemia is defined as acute renal failure that results from a structural or functional impediment to urine flow, affecting any portion of the urinary tract from the tubules to the urethra. In order to develop acute renal failure from urinary tract obstruction, the obstruction must be at the level of the urethra or bladder neck, or involve both ureters. Obstruction of one ureter will not lead to acute renal failure, because one functioning kidney can compensate for the other. Unilateral ureteral obstruction can, however, lead to acute renal failure in the patient with a solitary kidney or in the setting of pre-existing chronic renal insufficiency.

Clinical Features Suggestive of Postrenal Azotemia

Clues in the history that should prompt consideration of postrenal azotemia are listed in the following box.

POSTRENAL AZOTEMIA HISTORICAL FEATURES	
EXTREMES OF AGE	SUPRAPUBIC / FLANK PAIN
DECREASED FORCE OF URINARY STREAM	NEPHROLITHIASIS
	ANURIA
HISTORY OF CANCER	FLUCTUATING URINE VOLUMES
Bladder	MEDICATIONS
Prostate	Anticholinergics
Intra-abdominal	α-adrenergic agonists
Pelvic	Medication-induced crystalluria*

*Includes sulfonamides, methotrexate, acyclovir, triamterene, and protease inhibitors.

Physical examination findings that should prompt consideration of postrenal azotemia include an enlarged or indurated prostate, distended bladder, and abnormal pelvic (eg, pelvic mass) or rectal exam.

Causes of Postrenal Azotemia

The causes of postrenal azotemia are listed in the following box.

ACUTE RENAL FAILURE POSTRENAL CAUSES
URETERAL OBSTRUCTION
Calculus
Sloughed papilla
Blood clots
Malignancy
Uric acid, acyclovir, antiretroviral agent, or sulfonamide crystals
Extrinsic compression
Malignancy / abscess / retroperitoneal fibrosis / inadvertent surgical ligature / pelvic hematoma / endometriosis
BLADDER NECK OBSTRUCTION
Neurogenic bladder
Benign prostatic hypertrophy
Calculus
Blood clot
Sloughed papilla
Malignancy (bladder, prostate)
Medications (anticholinergics, α-adrenergic blockers)
URETHRAL OBSTRUCTION
Stricture
Congenital valves
Tumor
Diverticulum
Stones
Obstructed indwelling catheter
Phimosis

In young men, the most common cause of postrenal azotemia and urinary tract obstruction is nephrolithiasis. BPH and prostate cancer are major causes in elderly men, whereas, ovarian cancer is a major concern in elderly women.

Establishing the Diagnosis

Placing a Foley catheter and obtaining a renal ultrasound are invaluable tools in establishing the diagnosis of postrenal azotemia. Measuring a postvoid residual by the placement of a Foley catheter will determine if a lower urinary tract obstruction exists. If a large amount of residual urine (>100 mL) is obtained, a lower urinary tract obstruction is the likely cause of the acute renal failure.

If a large residual urine volume is not obtained, a renal ultrasound should be performed to evaluate for the possibility of an upper urinary tract obstruction. In general, ultrasound should be obtained in acute renal failure patients unless the etiology of the renal failure is quite clear. Dilatation of the urinary tract is characteristic of urinary tract obstruction. The clinician should realize, however, that the renal ultrasound is not considered a highly sensitive and specific test for obstructive uropathy. The sensitivity of the renal ultrasound is reported to be about 80% to 85%. Ultrasound may give a false-negative result because of dehydration or encasement of the collecting system by retroperitoneal fibrosis. In addition, recent obstruction (within the last several days) may not be demonstrated by ultrasound because sufficient time has not elapsed for dilatation to have occurred. When there is high clinical suspicion for urinary tract obstruction but the renal ultrasound is unremarkable, serial ultrasound studies should be considered.

The use of duplex Doppler ultrasound detecting a high resistive index diminishes the false negativity rate of ultrasound in patients with acute or chronic obstruction. CT scan, intravenous pyelography, and retrograde pyelography can also be helpful. However, there is a significant risk of exacerbating azotemia because of the radiocontrast used with CT and IVP studies. If urolithiasis is being considered, the clinician may wish to perform spiral CT without contrast. Retrograde pyelography should be considered in patients with poor kidney function, as well as in those who are allergic to contrast dye.

If the patient has postrenal azotemia, ***stop here***.

If the patient does not have postrenal azotemia, ***proceed to Step 4.***

STEP 4 – *Does the Patient Have Prerenal or Renal Azotemia?*

Once postrenal azotemia has been excluded, the clinician can focus on efforts to distinguish prerenal from renal azotemia. There is no single laboratory test that definitively distinguishes between prerenal and intrarenal causes of acute renal failure; however, the following laboratory values, when examined together (in combination with a thorough history and physical examination), can be quite helpful.

- Serum BUN and creatinine
- Urine osmolality
- Fractional excretion of sodium
- Urine sodium
- Urine microscopic examination

These tests are discussed in further detail in the remainder of this step.

BUN:Creatinine Ratio

A serum BUN to creatinine ratio >20:1 is very suggestive of prerenal azotemia, particularly if the patient has no reason for increased urea production (increased protein intake, corticosteroid use, blood in the gastrointestinal tract). In contrast, patients with acute tubular necrosis (ATN), the major cause of renal azotemia, often have a ratio between 10 and 15.

On occasion, patients with prerenal azotemia may present with a ratio less than 20 to 1. Examples include patients on a low-protein diet and those with liver disease. The clinician should also realize that acute tubular necrosis patients with an increased catabolic rate may present with an elevated ratio. It is important to recognize these limitations of the BUN to creatinine ratio.

The disproportionate increase in the BUN (as compared to creatinine) seen in patients with prerenal azotemia is more easily understood if one considers the renal handling of BUN and creatinine. Creatinine is freely filtered at the glomerulus with some tubular secretion. Creatinine is not reabsorbed. Urea is also freely filtered but, in contrast to creatinine, it is reabsorbed by the tubules. Tubular reabsorption of urea is linked to salt and water reabsorption. In states of renal hypoperfusion leading to prerenal azotemia, there is salt and water reabsorption because the kidneys sense volume depletion. As a result, urea is reabsorbed as well, leading to an increased ratio. This accounts for the disproportionate increase in BUN as compared to creatinine in prerenal azotemia.

Urine Osmolality

The ability to generate a high osmolality requires normal tubular function. Because prerenal azotemia is characterized by normal tubular function, the kidneys are able to produce urine with an osmolality >500 mOsm/kg. In ATN, there is considerable damage to the tubules. As a result, the kidneys often produce urine having an osmolality <350 mOsm/kg.

Urine Sodium Concentration

Urine sodium <20 mEq/L is consistent with prerenal azotemia, while a value >40 mEq/L argues for acute tubular necrosis. Compared to the fractional excretion of sodium (FENa), however, urine sodium is a less sensitive and specific test to differentiate between the two types of acute renal failure.

Fractional Excretion of Sodium (FENa)

The fractional excretion of sodium is very useful in differentiating prerenal azotemia from renal azotemia, particularly acute tubular necrosis. The FENa is calculated by measuring urine sodium and creatinine, as well as serum sodium and creatinine, as shown in the following formula.

FRACTIONAL EXCRETION OF SODIUM
$$\text{FENa} = \left[\frac{\text{urine}_{\text{Na}} \times \text{plasma}_{\text{creatinine}}}{\text{plasma}_{\text{Na}} \times \text{urine}_{\text{creatinine}}}\right] \times 100$$

Prerenal (FENa <1%): In patients with acute renal failure due to prerenal azotemia, the fractional excretion of sodium is <1%. Remember that in prerenal azotemia, either an absolute or effective decrease in arterial blood volume is sensed by the kidneys. The kidneys respond by conserving sodium, leading to a low FENa.

Intrarenal (FENa >2%): When the fractional excretion of sodium is >2%, a renal etiology for acute renal failure is likely. Recall that ATN is characterized by tubular damage resulting in the inability to conserve sodium and hence an increased FENa.

Values that fall between 1% and 2% reflect an area of overlap between prerenal azotemia and acute tubular necrosis.

Limitations of the Fractional Excretion of Sodium

Although the FENa is very useful, the clinician should recognize prerenal conditions that present with a high FENa and intrarenal conditions that can result in a low FENa. Conditions characterized by prerenal azotemia and a FENa >1% are listed in the following box.

PRERENAL AZOTEMIA DISORDERS ASSOCIATED WITH A FENa >1%
DIURETIC USE
BICARBONATURIA
PRE-EXISTING CHRONIC RENAL FAILURE COMPLICATED BY SALT WASTING
ADRENAL INSUFFICIENCY
ACUTE VOLUME EXPANSION

Some conditions that cause renal azotemia are associated with a FENa <1%. If these conditions are severe enough to cause tubular damage, the FENa may later rise in the disease course. These conditions are listed in the following box.

RENAL AZOTEMIA DISORDERS ASSOCIATED WITH A FENa <1%	
RADIOCONTRAST	ACUTE GLOMERULONEPHRITIS
NSAIDs	VASCULITIS
SEVERE BURNS	RHABDOMYOLYSIS
SEPSIS	ACUTE INTERSTITIAL NEPHRITIS

Urinalysis

Urinalysis should be obtained in every patient presenting with acute renal failure. One study revealed that urinalysis provided diagnostically useful information in approximately 75% of acute renal failure cases. As a general rule, an unremarkable urinalysis, except for an occasional hyaline cast, is suggestive of prerenal azotemia. The clinician should realize, however, that postrenal azotemia may also present with a normal urinalysis. An abnormal urinalysis should prompt the clinician to seriously consider renal azotemia, as shown in the following table.

Use of the Urinalysis in the Evaluation of Acute Renal Failure

Urinalysis Finding	Clinical Significance
Normal	Prerenal azotemia Postrenal azotemia
Positive dipstick for blood but no red blood cells present on microscopic analysis	Renal azotemia (hemoglobinuria, myoglobinuria)
Hematuria (positive dipstick for blood and red blood cells present on microscopic analysis)	Renal azotemia (glomerular, vascular, interstitial, or tubular disease) Postrenal azotemia (tumor, stone, blood clots)
Red blood cell casts	Renal azotemia (glomerular disease, vascular disease)
Dysmorphic red blood cells	Renal azotemia (glomerular disease)
White blood cells White blood cell casts	Renal azotemia (pyelonephritis, interstitial disease)
Renal tubular epithelial cells Muddy brown broad tubular cell casts Pigmented casts	Renal azotemia (acute tubular necrosis, myoglobinuria, hemoglobinuria)

Summary Table Highlighting the Differences Between Prerenal and Renal Azotemia

USING THE URINARY DIAGNOSTIC INDICES TO DIFFERENTIATE PRERENAL FROM RENAL AZOTEMIA		
Test	**Prerenal Azotemia**	**Renal Azotemia**
BUN:Cr ratio*	>20	10-15
Urine specific gravity	>1.020	1.010
Uosm (mOsm/kg)	>500	<350
Urine sodium (mEq/L)	<20	>40
FENa (%)†	<1	>2
UCr:PCr ratio	≥40	≤20
Fractional excretion of uric acid (%)	<7	>15
Fractional excretion of lithium (%)	<7	>20
Urine microscopy	Normal except for occasional hyaline casts	Abnormal

Note: Cr = creatinine; UCr = urine creatinine; PCr = plasma creatinine; Uosm = urine osmolality

*The elevated BUN:creatinine ratio is indicative of prerenal azotemia as long as GI bleed, tissue breakdown, increased protein intake, and steroid treatment are excluded. A normal BUN:creatinine ratio may occur in prerenal azotemia if protein intake is decreased or liver synthesis of urea is impaired.

†There are certain prerenal conditions associated with an increased FENa. These include diuretic use, bicarbonaturia, pre-existing chronic renal insufficiency complicated by salt wasting, acute volume expansion, and adrenal insufficiency. There are some causes of renal azotemia that are associated with a FENa <1%. These include radiocontrast induced renal failure, NSAIDs, severe burns, sepsis, acute glomerulonephritis, vasculitis, acute interstitial nephritis, and rhabdomyolysis.

Limitations of the above tests in differentiating prerenal from renal azotemia include the following.

- None of the above laboratory findings are completely sensitive or specific in differentiating prerenal from intrarenal causes.
- Data included in the above table were collected from patients with ARF having creatinine levels of 3-5 mg/dL. Therefore, the above criteria may not apply to creatinine values outside this range.
- In addition, a large gray area exists in which laboratory tests do not give definitive results.
- These values are most useful in the oliguric patient, because in nonoliguric ATN there is less tubular damage and the laboratory findings are often more consistent with prerenal azotemia.

If the laboratory values are consistent with prerenal azotemia, ***proceed to Step 5.***

If the laboratory values are consistent with renal azotemia, ***proceed to Step 6.***

STEP 5 – *What Is the Approach to Prerenal Azotemia?*

Prerenal azotemia is the most common form of acute renal failure. It is characterized by renal hypoperfusion. Acute renal failure in prerenal azotemia is reversible if perfusion to the kidneys is restored. Renal function normalizes within 24-48 hours if the cause of the impairment in renal perfusion is corrected. However, acute renal failure may not resolve in cases of prolonged or severe hypoperfusion. In these instances, ischemic damage to the kidneys resulting in acute tubular necrosis may develop.

Clinical Features Suggestive of Prerenal Azotemia

Historical features suggestive of prerenal azotemia are listed in the following box.

PRERENAL AZOTEMIA HISTORICAL FEATURES
DIZZINESS / LIGHTHEADEDNESS WITH STANDING THIRST OLIGURIA SYMPTOMS OF CONGESTIVE HEART FAILURE APPARENT VOLUME LOSS FROM SKIN / GI / RENAL SOURCE

Physical examination findings suggestive of prerenal azotemia are listed in the following box.

PRERENAL AZOTEMIA PHYSICAL EXAMINATION
ORTHOSTATIC HYPOTENSION TACHYCARDIA DRY MUCOUS MEMBRANES LACK OF AXILLARY MOISTURE DECREASED SKIN TURGOR EVIDENCE OF CONGESTIVE HEART FAILURE EDEMA

Causes of Prerenal Azotemia

The cause of prerenal azotemia is usually apparent from the history and physical exam. These causes are listed in the following box.

CAUSES OF PRERENAL AZOTEMIA
ABSOLUTE DECREASE IN EFFECTIVE BLOOD VOLUME HEMORRHAGE DEHYDRATION BURNS RENAL LOSS OF FLUID Diuretics Osmotic diuretics Adrenal insufficiency THIRD SPACE SEQUESTRATION Peritonitis Pancreatitis Muscle-crush injury Hypoalbuminemia GASTROINTESTINAL FLUID LOSS Vomiting Diarrhea Nasogastric suction

(continued)

CAUSES OF PRERENAL AZOTEMIA *(continued)*
INEFFECTIVE BLOOD VOLUME
DECREASED CARDIAC OUTPUT
Congestive heart failure
Cardiogenic shock
Tamponade
Pulmonary embolism (massive)
SYSTEMIC VASODILATION
Sepsis
Anaphylaxis
Anesthesia
Antihypertensive therapy (if blood pressure is lowered excessively)
Liver failure
RENAL VASOCONSTRICTION
Hypercalcemia
Cyclosporine
Amphotericin B
Norepinephrine
Sepsis
Liver disease (hepatorenal syndrome)
OTHERS
NSAIDs*
ACE INHIBITORS†

*Renal prostaglandins are not essential in maintaining the glomerular filtration rate (GFR) in normal individuals. Prostaglandins are, however, integral in maintaining renal blood flow when there is underlying glomerular disease, renal insufficiency, and in states characterized by the presence of increased vasoconstrictors, such as angiotensin II and norepinephrine. Risk factors for NSAID-induced acute renal failure include anesthesia, advanced age, CHF, nephrotic syndrome, cirrhosis, chronic renal failure, hypovolemia, ACE inhibitor use, and severe atherosclerotic disease of the renal arteries. In these conditions, maintaining GFR is dependent on prostaglandin mediated afferent arteriolar vasodilation. When NSAIDs are given to such patients, prostaglandin synthesis is inhibited, leading to acute renal failure. The increase in serum creatinine usually occurs within the first 3-7 days of therapy.

†In certain patients, ACE inhibitor therapy can cause acute renal failure that is typically reversible. Conditions in which acute renal failure may develop after starting ACE inhibitor therapy include significant bilateral renal artery stenosis (>70%), renal artery stenosis in the patient with a solitary kidney, any condition in which cardiac output is low or there is intense vasoconstriction, and severe small vessel disease of the kidney as in severe nephrosclerosis. The development of acute renal failure following the institution of ACE inhibitor therapy should prompt the clinician to perform testing to exclude bilateral renal artery stenosis or severe renal artery stenosis in the patient with a solitary kidney.

Other medications that can cause prerenal azotemia include COX-2 inhibitors, tacrolimus, interleukin-2, and interferon.

End of Section.

STEP 6 – *What Is the Approach to Renal Azotemia?*

Once prerenal and postrenal causes of acute renal failure have been excluded, the clinician should focus on renal causes of azotemia. The causes of renal azotemia are listed in the following box.

ACUTE RENAL FAILURE – RENAL CAUSES
DISEASES OF THE LARGE RENAL VESSELS
Renal artery / vein obstruction
Vasculitis
Atheroembolic disease
DISEASES OF THE GLOMERULI AND SMALL RENAL VESSELS
Glomerulonephritis (acute or rapidly progressive)
Vasculitis
Malignant hypertension
Scleroderma renal crisis
Hemolytic-uremic syndrome
Thrombotic thrombocytopenic purpura
Disseminated intravascular coagulation
ACUTE TUBULAR NECROSIS
Ischemic
Nephrotoxic
Radiocontrast
Antibiotics (aminoglycosides, amphotericin B, foscarnet, pentamidine, acyclovir)
Immunosuppressive (cyclosporine)
Chemotherapeutic (cisplatin, ifosfamide)
Tubular obstruction (indinavir, acyclovir, calcium oxalate)
Rhabdomyolysis (myoglobinuria)
Hemolysis (hemoglobinuria)
Malignancy
Lymphoma
Multiple myeloma
Tumor lysis syndrome
INTERSTITIAL DISEASES
Drug-induced allergic interstitial nephritis
Infectious nephritis
Connective tissue disease (systemic lupus erythematosus, Sjögren's syndrome)
Infiltrative nephritis (hematologic or solid malignancy)

For further information regarding the evaluation of patients with renal azotemia, please proceed to the chapter, ***Approach to the Patient With Renal Azotemia on page 511***.

References

Agrawal M and Swartz R, "Acute Renal Failure," *Am Fam Physician*, 2000, 61(7):2077-88.

Albright RC Jr, "Acute Renal Failure: A Practical Update," *Mayo Clin Proc*, 2001, 76(1):67-74.

Brown WW and Schmitz PG, "Acute and Chronic Kidney Disease," *Clin Geriatr Med*, 1998, 14(2):211-36.

Esson ML and Schrier RW, "Diagnosis and Treatment of Acute tubular Necrosis," *Ann Intern Med*, 2002, 137(9):744-52.

Gesualdo L, Grandaliano G, Mascia L, et al, "Acute Renal Failure in Critically Ill Patients," *Intensive Care Med*, 1999, 25(10):1188-90.

Klahr S, "Urinary Tract Obstruction," *Semin Nephrol*, 2001, 21(2):133-45.

Klahr S and Miller SB, "Acute Oliguria," *N Engl J Med*, 1998, 338(10):671-5.

Lameire N, Nelde A, Hoeben H, et al, "Acute Renal Failure in the Elderly," *Geriatr Nephrol Urol*, 1999, 9(3):153-65.

Nally JV Jr, "Acute Renal Failure in Hospitalized Patients," *Cleve Clin J Med*, 2002, 69(7):569-74.

Nissenson AR, "Acute Renal Failure: Definition and Pathogenesis," *Kidney Int Suppl*, 1998, 66:S7-10.

Nolan CR and Anderson RJ, "Hospital-Acquired Acute Renal Failure," *J Am Soc Nephrol*, 1998, 9(4):710-8.

Perazella MA, "Crystal-Induced Acute Renal Failure," *Am J Med*, 1999, 106(4):459-65.

Rabb H, "Evaluation of Urinary Markers in Acute Renal Failure," *Curr Opin Nephrol Hypertens*, 1998, 7(6):681-5.

Sadovnikoff N, "Perioperative Acute Renal Failure," *Int Anesthesiol Clin*, 2001, 39(1):95-109.

Shokeir AA, "The Diagnosis of Upper Urinary Tract Obstruction," *BJU Int*, 1999, 83(8):893-900, quiz 900-1.

Singri N, Ahya SN, and Levin ML, "Acute Renal Failure," *JAMA*, 2003, 289(6):747-51.

Solez K and Racusen LC, "Role of the Renal Biopsy in Acute Renal Failure," *Contrib Nephrol*, 2001, 132:68-75.

ACUTE RENAL FAILURE

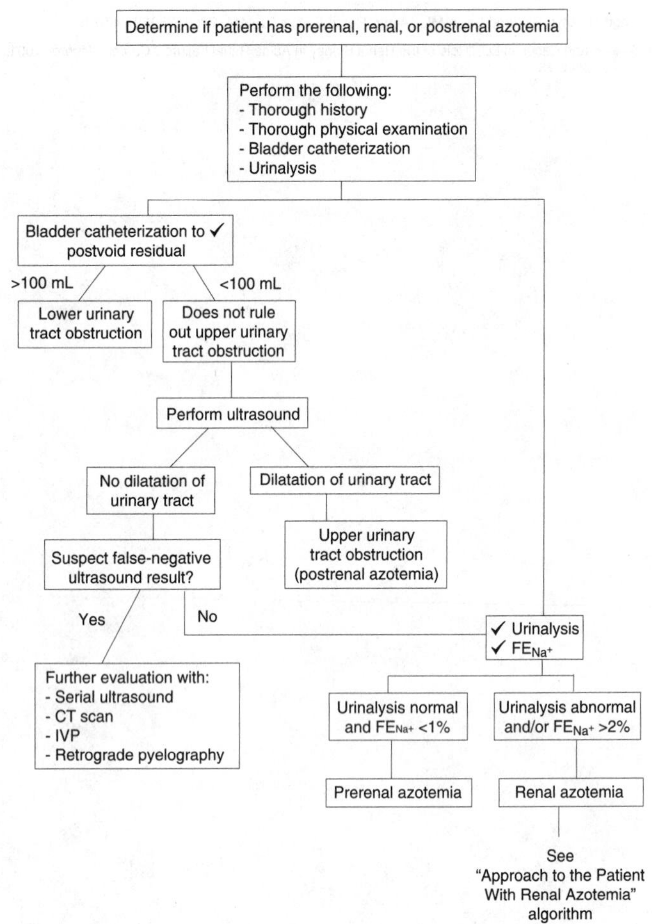
Determine if patient has prerenal, renal, or postrenal azotemia
Perform the following:
- Thorough history
- Thorough physical examination
- Bladder catheterization
- Urinalysis
Bladder catheterization to ✓ postvoid residual
>100 mL
<100 mL
Lower urinary tract obstruction
Does not rule out upper urinary tract obstruction
Perform ultrasound
No dilatation of urinary tract
Dilatation of urinary tract
Upper urinary tract obstruction (postrenal azotemia)
Suspect false-negative ultrasound result?
Yes
No
Further evaluation with:
- Serial ultrasound
- CT scan
- IVP
- Retrograde pyelography
✓ Urinalysis
✓ FENa+
Urinalysis normal and FENa+ <1%
Urinalysis abnormal and/or FENa+ >2%
Prerenal azotemia
Renal azotemia
See "Approach to the Patient With Renal Azotemia" algorithm

APPROACH TO THE PATIENT WITH RENAL AZOTEMIA

STEP 1 – *Does the Patient Have Renal Azotemia?*

The causes of acute renal failure can be categorized into one of the three following groups:

- Prerenal azotemia
- Postrenal azotemia
- Renal azotemia

Renal azotemia is defined as acute renal failure resulting from disease affecting the renal vasculature, glomeruli, tubules, or interstitium. The following approach assumes the diagnosis of renal azotemia has been established with confidence. This requires excluding prerenal and postrenal azotemia.

If the diagnosis of renal azotemia is not certain, ***proceed to the chapter, Acute Renal Failure*** *on page 499.*

If the patient has renal azotemia, ***proceed to Step 2.***

STEP 2 – *What Are the Different Types of Renal Azotemia?*

Once prerenal and postrenal causes of acute renal failure have been excluded, the clinician should focus on the causes of renal azotemia. The causes of renal azotemia are listed in the following box.

ACUTE RENAL FAILURE - RENAL CAUSES	
DISEASES OF THE LARGE RENAL VESSELS	
Renal artery / vein obstruction	Vasculitis
DISEASES OF THE GLOMERULI AND SMALL RENAL VESSELS	
Vasculitis	Scleroderma renal crisis
Malignant hypertension	Hemolytic-uremic syndrome
Thrombotic thrombocytopenic purpura	Atheroembolic disease
Glomerulonephritis (acute or rapidly progressive)	
ACUTE TUBULAR NECROSIS	
Ischemic	
Nephrotoxic	
Radiocontrast	Hemolysis (hemoglobinuria)
Poisons (ethylene glycol, toluene)	Myeloma kidney
Rhabdomyolysis (myoglobinuria)	Ethylene glycol intoxication
Organic solvents (carbon tetrachloride)	Tumor lysis syndrome
Immunosuppressive (cyclosporine)	Anesthetics (enflurane)
Chemotherapeutic (cisplatin, methotrexate, ifosfamide)	
Antibiotics (aminoglycosides, amphotericin B, foscarnet, pentamidine, acyclovir)	
INTERSTITIAL DISEASES	
Drug-induced allergic interstitial nephritis	
Infectious nephritis	
Connective tissue disease (systemic lupus erythematosus, Sjögren's syndrome)	
Infiltrative nephritis (hematologic or solid malignancy)	

Proceed to Step 3.

STEP 3 – *What Type of Renal Azotemia Does the Patient Have?*

As shown in the box in Step 2, the causes of renal azotemia are numerous. One approach to establishing the cause involves dividing the kidney into its anatomic components and considering the diseases that may affect these components. The four anatomic components of the kidney include the following:

- Large renal vessels
- Glomeruli / small renal vessels
- Tubules (acute tubular necrosis)
- Interstitium (acute interstitial nephritis)

Proceed to Step 4.

STEP 4 – *Does the Patient Have Renal Azotemia Due to a Disease of the Large Renal Vessels?*

Disease of the large renal vessels (arteries or veins) is an uncommon cause of renal azotemia. This is because occlusion of the large renal vessels can only result in acute renal failure if one of the following situations occur:

- Bilateral occlusion of the large renal vessels
- Unilateral occlusion of a large renal vessel in the patient with underlying chronic renal failure
- Unilateral occlusion of a large renal vessel in the patient with unilateral functioning kidney

Diseases to consider within this category include thromboembolism, thrombosis, and dissection. On occasion, vasculitis of large renal vessels (ie, Takayasu's arteritis) may present with acute renal failure. The major causes of acute renal failure due to disease of the large renal vessels are considered in the following table.

Major Causes of Acute Renal Failure Due to Disease of the Large Renal Vessels

Clinical Features	Urinalysis Findings	Condition Suggested
Sudden onset of abdominal or flank pain Source of embolus (ie, atrial fibrillation)	Mild proteinuria Occasional red blood cells	Renal artery thromboembolism
Flank pain History of nephrotic syndrome or pulmonary embolism	Proteinuria Hematuria	Renal vein thrombosis

If the patient has a clinical presentation consistent with a disease of the large renal vessels, ***proceed to Step 5.***

If the patient does not have a clinical presentation consistent with a disease of the large renal vessels, ***proceed to Step 6.***

STEP 5 – *What Type of Disease of the Large Renal Vessels Does the Patient Have?*

The major causes of acute renal failure due to a disease of the large renal vessels include thromboembolic disease of the renal artery and renal vein thrombosis. These former two are discussed in more detail in the remainder of this step.

THROMBOEMBOLIC DISEASE OF THE RENAL ARTERY

The causes of thromboembolic occlusion of the renal artery are listed in the following box.

CAUSES OF RENAL ARTERY THROMBOEMBOLIC OCCLUSION	
THROMBOSIS	***EMBOLISM***
TRAUMA	ATRIAL FIBRILLATION
ATHEROSCLEROSIS	ENDOCARDITIS
DISSECTION	MURAL THROMBUS
PROCEDURAL COMPLICATIONS	PARADOXICAL EMBOLI
Angioplasty	PROSTHETIC HEART VALVE
Angiography	ATRIAL MYXOMA
INFLAMMATORY DISORDER	
Takayasu arteritis	
Thromboangiitis obliterans	
Other vasculitides	
HYPERCOAGULABLE STATE	
ACUTE VASCULAR TRANSPLANT REJECTION	
RENAL ARTERY ANEURYSM	

Clinical Presentation

The clinical presentation varies depending on the course and extent of occlusion. Acute thrombosis or embolism leading to infarction often presents with sudden flank pain, nausea, vomiting, and fever. Pain may be absent in some patients. A minority of patients may have gross hematuria.

Laboratory Test Findings

If thrombosis or embolism leads to infarction, leukocytosis may be appreciated. In addition, AST, LDH, and alkaline phosphatase are often increased with infarction. Quite often, the LDH is markedly increased in the setting of minimally elevated transaminase levels. While this type of pattern is not specific for renal infarction, such a finding should at least prompt the clinician to consider it as a possibility. The urinalysis may reveal microscopic hematuria. With unilateral thrombosis or embolism, there may be a transient increase in the BUN and creatinine, but the rise may be marked and sustained with bilateral occlusion.

Establishing the Diagnosis

Establishing the diagnosis requires consideration of the disease. To confirm the diagnosis, a radioisotope renogram may be performed. Demonstration of a segmental or generalized decrease in renal perfusion corroborates the diagnosis. This finding may obviate the need for angiogram or contrast enhanced CT, both of which may exacerbate renal failure.

RENAL VEIN THROMBOSIS

Renal vein thrombosis typically occurs in the setting of the nephrotic syndrome. Although it has been reported in patients who do not have the nephrotic syndrome, this type of presentation is rare.

Clinical Presentation

Most commonly, renal vein thrombosis presents as an insidious illness with few if any symptoms suggestive of kidney disease. Symptomatic cases may present with flank pain, hematuria (gross or microscopic), and high serum LDH levels. Pulmonary embolism may also occur in renal vein thrombosis patients.

Laboratory Findings

Since the nephrotic syndrome is usually present, the urinalysis abnormalities seen in patients with renal vein thrombosis are those of the underlying glomerular disorder. However, proteinuria and hematuria can occur due to renal vein thrombosis itself.

Establishing the Diagnosis

Doppler ultrasound is a useful noninvasive method to establish the diagnosis. However, false negative and positive test results can occur. Other imaging methods that can be used include CT scanning and MRI. Inferior vena cava venography is the gold standard test for establishing the diagnosis of renal vein thrombosis.

End of Section.

STEP 6 – *Does the Patient Have Renal Azotemia Due to a Disease of the Glomeruli or Small Renal Vessels?*

Diseases of the glomeruli and small renal vessels include the following:

- Glomerulonephritis
- Vasculitis
- Malignant hypertension
- Thrombotic microangiopathy (ie, HUS, TTP)
- Atheroembolic disease

The major causes of acute renal failure due to disease of the glomeruli or small renal vessels are considered in the following table.

Major Causes of Acute Renal Failure Due to Disease of the Glomeruli or Small Renal Vessels

Clinical Features	Urinalysis Findings	Condition Suggested
Markedly elevated blood pressure Cardiac decompensation Retinopathy Encephalopathy Papilledema	Red blood cells; red blood cell casts; proteinuria	Malignant hypertension
Risk factor or precipitant for HUS MAHA Thrombocytopenia	Sometimes normal; red blood cells; mild proteinuria; occasional red blood cell or granular casts	HUS
Risk factor or precipitant for TTP MAHA Thrombocytopenia Neurologic dysfunction Fever	Sometimes normal; red blood cells; mild proteinuria; occasional red blood cell or granular casts	TTP
History of scleroderma MAHA	Sometimes normal; red blood cells; mild proteinuria; occasional red blood cell or granular casts	Scleroderma renal crisis
Unexplained constitutional symptoms (ie, fever, malaise, arthralgias, myalgias) Mononeuropathy multiplex Skin lesions (palpable purpura)	Red blood cell casts; granular casts; red blood cells; white blood cells; proteinuria	Vasculitis
Systemic condition associated with glomerulonephritis Hypertension Edema Hematuria	Red blood cell casts; granular casts; red blood cells; white blood cells; proteinuria	Glomerulonephritis
Older patient Evidence of atherosclerosis Recent angiography Hollenhorst plaques Livedo reticularis Palpable purpura	Often normal May show eosinophiluria	Atheroembolic disease

MAHA = mictoangiopathic hemolytic anemia; HUS = hemolytic-uremic syndrome; TTP = thrombotic thrombocytopenic purpura.

If the patient has a clinical presentation consistent with a disease of the glomeruli or small renal vessels, ***proceed to Step 7***.

If the patient does not have a clinical presentation consistent with a disease of the glomeruli or small renal vessels, ***proceed to Step 8.***

STEP 7 – *What Type of Disease of the Glomeruli or Small Renal Vessels Does the Patient Have?*

The major causes of acute renal failure due to a disease of the glomeruli or small renal vessels are listed in the following box.

MAJOR CAUSES OF ACUTE RENAL FAILURE DUE TO DISEASE OF THE GLOMERULI OR SMALL RENAL VESSELS
GLOMERULONEPHRITIS / VASCULITIS
HEMOLYTIC-UREMIC SYNDROME
THROMBOTIC THROMBOCYTOPENIC PURPURA
MALIGNANT HYPERTENSION
SCLERODERMAL RENAL CRISIS
ATHEROEMBOLIC DISEASE

These causes will be discussed in more detail in the remainder of this step.

ATHEROEMBOLIC DISEASE

Cholesterol emboli may dislodge from atherosclerotic plaques causing occlusion of blood vessels throughout the body, including the kidney. Spontaneous atheroembolism has been described; however, in most cases, it follows a procedure such as cardiac catheterization. The typical patient is an elderly individual with atherosclerotic vascular disease affecting the coronary, cerebral, and peripheral vasculature. Atheroembolic disease continues to be an underdiagnosed cause of acute renal failure.

Risk Factors for Atheroembolic Disease

Risk factors for atheroembolic disease are listed in the following box.

ATHEROEMBOLIC DISEASE RISK FACTORS	
AORTIC ANEURYSM REPAIR	ANGIOPLASTY
CARDIAC VALVE SURGERY	AORTIC BALLOON PUMP
ANGIOGRAPHY	ANTICOAGULATION
CORONARY ARTERY BYPASS GRAFTING	THROMBOLYTIC TREATMENT
SPONTANEOUS (from severe atherosclerotic disease)	

Clinical Presentation

Atheroembolic disease is a systemic process. The decline in renal function is often, but not invariably, accompanied by other organ manifestations. The decline in renal function typically occurs within days to weeks following a vascular procedure. It is important to realize, however, that the decline in renal function can be abrupt and marked.

The most common manifestation of atheroembolic disease is painful ischemic changes of the feet. Purple, blue, or gangrenous toes found in a patient with palpable distal arterial pulses should prompt the clinician to consider this diagnosis. Other common findings include livedo reticularis and palpable purpura. Transient ischemic attack, stroke, pancreatitis, and ischemic bowel are some of the other manifestations of this disease.

Laboratory Test Findings

Quite often, the urinalysis is unremarkable. In other cases, however, hematuria may be present. Red blood cell casts have been reported but are not a common finding. When present, it can be difficult to distinguish atheroembolic disease from glomerulonephritis or vasculitis. Proteinuria, if present, is typically modest but nephrotic range proteinuria has been described.

Peripheral eosinophilia and hypocomplementemia may occasionally be noted, however, these findings usually resolve in 1 week. If the urine is examined soon after the atheroembolic event, eosinophiluria may be detected. Urine eosinophils are best detected using Hansel's stain. Of note, eosinophiluria can also be demonstrated in other causes of acute renal failure such as acute interstitial nephritis. It is important to realize that eosinophilia, hypocomplementemia, and eosinophiluria usually resolve within one week. The clinician should consider persistent atheroembolic disease if peripheral eosinophilia and hypocomplementemia persist.

Since the above laboratory findings are nonspecific, the diagnosis of atheroembolism is usually a clinical one.

Establishing the Diagnosis

In classic cases of atheroembolic disease, a clinical diagnosis suffices. In nonclassic cases, the clinician may wish to confirm the diagnosis by biopsying affected tissue, such as skin or muscle. A more invasive alternative is kidney biopsy. The presence of intra-arterial cholesterol crystal clefts establishes the diagnosis.

MALIGNANT HYPERTENSION

Malignant HTN should be suspected in the patient who develops a sudden elevation of blood pressure along with signs and symptoms of organ decompensation. The typical patient has marked HTN with a diastolic blood pressure often >130 mm Hg. Most patients have a history of HTN, although malignant HTN may be the initial manifestation in a minority. Common complaints include throbbing headaches, blurred vision, nausea, vomiting, and decreased urine output. Signs and symptoms of encephalopathy often accompany these findings.

There is often an abrupt decline in renal function, characterized by hematuria and proteinuria. Examination of urine sediment may reveal the presence of red or white blood cell casts. In early malignant HTN, hypokalemic metabolic alkalosis may be appreciated. With worsening renal function, metabolic alkalosis may be replaced by metabolic acidosis. Microangiopathic hemolytic anemia is often present on inspection of the peripheral blood smear.

HEMOLYTIC-UREMIC SYNDROME (HUS) / THROMBOTIC THROMBOCYTOPENIC PURPURA (TTP)

HUS and TTP are uncommon disorders that are related to one another. The clinical features of HUS and TTP overlap. HUS is characterized by microangiopathic hemolytic anemia, renal failure, and thrombocytopenia. In addition to these clinical features, patients with TTP also have neurologic dysfunction and fever. Both disorders are characterized by occlusion of arteries and arterioles with platelet and fibrin thrombi.

Causes of HUS / TTP

The causes of HUS and TTP are listed in the following box.

CAUSES OF HUS / TTP	
INFECTION (viral, bacterial)*	IMMUNOLOGIC DISEASES
MEDICATIONS	Systemic lupus erythematosus
Mitomycin C	Sjögren's syndrome
Cisplatin	Rheumatoid arthritis
Bleomycin	Ankylosing spondylitis
Cyclosporine	Antiphospholipid antibody syndrome
Oral contraceptives	MISCELLANEOUS
Quinine	Pregnancy / postpartum
Clopidogrel	After renal or bone marrow transplantation
Ticlopidine	
Tacrolimus	
Valacyclovir	

*A wide variety of infectious agents have been associated with HUS and TTP. Viral causes include enterovirus, hepatitis A virus, coxsackie virus, influenza virus, and HIV. Bacterial causes include *E. coli*, *Shigella*, *Yersinia*, *Campylobacter*, and *Salmonella*.

Laboratory Test Findings

The laboratory test findings in HUS and TTP are listed in the following box.

HUS / TTP LABORATORY FEATURES	
THROMBOCYTOPENIA	ELEVATED LDH
MICROANGIOPATHIC HEMOLYTIC ANEMIA*	ELEVATED BILIRUBIN
INCREASED WBC COUNT	PT / PTT NORMAL
ELEVATED RETICULOCYTE COUNT	URINALYSIS ABNORMALITIES†

*Microangiopathic hemolytic anemia, a form of nonimmune hemolysis (negative direct Coombs test), is characterized by the presence of schistocytes and red cell fragmentation in the peripheral smear.

†The urinalysis may be fairly unremarkable in HUS and TTP patients. If present, proteinuria is typically mild (<2 g/day). Occasionally, red blood cell casts may be present. In these cases, it can be difficult to differentiate HUS and TTP from glomerulonephritis and vasculitis.

Differentiating HUS From TTP

As described above, there is some clinical overlap between patients with TTP and HUS. A comparison of the two entities is shown below.

Comparison of Clinical Features of HUS and TTP

	HUS	TTP
Neurologic abnormalities	Mild to absent	Severe
Hypertension	Moderate to severe	Mild to absent
Renal insufficiency	Moderate to severe	Mild
Preceded by enteric infection	Often	Rare
Oliguria / anuria	Common	Occasional
Fever	Uncommon	Common

Recently, TTP patients have been found to have deficiency of vWF-clearing protease. This abnormality has not been noted in HUS. An assay is now available to detect this abnormality, which will be of use to clinicians in their efforts to distinguish between these two disorders. One limitation of current testing is that results are not available at a time when treatment decisions need to be made.

Renal Biopsy in HUS and TTP

Tissue biopsy is not required in most cases of TTP or HUS, as the clinical presentation usually suffices. However, biopsy may be required in atypical cases. In these cases, biopsy of petechial skin lesions, gingiva, bone marrow, or kidney may show the characteristic hyaline microthrombi.

Monitoring the Response to Therapy

Lab testing is also useful in following the response to therapy. Platelet counts and LDH levels can be monitored with the institution of therapy such as plasma exchange. Within a few days of starting plasma exchange therapy, serum LDH levels decrease and the platelet count improves. Typically, the LDH level declines first. Renal function may also improve but is unpredictable. While complete recovery can occur, some renal dysfunction may persist after therapy. Some patients who require dialysis are able to discontinue dialysis but many of these patients will be left with some degree of renal dysfunction. When the platelet count returns to normal, the duration between plasma exchange treatments can be increased. With tapering or cessation of therapy, some patients may experience recurrent hemolysis and thrombocytopenia. These patients are said to have an exacerbation of HUS and TTP. They should be distinguished from patients who relapse. Relapsing HUS or TTP is said to be present if the disease recurs after at least 30 days have passed since the last treatment.

SCLERODERMA RENAL CRISIS

Scleroderma can present with slowly worsening chronic renal insufficiency or as scleroderma renal crisis. Scleroderma renal crisis is characterized by sudden onset of malignant hypertension, along with rapid decline in renal function. The frequency of this complication is 5% to 15% in patients with scleroderma. It most commonly occurs within the first 5 years following diagnosis. Laboratory test findings of sclerodermal renal crisis are listed in the following box.

SCLERODERMA RENAL CRISIS LABORATORY FEATURES
RAPID DECREASE IN RENAL FUNCTION
SUDDEN ONSET OF HTN
URINALYSIS
Proteinuria (<3.5 g/day)
Microscopic hematuria
Granular casts
MICROANGIOPATHIC HEMOLYTIC ANEMIA
DECREASED PLATELETS

If treatment for scleroderma renal crisis is not started, patients typically develop end-stage renal disease within 1-2 months.

VASCULITIS / GLOMERULONEPHRITIS

Because vasculitis affecting the small renal vessels often causes glomerular inflammation, vasculitis and glomerulonephritis will be discussed together.

Clinical Presentation

Clinical features of vasculitis are listed in the following box.

VASCULITIS CLINICAL FEATURES
MULTISYSTEM DISEASE FEVER OF UNKNOWN ORIGIN UNEXPLAINED CONSTITUTIONAL SYMPTOMS Fever Weakness Myalgia Arthralgia ISCHEMIC SYMPTOMS (especially in the young) MONONEUROPATHY MULTIPLEX SKIN LESIONS Palpable purpura Livedo reticularis Subcutaneous nodules Ulcers Digital infarcts Urticaria

Vasculitis is usually systemic in nature. As such, renal manifestations are often accompanied by other signs and symptoms. Constitutional symptoms include fever, weakness, arthralgia and myalgia. Palpable purpura and mononeuropathy multiplex on physical exam should prompt the clinician to suspect the diagnosis.

The clinical features of acute glomerulonephritis are listed in the following box.

ACUTE GLOMERULONEPHRITIS CLINICAL FEATURES
HYPERTENSION EDEMA HEMATURIA AZOTEMIA NON-NEPHROTIC RANGE PROTEINURIA

Types of Vasculitis Causing Glomerular Inflammation

Vasculitis can be divided into large, medium, and small vessel types. While any of these may result in renal insufficiency, small vessel vasculitis is the form that most often affects renal vessels. The different types of small vessel vasculitis are listed in the following box.

SMALL VESSEL VASCULITIS
WEGENER'S GRANULOMATOSIS CHURG-STRAUSS SYNDROME MICROSCOPIC POLYARTERITIS SYSTEMIC LUPUS ERYTHEMATOSUS HENOCH-SCHÖNLEIN PURPURA

Polyarteritis nodosa (PAN), a disorder of medium sized vessels, also has a predilection for renal vessels.

Urinalysis Findings in Vasculitis / Glomerulonephritis

The diagnosis should be suspected when examination of the urinary sediment reveals the presence of red blood cell casts, dysmorphic red blood cells, and hematuria accompanied by proteinuria.

Laboratory Testing to Elucidate the Etiology

It is essential to not only establish the diagnosis, but to institute treatment for a rapidly progressive or acute glomerulonephritis, in order to prevent the development of irreversible renal failure. Renal biopsy is the gold standard. Tissue obtained at the time of biopsy can be subjected to immunofluorescent microscopy. With the use of this technique, three major patterns of immune complex (IC) deposition may be identified. These patterns include:

- Granular deposition of IC (characteristic of IC glomerulonephritis)
- Absence or paucity of IC (characteristic of pauci-immune glomerulonephritis)
- Linear deposition of IC along the glomerular basement membrane (characteristic of antiglomerular basement membrane disease)

Percentage of Patients With AGN or RPGN Presenting With a Particular Pattern of Immune Complex Deposition

Pattern of IC Deposition	Class of GN	AGN	Rapidly Progressive GN
Granular deposition	Immune complex GN	70%	45%
Absence or paucity of IC	Pauci-immune GN	30%	45%
Linear deposition	Anti-GBM disease	<1%	10%

While renal biopsy is the gold standard, there are three laboratory tests that may help establish a diagnosis and obviate the need for a renal biopsy. These tests are:

- C3 level
- Anti-GBM Ab
- ANCA

Laboratory Tests That Can Predict the Immune Complex Deposition in AGN

Pattern of IC Deposition	Class of GN	C3	Anti-GBM Antibody	ANCA
Granular deposition	IC GN	↓*	(-)	(-)
Absence or paucity of IC	Pauci-immune GN	Normal	(-)	(+)
Linear deposition	Anti-GBM disease	Normal	(+)†	(-)‡

*It must be noted that some cases of IC GN have normal C3 levels. These include HSP and IgA nephropathy.

†90% to 95% of patients have elevated titers of anti-GBM antibody, while C3 and ANCA levels are typically normal.

‡It should be noted that 20% of patients with anti-GBM disease have a positive ANCA.

Patterns of Immune Complex Deposition and Associated Diseases

Pattern of IC Deposition	Associated Diseases
Granular deposition	Postinfectious GN Lupus nephritis Cryoglobulinemia Bacterial endocarditis Shunt nephritis IgA nephropathy HSP Membranoproliferative GN
Absence or paucity of IC	Microscopic polyarteritis Wegener's granulomatosis Idiopathic renal limited crescentic GN
Linear deposition	Anti-GBM disease Goodpasture's syndrome

End of Section.

STEP 8 – *Does the Patient Have Acute Interstitial Nephritis (AIN)?*

The major cause of acute interstitial nephritis is allergic drug-induced interstitial nephritis. The classic history is the onset of acute renal failure several days after starting a new medication. Acute interstitial nephritis may also occur due to immunologic disease (systemic lupus erythematosus, Sjögren's syndrome), sarcoidosis, lymphoma, or leukemia.

Clinical features suggestive of allergic drug-induced interstitial nephritis include fever, rash, and arthralgias. Urinalysis findings consistent with acute interstitial nephritis include the following:

- White blood cells (frequently eosinophils)
- White blood cell casts
- Red blood cells (rarely casts are present)
- Proteinuria (occasionally nephrotic range)

Although urine eosinophils are found in some patients with acute interstitial nephritis, their presence is not specific for the illness. Urine eosinophils have been reported in a variety of renal diseases. They are commonly found in atheroembolic disease, acute prostatitis, and rapidly progressive glomerulonephritis. If the clinical presentation is consistent with acute interstitial nephritis and other causes of eosinophiluria are not present, then the presence of urine eosinophils should be considered supportive of the diagnosis.

If the clinical presentation is consistent with acute interstitial nephritis, ***proceed to Step 9.***

If the clinical presentation is not consistent with acute interstitial nephritis, ***proceed to Step 10.***

STEP 9 – *What Type of Acute Interstitial Nephritis Does the Patient Have?*

The causes of AIN are listed in the following box.

CAUSES OF ACUTE INTERSTITIAL NEPHRITIS

MEDICATIONS

INFECTION

- Bacterial
  - Streptococci
  - Staphylococci
  - *Legionella*
  - *Brucella*
  - Diphtheria
  - *Salmonella typhi*
  - *M. tuberculosis*
- Viral
  - Measles
  - Epstein-Barr virus
  - Cytomegalovirus
  - HIV
  - Hanta
  - Herpes simplex virus type I
- Fungal
  - Histoplasmosis
  - *Candida*
- Others
  - Toxoplasmosis
  - Leishmaniasis
  - Schistosomiasis
  - Rocky Mountain spotted fever
  - Malaria
  - *Mycoplasma*
  - Leptospirosis
  - Syphilis

SYSTEMIC DISEASE

- Malignancy
  - Solid
  - Lymphoma
  - Leukemia
- Systemic lupus erythematosus
- Sjögren's syndrome
- Sarcoidosis

IDIOPATHIC

There are no clinical findings or laboratory tests that can definitively diagnose acute interstitial nephritis. The definitive diagnosis can only be made at the time of kidney biopsy. However, there may be clues in the patient's clinical presentation that suggest the diagnosis. The presence of fever, rash, or eosinophilia should prompt the clinician to consider drug-induced interstitial nephritis. The absence of these clinical features, however, does not exclude the diagnosis. With discontinuation of the offending medication, renal function typically returns to baseline with an improvement being seen within one week of stopping the medication. Renal biopsy should be considered if the renal failure persists or worsens despite discontinuation of the offending medication. Causes of drug-induced allergic interstitial nephritis are listed in the following box.

MEDICATIONS CAUSING DRUG-INDUCED ALLERGIC INTERSTITIAL NEPHRITIS

ANTIBIOTICS	OTHERS
β-lactams*	α-methyldopa
Ampicillin	Allopurinol
Amoxicillin	Azathioprine
Carbenicillin	Captopril
Methicillin	Carbamazepine
Nafcillin	Chinese herbs
Oxacillin	Cimetidine
Penicillin G	Clofibrate
Cephalexin	Diphenylhydantoin
Cephalothin	Gold
Cephradine	Indinavir
Cefotaxime	Interferon-alpha
Others	Lithium
Ethambutol	Omeprazole
Rifampin	Penicillamine
Sulfonamides	Phenindione
Trimethoprim-sulfamethoxazole	Phenobarbital
Ciprofloxacin	Phenylpropanolamine
NSAIDs†	Phenytoin
DIURETICS	Ranitidine
Chlorthalidone	Streptokinase
Furosemide	Sulfinpyrazone
Thiazides	Valproic acid
Ticrynafen	

*Any penicillin or cephalosporin can cause AIN. The average duration of medication use prior to the onset of clinical disease is about 10 days. However, some patients have developed renal insufficiency as early as 2-3 days after taking the medication. Approximately 30% of patients have the classic features of hypersensitivity. The absence of hypersensitivity features does not exclude the diagnosis. The diagnosis should be suspected in any patient who develops renal failure of unknown etiology while taking an antibiotic. The presence of any hypersensitivity feature lends strong support to the diagnosis. Although the definitive diagnosis requires kidney biopsy, in most cases, the clinical presentation suffices. Most patients have improvement in renal function after withdrawal of the antibiotic.

†While almost any NSAID can cause AIN, derivatives of propionic acid such as fenoprofen, ibuprofen, and naproxen, are the most common offenders. There are some notable differences in the presentation of NSAID-induced AIN as compared to antibiotic-induced AIN. For NSAID-induced AIN, the following features should be noted:

- Duration of exposure to medications is longer with NSAIDs (several months)
- Systemic hypersensitivity features, such as fever and rash, are usually absent
- Eosinophilia is usually absent
- Proteinuria is found in 75% of cases
- FENa <1%

The diagnosis should be suspected in any patient taking an NSAID who develops features consistent with AIN. Heavy proteinuria and a low FENa are clues to the diagnosis. While renal biopsy is definitive, it is not required if renal function improves after withdrawal of the medication.

Adapted from *Brenner and Rector's The Kidney,* Brenner BM, ed, Philadelphia, PA: WB Saunders Co, 2000, 1206.

End of Section.

STEP 10 – *Does the Patient Have Acute Tubular Necrosis (ATN)?*

Once glomerular, vascular, and interstitial causes of renal azotemia are excluded, the clinician should focus on the possibility of acute tubular necrosis. Although ATN is a diagnosis of exclusion, it is the most common cause of renal azotemia. ATN may be divided into nephrotoxic and ischemic types. The causes of nephrotoxic ATN are listed in the following box.

CAUSES OF NEPHROTOXIC ATN

ENDOGENOUS
- Pigment-induced nephropathy
  - Myoglobinuria
  - Hemoglobinuria
- Tumor lysis syndrome
- Myeloma kidney

EXOGENOUS
- Radiocontrast-induced nephropathy
- Ethylene glycol intoxication
- Medication-induced
  - Aminoglycosides
  - Cephalosporins
  - Vancomycin
  - Amphotericin B
  - Foscarnet
  - Pentamidine
  - Cisplatin
  - Acetaminophen
  - Ifosfamide
  - Mitomycin C
  - Methotrexate
  - Interleukin-2

Ischemic and nephrotoxic ATN account for >90% of renal azotemia. While the causes of nephrotoxic ATN are many, the history, physical exam, and laboratory data will often identify the etiology. The steps that follow will help the clinician sort through the many causes listed above.

Proceed to Step 11.

STEP 11 – *What Is the Cause of the Acute Tubular Necrosis?*

The clinical presentation will often allow the clinician to establish the etiology of the acute tubular necrosis, as shown in the following box. The clinician should realize, however, that it is common to have more than one cause present. That is, acute tubular necrosis is often multifactorial.

Clinical Features	Condition Suggested	Proceed to...
History suggestive of rhabdomyolysis Significantly increased CK* level	Myoglobinuria	Step 12
History suggestive of hemolysis Increased LDH Increased unconjugated bilirubin Decreased haptoglobin Spherocytes or schistocytes on peripheral blood smear	Hemoglobinuria	Step 13
Recent administration of radiocontrast	Radiocontrast-induced renal failure	Step 14

(continued)

Clinical Features	Condition Suggested	Proceed to...
Recent treatment of malignancy Marked hyperuricemia	Tumor lysis syndrome	Step 15
Administration of antibiotics	Antibiotic-induced ARF	Step 16
Administration of chemotherapeutic or immunosuppressive agents	ARF secondary to chemotherapeutic or immunosuppressive agents	Step 17
Anemia Back pain Osteoporosis Osteolytic lesions Spontaneous fracture Hypercalcemia Recurrent infections	Multiple myeloma	Step 18
History of ethylene glycol intoxication	Ethylene glycol intoxication	Step 19
Recent hemorrhage, surgery, or hypotension	Ischemic acute tubular necrosis	Step 20

*CK = creatinine kinase.

STEP 12 – *Does the Patient Have Rhabdomyolysis?*

Rhabdomyolysis should be suspected in the acute renal failure patient who has a significantly elevated CK-MM level. CK levels should be obtained in patients who have signs and symptoms of rhabdomyolysis such as muscle pain, swelling, bruising, weakness, or tenderness. Other laboratory test findings in rhabdomyolysis are listed in the following box.

RHABDOMYOLYSIS LABORATORY FEATURES	
ELEVATED CK-MM*	INCREASED SERUM POTASSIUM
BUN:Cr <5†	DECREASED SERUM CALCIUM§
INCREASED SERUM URIC ACID‡	LEUKOCYTOSIS
INCREASED SERUM PHOSPHORUS	FENa VARIABLE

*CK-MM, the most sensitive test for diagnosis of rhabdomyolysis, may range from 500 to >100,000 units/L. Most often, the CK-MM level is >16,000 units/L in acute renal failure patients with rhabdomyolysis. Serum CK levels typically reach their maximum within 24-36 hours of the insult. Thereafter, there is a fall in levels by about 40% per day. Because patients may delay seeking medical attention, some patients may be seen at a time when CK levels are elevated but perhaps not impressively so. In these patients, the diagnosis should not be discarded. The degree of CK elevation roughly correlates with the risk and severity of renal failure. With significant muscle injury, there may be an increase in the CK-MB fraction, but it rarely exceeds 3% to 5% of the total CK. Levels exceeding this should prompt consideration of acute myocardial infarction.

†The serum creatinine elevation may be disproportionate to the elevation in BUN. The normal BUN:creatinine ratio is about 10 but in patients with rhabdomyolysis, the ratio may be ≤5. This is because the creatine phosphate that is released from damaged muscle is converted into creatinine. Many suggest that the serum creatinine increases more rapidly in patients with rhabdomyolysis than in other causes of acute renal failure. Elevations in the serum creatinine >2.5 mg/dL/day are not unusual.

‡Hyperuricemia is a feature of rhabdomyolysis with impressive uric acid elevations seen in some patients. Indeed, uric acid levels >40 mg/dL have been appreciated in these patients.

§Hypocalcemia is the result of the hyperphosphatemia as well as calcium precipitation in injured muscle. Hypercalcemia may be appreciated during the recovery phase of this disease.

The clinician should also realize that one complication of rhabdomyolysis is disseminated intravascular coagulation in which case the characteristic lab test findings will be present. Once the presence of rhabdomyolysis has been established, the clinician should focus on elucidating the etiology. The causes of rhabdomyolysis are listed in the following box.

CAUSES OF RHABDOMYOLYSIS	
MEDICATIONS	TRAUMA
HMG-CoA reductase inhibitors*	Electrical shock
Gemfibrozil	Burns (extensive)
Cyclosporine	Crush injury
Colchicine	IMMOBILIZATION
Zidovudine	HEATSTROKE
Erythromycin	MALIGNANT HYPERTHERMIA
Itraconazole	NEUROLEPTIC MALIGNANT SYNDROME
ILLICIT DRUGS	EXERTION
Cocaine	Overexertion
Amphetamines	Marathon running
LSD	METABOLIC
Ecstasy (MDMA)	Hyponatremia
Opiates	Hypernatremia
ALCOHOL	Hypokalemia
INFECTION	Hypocalcemia
Viral	Hyperphosphatemia
Adenovirus	ENDOCRINE
Coxsackievirus	Hypothyroidism
Cytomegalovirus	Hyperthyroidism
Echovirus	Diabetic ketoacidosis
EBV	Nonketotic hyperosmolar syndrome
Herpes simplex virus	INFLAMMATORY
HIV	Polymyositis
Influenza B	Dermatomyositis
Parainfluenza	OTHER
Bacterial	Snake bites
Legionella	Seizure
Listeria	Ethylene glycol
Salmonella	Toluene
Streptococcus	INHERITED
Staphylococcus	

*Medications that increase the risk for statin-associated myopathy include niacin, fibric acid derivatives (gemfibrozil), macrolide antibiotics, verapamil, diltiazem, amiodarone, nefazodone, protease inhibitors, cyclosporine, and azole antifungals.

End of Section.

STEP 13 – *Does the Patient Have Hemolysis?*

Hemoglobinuria only occurs in the setting of serious intravascular hemolysis. Elevation in LDH, bilirubin, and potassium, as well as a decrease in haptoglobin, support the diagnosis. The urinalysis may reveal a discrepancy between the amount of blood and the number of red blood cells. The finding of a large amount of blood, but a small amount of red blood cells, should prompt the clinician to consider hemoglobinuria or myoglobinuria.

To differentiate between the two, blood should be centrifuged and serum examined. Since hemoglobin is poorly filtered at the glomerulus because of its large size, as well as its binding to haptoglobin, it imparts a red to brown color to plasma. On the other hand, myoglobin is much smaller and does not bind to plasma protein. As a result, it is freely filtered and does not accumulate in the plasma. Therefore, plasma of patients with myoglobinuria has a normal color.

Causes of hemolysis and hemoglobinuria are listed in the following box.

CAUSES OF HEMOLYSIS AND HEMOGLOBINURIA
TRANSFUSION REACTION
INFECTION: Malaria, clostridia
SPIDER OR SNAKE BITE
MEDICATIONS
G6PD DEFICIENCY
PAROXYSMAL NOCTURNAL HEMOGLOBINURIA
VALVULAR PROSTHESIS
MICROANGIOPATHIC HEMOLYTIC ANEMIA

End of Section.

STEP 14 – *Does the Patient Have Radiocontrast-Induced Renal Failure?*

This is a relatively common cause of acute renal failure in hospitalized patients. A small increase in serum creatinine averaging 0.2 mg/dL is a frequent observation after radiocontrast administration. A more severe decrease in renal function can be appreciated as well, particularly in those with risk factors for the development of radiocontrast-induced renal failure. Risk factors for radiocontrast-induced ARF are listed in the following box.

RADIOCONTRAST NEPHROTOXICITY RISK FACTORS FOR DEVELOPING ARF
PRE-EXISTING RENAL INSUFFICIENCY
DIABETIC NEPHROPATHY
SEVERE CONGESTIVE HEART FAILURE
VOLUME DEPLETION
HYPOTENSION
ELDERLY PATIENT (age >55)
ACUTE LIVER FAILURE
PROTEINURIA
INCREASED VOLUME / DOSE / FREQUENCY OF RADIOCONTRAST
CONCOMITANT TREATMENT WITH ACE INHIBITORS / NSAIDs / OTHER NEPHROTOXINS

Renal insufficiency typically develops 1-2 days after administration. It is usually mild and transient, however, some patients develop renal insufficiency of sufficient severity that dialysis is required. Most cases are mild and not clinically apparent. Persistent renal insufficiency is not common, but can occur, especially in those with advanced renal disease.

End of Section.

STEP 15 – *Does the Patient Have the Tumor Lysis Syndrome?*

Classically, the tumor lysis syndrome occurs in patients who are given chemotherapy for the treatment of lymphoma or leukemia. Chemotherapy results in the destruction of tumor cells and the rapid rate of cell turnover results in metabolic derangements such as hyperuricemia, hyperkalemia, hyperphosphatemia, and hypocalcemia. Although many patients are asymptomatic, some may report flank pain if renal pelvic or ureteral obstruction occurs.

Risk factors for the tumor lysis syndrome are listed in the following box.

RISK FACTORS FOR ACUTE TUMOR LYSIS SYNDROME
High-risk tumor types
Burkitt's lymphoma
Lymphoblastic lymphoma
Undifferentiated lymphoma
Diffuse large cell lymphoma
Leukemias
Extensive disease
Bulky (>10 cm) tumors
Severe LDH elevation
Severe leukocytosis
Impaired renal function
Pre-existing chronic renal failure
Oliguria
Current acute renal failure

From Flombaum CD, "Metabolic Emergencies in the Cancer Patient," *Semin Oncol*, 2000, 27:322-34 and from Krimsky WS, Behrens RJ, and Kerkvliet GJ, "Oncologic Emergencies for the Internist," *Cleveland Clinic Journal of Medicine*, Vol 69, March 2002.

The diagnosis should be suspected when acute renal failure develops in the above setting, along with an elevated uric acid level. Usually, the uric acid level exceeds 15 mg/dL. In most other causes of acute renal failure, the uric acid level is <12 mg/dL, except in prerenal disease. If there is any doubt, a uric acid:creatinine ratio can be calculated on a random urine specimen. Patients with acute uric acid nephropathy have a ratio that exceeds 2.

The urinalysis may be normal. In some cases, uric acid crystals may be appreciated. Other laboratory abnormalities include hyperkalemia, hyperphosphatemia, and hypocalcemia.

End of Section.

STEP 16 – *Is the Patient Taking Any Nephrotoxic Antibiotics?*

Antibiotics are the most common cause of drug-induced renal failure. Antibiotics that may result in ATN are listed in the following box.

ANTIBIOTIC-INDUCED ATN	
AMINOGLYCOSIDES*	ACYCLOVIR
CEPHALOSPORINS	PENTAMIDINE
VANCOMYCIN	FOSCARNET
AMPHOTERICIN B†	

*Risk factors for acute tubular necrosis due to aminoglycosides include advanced age, volume depletion, pre-existing renal disease, concomitant use of other nephrotoxic medications (eg, diuretics, amphotericin B, cyclosporine), prolonged therapy, malnutrition, liver disease, and high trough concentration. Even with careful monitoring of serum drug levels, nephrotoxicity can still occur. It typically presents with nonoliguric acute tubular necrosis. Although the serum creatinine usually rises 5-10 days after starting treatment, acute renal failure can occur earlier, especially if the patient is being treated with other nephrotoxic agents or has sepsis or hypotension.

†Amphotericin B therapy is commonly complicated by acute renal failure and electrolyte abnormalities. Therapy results in urinary magnesium and potassium wasting which can lead to hypomagnesemia and hypokalemia, respectively. Other renal manifestations include renal tubular acidosis and nephrogenic diabetes insipidus. The renal failure is typically reversible with discontinuation of the amphotericin therapy. Nephrotoxicity is less common with liposomal amphotericin B.

End of Section.

STEP 17 – *Is the Patient Receiving Any Nephrotoxic Chemotherapeutic or Immunosuppressive Medications?*

Cancer chemotherapeutic and immunosuppressive medications that can cause ATN are listed in the following box.

CANCER CHEMOTHERAPY / IMMUNOSUPPRESSIVE MEDICATIONS THAT CAUSE ATN	
CYCLOSPORINE	MITOMYCIN C
TACROLIMUS	MITHRAMYCIN
CISPLATIN	IFOSFAMIDE
STREPTOZOCIN	BIOLOGIC RESPONSE MODIFIERS
METHOTREXATE	(Interleukin-2)

End of Section.

STEP 18 – *Does the Patient Have Myeloma Kidney?*

The diagnosis of multiple myeloma is apparent when patients present with chronic back pain, pathologic fractures, and hypercalcemia along with proteinuria and renal failure. Twenty-five percent to 50% of patients with multiple myeloma develop renal failure. The major cause of ARF is myeloma kidney, in which the urinary excretion of immunoglobulin light chains plays a large role. The freely filtered light chains cause renal tubular damage due to precipitation and formation of casts (obstructing lumen), as well as by causing injury as a result of the reabsorption of light chains (toxic to tubular cells). Hypercalcemia and dehydration can also contribute to ARF.

Urine dipstick testing does not detect the presence of urine light chains. Sulfosalicylic acid (or SSA) testing, however, detects all proteins. A positive SSA with a negative dipstick for protein indicates the presence of nonalbumin proteins, such as light chains. A negative SSA does not exclude the diagnosis, since the test is not positive unless the light chain concentration exceeds 1-1.5 g/day. The definitive test to establish the diagnosis is urine protein electrophoresis and immunofixation.

End of Section.

STEP 19 – *Does the Patient Have Ethylene Glycol Intoxication?*

Ethylene glycol is a component of antifreeze and other solvents. Intoxication with ethylene glycol may result in damage to the CNS, kidney, and cardiopulmonary system. A high anion gap metabolic acidosis with calcium oxalate crystalluria is the hallmark of ethylene glycol intoxication. Another clue to the diagnosis is the presence of an elevated osmolal gap. For more information regarding the diagnosis of ethylene glycol intoxication, proceed to the chapter, ***Approach to the Patient With High Anion Gap Metabolic Acidosis*** *on page 287.*

End of Section.

STEP 20 – *Does the Patient Have Ischemic ATN?*

The only difference between prerenal azotemia and ischemic ATN is that the underlying hypoperfusion is more severe and/or more prolonged in ischemic ATN. As a result, there is damage to the tubular epithelium. Risk factors for the development of ischemic ATN are listed in the following box.

RISK FACTORS FOR DEVELOPING ISCHEMIC ATN	
MAJOR CARDIOVASCULAR SURGERY	SEPSIS
SEVERE TRAUMA	VOLUME DEPLETION
HEMORRHAGE	

End of Section.

References

Agrawal M and Swartz R, "Acute Renal Failure," *Am Fam Physician*, 2000, 61(7):2077-88.

Albright RC Jr, "Acute Renal Failure: A Practical Update," *Mayo Clin Proc*, 2001, 76(1):67-74.

Alexopoulos E, "Drug-Induced Acute Interstitial Nephritis," *Ren Fail*, 1998, 20(6):809-19.

Allison RC and Bedsole DL, "The Other Medical Causes of Rhabdomyolysis," *Am J Med Sci*, 2003, 326(2):79-88.

Esson ML and Schrier RW, "Diagnosis and Treatment of Acute Tubular Necrosis," *Ann Intern Med*, 2002, 137(9):744-52.

Gesualdo L, Grandaliano G, Mascia L, et al, "Acute Renal Failure in Critically Ill Patients," *Intensive Care Med*, 1999, 25(10):1188-90.

Guo X and Nzerue C, "How to Prevent, Recognize, and Treat Drug-Induced Nephrotoxicity," *Cleve Clin J Med*, 2002, 69(4):289-90, 293-4, 296-7 passim.

Kodner CM and Kudrimoti A, "Diagnosis and Management of Acute Interstitial Nephritis," *Am Fam Physician*, 2003, 67(12):2527-34.

Madaio MP and Harrington JT, "The Diagnosis of Glomerular Diseases: Acute Glomerulonephritis and the Nephrotic Syndrome," *Arch Intern Med*, 2001, 161(1):25-34.

Michel DM and Kelly CJ, "Acute Interstitial Nephritis," *J Am Soc Nephrol*, 1998, 9(3):506-15.

Modi KS and Rao VK, "Atheroembolic Renal Disease," *J Am Soc Nephrol*, 2001, 12(8):1781-7.

Perazella MA, "Acute Renal Failure in HIV-Infected Patients: A Brief Review of Common Causes," *Am J Med Sci*, 2000, 319(6):385-91.

Quader MA, Sawmiller C, and Sumpio BA, "Contrast-Induced Nephropathy: Review of Incidence and Pathophysiology," *Ann Vasc Surg*, 1998, 12(6):612-20.

Ruggenenti P, Noris M, and Remuzzi G, "Thrombotic Microangiopathy, Hemolytic Uremic Syndrome, and Thrombotic Thrombocytopenic Purpura," *Kidney Int*, 2001, 60(3):831-46.

Scolari F, Tardanico R, Zani R, et al, "Cholesterol Crystal Embolism: A Recognizable Cause of Renal Disease," *Am J Kidney Dis*, 2000, 36(6):1089-109.

Solomon R, "Radiocontrast-Induced Nephropathy," *Semin Nephrol*, 1998, 18(5):551-7.

Steen VD, "Scleroderma Renal Crisis," *Rheum Dis Clin North Am*, 2003, 29(2):315-33.

Vanholder R, Server MS, Erek E, et al, "Rhabdomyolysis," *J Am Soc Nephrol*, 2000, 11(8):1553-61.

Yoshizawa N, "Acute Glomerulonephritis," *Intern Med*, 2000, 39(9):687-94.

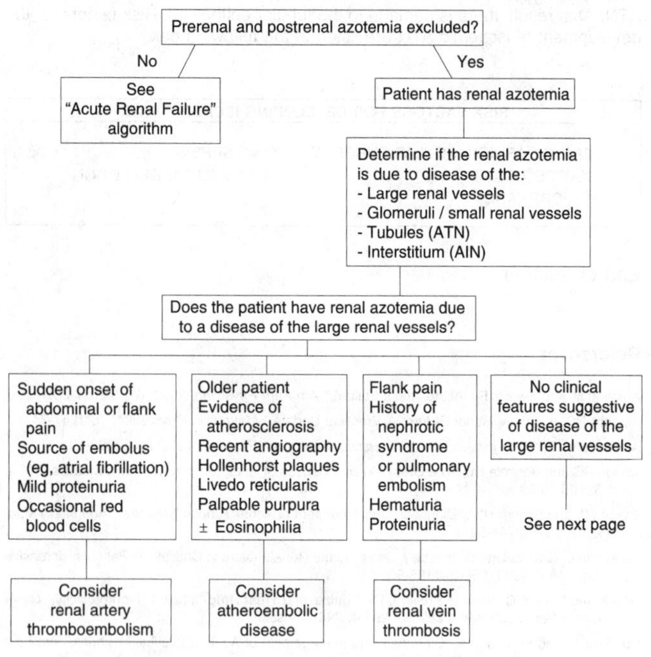
APPROACH TO THE PATIENT WITH RENAL AZOTEMIA
Prerenal and postrenal azotemia excluded?
No
Yes
See "Acute Renal Failure" algorithm
Patient has renal azotemia
Determine if the renal azotemia is due to disease of the:
- Large renal vessels
- Glomeruli / small renal vessels
- Tubules (ATN)
- Interstitium (AIN)
Does the patient have renal azotemia due to a disease of the large renal vessels?
Sudden onset of abdominal or flank pain
Source of embolus (eg, atrial fibrillation)
Mild proteinuria
Occasional red blood cells
Older patient
Evidence of atherosclerosis
Recent angiography
Hollenhorst plaques
Livedo reticularis
Palpable purpura
± Eosinophilia
Flank pain
History of nephrotic syndrome or pulmonary embolism
Hematuria
Proteinuria
No clinical features suggestive of disease of the large renal vessels
See next page
Consider renal artery thromboembolism
Consider atheroembolic disease
Consider renal vein thrombosis

APPROACH TO THE PATIENT WITH RENAL AZOTEMIA *(continued)*

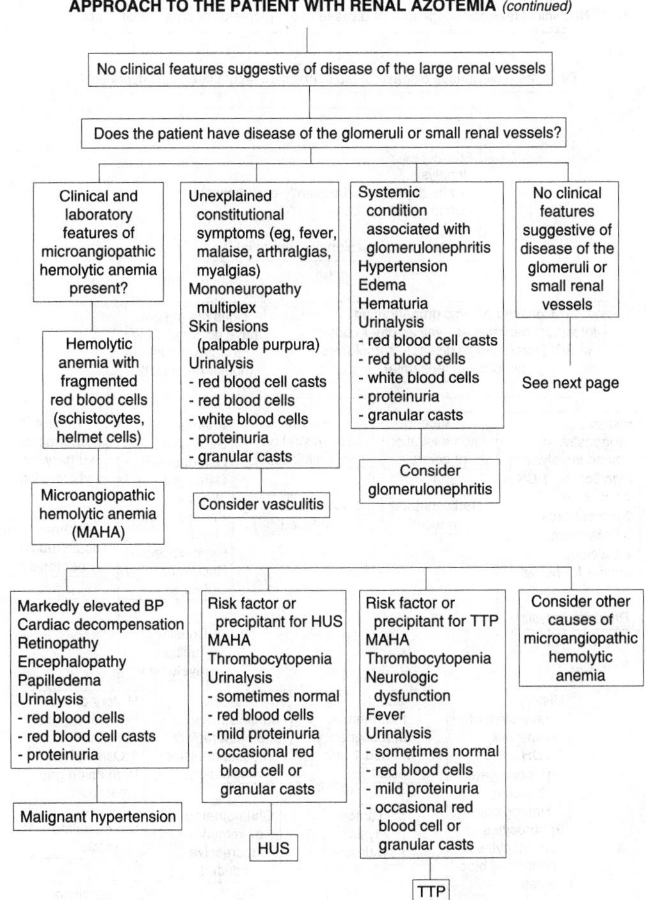

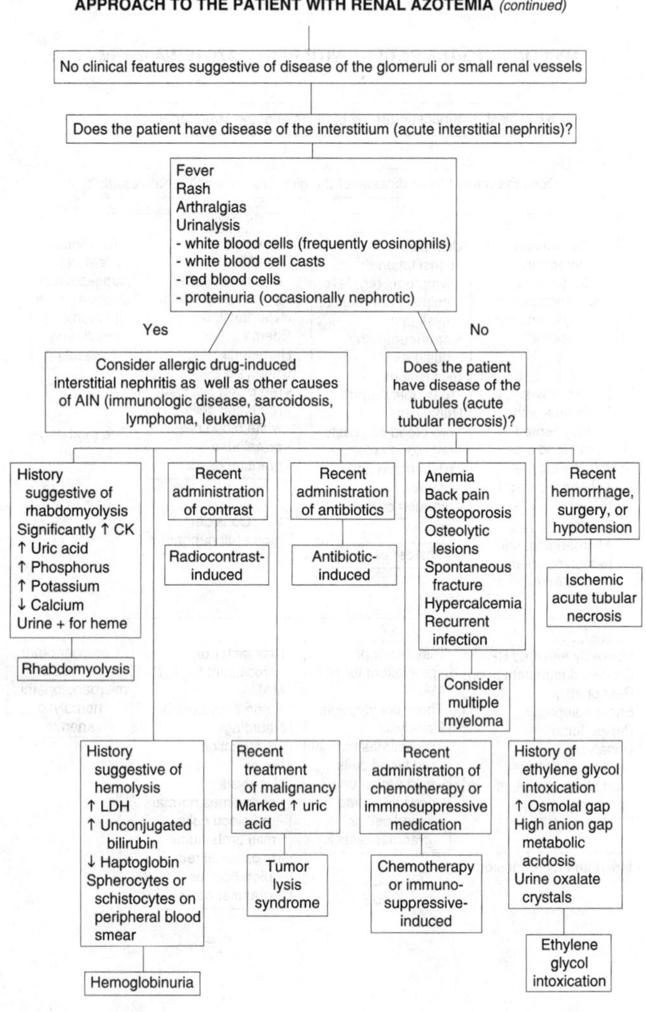
APPROACH TO THE PATIENT WITH RENAL AZOTEMIA (continued)
No clinical features suggestive of disease of the glomeruli or small renal vessels
Does the patient have disease of the interstitium (acute interstitial nephritis)?
Fever
Rash
Arthralgias
Urinalysis
- white blood cells (frequently eosinophils)
- white blood cell casts
- red blood cells
- proteinuria (occasionally nephrotic)
Yes
No
Consider allergic drug-induced interstitial nephritis as well as other causes of AIN (immunologic disease, sarcoidosis, lymphoma, leukemia)
Does the patient have disease of the tubules (acute tubular necrosis)?
History suggestive of rhabdomyolysis
Significantly ↑ CK
↑ Uric acid
↑ Phosphorus
↑ Potassium
↓ Calcium
Urine + for heme
Rhabdomyolysis
Recent administration of contrast
Radiocontrast-induced
Recent administration of antibiotics
Antibiotic-induced
Anemia
Back pain
Osteoporosis
Osteolytic lesions
Spontaneous fracture
Hypercalcemia
Recurrent infection
Consider multiple myeloma
Recent hemorrhage, surgery, or hypotension
Ischemic acute tubular necrosis
History suggestive of hemolysis
↑ LDH
↑ Unconjugated bilirubin
↓ Haptoglobin
Spherocytes or schistocytes on peripheral blood smear
Hemoglobinuria
Recent treatment of malignancy
Marked ↑ uric acid
Tumor lysis syndrome
Recent administration of chemotherapy or immnosuppressive medication
Chemotherapy or immuno-suppressive-induced
History of ethylene glycol intoxication
↑ Osmolal gap
High anion gap metabolic acidosis
Urine oxalate crystals
Ethylene glycol intoxication

CHRONIC RENAL FAILURE

Chronic renal failure (CRF) refers to a decline in kidney function over an extended period of time. The loss of renal function is often permanent and is usually progressive. It can be classified as mild, moderate, or severe based upon the reduction in the glomerular filtration rate (GFR), as shown in the following table.

Renal Failure	Glomerular Filtration Rate (mL/min)	Typical Serum Creatinine in a 65 kg Subject (mg/dL)
Mild	30-50	2
Moderate	10-29	4
Severe	<10	8
End stage	<5	17

Adapted from Johnson R and Feehally J, *Comprehensive Clinical Nephrology*, Harcourt Publishers Ltd, 2000, 14.68.1.

Not uncommonly, the terms "chronic renal failure" and "end-stage renal disease" are used interchangeably. However, these two terms should not be used synonymously. They refer to different degrees of renal failure. End-stage renal disease should only be used to describe renal failure that is not compatible with life if renal replacement therapy (eg, dialysis) is not initiated or maintained.

In 2002, the National Kidney Foundation published guidelines to help clinicians stratify patients with chronic kidney disease into one of 5 groups.

Stages of Chronic Kidney Disease*

Stage	Description	GFR
1	Kidney damage with normal or ↑ GFR	≥90
2	Kidney damage with mild ↓ GFR	60-89
3	Moderate ↓ GFR	30-59
4	Severe ↓ GFR	15-29
5	Kidney failure	<15 (or dialysis)

*Chronic kidney disease is defined as either kidney damage or GFR <60 mL/min/1.73 m^2 for ≥3 months. Kidney damage is defined as pathological abnormalities or markers of damage including abnormalities in blood or urine tests or imaging studies.

From National Kidney Foundation. "KIDOQI Clinical Practice Guidelines for Chronic Kidney Disease: Evaluation, Classification, and Stratification. Part 4. Definition and Stages of Chronic Kidney Disease," *Am J Kidney Dis*, 2002, 39.

Distinguishing Chronic From Acute Renal Failure (ARF)

Features noted in the following table help distinguish between CRF and ARF.

Comparison of ARF vs CRF

	History	Kidney Size	Bone X-ray	Hgb*	Broad Casts
ARF	Normal renal function	Normal†	Normal	Normal*	Absent
CRF	Increased BUN and Cr	Small bilaterally‡	Renal osteodystrophy	↓*	Present

*Remember that anemia can complicate acute renal failure (irrespective of the etiology) if a sufficient period of time passes. It is also important to realize that anemia may not be a feature of certain chronic renal diseases, such as polycystic kidney disease.

†The kidney may be enlarged in ARF secondary to obstructive uropathy.

‡Chronic renal failure secondary to multiple myeloma, autosomal dominant polycystic kidney disease, diabetic nephropathy, and amyloidosis may be associated with normal or enlarged kidneys.

Of the features listed in the above table, the most useful in differentiating chronic from acute renal failure is the renal ultrasound. In adults, normal kidney size ranges from 9-12 cm in length. In contrast to acute renal failure, most cases of chronic renal failure are characterized by a reduction in kidney size. Other features of a chronic process include reduction of cortical thickness, increased echo density, and scarring.

The presence of a normocytic, normochromic anemia is common in patients with chronic renal failure. Although it is uncommon in acute renal failure, it can be seen, especially if the acute renal failure is prolonged or is a feature of a systemic illness.

Although radiologic findings consistent with renal osteodystrophy are indicative of chronic renal failure, these findings are usually a manifestation of severe chronic renal failure. Therefore, milder degrees of chronic renal failure may not present with these radiologic changes (ie, erosion of lateral end of clavicle or radial edge of 2nd phalanx).

In most cases, the degree of BUN and creatinine elevation does not allow the clinician to differentiate chronic from acute renal failure. On occasion, patients appear well despite marked increases in BUN (>300 mg/dL) and creatinine (>13.5 mg/dL). In these patients, chronic renal failure is more likely to be present. Patients with acute renal failure who present with BUN and creatinine elevations to this extent usually do not appear well because they have not had time to adapt to the renal failure.

Acute on Chronic Renal Failure

Not uncommonly, patients with chronic renal failure develop a worsening of their BUN and creatinine levels beyond that which is expected from the natural history of their kidney disease. These patients are said to have acute on chronic renal failure. Every effort should be made to identify the cause of the acute on chronic renal failure. The causes of acute on chronic renal failure are listed in the following box.

FACTORS CONTRIBUTING TO ACUTE ON CHRONIC RENAL FAILURE	
VOLUME DEPLETION / DEHYDRATION	DISEASE RELAPSE
HYPOTENSION	DISEASE ACCELERATION
URINARY TRACT OBSTRUCTION	HYPERTENSION
INFECTION	INTERSTITIAL NEPHRITIS
DRUG TOXICITY / NEPHROTOXINS	HYPERCALCEMIA
CONGESTIVE HEART FAILURE	PERICARDIAL TAMPONADE

Reversible factors should be suspected whenever there is a greater than expected deterioration in renal function. This can be determined by plotting the inverse of serum creatinine (1/serum Cr) versus time. In most patients, the plot reveals a straight line, as long as the above factors are not present. If the slope of this line declines, the clinician should aggressively search for an exacerbating factor.

Causes of Chronic Renal Failure

Once chronic renal failure is confirmed and exacerbating factors have been excluded, the clinician should focus on determining the etiology. This requires a thorough history and physical exam.

In many cases, the cause of chronic renal failure is evident from the history and physical examination. In other instances, a renal biopsy done at some time during the course of the patient's renal disease establishes the diagnosis. In some cases, however, the etiology is never established, because renal insufficiency is discovered at an advanced stage. When renal insufficiency is discovered at a late stage, a renal biopsy is not often performed because of the low probability of finding a reversible lesion.

CAUSES OF CHRONIC RENAL FAILURE	
HEREDITARY DISEASES	TUBULOINTERSTITIAL DISEASES
Polycystic kidney disease	Reflux nephropathy
Alport's syndrome	Analgesic abuse nephropathy
Medullary cystic disease	Hypercalcemic nephropathy
Fabry disease	Heavy metal nephropathy
Cystinosis	(copper, lead, uranium, cadmium)
Familial amyloidosis	Myeloma kidney
PRIMARY GLOMERULAR DISEASES	Gouty nephropathy
Membranous nephropathy	Oxalate deposition
Membranoproliferative	OBSTRUCTIVE UROPATHY
glomerulonephritis	VASCULAR DISEASE
Focal segmental glomerulosclerosis	Hypertensive nephropathy
IgA nephropathy	Renal artery stenosis (bilateral)
SECONDARY GLOMERULAR DISEASES	Atheroembolic disease
Diabetic nephropathy	
Amyloidosis	
Heroin abuse	
HIV	
Postinfectious glomerulonephritis	
Collagen vascular diseases	
Sickle cell nephropathy	

Diabetic nephropathy, hypertensive nephropathy, and chronic glomerulonephritis account for 60% to 90% of cases. Polycystic kidney disease and obstructive uropathy make up a considerable proportion of the remaining cases.

In the majority of patients, discovery of chronic renal failure implies that a progressive decline in the GFR is inevitable. As a result, most clinicians do a limited evaluation. Nonetheless, it is important to realize that there are several diseases which should be excluded. These deserve mention because appropriate treatment of these conditions may stabilize or even reverse the decline in the GFR. These diseases include renal artery stenosis, chronic obstructive uropathy, analgesic nephropathy, chronic hypercalcemia, SLE, amyloidosis, tuberculosis, systemic vasculitis, membranous nephropathy, multiple myeloma, and atheroembolic disease.

Laboratory testing can provide clues to the etiology of the chronic renal failure, as shown in the following box.

Laboratory Findings in CRF

Laboratory Findings	Suggested Etiology of CRF
Heavy proteinuria (>3.0 g/day)	Glomerular disease
Mild proteinuria (<1.5 g/day)	Tubulointerstitial disease
Urine RBC casts	Glomerular disease
Urine WBC casts	Tubulointerstitial disease
(+) Urine immunoelectrophoresis	Multiple myeloma Light chain deposition disease
(+) ANA	Systemic lupus erythematosus
(+) ANCA	Wegener's granulomatosis Other small vessel vasculitis
↓ Complement	Systemic lupus erythematosus Membranoproliferative glomerulonephritis
↑ Calcium	Hypercalcemia-induced nephropathy

Other nonspecific laboratory abnormalities that may be appreciated in patients with chronic renal failure are found in the following box.

CHRONIC RENAL FAILURE COMMON LABORATORY FEATURES	
DECREASED SERUM CALCIUM*	INCREASED SERUM URIC ACID
INCREASED SERUM PHOSPHORUS*	INCREASED PARATHYROID HORMONE
INCREASED SERUM POTASSIUM†	ANEMIA
METABOLIC ACIDOSIS‡	INCREASED SERUM MAGNESIUM§

*The serum calcium level is typically normal in patients with mild chronic renal failure. As the renal dysfunction progresses, hypocalcemia becomes common. Factors contributing to hypocalcemia include hyperphosphatemia, resistance to the effects of PTH on bone, and decreased 1,25 dihydroxyvitamin D3 levels. Plasma phosphate levels remain in the normal range until the GFR falls below 25 mL/minute.

†The potassium level usually remains within the normal range until the GFR falls below 10 mL/minute. In patients who have higher glomerular filtration rates, hyperkalemia may ensue if they are given potassium-sparing diuretics, ACE inhibitors, or NSAIDs. Other factors that may predispose to hyperkalemia include hypercatabolism and acidosis. In milder degrees of chronic renal failure, hyperkalemia may be a manifestation of hyporeninemic hypoaldosteronism. Chronic renal failure patients may also present with hypokalemia. Some causes of hypokalemia in this population include poor dietary potassium intake, diuretic treatment, diarrhea, and renal tubular defects (type 1 or 2 RTA).

‡Acidosis, which is usually absent in mild chronic renal failure, becomes more common as the renal dysfunction advances. In early renal failure, patients may have a hyperchloremic metabolic acidosis with normal anion gap. With advancing disease, the plasma chloride level normalizes and a high anion gap metabolic acidosis is the usual finding.

§Plasma magnesium levels remain normal until the GFR falls below 25 mL/minute. Mildly elevated levels tend to be the rule unless the patient takes magnesium-containing laxatives or antacids.

Ultrasound Findings in Chronic Renal Failure

Earlier, the role of ultrasound in distinguishing acute from chronic renal failure was discussed. Ultrasound may also provide clues as to the etiology of the chronic renal failure. Ultrasound findings that should prompt the clinician to consider certain causes of chronic renal failure are listed in the following table.

Ultrasound Findings in CRF

Ultrasound Finding	Diagnosis Suggested
Dilatation of the urinary tract	Obstructive uropathy
Multiple cysts in the kidney	Polycystic kidney disease
Papillary necrosis	Analgesic nephropathy

Estimating the Severity of the CRF

The severity of the chronic renal failure may be estimated by calculating the creatinine clearance. This calculation, however, requires performing a 24-hour urine collection. Many patients find the 24-hour urine collection cumbersome, which can lead to inaccurate estimation of the severity of the chronic renal failure. Because of this, many clinicians turn to the Cockcroft-Gault formula for calculation of the creatinine clearance, as shown in the following box.

COCKROFT-GAULT EQUATION

Creatinine clearance = $\frac{[(140 - \text{age}) \times \text{wt (kg)}]}{(72 \times \text{serum creatinine})}$

For women, multiply the result by 0.85

Recently, the National Kidney Foundation has recommended the use of simplified GFR prediction equations that are more accurate and precise than the Cockcroft-Gault equation in the quantification of renal function. One that is widely used is the modification of Diet in Renal Disease (MDRD) equation. This equation is not as easy to remember but is available at a number of internet sites.

When the creatinine clearance falls below 30 mL/minute, the clinician should discuss issues regarding renal replacement therapy (ie, dialysis). In addition, this is an appropriate time to discuss the possibility of renal transplantation.

If hemodialysis is planned, issues related to dialysis access should be addressed. There are many others who feel that hemodialysis access should be created when the clinician estimates that the need for dialysis is likely within 6 months. This is because 3-6 months are usually required for maturation of a native arteriovenous fistula. In contrast, an arteriovenous synthetic graft can be used 2-4 weeks after placement. If peritoneal dialysis is planned, 4-6 weeks are required for healing before the catheter can be used on a regular basis.

Other management decisions are often based upon the severity of the chronic renal failure, as shown in the following table.

Guidelines for Management of Chronic Renal Failure Based Upon GFR

Degree of Renal Failure	GFR (mL/min)	Protein (g/kg/ day)	Sodium (mEq/ day)	Potassium (mEq/day)	Phosphorus (mg/day)	Fluid (mL/day)	Other
Mild	30-50	1.0	90	Normal dietary intake	Normal dietary intake	Normal dietary intake	Begin phosphate restriction and vitamin D analogs
Moderate	10-29	0.8-1.0	90	60-90	1000	Normal dietary intake*	Plan renal replacement including vascular access
Severe	<10	0.6-0.8†	60-90	60	800	24-hour urine output + 1000 mL‡	Plan elective start of dialysis or pre-emptive transplant
Dialysis	<5	1.0-1.2	90	60-90	800-1000	24-hour urine output + 1000 mL‡	

*May need restriction in some patients.

†Severe restriction of 0.6 g/kg/day is difficult for patients to follow and may cause protein malnutrition. Prolonged use of such a diet is not feasible.

‡Sodium and potassium restriction may differ for patients with good urinary output or "salt-wasting".

Adapted from Johnson R and Feehally J, *Comprehensive Clinical Nephrology*, Harcourt Publishers Ltd, 2000, 14.68.1.

Anemia of Chronic Renal Failure

The anemia of chronic renal failure is typically not encountered until the creatinine clearance falls below 35-40 mL/minute. It should be realized, however, that there is no absolute level at which anemia develops in patients with chronic renal failure. In general, the severity of the anemia is proportional to the degree of renal dysfunction. It is not common, however, for the hematocrit to fall below 25% in uncomplicated anemia of chronic renal failure. Hematocrit levels below 25% should prompt consideration of bleeding, hemolysis, or another factor superimposed on the anemia of chronic renal failure.

It is due, in most part, to a decline in erythropoietin production from the failing kidneys. The availability of recombinant human erythropoietin has significantly reduced the morbidity and mortality of patients with chronic renal failure. Despite the fact that it is readily available, many patients with advanced chronic renal failure are not receiving erythropoietin therapy.

The mere documentation of anemia in patients with chronic renal failure does not definitively establish the diagnosis of the anemia of renal failure. Since there are other causes of anemia in patients with chronic renal failure, every effort should be made to determine the precise etiology of the anemia. Other causes of anemia in patients with chronic renal failure are listed in the following box.

CAUSES OF ANEMIA IN PATIENTS WITH CHRONIC RENAL FAILURE
ANEMIA OF CHRONIC RENAL FAILURE (decreased erythropoietin production)
IRON DEFICIENCY ANEMIA
FOLIC ACID DEFICIENCY
HEMOLYSIS (decreased RBC survival)
HEMORRHAGE
BONE MARROW FIBROSIS FROM ADVANCED OSTEITIS FIBROSA CYSTICA
ALUMINUM EXCESS

To exclude these other causes of anemia, the clinician should obtain the following tests:

- Serum iron studies (iron, ferritin, total iron binding capacity, transferrin saturation)
- MCV
- Reticulocyte count
- Review of peripheral blood smear
- Serum vitamin B_{12} level
- Serum folate level
- Fecal occult blood test

At the current time, measurement of erythropoietin levels are not recommended in the evaluation of these patients. This is because there is considerable difficulty in interpreting these levels in patients with renal failure. If no other causes of anemia are present, deciding when to begin erythropoietin therapy for anemia of chronic renal failure is based on the answers to the following questions:

- Is the patient symptomatic?
- Does the patient have angina?
- Is the hematocrit <30% (hemoglobin <10 g/dL)

If the answer to any of the above questions is yes, the clinician should consider starting erythropoietin therapy. Before starting therapy, the clinician should assess the patient's iron status. Studies have shown that iron deficiency may be present in up to 33% of patients with the anemia of chronic renal failure. Serum ferritin <100 ng/mL and/or transferrin saturation <20% are consistent with the diagnosis of iron deficiency. Iron deficient patients should be started on iron replacement therapy prior to erythropoietin administration.

After erythropoietin therapy is started, the patient's hemoglobin, hematocrit, and iron studies need to be monitored periodically, as shown in the following box.

SERIAL MONITORING OF HEMOGLOBIN / HEMATOCRIT / IRON STUDIES IN CHRONIC RENAL FAILURE PATIENTS TREATED WITH ERYTHROPOIETIN
Hemoglobin or hematocrit should be measured each week during induction of therapy and every 2 weeks thereafter.
Serum iron, total iron binding capacity, and ferritin should be checked monthly for 3 months and every 2-3 months thereafter.

Adapted from Ad Hoc Committee for the National Kidney Foundation, "Statement of the Clinical Use of Recombinant Erythropoietin in Anemia of End-Stage Renal Disease," *Am J Kid Dis*, 1989, 14:163-9.

Some patients, despite erythropoietin therapy, fail to reach the target hematocrit (33% to 36%). One of the common causes of hyporesponsiveness to erythropoietin therapy is iron deficiency. Iron stores can quickly become depleted during erythropoietin therapy due to the stimulation of red blood cell production. Although the presence of iron deficiency is most accurately determined by Prussian blue staining of a bone marrow aspirate for iron, clinicians usually turn to noninvasive measurements of serum iron, transferrin saturation (serum iron/total iron binding capacity), and ferritin to establish the diagnosis of iron deficiency.

Studies have revealed that the serum ferritin and transferrin saturation are superior to the serum iron level in the detection of iron deficiency. In end-stage renal disease patients, iron deficiency is likely to be present when the serum ferritin is <100 ng/mL or transferrin saturation is <20%. Because the diagnosis of iron deficiency anemia can be challenging in end-stage renal disease patients, in recent years, much work has focused on other markers of iron deficiency, such as the percentage of circulating hypochromic red blood cells and reticulocyte hemoglobin content. It remains to be seen what the precise role for these tests will be.

If the target hematocrit cannot be reached with erythropoietin therapy and the patient does not have iron deficiency anemia, other causes of erythropoietin resistance should be considered such as chronic inflammation, folate deficiency, aluminum accumulation in bone, malnutrition, and bone marrow fibrosis due to secondary hyperparathyroidism.

References

Bolton WK and Kliger AS, "Chronic Renal Insufficiency: Current Understandings and Their Implications," *Am J Kidney Dis*, 2000, 36(6 Suppl 3):S4-12.

Bourgoignie JJ, Jacob AI, Sallman AL, et al, "Water, Electrolyte, and Acid-Base Abnormalities in Chronic Renal Failure," *Semin Nephrol*, 1981, 1:91-111.

Delmez JA and Slatoplosky E, "Hyperphosphatemia: Its Consequences and Treatment in Patients With Chronic Renal Disease," *Am J Kidney Dis*, 1992, 19(4):303-17 (review).

Jacobs C, "At Which Stage of Renal Failure Should Dialysis Be Started?" *Nephrol Dial Transplant*, 2000, 15(3):305-7.

Kausz AT and Levey AS, "The Care of Patients With Chronic Kidney Disease," *J Gen Intern Med*, 2002, 17(8):658-62.

Klahr S, "Chronic Renal Failure: Management," *Lancet*, 1991, 338(8764):423-7 (review).

Levey AS, "Clinical Practice. Nondiabetic Kidney Disease," *N Engl J Med*, 2002, 347(19):1505-11.

McCarthy JT, "A Practical Approach to the Management of Patients With Chronic Renal Failure," *Mayo Clin Proc*, 1999, 74(3):269-73.

Parmar MS, "Chronic Renal Disease," *BMJ*, 2002, 325(7355):85-90.

Patel SS, Kimmel PL, and Singh A, "New Clinical Practice Guidelines for Chronic Kidney Disease: A Framework for K/DOQI," *Semin Nephrol*, 2002, 22(6):449-58.

Rahman M and Smith MC, "Chronic Renal Insufficiency: A Diagnostic and Therapeutic Approach," *Arch Intern Med*, 1998, 158(16):1743-52.

Reikes ST, "Trends in End-Stage Renal Disease. Epidemiology, Morbidity, and Mortality," *Postgrad Med*, 2000, 108(1):124-6, 129-31, 135-6 passim.

Ruggenenti P, Schieppati A, and Remuzzi G, "Progression, Remission, Regression of Chronic Renal Diseases," *Lancet*, 2001, 357(9268):1601-8.

Schmitz PG, "Progressive Renal Insufficiency. Office Strategies to Prevent or Slow Progression of Kidney Disease," *Postgrad Med*, 2000, 108(1):145-8, 151-4.

Tong EM and Nissenson AR, "Erythropoietin and Anemia," *Semin Nephrol*, 2001, 21(2):190-203.

Van Wyck DB, "Management of Early Renal Anaemia: Diagnostic Workup, Iron Therapy, Epoetin Therapy," *Nephrol Dial Transplant*, 2000, 15(Suppl 3):36-9.

NEPHROTIC SYNDROME

Nephrotic-range proteinuria is said to be present when urinary protein excretion exceeds 3.5 g/1.73 m^2 in a 24-hour period. This degree of proteinuria is the hallmark of the nephrotic syndrome. The characteristic pentad of the nephrotic syndrome is listed in the following box.

FEATURES OF THE NEPHROTIC SYNDROME
NEPHROTIC RANGE PROTEINURIA (>3.5 g/1.73 m^2 in 24 hours) HYPOALBUMINEMIA HYPERLIPIDEMIA EDEMA LIPIDURIA Fat droplets Oval fat bodies Fatty / waxy casts

Not all patients with the nephrotic syndrome have all elements of the pentad. For example, hypoalbuminemia may be absent in some patients with the nephrotic syndrome. In these cases, the liver is able to compensate for the increased urinary protein loss by increasing synthesis of albumin. The presence of edema is also variable.

Renal Function at the Time of Clinical Presentation

The characteristic pentad of the nephrotic syndrome does not include renal insufficiency. This is because many patients with the nephrotic syndrome have preserved renal function at the time of diagnosis. This group is, however, at increased risk of developing both acute and chronic renal failure. The risk of developing chronic renal failure increases in proportion to the severity of the proteinuria.

When acute renal failure develops in nephrotic syndrome patients, evaluation to elucidate the etiology does not differ from other patients who develop acute renal failure. The clinician should realize, however, that nephrotic syndrome patients are at increased risk of developing acute renal failure due to the following causes:

- Volume depletion
- Sepsis
- Transformation of underlying disease (eg, development of crescentic glomerulonephritis in patient with membranous glomerulopathy)
- Bilateral renal vein thrombosis

  Renal vein thrombosis is a complication of nephrotic syndrome. Reported to occur in 8% of patients, the frequency increases to 10% to 50% if all nephrotic syndrome patients are screened for renal vein thrombosis by ultrasound, irrespective of the presence or absence of symptoms. Acute renal failure may develop if the renal vein thrombosis is bilateral. Manifestations include flank pain and hematuria.
- NSAIDs
- ACE inhibitor therapy
- Acute interstitial nephritis due to drugs

Causes of the Nephrotic Syndrome

There are numerous causes of the nephrotic syndrome. Many of these causes are firmly associated with the nephrotic syndrome while others are based on single or small case reports. The major causes of nephrotic syndrome are listed in the following box.

MAJOR CAUSES OF THE NEPHROTIC SYNDROME
PRIMARY RENAL DISEASE
MEMBRANOUS NEPHROPATHY
FOCAL GLOMERULOSCLEROSIS
IgA NEPHROPATHY
MINIMAL CHANGE DISEASE
MEMBRANOPROLIFERATIVE GLOMERULONEPHRITIS
OTHER
SYSTEMIC DISEASES
DIABETES MELLITUS
AMYLOIDOSIS
SYSTEMIC LUPUS ERYTHEMATOSUS
DYSPROTEINEMIA
Multiple myeloma
Immunotactoid / fibrillary glomerulonephritis
Light chain deposition disease
Heavy chain deposition disease
INFECTIONS
Human immunodeficiency virus
Hepatitis B
Hepatitis C
Syphilis
Schistosomiasis
Tuberculosis
Leprosy
MALIGNANCY
Solid adenocarcinomas (eg, lung, breast, colon)
Hodgkin's lymphoma
Other malignant neoplasms
DRUGS OR TOXINS
NSAIDs
Gold
Penicillamine
Probenecid
Mercury
Captopril
Heroin
OTHER
Pre-eclampsia
Chronic allograft rejection
Vesicoureteral reflux
Bee sting

Adapted from Madaio MP and Harrington JT, "The Diagnosis of Glomerular Diseases," *Arch Intern Med*, 2001, 161:30.

As shown in the preceding box, the causes of the nephrotic syndrome may be categorized as primary or systemic. In primary nephrotic syndrome, there is no evidence of a systemic disease. Some of the more common systemic causes of the nephrotic syndrome are described below.

- Diabetes mellitus

  In the United States, diabetes mellitus is the most common cause of the nephrotic syndrome. Approximately 33% of patients with type I diabetes mellitus go on to develop diabetic nephropathy. In these patients, one of the earliest manifestations of diabetic nephropathy is the appearance of microalbuminuria 5-10 years after disease onset. If left untreated, overt proteinuria may be detected 13-20 years after disease onset. Several years thereafter, nephrotic-range proteinuria may be noted.

  Merely demonstrating the presence of nephrotic-range proteinuria in a diabetic patient does not signify causality. To support the diagnosis of diabetic nephropathy, the clinician should perform a thorough eye examination, looking carefully for findings consistent with diabetic retinopathy. Over 90% of type I diabetic patients with diabetic nephropathy have diabetic retinopathy. Therefore, the absence of diabetic retinopathy should prompt the clinician to question the diagnosis. Most patients (50% to 80%) with type II diabetes who have diabetic nephropathy will also have diabetic retinopathy.

- Lupus nephritis

  While most patients with lupus nephritis have other signs and symptoms of systemic lupus erythematosus, on occasion, the renal manifestations of this disease dominate the clinical picture or precede other manifestations of lupus. For these reasons, appropriate testing for lupus nephritis is recommended in all patients with unexplained nephrotic syndrome. Of note, serologic testing may be negative in patients with lupus nephritis because of the loss of autoantibodies in the urine. These are factors that may delay the diagnosis of lupus pleuritis. In these cases, a clue to the diagnosis is the presence of low serum complement levels.

- Amyloidosis

  Amyloidosis should be a consideration in patients with the nephrotic syndrome, especially those older than 40 years of age. The nephrotic syndrome occurs in 33% of amyloidosis cases. Although amyloidosis may be the result of chronic infection or inflammation (eg, longstanding rheumatoid arthritis), in recent years, the majority of cases in the United States are due to immunoglobulin light chain associated disease. While amyloidosis may present with renal manifestations alone, in other cases, there is evidence of other organ involvement. In these latter cases, signs and symptoms of cardiac involvement may be present. Other clues that should prompt consideration of the diagnosis include easy bruising, autonomic neuropathy, unexplained hepatomegaly, and carpal tunnel syndrome. Electrophoresis of the serum or urine will reveal a monoclonal protein in >90% of amyloidosis patients who present with the nephrotic syndrome. Abdominal fat-pad biopsy has a diagnostic yield of about 75% and should be considered when the cause of nephrotic syndrome remains unclear, especially if serum or urine electrophoresis does not reveal the presence of a monoclonal gammopathy.

- Malignancy

  Malignancy is always a concern in patients with the nephrotic syndrome. A number of different malignancies have been associated with glomerular disease. While the diagnosis of malignancy is usually suggested by signs and symptoms elicited by a thorough history and physical examination, on occasion, the nephrotic syndrome may be the initial manifestation of an occult malignancy.

- Drug-induced

  Drug-induced nephrotic syndrome always deserves consideration in patients with the nephrotic syndrome. NSAIDs are the medications most commonly associated with development of the nephrotic syndrome. The diagnosis of drug-induced disease can be a difficult one, mainly because resolution of the nephrotic syndrome features may take weeks to months following withdrawal of the suspect medication.

- Infection

  Many infections are associated with the nephrotic syndrome. A wide variety of glomerular diseases have been described in AIDS patients. These diseases may manifest clinically at any stage of HIV infection. Most HIV patients with the nephrotic syndrome are found to have focal segmental glomerulosclerosis. Patients with a history of intravenous drug abuse or blood transfusion are at increased risk of hepatitis B or C viral infection, both of which are associated with the nephrotic syndrome. Other infections that are associated with the nephrotic syndrome include syphilis, malaria, tuberculosis, leprosy, and schistosomiasis.

Establishing the Etiology of the Nephrotic Syndrome

Once the presence of the nephrotic syndrome has been established, further evaluation is geared towards identifying its etiology. Of key importance is the performance of a thorough history and physical examination to assess for the presence of systemic disease. The information in the following box provides guidance in the evaluation of adult patients with the nephrotic syndrome.

EVALUATION OF NEPHROTIC SYNDROME IN ADULTS

HISTORY
- Family history and history of drug or toxin exposure

PHYSICAL EXAMINATION
- If patient is >50 years, usual recommendations for age, including stool examination (hemoccult testing 3x)
  - If stool examination is negative, perform flexible sigmoidoscopy
  - If stool examination is positive, perform standard GI tract workup

LABORATORY TESTING

CBC	Lactate dehydrogenase
Serum BUN	Alkaline phosphatase
Serum creatinine	Albumin
Glucose	Lipid profile
AST	Chest radiograph
ALT	

CONSIDER SYSTEMIC DISEASES
- Fluorescein angiography (for diabetes mellitus)
- Antinuclear antibodies (for systemic lupus erythematosus)

CONSIDER MALIGNANT NEOPLASM (eg, amyloid or light chain disease or myeloma)
- If either patient >50 years or initial evaluation raises suspicion, perform:
  - Serum protein electrophoresis
  - Serum immunoelectrophoresis
  - Urine protein electrophoresis
  - Abdominal fat-pad biopsy

CONSIDER INFECTION
- Perform the following: Hepatitis B serology, hepatitis C serology, HIV testing

RENAL BIOPSY
- Distinguish primary glomerular disease
- Diagnosis of unsuspected secondary glomerular disease (eg, amyloid)
- Determine disease severity

Adapted from Madaio MP and Harrington JT, "The Diagnosis of Glomerular Diseases," *Arch Intern Med*, 2001, 161:32.

Indications for Renal Biopsy

When a thorough evaluation does not reveal the presence of a systemic cause of the nephrotic syndrome, the patient is likely to have idiopathic nephrotic syndrome. Only with the use of renal biopsy will the clinician be able to identify the primary renal disease. The incidence of the various causes of the idiopathic nephrotic syndrome is listed in the following table.

Causes of the Idiopathic Nephrotic Syndrome

Histologic Type	Incidence (%)
Minimal change disease	10-15
Membranous glomerulopathy	20-25
Focal segmental glomerulosclerosis	25-30
Membranoproliferative glomerulonephritis	5
Other proliferative and sclerosing glomerulonephritides	15-30

Adapted from Goldman L and Bennett JC, *Cecil Textbook of Medicine,* Philadelphia, PA: WB Saunders Co, 2000, 588.

On occasion, patients thought to have the idiopathic nephrotic syndrome may be diagnosed with a systemic disease based upon the results of the renal biopsy.

Renal biopsy is not indicated in most patients who have a clinical presentation consistent with diabetic nephropathy. It should be considered, however, if any of the following hold true:

- Atypical history
- Absence of retinopathy
- Clinical course atypical for diabetic nephropathy (early-onset renal failure, rapid progression of renal failure)
- Active urinary sediment (red blood cells, red blood cell casts)

Renal biopsy is usually recommended in patients with lupus nephritis to gauge disease activity and extent of fibrosis. These factors are important in guiding the therapy of lupus nephritis.

In summary, renal biopsy is recommended in nephrotic syndrome patients who meet one or more of the following criteria:

- Diagnosis is uncertain
- Therapy of the patient's condition is likely to be affected by knowing the severity of the disease

Nephrology Referral

Although nephrology referral is warranted in the majority of patients with the nephrotic syndrome, there is no need for urgent referral unless the patient has one of the following:

- Abnormal GFR
- Rapid decline in kidney function

In the absence of both of these findings, it is reasonable to perform the workup listed above. After the results are obtained, then the clinician may wish to refer the patient to nephrology for further evaluation and management.

References

Abrass CK, "Clinical Spectrum and Complications of the Nephrotic Syndrome," *J Investig Med* 1997, 45(4):143-53.

Cameron JS, "Nephrotic Syndrome in the Elderly," *Semin Nephrol*, 1996, 16(4):319-29.

Cunard R and Kelly CJ, "Immune-Mediated Renal Disease," *J Allergy Clin Immunol*, 2003, 111(2 Suppl):S637-44.

Eddy AA and Schnaper HW, "The Nephrotic Syndrome: From the Simple to the Complex," *Semin Nephrol*, 1998, 18(3):304-16.

Glassock RJ and Cohen AH, "The Primary Glomerulopathies," *Dis Mon*, 1996, 42(6):329-83.

Jennette JC and Falk RJ, "Diagnosis and Management of Glomerular Diseases," *Med Clin North Am*, 1997, 81(3):653-77.

Kashtan CE, "Glomerular Disease," *Semin Nephrol*, 1999, 19(4):353-63.

Madaio MP and Harrington JT, "The Diagnosis of Glomerular Diseases: Acute Glomerulonephritis and the Nephrotic Syndrome," *Arch Intern Med*, 2001, 161(1):25-34.

Orth SR and Ritz E, "The Nephrotic Syndrome," *N Engl J Med*, 1998, 338(17):1202-11.

Sezer O, Eucker J, Jakob C, et al, "Diagnosis and Treatment of AL Amyloidosis," *Clin Nephrol* 2000, 53(6):417-23.

ACUTE GLOMERULONEPHRITIS

Acute glomerulonephritis is a syndrome characterized by the sudden onset of the features listed in the following box.

FEATURES OF ACUTE GLOMERULONEPHRITIS	
HEMATURIA	ACUTE RENAL FAILURE
RED BLOOD CELL CASTS*	HYPERTENSION
PROTEINURIA†	EDEMA
OLIGURIA	

*Red blood cell casts are considered to be diagnostic of glomerular disease. Not uncommonly, however, red blood cell casts may be difficult to find. In these cases, visualization of dysmorphic red blood cells using phase contrast microscopy can be used as a surrogate to red blood cell casts in establishing the presence of glomerular disease.

†In most cases, proteinuria is modest, ranging from 500 mg/day to 3 g/day. On occasion, however, nephrotic range proteinuria (>3.5 g/day) may be encountered.

Causes of Acute Glomerulonephritis

Although there are many causes of acute glomerulonephritis, most patients present with one of the causes listed in the following box.

MAJOR CAUSES OF ACUTE GLOMERULONEPHRITIS
SYSTEMIC DISEASE
SYSTEMIC LUPUS ERYTHEMATOSUS
CRYOGLOBULINEMIA
SUBACUTE BACTERIAL ENDOCARDITIS
SHUNT NEPHRITIS
POLYARTERITIS NODOSA
WEGENER'S GRANULOMATOSIS
HYPERSENSITIVITY VASCULITIS
HENOCH-SCHÖNLEIN PURPURA
GOODPASTURE'S SYNDROME
VISCERAL ABSCESS
RENAL DISEASE
ACUTE POSTSTREPTOCOCCAL GLOMERULONEPHRITIS
MEMBRANOPROLIFERATIVE GLOMERULONEPHRITIS
IGA NEPHROPATHY
IDIOPATHIC RAPIDLY PROGRESSIVE GLOMERULONEPHRITIS
Anti-GBM disease
Pauci-immune
Immune-deposit disease

As shown in the preceding box, the causes of acute glomerulonephritis may be classified as systemic or renal. Every effort should be made to differentiate systemic from renal causes of acute glomerulonephritis. Making this distinction begins with a thorough history and physical examination, which may provide clues to the presence of a systemic condition.

Establishing the Etiology

In some cases, clues present in the patient's history and physical examination may point to a particular etiology. In these cases, the clinician should perform the appropriate laboratory testing to confirm the diagnosis.

In other cases, the etiology of the acute glomerulonephritis remains unclear. In these cases, serologic evaluation is necessary to elucidate the cause. Serologic testing that is recommended in patients with acute glomerulonephritis is listed in the following box.

SEROLOGIC TESTING RECOMMENDED IN PATIENTS WITH ACUTE GLOMERULONEPHRITIS*	
COMPLEMENT LEVELS	HEPATITIS B SEROLOGY
C3, C4, CH50	HEPATITIS C SEROLOGY
ANTI-DNA ANTIBODIES	BLOOD CULTURES†
ANCA	ANTI-GBM ANTIBODIES
CRYOGLOBULINS	STREPTOZYME

*If rapidly progressive glomerulonephritis is present, empiric therapy (eg, pulse steroids) is indicated before definitive diagnosis, to prevent irreversible scarring.

†Blood cultures are indicated if endocarditis or abscess is suspected.

Adapted from Madaio MP and Harrington JT, "The Diagnosis of Glomerular Diseases," *Arch Intern Med*, 2001, 161:26.

Particularly useful in the evaluation of these patients are complement levels. The major causes of acute glomerulonephritis can be divided into two groups based upon the serum complement level, as shown in the following table.

Serum Complement Levels in the Major Causes of Acute Glomerulonephritis

Serum Complement Level*	Causes of Acute Glomerulonephritis to Consider
Low	Systemic disease
	Systemic lupus erythematosus
	Cryoglobulinemia
	Subacute bacterial endocarditis
	Shunt nephritis
	Renal disease
	Acute poststreptococcal glomerulonephritis
	Membranoproliferative glomerulonephritis
	Type I, Type II
Normal	Systemic disease
	Polyarteritis nodosa
	Wegener's granulomatosis
	Hypersensitivity vasculitis
	Henoch-Schönlein purpura
	Goodpasture's syndrome
	Visceral abscess
	Renal disease
	IgA nephropathy
	Idiopathic rapidly progressive
	Anti-GBM disease
	Pauci-immune
	Immune-deposit disease

*Repeated measurements are useful (2-3 times, 1 week apart). Consistently normal serum levels are useful in narrowing the diagnostic possibilities

Adapted from Madaio MP and Harrington JT, "The Diagnosis of Glomerular Diseases," *Arch Intern Med*, 2001, 161:26.

Acute Glomerulonephritis With Hypocomplementemia

The causes of acute glomerulonephritis with hypocomplementemia can be categorized as systemic or renal, as shown in the preceding table. A thorough history and physical examination along with appropriate laboratory testing usually allows the clinician to distinguish systemic from renal causes, as shown in the following table.

Systemic Causes of Acute Glomerulonephritis Associated With Hypocomplementemia

Systemic Cause of Acute Glomerulonephritis	Clinical Findings	Laboratory Testing
Systemic lupus erythematosus	Arthritis Skin rash	ANA Anti-double stranded DNA antibodies
Subacute bacterial endocarditis	Symptoms Fever (80% to 85%) Chills (42% to 75%) Sweats (25%) Anorexia (25% to 55%) Weight loss (25% to 35%) Malaise (25% to 40%) Signs Fever (80% to 90%) Murmur (85% to 85%) Changing new murmur (10% to 40%) Neurologic abnormalities (30% to 40%)	Blood cultures Echocardiography
Cryoglobulinemia	Purpura Arthralgias Other signs of vasculitis	Rheumatoid factor positivity (70%) Cryoglobulin positivity (75%) Hepatitis C testing*
Shunt nephritis		Blood cultures CSF cultures

*Since many cases of cryoglobulinemia-associated acute glomerulonephritis are associated with hepatitis C infection, testing for hepatitis C viral infection is also recommended. Available tests include anti-HCV and hepatitis C viral RNA. Of note, anti-HCV tests are not always positive in patients with cryoglobulinemia and hepatitis C. It is also important to realize that liver function tests may be normal in these patients.

In the absence of one of the above systemic diseases, renal causes of acute glomerulonephritis and hypocomplementemia must be considered. These include acute poststreptococcal glomerulonephritis and membranoproliferative glomerulonephritis.

In acute poststreptococcal glomerulonephritis, a history of recent streptococcal skin or throat infection is often elicited but is not invariably present. The onset of renal involvement typically occurs 2-3 weeks after the streptococcal infection. The diagnosis is based on a characteristic history and physical exam along with evidence of a recent streptococcal infection. Streptococcal antibodies (streptolysin O, streptokinase, hyaluronidase, and nicotinamide dinucleotidase) are usually measured to establish the diagnosis of recent streptococcal infection.

Although many patients with acute poststreptococcal glomerulonephritis have depressed renal function, recovery of kidney function is the rule, with serum creatinine usually returning to normal within 4 weeks. Although hematuria typically resolves within 6 months, proteinuria may take years to resolve. Serum complement levels typically return to normal in 6-8 weeks. Persistently low serum complement levels should prompt consideration of other diagnoses, particularly systemic lupus erythematosus and membranoproliferative glomerulonephritis.

Membranoproliferative glomerulonephritis is the other renal cause of acute glomerulonephritis that presents with hypocomplementemia. The illness is characterized by recurrent episodes of acute glomerulonephritis, often with progression over time to end-stage renal disease. In cases where it is difficult to differentiate membranoproliferative from acute poststreptococcal glomerulonephritis, repeated measurement of serum complement levels and renal biopsy may be indicated.

Acute Glomerulonephritis With Normocomplementemia

Causes of acute glomerulonephritis and normocomplementemia can be categorized as systemic or renal. History, physical examination, and appropriate laboratory testing can establish the presence of a systemic cause, as shown in the following table.

Systemic Causes of Acute Glomerulonephritis Associated With Normocomplementemia

Systemic Cause of Acute Glomerulonephritis	Clinical Findings	Laboratory Testing
Polyarteritis nodosa	Weight loss	Hb_sAg
	Livedo reticularis	Anti-HCV
	Testicular pain/tenderness	
	Myalgia / weakness / leg tenderness	
	Mononeuropathy / mononeuropathy multiplex / polyneuropathy	
Wegener's granulomatosis	Painful or painless oral ulcers	ANCA*
	Purulent or bloody nasal discharge	
	Abnormal chest radiograph	
	Nodules	
	Fixed infiltrates	
	Cavities	
Henoch-Schönlein purpura	Purpura	—
	Abdominal pain	
	Nausea/vomiting	
	Arthritis	
Goodpasture's syndrome	Pulmonary hemorrhage	Anti-GBM antibodies
Visceral abscess	Signs and symptoms vary depending upon location of abscess	Blood cultures Imaging

*85% to 95% of patients with Wegener's granulomatosis have detectable serum ANCA (most common pattern is cANCA).

The renal causes of acute glomerulonephritis with normocomplementemia include IgA nephropathy and idiopathic rapidly progressive glomerulonephritis. The clinical presentation of IgA nephropathy, the most common primary glomerulopathy in the world, is varied. Asymptomatic hematuria, nephrotic syndrome, and rapidly progressive glomerulonephritis have all been described.

Although rapidly progressive glomerulonephritis (RPGN) may present with low serum complement levels, over 95% have normocomplementemia. RPGN is a clinical syndrome characterized by features of acute glomerulonephritis but differs from most cases of acute glomerulonephritis in that there is a rapid decline in renal function. Left untreated, patients may develop end-stage renal disease within days to weeks.

When idiopathic rapidly progressive glomerulonephritis is a consideration, further evaluation includes testing for ANCA and anti-GBM antibodies. Most patients with idiopathic RPGN are ANCA positive (most common pattern is pANCA). A fewer number (10% to 20%) have anti-GBM disease. Both ANCA and anti-GBM antibodies are present together in up to 10% of RPGN cases.

Renal Biopsy

Not all patients with acute glomerulonephritis require renal biopsy. For example, most cases of acute glomerulonephritis secondary to systemic disease can be diagnosed with a thorough history and physical examination followed by serologic testing to confirm the diagnosis. If serologic testing is inconclusive or unavailable, renal biopsy is required to establish the diagnosis. Even when a renal biopsy is performed in this setting, the histopathologic findings may not be pathognomonic of a particular condition but the findings may serve to narrow the differential diagnosis. Histopathologic examination of the kidneys may also provide information regarding the degree of inflammation and extent of fibrosis, two factors that play a role in selecting appropriate therapy.

Renal biopsy should also be a consideration in patients with RPGN. In these patients, prompt diagnosis and treatment are important in renal survival. A delay in diagnosis and treatment increases the risk of irreversible end-stage renal disease. Although renal biopsy can provide important information regarding the etiology of the RPGN, in recent years, noninvasive serologic testing (anti-GBM, ANCA) has been used as a surrogate. In fact, the results of serologic testing often obviate the need for renal biopsy and are also helpful in guiding initial therapy. However, if the results of serologic testing are not rapidly available, consideration of renal biopsy is warranted. Renal biopsy will not only help establish the etiology of RPGN but also provide information regarding the extent of disease activity, a factor that is useful in making treatment decisions.

The clinician should realize that the yield of renal biopsy in patients with small kidneys is decreased. This is because small kidneys suggest the presence of a more chronic process. Histologic examination is more likely to reveal irreversible glomerulosclerosis and interstitial fibrosis. These findings are nonspecific and therefore of limited value in elucidating the cause of the glomerular disease. In addition, these findings suggest that the patient will have a poor response to therapy.

Indications for Nephrology Referral

In general, it is reasonable to delay nephrology referral while proceeding with serologic testing in most patients with acute glomerulonephritis, especially if renal function is normal and stable. Renal function should be followed closely while awaiting the results of serologic testing.

If the GFR is decreased, renal function is declining rapidly, or the patient has systemic symptoms, the clinician should arrange for immediate nephrology consultation so that decisions regarding biopsy, treatment, and need for dialysis can be made expeditiously.

References

Andreoli SP, "Renal Manifestations of Systemic Diseases," *Semin Nephrol*, 1998, 18(3):270-9.

Berden JH, "Lupus Nephritis," *Kidney Int*, 1997, 52(2):538-58.

Blatt NB and Glick GD, "Anti-DNA Autoantibodies and Systemic Lupus Erythematosus," *Pharmacol Ther*, 1999, 83(2):125-39.

Cameron JS, "Lupus Nephritis," *J Am Soc Nephrol*, 1999, 10(2):413-24.

Cunard R and Kelly CJ, "Immune-Mediated Renal Disease," *J Allergy Clin Immunol*, 2003, 111(2 Suppl):S637-44.

Jennette JC and Falk RJ, "Diagnosis and Management of Glomerular Diseases," *Med Clin North Am*, 1997, 81(3):653-77.

Kashtan CE, "Glomerular Disease," *Semin Nephrol*, 1999, 19(4):353-63.

Madaio MP and Harrington JT, "The Diagnosis of Glomerular Diseases: Acute Glomerulonephritis and the Nephrotic Syndrome," *Arch Intern Med*, 2001, 161(1):25-34.

Vinen CS and Oliveira DB, "Acute Glomerulonephritis," *Postgrad Med J*, 2003, 79(930):206-13; quiz 212-3.

Yoshizawa N, "Acute Glomerulonephritis," *Intern Med*, 2000, 39(9):687-94.

MINIMAL CHANGE DISEASE

Minimal change disease, also known as nil disease or lipoid nephrosis, is the most common cause of nephrotic syndrome in children, accounting for about 80% of cases. In adults, it is less common but still accounts for 20% to 30% of nephrotic syndrome cases.

Clinical Presentation

It typically presents with the features of the nephrotic syndrome, with edema being a prominent complaint. Some patients may present with anasarca.

Causes

Although most cases are idiopathic, a thorough evaluation should be performed looking for one of the causes of the disease. Treatment of the underlying etiology can result in resolution of the minimal change disease. Causes of the disease are listed in the following box.

CAUSES OF MINIMAL CHANGE DISEASE	
IDIOPATHIC	IMMUNIZATIONS
MEDICATIONS	MALIGNANCY†
NSAIDs*	Hodgkin's lymphoma
Ampicillin	Non-Hodgkin's lymphoma
Rifampin	Leukemia
α-interferon	HEAVY METALS
Lithium	Mercury
Tiopronin	Lead
INFECTION	FOOD ALLERGY
HIV	

*Most patients with minimal change disease due to NSAID use have a concomitant interstitial nephritis. The urinalysis typically reveals hematuria and pyuria. Renal insufficiency is not uncommon in these patients.

†Most patients with minimal change disease due to malignancy will present with a known diagnosis of malignancy. Some may present with minimal change disease being the initial manifestation but, in these cases, signs and symptoms of the underlying malignancy are usually present. With effective treatment of the disease, minimal change disease usually improves or resolves.

Laboratory Testing

In patients suspected of having minimal change disease, lab tests that should be obtained include chemistry profile (to assess renal function), urinalysis (to assess for hematuria and proteinuria), 24-hour urine collection (to quantify the degree of proteinuria and determine glomerular filtration rate), lipid profile, and serum albumin. Testing will usually confirm the presence of the nephrotic syndrome. Young patients with minimal change disease usually present with normal renal function. In adults, however, an elevated serum creatinine is not unusual at the time of diagnosis. In most cases, the urinalysis is bland other than the presence of protein. In a minority of patients, hematuria may be present.

Establishing the Diagnosis

Because minimal change disease is such a common cause of the nephrotic syndrome in children, in this age group, the diagnosis is based on a compatible clinical presentation as well as a response to corticosteroid therapy. Renal biopsy is usually not performed. It should be considered, however, if there are features in the patient's clinical presentation considered atypical for the disease. These features include older age, abnormal serum creatinine, microscopic or macroscopic hematuria, and hypertension.

In adults, minimal change disease accounts for a lesser percentage of nephrotic syndrome cases. Therefore, renal biopsy is usually required to establish the definitive diagnosis. The renal biopsy findings of minimal change disease are summarized in the following table.

Renal Biopsy Findings in Minimal Change Disease

Renal Biopsy Study	Finding
Light microscopy	Normal
Immunofluorescence	Normal
Electron microscopy	Effacement and widening of epithelial foot processes

MEMBRANOUS NEPHROPATHY

Membranous nephropathy, also known as membranous glomerulopathy or membranous glomerulonephritis, is characterized by subepithelial immune complex deposition. Membranous nephropathy accounts for about 20% of adult idiopathic nephrotic syndrome cases. In children, it is much less common, accounting for <5% of cases.

Clinical Presentation

Most patients present with the typical features of the nephrotic syndrome. Twenty percent, however, present with non-nephrotic range proteinuria, with many of these patients being asymptomatic.

Causes of Membranous Nephropathy

Most cases of membranous nephropathy are primary or idiopathic but 15% to 30% of cases in adults are secondary. Primary and secondary causes of membranous nephropathy are listed in the following box.

CAUSES OF MEMBRANOUS NEPHROPATHY

IDIOPATHIC OR PRIMARY

SECONDARY

- Malignancy*
  - Lung
  - Colon
  - Breast
  - Stomach
  - Melanoma
  - Esophagus
  - Carotid body
  - Bladder
  - Prostate
  - Thyroid
  - Pancreas
  - Leukemia
  - Lymphoma
  - Others
- Connective tissue disease / autoimmune
  - Systemic lupus erythematosus†
  - Rheumatoid arthritis
  - Dermatomyositis / polymyositis
  - Sjögren's syndrome
  - Sarcoidosis
  - Mixed connective tissue disease
  - Ankylosing spondylitis
  - Myasthenia gravis
  - Hashimoto's thyroiditis
  - Graves' disease
  - Graft-versus-host disease
  - Bullous pemphigus
  - Pemphigus
  - Dermatitis herpetiformis
  - Guillan-Barre syndrome
  - Crohn's syndrome
- Medications
  - Gold
  - Mercury
  - Probenecid
  - Captopril
  - Penicillamine
  - NSAIDs
  - Trimethadione
  - Tiopronin
  - Bucillamine
- Infection
  - Syphilis
  - Hepatitis B
  - Hepatitis C
  - Filariasis
  - Leprosy
  - Malaria
  - Schistosomiasis

*Malignancy is a concern in patients found to have membranous nephropathy. Malignancies that are most commonly associated with membranous nephropathy include carcinomas of the lung, colon, breast, and stomach. In most cases, the patient will be known to have a malignancy at the time the diagnosis of membranous nephropathy is established. In some cases, signs and symptoms of malignancy will be present in a patient who has no history of neoplasm. In a minority of patients (<1% to 2%), membranous nephropathy will be an occult manifestation of malignancy.

†Membranous nephropathy is the histologic finding found in 10% to 20% of lupus nephritis cases. Interestingly, membranous nephropathy may be the initial manifestation of lupus nephritis, even before there are symptoms or serologic findings of systemic lupus erythematosus.

Laboratory Testing

In patients suspected of having membranous nephropathy, lab tests that should be obtained include chemistry profile (to assess renal function), urinalysis (to assess for hematuria and proteinuria), 24-hour urine collection (to quantify the degree of proteinuria and determine the glomerular filtration rate), lipid profile, and serum albumin. Testing will confirm the presence of the nephrotic syndrome in 75% to 80% of patients with membranous nephropathy. In the remainder, non-nephrotic range proteinuria is present. Up to 50% of patients will be found to have microscopic hematuria. Renal insufficiency is present in 5% to 10% of patients at the time of diagnosis.

Serum complement levels are normal unless the membranous nephropathy is due to systemic lupus erythematosus or hepatitis B infection. Other tests may be indicated depending upon whether the patient has signs or symptoms of some of the secondary causes of membranous nephropathy listed in the above box.

Poor prognostic factors include hypertension, heavy proteinuria, older age, male gender, and decreased renal function at the time of presentation. The course of the disease is variable but the rule of 1/3s applies to these patients:

- The disease remits spontaneously in 1/3 of patients. Remission may be partial or complete and tends to occur within the first two years after diagnosis. Relapses can occur, however.
- Proteinuria persists in 33% of patients but with no decline in renal function.
- Progression to end-stage renal disease occurs in 33% of patients.

Establishing the Diagnosis

Renal biopsy is required to establish the definitive diagnosis. Immunofluorescence will reveal the presence of granular IgG deposits along the peripheral capillary walls. Electron microscopy will demonstrate subepithelial electron-dense deposits. With advancing disease, spikes will be present. The term "spikes" refers to projections of basement membrane material, which may be present in between the electron-dense deposits or encircle them completely.

References

Glassock RJ, "Diagnosis and Natural Course of Membranous Nephropathy," *Semin Nephrol*, 2003, 23(4):324-32.

FOCAL SEGMENTAL GLOMERULOSCLEROSIS

Focal segmental glomerulosclerosis, also known as focal glomerulosclerosis, is found in 10% to 20% of patients with the idiopathic nephrotic syndrome. However, some studies have found it to be the most common glomerulopathy among patients with the nephrotic syndrome. Of note, it is the most common cause of idiopathic nephrotic syndrome in African Americans. It is characterized by scarring (sclerosis) affecting parts of some glomeruli.

Clinical Presentation

Focal segmental glomerulosclerosis classically presents with features of the nephrotic syndrome although some patients may present with non-nephrotic range proteinuria.

Causes of Focal Segmental Glomerulosclerosis

Focal segmental glomerulosclerosis can be primary (idiopathic) or secondary. Secondary forms of the disease are said to be present when one of the causes listed in the following box is identified.

CAUSES OF FOCAL SEGMENTAL GLOMERULOSCLEROSIS
IDIOPATHIC OR PRIMARY
SECONDARY
Sickle cell disease
Heroin nephropathy
HIV infection
Chronic vesicoureteral reflux
Morbid obesity
Hematologic malignancies
Chronic transplant rejection
Diabetes mellitus (rare)
Healing of prior inflammatory injury
Unilateral renal agenesis
Type I glycogen storage diseases

Laboratory Testing

In patients suspected of having focal segmental glomerulosclerosis, lab tests that should be obtained include chemistry profile (to assess renal function), urinalysis (to assess for hematuria and proteinuria), 24-hour urine collection (to quantify the degree of proteinuria and determine the glomerular filtration rate), lipid profile, and serum albumin. Testing will usually confirm the presence of the nephrotic syndrome although some patients may present with non-nephrotic range proteinuria. Over 50% of patients have hematuria. Thirty-three percent of patients are found to have hypertension at the time of diagnosis. Renal insufficiency is not uncommon, affecting 33% of patients at the time of diagnosis. Laboratory testing also plays a role in the identification of secondary causes of focal segmental glomerulosclerosis (eg, HIV - see box above).

The prognosis of the disease depends upon the severity of the proteinuria. Ten years after the initial diagnosis, the prevalence of end-stage renal disease is >50% in patients who have heavy proteinuria and renal insufficiency. Focal segmental glomerulosclerosis patients with the collapsing variant have a more aggressive disease course with patients progressing to end-stage renal disease months to several years after the diagnosis is established.

Establishing the Diagnosis

Renal biopsy is required to establish the diagnosis. Light microscopy may reveal mesangial collapse and sclerosis in parts of the glomerular capillary tufts. Immunofluorescent studies are typically unremarkable. Foot process effacement, especially in those with heavy proteinuria, is the typical finding on electron microscopy. The clinician should be aware of two variants of focal segmental glomerulosclerosis. One variant, termed the "glomerular tip lesion," tends to be a more benign disease. Patients with this type of histology tend to be more responsive to therapy. In contrast, another variant, termed the "collapsing" variant, has a more aggressive course. It is seen more commonly in the African American and HIV populations.

References

Schnaper HW, "Idiopathic Focal Segmental Glomerulosclerosis," *Semin Nephrol*, 2003, 23(2):183-93.

Schwimmer JA, Markowitz GS, Valeri A, et al, "Collapsing Glomerulopathy," *Semin Nephrol*, 2003, 23(2):209-18.

HEMATURIA

STEP 1 – *What Is Hematuria?*

Hematuria is defined as the presence of blood in the urine. It may either be gross or microscopic. When it is gross, it understandably causes considerable anxiety in both patients and clinicians alike. In particular, there is concern that the hematuria may be caused by a serious condition (ie, malignancy). It is important to realize, however, that the causes of gross and microscopic hematuria are the same. Therefore, a thorough evaluation is necessary regardless of whether the patient presents with gross or microscopic hematuria.

If the patient complains of gross hematuria, ***proceed to Step 2.***

If the patient has microscopic hematuria, ***proceed to Step 3.***

STEP 2 – *Does the Patient Truly Have Gross Hematuria?*

Because there are other causes of a red or brown urine, the clinician must verify the presence of hematuria prior to embarking on an evaluation, which, at times, can be very extensive. A variety of substances may cause urine discoloration that mimics gross hematuria. This is known as pseudohematuria, the causes of which are listed in the following box.

CAUSES OF PSEUDOHEMATURIA	
MEDICATIONS	VEGETABLE DYES
Analgesics	Beets
Phenacetin	Blackberries
Phenazopyridine	Paprika
Antimicrobials	Rhubarb
Rifampin	
Antimalarials	ANTISEPTICS
Laxatives	Cresols
Anthraquinone (cascara, senna)	Mercurochrome
Chemotherapeutic agents	Phenols
Daunorubicin	Povidone-iodine
Doxorubicin	
Miscellaneous	METABOLIC
Deferoxamine	Porphyrins
Dilantin	Urate crystalluria
Levodopa	
Methyldopa	
Phenothiazines	

To distinguish between pseudohematuria and gross hematuria, it is necessary to obtain a urinalysis.

Proceed to Step 3.

STEP 3 – *What Are the Results of the Urine Dipstick for Blood?*

A positive urine dipstick test for blood is usually noted in both gross and microscopic hematuria. False-negative test results may be seen in the following situations:

- Ingestion of large amounts of vitamin C (>200 mg/day)
- Contamination of the urine specimen container with formaldehyde

It is important to realize, however, that a positive urine dipstick test for blood is not synonymous with hematuria because there are other causes of a positive test. The causes of a positive urine dipstick test for blood are listed in the following box.

CAUSES OF A POSITIVE URINE DIPSTICK TEST FOR BLOOD	
FALSE-POSITIVE REACTION	HEMOGLOBINURIA (hemolysis)
HEMATURIA	MYOGLOBINURIA (muscle injury)

To distinguish between these possibilities, it is necessary to perform urine microscopy.

Proceed to Step 4.

STEP 4 – *What Are the Results of Urine Microscopy?*

To differentiate between the causes of a positive urine dipstick test for blood, it is necessary to perform urine microscopy. Hematuria is present when microscopic analysis of the urine reveals the presence of red blood cells. Normal urine contains a small number of red blood cells. Just what constitutes the upper limit of normal, however, is widely debated. Although a consensus definition of hematuria is lacking, many authorities consider the presence of >3 red blood cells per high power field to be abnormal.

When the urine dipstick test is positive for blood but urine microscopy is negative for red blood cells, the clinician should suspect one of the following:

- Hemoglobinuria
- Myoglobinuria
- Lysis of red blood cells in the urine

When a patient with a positive urine dipstick test for blood but negative urine microscopy for red blood cells is encountered, it is essential to exclude hemoglobinuria (hemolysis) and myoglobinuria. The following table provides information in differentiating myoglobinuria and hemoglobinuria from hematuria.

	Urine Dipstick	Urine RBC	Serum Supernatant	LDH	Bilirubin	CPK
Hematuria	(+)	(+)	Clear	NL	NL	NL
Hemoglobinuria	(+)	(–)	Pink	Increased	Increased	NL
Myoglobinuria	(+)	(–)	Clear	NL	NL	Increased

Once hemoglobinuria and myoglobinuria have been excluded, the clinician should consider the possibility that the discrepancy between the urine dipstick test result and the number of red blood cells seen during microscopy reflects red blood cell lysis. Red blood cells are more likely to lyse in hypotonic urine (specific gravity <1.008) or highly alkaline urine (pH >6.5). Red blood cell lysis should not be ignored because it may signify the presence of true hematuria.

Because of the limitations of the urine dipstick test for blood, every patient thought to have hematuria, whether gross or microscopic, should have microscopic analysis of the urine to verify the presence of hematuria.

If the patient has hemoglobinuria or myoglobinuria, ***stop here.***

If the patient has hematuria, ***proceed to Step 5.***

STEP 5 – *What Are the Causes of Hematuria?*

The causes of hematuria are either intrarenal or extrarenal. Intrarenal hematuria can be of glomerular or nonglomerular origin. The nonglomerular causes of intrarenal hematuria are listed in the following box.

INTRARENAL CAUSES OF NONGLOMERULAR HEMATURIA	
FAMILIAL	PAPILLARY NECROSIS
Medullary cystic or sponge disease	Analgesic abuse
Polycystic kidney disease	Diabetes mellitus
HYDRONEPHROSIS	Obstructive uropathy
MALIGNANCY	Sickle cell disease or trait
METABOLIC	TRAUMA
Hypercalciuria	VASCULAR
Hyperuricosuria	Malignant hypertension
	Renal infarct
	Renal vein thrombosis

The glomerular causes of intrarenal hematuria are listed in the following box.

INTRARENAL CAUSES OF GLOMERULAR HEMATURIA	
PRIMARY	SECONDARY
Alport's syndrome	Anti-GBM disease
Focal segmental glomerulosclerosis	Hemolytic-uremic syndrome
IgA nephropathy	Henoch-Schönlein purpura
Membranous nephropathy	Mixed essential cryoglobulinemia
Membranoproliferative glomerulonephritis	Postinfectious glomerulonephritis
Minimal change disease	Systemic lupus erythematosus
Rapidly progressive glomerulonephritis	Vasculitis
Thin basement membrane disease	

The extrarenal causes of hematuria are listed in the following box.

EXTRARENAL CAUSES OF HEMATURIA	
BLEEDING DISORDER	MALIGNANCY
INFECTION	Prostatic adenocarcinoma
Cystitis	Transitional cell cancer of the urinary tract
Prostatitis	MEDICATIONS
Schistosomiasis	Anticoagulants
Tuberculosis	Cyclophosphamide
Urethritis	STONES
	TRAUMA

Proceed to Step 6.

STEP 6 – *Are There Any Clinical Clues to Suggest the Etiology of the Hematuria?*

While there are many causes of hematuria, a thorough history and physical examination can be invaluable in elucidating the etiology.

Historical Clues	Condition Suggested
Burning, urgency, frequency	Urinary tract infection
Painless gross hematuria	Noninfectious origin Urinary tract malignancy
Initial gross hematuria that clears with voiding	Anterior urethral source
Initial clear urine followed by terminal gross hematuria	Prostatic source of bleed
Urinary blood clots	Nonglomerular hematuria
Weight loss	Urinary tract malignancy
Recurrent loin or lumbar pain in female	Loin pain – hematuria syndrome
Hemoptysis	Goodpasture's syndrome SLE
Arthritis / arthralgia	Vasculitis Henoch-Schönlein purpura SLE
Rash	Vasculitis Henoch-Schönlein purpura SLE
Flank pain	Upper urinary tract calculi Ureteral colic from blood clots Ureteral colic from sloughed renal papillae (papillary necrosis) Renal infarction
Medication history	Anticoagulant therapy Aspirin NSAIDs Cyclophosphamide

(Continued)

Historical Clues	Condition Suggested
Radiation therapy	Hemorrhagic cystitis
Recent contact or noncontact sports	Exercise-related hematuria
Foreign travel	Schistosomiasis; malaria
Recent upper respiratory infection	Poststreptococcal glomerulonephritis IgA nephropathy MPGN
African-American background	Sickle cell trait
Family history of hematuria and/or renal disease	Sickle cell hemoglobinopathy Alport's syndrome Benign familial hematuria Polycystic kidney disease
Family history of deafness and/or ocular defects	Alport's syndrome

Clues in the physical examination that point to the etiology of the hematuria are listed in the following table.

Physical Exam Finding	Condition Suggested
Elevated blood pressure	Glomerular disease
Fever	Infectious origin Acute prostatitis Acute cystitis Acute pyelonephritis
Palpable kidney	Renal cell cancer
Flank tenderness	Acute pyelonephritis Ureteral calculi
Palpable bladder after voiding	Incomplete bladder emptying from outflow obstruction BPH Urethral stricture Prostate cancer Acute prostatitis
Peripheral edema	Glomerular disease
Mass on pelvic examination	Cancer of vagina or uterus invading the bladder
Tenderness on rectal examination	Acute prostatitis
Mass on rectal examination	Prostate cancer Rectal cancer invading the bladder

If clinical clues are suggestive of a particular disease, the clinician can tailor the investigation accordingly.

If clinical clues are not present, ***proceed to Step 7***.

STEP 7 – *Does the Patient Have a Urinary Tract Infection?*

Dysuria, urinary frequency, and fever are common complaints in patients with a urinary tract infection. However, urinary tract infections may be asymptomatic as well. As a result, in every patient presenting with gross or microscopic hematuria, the possibility of a urinary tract infection should be entertained. The presence of pyuria and bacteriuria supports the diagnosis. A urine culture is not needed in every case of urinary tract infection. For example, it is not necessary in the female presenting with an uncomplicated urinary tract infection.

If obtained, a urine culture usually reveals growth of a single organism. A negative urine culture, in the presence of pyuria, should prompt consideration of tuberculosis or urethritis.

At the completion of a course of antibiotic therapy, urinalysis should be repeated several times to ensure resolution of the hematuria.

If hematuria resolves after appropriate antibiotic therapy, ***stop here***.

If hematuria persists, ***proceed to Step 8***.

STEP 8 – *What Are the Results of the PT and PTT?*

If the PT and PTT are normal, ***Proceed to Step 9***.

Hematuria may be the result of a systemic bleeding disorder. In most cases, there will be manifestations of bleeding elsewhere. Documentation of a normal PT and PTT will help exclude this possibility.

Hematuria that develops during anticoagulation also deserves mention here. Hematuria is not uncommon in patients being treated with heparin or Coumadin®, but other etiologies must be ruled out before attributing hematuria solely to anticoagulation therapy.

Proceed to Step 9.

STEP 9 – *Does the Patient Have Sickle Cell Trait / Disease?*

Patients with sickle cell trait are usually asymptomatic, but occasionally, painless hematuria may occur. A hemoglobin electrophoresis should be performed to exclude this diagnosis in African-American patients presenting with hematuria. Of note, in the older patient with sickle cell trait, hematuria should not be merely attributed to the sickle cell trait. Rather, an investigation (outlined below) should be done to exclude other more serious etiologies.

Proceed to Step 10.

STEP 10 – *Is the Hematuria of Glomerular or Nonglomerular Origin?*

The following support a glomerular origin of the hematuria:

- Red blood cell casts
- Dysmorphic or "distorted" red blood cells
- Protein excretion >500 mg/day

It is important to note that the absence of these features does not exclude hematuria of glomerular origin.

If the hematuria is glomerular in origin, ***proceed to Step 11***.

If the hematuria is nonglomerular in origin, ***proceed to Step 12***.

STEP 11 – *What Tests Should Be Obtained to Determine the Etiology of Glomerular Hematuria?*

The differential diagnosis of glomerular hematuria is long and has been described earlier in this section. Definitive diagnosis can only be established by renal biopsy. However, the need for renal biopsy is controversial. There is no evidence to suggest that renal biopsy will alter treatment or prognosis in this group of patients unless the patient has hypertension, decreased renal function, or proteinuria. In the absence of these features, the clinician should evaluate the patient periodically with the following tests:

- Blood pressure
- Serum BUN and creatinine
- Creatinine clearance
- 24-hour urine collection for protein

The development of hypertension, renal insufficiency, or worsening proteinuria should prompt consideration of a renal biopsy.

Depending on the patient's clinical presentation, other tests may be helpful in elucidating the etiology of the hematuria. These laboratory abnormalities and their associated disease states are listed in the following table.

Laboratory Abnormalities	Condition Suggested
Decreased C3 level	SLE Cryoglobulinemia Poststreptococcal glomerulonephritis Postinfectious glomerulonephritis Membranoproliferative glomerulonephritis
Positive ANA	SLE
Positive antistreptolysin O (ASO) Positive anti-DNase B Positive antihyaluronidase Positive antistreptokinase	Poststreptococcal glomerulonephritis
Positive ANCA	Wegener's glomerulonephritis Microscopic polyarteritis Idiopathic crescentic necrotizing glomerulonephritis
Positive anti-GBM	Anti-GBM nephritis Goodpasture's syndrome
Increased cryoglobulins	Cryoglobulinemia
Positive hepatitis C antibody	Hepatitis C associated membranoproliferative glomerulonephritis

End of Section.

STEP 12 – *What Are the Results of the Intravenous Pyelography Study (IVP)?*

Intravenous pyelography (IVP) is the test of choice in evaluating the patient with nonglomerular hematuria. There are, however, some investigators who argue that the sensitivity of ultrasound is equivalent to that of IVP in the detection and characterization of masses in the renal parenchyma, and that it should replace IVP as the gold standard. However, IVP appears to be superior in detection of subtle abnormalities in the renal collecting system, and in the detection of urothelial malignancies of the upper urinary tract. As a result, IVP continues to be the initial test of choice. If IVP is contraindicated, it is reasonable to perform ultrasound. Patients with a normal IVP may need further radiologic imaging.

The age of the patient is often used to help decide whether further imaging is necessary. Older patients with normal IVP study should undergo CT or ultrasonography since these studies may detect small renal tumors not visualized by IVP. In younger patients, these studies are not necessary.

If the IVP is positive, ***stop here***.

If the IVP is negative, ***proceed to Step 13***.

STEP 13 – *Which Patients Should Have a Cystoscopy?*

Many investigators have questioned the role of cystoscopy in the younger patient with nonglomerular hematuria. While there is no doubt that cystoscopy is the gold standard in the detection of bladder malignancy, the likelihood of finding a malignant lesion in the younger patient is quite low. As a result, cystoscopy is recommended in the younger patient (<40 years of age) only if one or more of the risk factors for bladder cancer listed in the following box are present.

RISK FACTORS FOR BLADDER CANCER	
CIGARETTE SMOKING	OCCUPATIONAL EXPOSURE
CYCLOPHOSPHAMIDE	Aniline dyes
PELVIC IRRADIATION	Aromatic amines
URINARY SCHISTOSOMIASIS	Benzidine

If these factors are not present in the patient <40 years of age, ***proceed to Step 15***.

Cystoscopy should be performed in the younger patient with risk factors for bladder cancer or in the older patient with nonglomerular hematuria.

If cystoscopy is positive, ***stop here***.

If cystoscopy is negative, ***proceed to Step 14***.

STEP 14 – *What Are the Results of the Urine Cytology?*

Diagnosis can be established in the majority of patients who receive a full evaluation (ie, IVP, cystoscopy). However, in a minority of patients, a diagnosis cannot be established. Unfortunately, there are no consensus guidelines as to how these patients should be further evaluated. Should cystoscopy and IVP be performed again? If so, when and how often should these tests be performed?

There are no easy answers to these questions. Some studies have found that hematuria can predate the diagnosis of urinary tract cancer by many years. It is possible, then, that patients with hematuria who have had a negative initial evaluation are at increased risk for urinary tract cancer in the future. It seems reasonable to manage these patients in consultation with a urologist. In most cases, these patients will have a repeat evaluation.

It is also important to send the urine for cytology in the patient with a negative evaluation. Occasionally, urine cytology may be positive in the patient with unexplained hematuria. Such a patient may have a very superficial bladder cancer or carcinoma *in situ*. These lesions may not have been grossly evident during cystoscopy. Multiple biopsies and washings may aid in establishing the diagnosis.

In the event that repeat evaluation is unrevealing, consideration should be given to hypercalciuria, hyperuricosuria, and mild glomerulopathy as the cause of hematuria. A 24-hour urine collection for uric acid and calcium can establish the diagnosis of hyperuricosuria and hypercalciuria, respectively. Treatment with thiazide diuretics or allopurinol for hypercalciuria or hyperuricosuria, respectively, may lead to the resolution of hematuria. If the 24-hour urine collection is unrevealing, then a mild glomerulopathy may be present. The most common glomerular diseases include IgA nephropathy, thin basement membrane disease, and Alport's syndrome.

End of Section.

STEP 15 – *What Are the Results of the 24-Hour Urine Collection for Calcium and Uric Acid?*

In younger patients without risk factors for bladder cancer, it is not necessary to do cystoscopy. In these patients, the most likely diagnoses include hypercalciuria, hyperuricosuria, or a mild glomerulopathy. Although these patients are at low risk for urothelial cancer, some clinicians recommend performing urine cytology with subsequent cystoscopy if the cytology reveals findings suspicious for malignancy.

Hypercalciuria and hyperuricosuria can be diagnosed with a 24-hour urine collection for calcium and uric acid, respectively. Treatment with thiazide diuretics and allopurinol can lead to resolution of hematuria if hypercalciuria and hyperuricosuria are the suspected etiologies. If the 24-hour urine collection is unrevealing, then the patient likely has a glomerular lesion. Glomerular diseases that often present with isolated hematuria include IgA nephropathy, thin basement membrane disease, and Alport's syndrome.

End of Section.

References

Ahmed Z and Lee J, "Asymptomatic Urinary Abnormalities. Hematuria and Proteinuria," *Med Clin North Am*, 1997, 81(3):641-52.

Bryden AA, Paul AB, and Kyriakides C, "Investigation of Haematuria," *Br J Hosp Med*, 1995, 54(9):455-8.

Cohen RA and Brown RS, "Clinical Practice. Microscopic Hematuria," *N Engl J Med*, 2003, 348(23):2330-8.

Desai SP and Isa-Pratt S, *Clinicians's Guide to Laboratory Medicine,* Hudson, OH: Lexi-Comp Inc, 2000, 525.

Fogazzi GB and Ponticelli C, "Microscopic Hematuria Diagnosis and Management," *Nephron*, 1996, 72(2):125-34 (review).

Grossfeld GD and Carroll PR, "Evaluation of Asymptomatic Microscopic Hematuria," *Urol Clin North Am*, 1998, 25(4):661-76.

Hall CL, "The Patient With Haematuria," *Practitioner*, 1999, 243(1600):564-6, 568, 570-1.

Mazhari R and Kimmel PL, "Hematuria: An Algorithmic Approach to Finding the Cause," *Cleve Clin J Med*, 2002, 69(11):870, 872-4, 876 passim.

McCarthy JJ, "Outpatient Evaluation of Hematuria: Locating the Source of Bleeding," *Postgrad Med*, 1997, 101(2):125-8, 131.

Rockall AG, Newman-Sanders AP, al-Kutabima, et al, "Haematuria," *Postgrad Med J*, 1997, 73(857):129-36.

Thaller TR and Wang LP, "Evaluation of Asymptomatic Microscopic Hematuria in Adults," *Am Fam Phys*, 1999, 60(4):1143-52, 1154.

Tomson C and Porter T, "Asymptomatic Microscopic or Dipstick Haematuria in Adults: Which Investigation for Which Patients? A Review of the Evidence," *BJU Int*, 2002, 90(3):185-98.

Webb JA, "Imaging in Haematuria," *Clin Radiol*, 1997, 52(3):167-71 (review).

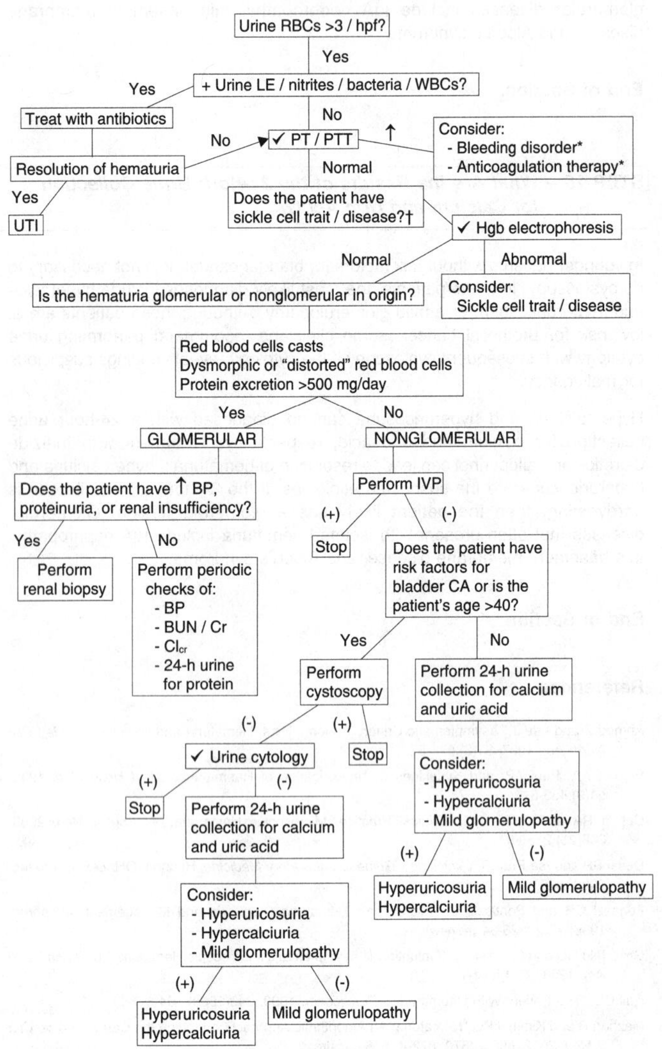
HEMATURIA
Urine RBCs >3 / hpf?
Yes
+ Urine LE / nitrites / bacteria / WBCs?
Yes
Treat with antibiotics
Resolution of hematuria
Yes
UTI
No
No
✓ PT / PTT
↑
Consider:
- Bleeding disorder*
- Anticoagulation therapy*
Normal
Does the patient have sickle cell trait / disease?†
✓ Hgb electrophoresis
Normal
Abnormal
Consider:
Sickle cell trait / disease
Is the hematuria glomerular or nonglomerular in origin?
Red blood cells casts
Dysmorphic or "distorted" red blood cells
Protein excretion >500 mg/day
Yes
No
GLOMERULAR
NONGLOMERULAR
Does the patient have ↑ BP, proteinuria, or renal insufficiency?
Yes
No
Perform renal biopsy
Perform periodic checks of:
- BP
- BUN / Cr
- Clcr
- 24-h urine for protein
Perform IVP
(+)
(-)
Stop
Does the patient have risk factors for bladder CA or is the patient's age >40?
Yes
No
Perform cystoscopy
(-)
(+)
Stop
✓ Urine cytology
(+)
(-)
Stop
Perform 24-h urine collection for calcium and uric acid
Consider:
- Hyperuricosuria
- Hypercalciuria
- Mild glomerulopathy
(+)
(-)
Hyperuricosuria
Hypercalciuria
Mild glomerulopathy
Perform 24-h urine collection for calcium and uric acid
Consider:
- Hyperuricosuria
- Hypercalciuria
- Mild glomerulopathy
(+)
(-)
Hyperuricosuria
Hypercalciuria
Mild glomerulopathy

*Hematuria that occurs in the patient with an elevated PT / PTT may be the result of anticoagulation therapy or a bleeding disorder. However, an underlying structural etiology cannot be excluded.

†Sickle cell trait/disease may be the sole cause of hematuria; however, this diagnosis must be one of exclusion.

PROTEINURIA

STEP 1 – *What Are the Mechanisms of Proteinuria?*

Normally, there is <150 mg of protein excreted in the urine over a 24-hour period. Excreted protein comes from plasma and the urinary tract. Plasma proteins include albumin and a globulin fraction. The major constituent of protein derived from the urinary tract is the Tamm-Horsfall protein, which is secreted by the cells of the ascending limb of the loop of Henle and the distal tubule.

Plasma protein must traverse the glomerular barrier to enter the urine. In general, proteins with a molecular weight >20,000 daltons have considerable difficulty passing through glomerular capillary walls. The glomerular basement membrane is also negatively charged, and therefore impedes the passage of negatively charged plasma proteins such as albumin. Much of the protein that does traverse the glomerular barrier is reabsorbed by the tubular cells. This is especially true if the protein is of low molecular weight.

Proteinuria can be classified as follows:

- Glomerular

  Glomerular proteinuria occurs as a result of increased glomerular permeability, which may be due to a variety of processes. The degree of proteinuria may vary from several hundred milligrams to over 100 grams of protein excreted per day.
- Tubular

  In normal healthy individuals, the proximal tubular epithelium almost completely reabsorbs freely filtered low molecular weight proteins. Any process that damages the proximal tubular epithelium will allow low molecular weight proteins to be excreted in the urine (tubular proteinuria).
- Overflow

  Overflow proteinuria is the result of overproduction of a particular protein. These proteins, which are of low molecular weight, are able to traverse the glomerular barrier. The increased amount of protein that is filtered overwhelms the ability of the proximal tubular epithelium to reabsorb and catabolize the protein, resulting in urinary excretion of excess protein. In clinical practice, this occurs in multiple myeloma.

Proceed to Step 2.

STEP 2 – *How Is Proteinuria Detected?*

In most instances, there are no signs pointing to the presence of proteinuria. In some cases, particularly when proteinuria is marked (exceeding several grams per day), the urine may become frothy. Edema may accompany proteinuria, but this is an unusual finding unless there is heavy proteinuria, as in the nephrotic syndrome. As a result, proteinuria typically comes to clinical attention through laboratory testing.

Because of widespread availability, urine dipstick examination usually first identifies proteinuria. Most urine dipsticks for protein use tetrabromophenol blue. Using this indicator, changes in color correspond to the degree of proteinuria if the urine contains negatively-charged proteins. How the results are reported varies, depending on the manufacturer of the dipstick. They are often reported on a scale of 0 to 4+ or as a range between 0 and >500 mg/dL.

It is important not to ignore proteinuria. While it is true that proteinuria may represent a benign finding, it may also indicate the presence of serious underlying renal or systemic disease.

Proceed to Step 3.

STEP 3 – *What Are the Causes of False-Positive and Negative Urine Dipstick Test Results?*

The urine dipstick is a useful screening test but, as is the case with other tests, it has some limitations. Both false-positive and false-negative test results may occur. In addition, there is great interobserver variability in the interpretation of the color change.

A urine dipstick test that is positive should be interpreted in the context of the patient's urine specific gravity. Specific gravity provides information as to how concentrated the urine is. A high specific gravity indicates a concentrated urine whereas a low specific gravity connotes dilute urine. When the urine is particularly concentrated, a dipstick may reveal significant proteinuria when, in fact, there may be little to no proteinuria. Other causes of false-positive test results include alkaline urine, bloody urine, and recent radiocontrast administration (within 24 hours).

In the patient with a very low specific gravity, a dipstick test that is negative for protein does not exclude the presence of proteinuria. A false-negative test result can also occur with mild degrees of proteinuria. In general, the urine dipstick is not positive until urinary protein excretion exceeds 300-500 mg/day. In patients with diabetic nephropathy, this degree of proteinuria is a relatively late finding, noted usually after significant structural kidney damage has occurred. For this reason, diabetic patients are screened for diabetic nephropathy using tests to detect microalbuminuria. Microalbuminuria simply refers to the presence of abnormal amounts of protein in the urine that is below the detection capability of the urine dipstick.

The urine dipstick may also fail to yield a positive test result when low molecular weight proteinuria is present. Low molecular weight proteinuria may be encountered in patients who have either tubular proteinuria or overflow proteinuria. In normal healthy individuals, low molecular weight proteins are filtered at the glomerulus and then almost completely reabsorbed by the tubules. With disease of the tubules, there is an impairment in the ability of the proximal tubules to reabsorb and catabolize the filtered protein. Overflow proteinuria is a type of low molecular weight proteinuria that is seen in patients with a condition associated with an excess production of proteins. Such an excess overwhelms the capacity of the proximal tubule to reabsorb and catabolize the filtered protein. In usual clinical practice, this situation is encountered in patients with multiple myeloma. In both tubular and overflow proteinuria, the urine dipstick may yield false-negative test results because the dipstick is relatively insensitive to the presence of low molecular weight proteins. If tubular or overflow proteinuria is suspected, the urine can be tested with sulfosalicylic acid, which is capable of detecting all types of protein. This test should be obtained in acute renal failure patients who present with a benign urinalysis and negative dipstick test for protein. In these cases, multiple myeloma is a major consideration. If the sulfosalicylic acid test is positive, an evaluation for multiple myeloma and other causes of tubular/overflow proteinuria is warranted.

Causes of False-Positive and Negative Urine Dipstick Test for Protein

False-Positive Urine Dipstick Test for Protein	False-Negative Urine Dipstick Test for Protein
Concentrated urine	Dilute urine
Alkaline urine	Mild proteinuria (microalbuminuria)
Bloody urine	Low molecular weight proteinuria (tubular or overflow)
Radiocontrast administration (within 24 hours)	

Proceed to Step 4.

STEP 4 – *Does the Patient Have Isolated Proteinuria?*

When proteinuria is noted on a urine dipstick test, it is important to look at the rest of the urinalysis test results. In addition, renal function tests should be obtained (serum BUN and creatinine). Isolated proteinuria is considered to be present if the patient has the following:

- Urine sediment is normal
- No evidence of a systemic or renal disease by history, physical exam, and laboratory tests (eg, normal serum BUN and creatinine)

If the patient has isolated proteinuria, ***proceed to Step 5.***

If the patient has proteinuria that is accompanied by other urinalysis abnormalities (hematuria) and/or renal dysfunction, ***proceed to Step 6.***

STEP 5 – *What Are the Results of the Repeat Urine Dipstick Test for Protein?*

In patients with isolated proteinuria, a repeat urine dipstick test for protein should be performed. In many cases, the repeat test will be negative. Presumably, the patient had transient proteinuria at the time of the test. Transient proteinuria, which is common, can be caused by any of the conditions listed in the following box.

CAUSES OF TRANSIENT PROTEINURIA
IDIOPATHIC FEVER STRENUOUS EXERCISE CONGESTIVE HEART FAILURE EXPOSURE TO COLD EMOTIONAL STRESS PREGNANCY OBSTRUCTIVE SLEEP APNEA SEIZURES

Transient proteinuria is a benign condition that requires no further evaluation. It typically resolves within several days. Patients with transient proteinuria need to be reassured that the abnormality does not reflect underlying structural kidney disease.

Transient proteinuria needs to be distinguished, however, from persistent proteinuria. When repeat urinalysis demonstrates proteinuria, the patient is said to have persistent proteinuria. Patients with persistent proteinuria are more likely to have some type of underlying systemic or renal disease. It is in these patients that a more thorough evaluation is warranted.

If the patient has transient proteinuria, ***stop here.***

If the patient has persistent proteinuria, ***proceed to Step 6.***

STEP 6 – *What Are the Results of the 24-Hour Urine Collection for Protein?*

Persistent proteinuria and proteinuria that is accompanied by hematuria and/or renal dysfunction (acute or chronic renal failure) always requires further evaluation. For patients who have acute or chronic renal failure, please proceed to the chapters on acute renal failure and chronic renal failure, respectively.

Quite often, the evaluation begins with a 24-hour urine collection to quantify the amount of protein that is excreted per day. The urine dipstick is not a quantitative test but rather a semiquantitative test, one that is influenced by urine volume. When performing a 24-hour urine collection for protein, creatinine should also be measured concurrently to ensure the adequacy of the collection. Normal urinary creatinine excretion over a 24-hour time period is shown in the following box.

24-HOUR CREATININE EXCRETION
Male: 20-25 mg/kg creatinine **Female:** 15-20 mg/kg creatinine

The 24-hour urine collection will quantify the proteinuria. Based on the results, proteinuria can be classified into two categories:

- <3 g/24 hours - glomerular or tubular disease may be present
- >3 g/24 hours - usually glomerular disease (nephrotic-range proteinuria)

Since this test is often difficult to do, many prefer to calculate the urine protein to creatinine ratio from a random spot urine specimen. This ratio has been found to be a relatively accurate approximation of the protein excreted over a 24-hour time period. The ratio is calculated by dividing the protein measured (mg/dL) by the creatinine measured (mg/dL). This ratio (mg/mg) will correlate to the total amount of protein excreted as determined by the 24-hour urine collection. For example, a urine protein to creatinine ratio of 4 corresponds to the excretion of 4 grams of protein over a 24-hour time period.

Before calculating the ratio, it is important to look closely at the units the urine creatinine concentration is reported in. If the urine creatinine concentration is reported in mmol/L rather than mg/dL, the following formula should be used:

Protein excretion = (urine protein x 0.088) / (urine creatinine)

Several limitations of the urine to protein creatinine ratio should be recognized. Underestimation and overestimation of the degree of protein excretion will occur in muscular and cachectic patients, respectively. Another limitation of the test is that it cannot be used to establish the diagnosis of orthostatic proteinuria.

Orthostatic proteinuria, a common cause of proteinuria in adolescents and young adults, is very uncommon in those older than 30 years of age. It is characterized by increased protein excretion in the upright position but normal protein excretion in the supine position. Orthostatic proteinuria is not accompanied by hematuria; therefore, the finding of hematuria strongly argues against the diagnosis. The diagnosis can be established by performing a split

24-hour urine collection for protein. In the split collection, the patient is instructed to collect the urine over a 16-hour time period between the hours of 7 AM and 11 PM (when the patient is primarily upright), as well as over an 8-hour time period between 11 PM and 7 AM (when the patient is primarily supine). Orthostatic proteinuria is present when excretion of protein during the 16-hour time period exceeds the normal range but remains normal during the supine overnight collection (supine 8-hour collection <50 mg). Since orthostatic proteinuria is a benign condition (no progression to renal insufficiency), no further evaluation is necessary.

If the patient has orthostatic proteinuria, ***stop here***.

If the patient does not have orthostatic proteinuria and the protein excretion is >3 g/day, then glomerular pathology is likely. ***Proceed to Step 9***.

If the patient does not have orthostatic proteinuria and the protein excretion is <3 g/day, ***proceed to Step 7***.

STEP 7 – *Does the Patient Have Glomerular Disease?*

Patients who excrete <3 g protein/day are generally considered to have non-nephrotic range proteinuria. In these cases, it can be difficult to differentiate between glomerular, tubular, and overflow types of proteinuria. If the urinalysis reveals the presence of red blood cell casts or dysmorphic red blood cells, however, then a glomerular etiology is very likely.

If the urinalysis does not reveal red blood cell casts or dysmorphic red blood cells, ***Proceed to Step 8***.

If the urinalysis reveals red blood cell casts and/or dysmorphic red blood cells, then the patient has glomerular disease. ***Proceed to Step 9***.

STEP 8 – *What Are the Results of the Urine Protein Electrophoresis?*

When urinary protein excretion is < 3 grams per day in the patient having no urinalysis abnormalities pointing to glomerular disease (ie, red blood cell casts, dysmorphic red blood cells), a urine protein electrophoresis should be performed to differentiate between glomerular, tubular, and overflow types of proteinuria. When albumin represents >70% of the total protein, the clinician can be confident of a glomerular source. When the urine protein electrophoresis reveals that the excretion of globulins exceeds that of albumin, a tubular or overflow type of proteinuria exists.

If the patient has glomerular proteinuria, ***Proceed to Step 9***.

If the patient has tubular or overflow proteinuria, ***proceed to Step 10***.

STEP 9 – *What Is the Etiology of the Glomerular Disease?*

Once glomerular proteinuria has been identified, the next step involves determining the etiology. For patients who have the nephrotic syndrome, the reader is referred to the chapter on nephrotic syndrome. The remainder of this step will focus on the determining the cause of non-nephrotic range glomerular proteinuria.

There are many causes of glomerular proteinuria, many of which are listed in the following box.

GLOMERULAR PROTEINURIA DIFFERENTIAL DIAGNOSIS	
PRIMARY KIDNEY DISEASES	
MINIMAL CHANGE DISEASE	
MEMBRANOUS NEPHROPATHY	
FOCAL SEGMENTAL GLOMERULOSCLEROSIS	
MEMBRANOPROLIFERATIVE GLOMERULONEPHRITIS	
IgA NEPHROPATHY	
SYSTEMIC DISEASES	
CONNECTIVE TISSUE DISEASES	INFECTION
Systemic lupus erythematosus	HIV
Vasculitis	Hepatitis B
Cryoglobulinemia	Hepatitis C
MALIGNANCY	Syphilis
Solid tumors	Subacute bacterial endocarditis
Lymphomas	Poststreptococcal glomerulonephritis
Multiple myeloma	Shunt nephritis
MEDICATIONS	Malaria
NSAIDs	DIABETES MELLITUS
Gold	SARCOIDOSIS
Penicillamine	AMYLOIDOSIS
Heavy metals	HEROIN USE
ACE inhibitors	

In some cases, the cause of the glomerular disease may be readily apparent, as in the patient with diabetic nephropathy. In other cases, the etiology is unclear even after a thorough history and physical examination. There are several laboratory tests that may help determine the etiology. Based on the patient's clinical presentation, one or more of the tests listed in the following box can be obtained.

GLOMERULAR DISEASE HELPFUL SELECTED LABORATORY TESTS	
ANTINUCLEAR ANTIBODY	HIV TESTING
HEPATITIS C SEROLOGY	COMPLEMENT LEVELS
HEPATITIS B SEROLOGY	CRYOGLOBULINS
SYPHILIS TESTING	SERUM / URINE PROTEIN ELECTROPHORESIS*

*Patients with glomerular proteinuria should also have testing to exclude multiple myeloma because, in some cases of multiple myeloma, there may be concomitant glomerular damage. When glomerular damage is present, proteinuria is due to both overflow and increased glomerular permeability. This explains why some patients with multiple myeloma have heavy proteinuria.

In patients who have non-nephrotic range glomerular proteinuria, renal biopsy is often considered. However, renal biopsy is not indicated in all patients. Decisions regarding renal biopsy are usually based on the degree of proteinuria, blood pressure, renal function, and presence of hematuria. Most nephrologists recommend renal biopsy when 24-hour urine protein excretion exceeds 2 g/day. Renal biopsy is also recommended if the patient has hypertension, renal insufficiency, hematuria, or signs/symptoms of a disease affecting the kidney.

In the absence of these features, it is recommended that the patient have close follow-up. During periodic monitoring, patients should be assessed for the development of any of these clinical features (hypertension, renal insufficiency, hematuria, signs/symptoms of a disease affecting the kidney, 24-hour protein excretion >2 g). Should any of the features be present, renal biopsy should be considered.

End of Section.

STEP 10 – *Does the Patient Have Tubular or Overflow Proteinuria?*

To differentiate between these two causes of proteinuria, the clinician should look closely at the results of the electrophoresis. Overflow proteinuria primarily occurs in patients with a monoclonal gammopathy. In these patients, electrophoresis will reveal a single globulin peak. In contrast, tubular proteinuria will reveal multiple peaks, representing the excretion of many different globulins.

If the patient has tubular proteinuria, ***proceed to Step 11***.

If the patient has overflow proteinuria, then the patient likely has a monoclonal gammopathy. Proceed to the chapter ***Monoclonal Gammopathy*** *on page 181* for more information.

STEP 11 – *What Is the Etiology of the Tubular Proteinuria?*

Once tubular proteinuria has been identified, the next step involves determining the etiology. The causes of tubular proteinuria are listed in the following box.

CAUSES OF TUBULAR PROTEINURIA	
Hereditary	Fanconi syndrome
Polycystic kidney disease	Chronic pyelonephritis
Medullary cystic kidney disease	Kidney transplant rejection
Galactosemia	Radiation nephritis
Fructose intolerance	Heavy metal poisoning
Tyrosinemia	Lead
Glycogen storage disease	Mercury
Wilson's disease	Arsenic
Cystinosis	Cadmium
Oxalosis	Allergic interstitial nephritis
Hypercalcemic nephropathy	Acute tubular necrosis
Hypokalemic nephropathy	Sarcoidosis
Reflux nephropathy	Balan nephropathy
Obstructive uropathy	Systemic lupus erythematosus

A thorough history and physical examination, in most cases, establishes the etiology. Certain laboratory or radiologic testing may be quite helpful in elucidating the cause of tubular proteinuria, as shown in the following table.

Establishing the Etiology of Tubular Proteinuria

Cause of Tubular Proteinuria	Diagnostic Test Result
Adult polycystic kidney disease	Cystic kidneys on ultrasound
Fanconi syndrome	Proximal renal tubular acidosis Glucosuria Hypophosphatemia / phosphaturia Hypouricemia / uricosuria Hypokalemia Aminoaciduria
Reflux nephropathy	Abnormal IVP Abnormal voiding cystourethrography
Acute interstitial nephritis	Pyuria Peripheral blood eosinophilia Eosinophiluria
Hypercalcemia	Elevated serum calcium level
Lead nephropathy	Elevated serum lead level Urinary excretion of lead following administration of calcium disodium edetate
Wilson's disease	Decreased serum ceruloplasmin Anemia secondary to hemolysis Diagnostic liver biopsy
Transplant rejection	Diagnostic renal biopsy
Obstructive uropathy	Urinary obstruction on ultrasound

End of Section.

References

Ali H, "Proteinuria. How Much Evaluation Is Appropriate?" *Postgrad Med*, 1997, 101(4):173-5, 179-80.

Carroll MF and Temte JL, "Proteinuria in Adults: A Diagnostic Approach," *Am Fam Physician*, 2000, 15;62(6):1333-40.

Eknoyan G, "On Testing for Proteinuria: Time for a Methodical Approach," *Cleve Clin J Med*, 2003, 70(6):493, 496-7, 501.

Kashif W, Siddiqi N, Dincer AP, et al, "Proteinuria: How to Evaluate an Important Finding," *Cleve Clin J Med*, 2003, 70(6):535-7, 541-4, 546-7.

Keane WF, "Proteinuria: Its Clinical Importance and Role in Progressive Renal Disease," *Am J Kidney Dis*, 2000, 35(4 Suppl 1):S97-105.

Levinson SS, "Urine Protein Electrophoresis and Immunofixation Electrophoresis Supplement One Another in Characterizing Proteinuria," *Ann Clin Lab Sci*, 2000, 30(1):79-84.

Ralston SH, Caine N, Richards I, et al, "Screening for Proteinuria in a Rheumatology Clinic: Comparison of Dipstick Testing, 2-Hour Urine Quantitative Protein, and Protein/Creatinine Ratio in Random Urine Samples," *Ann Rheum Dis*, 1988, 47(9):759-63.

Wingo CS and Clapp WL, "Proteinuria: Potential Causes and Approach to Evaluation," *Am J Med Sci*, 2000, 320(3):188-94.

PROTEINURIA

- Repeat urine dipstick test for protein
- Proteinuria detected?
  - No → Transient proteinuria
  - Yes → Accompanying hematuria?
    - Yes → Glomerular cause likely
    - No → Orthostatic proteinuria?
      - Perform 24-hour urine split collection
      - Abnormal 16-hour upright protein? Normal supine protein?
        - Yes → Orthostatic proteinuria
        - No → What is total protein excreted in 24-hour urine collection?
          - >3 g → Glomerular cause likely
          - <3 g → ✓ Urine protein electrophoresis
            - Albumin >70% of total protein
              - Glomerular proteinuria
              - <2 g urine protein/day
                - Yes → Normal BP? Normal renal function? No hematuria?
                  - Yes → Serial follow-up
                  - No → Consider renal biopsy
                - No → Perform renal biopsy
            - Globulin excretion > albumin excretion
              - Tubulointerstitial vs overflow proteinuria
              - Single globulin peak on urine protein electrophoresis?
                - Yes → Overflow proteinuria
                  - Consider: Bence Jones proteinuria; Lysozymuria
                - No → Tubulointerstitial proteinuria

Glomerular cause likely:

- ✓ ANA
- ✓ Hepatitis C serology
- ✓ Hepatitis B serology
- ✓ Syphilis testing (VDRL)
- ✓ HIV testing
- ✓ Complement levels
- ✓ Cryoglobulins
- ✓ Serum / urine protein electrophoresis
  - (-) → Perform renal biopsy
  - (+) → Treat underlying disease

MICROALBUMINURIA

Microalbuminuria is really a misnomer. It does not refer to an abnormal structure of albumin; rather, it indicates urinary excretion of albumin that is below the detection capability of the urine dipstick, but above the upper limit of normal for healthy individuals.

Significance of Microalbuminuria

Testing for microalbuminuria is particularly important in diabetes mellitus patients. These patients are at risk for the development of diabetic nephropathy, the most common cause of end-stage renal disease. The presence of microalbuminuria is the earliest clinically recognizable indicator of nephropathy. If detected early, this stage of diabetic nephropathy is reversible. Once detected, clinicians can begin therapy to prevent the development of overt diabetic nephropathy and progression to end-stage renal disease. Recently, it has been shown that diabetes mellitus patients with microalbuminuria are at higher risk for cardiovascular disease.

Screening for Microalbuminuria

Patients with type I diabetes mellitus should have annual screening for microalbuminuria when 5 years have passed after the diagnosis of the diabetes. Patients with type II diabetes mellitus should be tested at the time of diagnosis, as well as yearly thereafter. It is important to note that up to 30% of newly diagnosed type II diabetics will have abnormally elevated urine albumin levels. Seventy-five percent of these patients will be found to have microalbuminuria while 25% have overt diabetic nephropathy. In older type II diabetes mellitus patients (>75 years) and in diabetics with short life expectancy (<20 years), there may not be enough time for clinically significant diabetic nephropathy to develop. In these patients, the role of screening for microalbuminuria is unclear.

Detection of Microalbuminuria

The urine dipstick test for protein will not reliably detect urine albumin <300 mg/day. If a patient with diabetes mellitus has a positive urine dipstick test result for protein (and no other etiology can explain the abnormality), then the patient is said to have overt diabetic nephropathy.

However, urine albumin excretion between 30-300 mg/day is abnormal and is termed microalbuminuria if it the test is abnormal on at least two of three urine specimens performed at intervals of 3-6 months.

There are a number of tests that are available for the detection of microalbuminuria. Although timed tests (12- or 24-hour urine collection) are available, in usual clinical practice, these tests are not often performed because of their inconvenience. Instead, clinicians usually rely on the albumin to creatinine ratio, which is determined from a first void urine specimen (ratio >30 mg/g consistent with microalbuminuria). This ratio has been shown to correlate well with the results of the timed collection.

Definitions of Microalbuminuria and Diabetic Nephropathy According to Urine Dipstick Test Results, Daily Urine Albumin Levels, and Albumin:Creatinine Ratios

Condition	Results of Urine Dipstick Test for Protein	Daily Urine Albumin Level (mg/day)	Urine Albumin:Creatinine Ratio (mg/mmol)
Normal	Negative	<30	Males: <2.0 Females: <2.8
Microalbuminuria	Negative	30-300	Males: 2.0-20 Females: 2.8-28
Overt diabetic nephropathy	Positive	>300	Males: >20 Females: >28

From Tobe SW, McFarlane PA, and Naimark DM, "Microalbuminuria in Diabetes Mellitus," *CMAJ*, 2002, 167(5).

When tests for microalbuminuria are positive, the clinician should look for other causes before attributing the increased urinary albumin excretion to diabetic nephropathy. Other causes include congestive heart failure, urinary tract infection, exercise, pregnancy, febrile state, inflammatory disorders, and urinary tract bleeding. To exclude these causes in the diabetic patient, a thorough history and physical examination should be performed. If other causes are absent and abnormal urinary albumin excretion is demonstrated on at least two of three urine specimens performed at intervals 3-6 months apart, microalbuminuria is diagnosed in the diabetic patient.

References

Bakris GL, "Microalbuminuria: What Is It? Why Is It Important? What Should Be Done About It?" *J Clin Hypertens (Greenwich)*, 2001, 3(2):99-102.

Bianchi S, Bigazzi R, and Campese VM, "Microalbuminuria in Essential Hypertension: Significance, Pathophysiology, and Therapeutic Implications," *Am J Kidney Dis*, 1999, 34(6):973-95.

Emancipator K, "Laboratory Diagnosis and Monitoring of Diabetes Mellitus," *Am J Clin Pathol*, 1999, 112(5):665-74.

Rosa TT and Palatini P, "Clinical Value of Microalbuminuria in Hypertension," *J Hypertens*, 2000, 18(6):645-54.

Scheid DC, McCarthy LH, Lawler FH, et al, "Screening for Microalbuminuria to Prevent Nephropathy in Patients With Diabetes: A Systematic Review of the Evidence," *J Fam Pract*, 2001, 50(8):661-8.

Tobe SW, McFarlane PA, and Naimark DM, "Microalbuminuria in Diabetes Mellitus," *CMAJ*, 2002, 167(5):499-503.

PROSTATE-SPECIFIC ANTIGEN (PSA)

Prostate cancer is the second leading cause of cancer deaths among males. In 1999, according to the American Cancer Society, prostate cancer accounted for over 30,000 deaths in the United States. Since the mid to late 1980s, the prostate-specific antigen (PSA) test has played a major role in the screening, diagnosis, staging, and management of patients with prostate cancer.

PSA, a glycoprotein produced by the prostatic epithelium, is secreted in the seminal fluid. It functions to liquefy the seminal coagulum. Nearly all of the PSA measured in the serum is derived from the prostate. Very small amounts, however, may be synthesized in other organs such as the kidney and breast. In usual clinical practice, an elevation in the serum PSA should prompt concern for a disease affecting the prostate. Of major concern is the possibility of prostate cancer.

Screening for Prostate Cancer

Prior to the arrival of serum PSA testing in the mid to late 1980s, clinicians relied on the digital rectal examination alone in the early detection of prostate cancer. It is now known, however, that the serum PSA level is superior to the digital rectal examination in the detection of prostate cancer. Studies have shown that serum PSA testing not only allows for the detection of more tumors but also leads to an earlier diagnosis.

Although the serum PSA level is more sensitive for the detection of early prostate cancer, not all patients with prostate cancer have an elevated serum PSA. In fact, about 25% of patients with prostate cancer have a normal PSA level. Many of these patients will be found to have an abnormal digital rectal examination. For this reason, at the current time, most screening guidelines recommend the combination of serum PSA testing and digital rectal examination for the detection of prostate cancer.

The American Cancer Society and the American Urological Association advocate yearly digital rectal examination and measurement of the serum PSA in asymptomatic men older than the age of 50. Annual screening at the age of 40 years is recommended in high-risk individuals (African-American men, men who have first-degree relatives with prostate cancer). Further management is based upon the results of the serum PSA test and the digital rectal examination, as shown in the following table.

Using the Serum PSA Level and Digital Rectal Examination to Screen for Prostate Cancer

Screening Test Result	Recommended Management
Negative digital rectal examination Elevated serum PSA level	Transrectal ultrasonography with biopsy
Suspicious digital rectal examination Normal serum PSA level	Transrectal ultrasonography with biopsy
Suspicious digital rectal examination Elevated serum PSA level	Transrectal ultrasonography with biopsy
Negative digital rectal examination Normal serum PSA level	Annual PSA and digital rectal examination

Other organizations, such as the U.S. Preventive Services Task Force, do not recommend the routine use of the PSA as a screening tool for the early detection of prostate cancer.

Controversy in the Use of the Serum PSA as a Screening Test for Prostate Cancer

There is much controversy over the role of the serum PSA in screening asymptomatic men for prostate cancer. Proponents for screening argue that serum PSA in conjunction with digital rectal examination allows the clinician to diagnose prostate cancer earlier. Earlier and more aggressive treatment can then be instituted, thus decreasing mortality. However, at the current time, no statistical or epidemiological evidence of mortality reduction is available with regards to the use of the serum PSA as a screening test. Those who do not favor the serum PSA as a screening test contend that early detection may be more harmful than beneficial. They argue that the early diagnosis of prostate cancer, in many patients, does not outweigh the morbidity and reduced quality of life that results from prostate cancer therapy. At the time of this writing, there is no definite answer to this issue. Currently, randomized trials are underway to address the problem.

Sensitivity of PSA in the Detection of Prostate Cancer

The upper limit of normal for PSA in many laboratories is about 4 ng/mL. Although most prostate cancers are associated with an elevated PSA, approximately 20% to 30% will present with a normal PSA level. As a result, 20% to 30% of prostate cancers will not be detected if the clinician relies on the serum PSA level alone.

Specificity of PSA in the Detection of Prostate Cancer

Any condition that leads to the disruption of the normal architecture of the prostate gland can result in an elevation of the serum PSA level. These conditions may be benign or malignant in nature. In addition, an increase in the serum PSA level may be iatrogenic. The causes of serum PSA elevation are listed in the following box.

CAUSES OF SERUM PSA ELEVATION	
PROSTATE CANCER	INFECTION
BENIGN PROSTATIC HYPERPLASIA (BPH)*	MEDICATIONS†
PROSTATITIS (acute, subclinical, chronic)	EJACULATION‡
PROSTATIC INFARCTION	DIGITAL RECTAL EXAM#
PROSTATIC MASSAGE	PROSTATE BIOPSY§
URINARY RETENTION	CYSTOSCOPY§
PHYSICAL ACTIVITY	

*33% of patients with BPH present with an elevated serum PSA. Most patients have levels between 4 and 10 ng/mL. However, 5% of patients may have serum PSA levels >10 ng/mL.

†It is essential to obtain a thorough medication history in all patients who present with an elevated serum PSA. Both prescription and over-the-counter medications, including herbal preparations, may cause a rise in the serum PSA level. Other medications may suppress PSA levels, which may lead to false-negative test results. For example, finasteride lowers serum PSA levels by an average of 50% after a 6-month course of therapy. In patients on finasteride, the 6 month PSA level should be used as the baseline. PC SPES, an herbal medication, can also lower serum PSA levels.

‡An increase in the serum PSA level has been reported after ejaculation. In some reports, the increase has been as much as twofold. Testing should be repeated if performed on blood that was drawn within 48 hours after ejaculation.

#An increase in the serum PSA level has been reported after digital rectal examination. Many of these studies, however, have shown that the increase is not clinically significant. As a result, many experts do not recommend delaying measurement of the serum PSA level in a patient who has recently had digital rectal examination.

§Significant elevations in the serum PSA level have been described following cystoscopy and prostate biopsy. For this reason, serum PSA testing should be delayed for at least 1 month after cystoscopy or prostate biopsy. Although serum PSA levels may be elevated for up to one month after prostate biopsy, in most patients, levels normalize 14-17 days after the procedure.

Studies have shown that the specificity of the PSA level in the detection of prostate cancer is about 60% to 70% when the serum PSA level is >4 ng/mL.

PSA Derivatives

Improving the sensitivity and specificity of the PSA in the detection of prostate cancer has been the focus of many investigators. A number of studies have investigated PSA derivatives in an effort to improve the diagnostic accuracy of PSA testing. PSA derivatives include the following:

- Age-adjusted PSA

  It is clear that adjusting the PSA for age increases the number of cancers detected in younger men. The basis behind the age-adjusted PSA is that younger males typically have lower serum PSA levels. Instead of using 4 ng/mL as the upper limit of normal, proponents of age-adjusted PSA testing recommend adjusting the upper limit of normal according to the age of the patient, as shown in the following table.

  Age-Specific Reference Range for Serum PSA (ng/mL)

Age (y)	Asians	African-Americans	Whites
40-49	0-2.0	0-2.0	0-2.5
50-59	0-3.0	0-4.0	0-3.5
60-69	0-4.0	0-4.5	0-4.5
70-79	0-5.0	0-5.5	0-6.5

  Adapted from Richardson TD and Oesterling JE, "Age-Specific Reference Ranges for Serum Prostate Specific Antigen," *Urol Clin North Am*, 1997, 24:339-51.

  By making this adjustment based on age, a white male in his 40s with a PSA of 3.0 is considered to have an elevated PSA. If age-adjusted PSA reference ranges were not used, this patient would be considered to have a normal PSA level.

  In one study using age-adjusted PSA reference ranges in men between the ages of 50 and 59, the cancer detection rate was increased by 15%. This was accompanied, however, by a 45% increase in the number of prostate biopsies that were performed.

  Adjusting the serum PSA for age can also improve test specificity. As shown in the previous table, using a higher upper limit for the "normal" serum PSA in older men will decrease the number of biopsies done. In one study of men over the age of 70 years, the use of the age specific PSA resulted in the performance of 44% fewer biopsies. Because of this, however, nearly 50% of organ-confined cancer cases were not detected. Although some argue that organ-confined cancer in this age group may not be significant, universal agreement on this is lacking. At the present time, age adjusted PSA testing is controversial in men over the age of 60.

- PSA velocity

  As with age-adjusted PSA testing, measurement of the PSA velocity (rate of serum PSA increase with time) has been shown to increase the numbers of cancers detected. The PSA velocity is determined by following the serum PSA values in an individual patient over a period of time. Some investigators maintain that a rise in the serum PSA level ≥0.75 ng/mL in 1 year should prompt concern for the possibility of prostate cancer. The PSA velocity can be determined by using the following formula:

PSA velocity = 1/2[(PSA2 - PSA1/time in years) + (PSA3 - PSA2/time in years)]

PSA1 = first serum PSA measurement

PSA2 = second serum PSA measurement

PSA3 = third serum PSA measurement

Widespread acceptance of the PSA velocity has been hampered by the day to day variations in PSA. This variation can be as high as 25%, even in the same individual. The test also requires three separate PSA measurements over at least a 2-year period, yet another factor that has limited its use.

It has a role, however, in deciding whether to perform a repeat biopsy in men with a negative initial prostate biopsy. Some have suggested that a repeat biopsy should be performed if the rate of rise of the serum PSA exceeds .4 ng/mL/year.

- PSA density

  The PSA density is calculated by adjusting the serum PSA level for the size of the prostate (serum PSA/gland volume as determined by transrectal ultrasound). The basis behind the use of the PSA density is that larger amounts of PSA are produced by larger prostates. Widespread acceptance of this PSA derivative has been limited by the variability in prostate volume measurement by transrectal ultrasound and the need to perform it in the first place. This PSA modification may have a role in deciding whether to rebiopsy men who have had a negative initial prostate biopsy.

Free:Total PSA Ratio (Percent Free PSA)

In the blood, PSA may circulate in one of two forms: protein-bound or free. It has become clear that prostate cancer is associated with lower free:total PSA ratios. In contrast, benign diseases of the prostate presenting with an elevated serum PSA usually present with higher free:total PSA ratios.

The free:total PSA ratio has been found to be useful in men with serum PSA levels between 4-10 ng/mL. In 1998, the results of a multicenter prospective trial investigating the utility of this ratio in men with serum PSA levels between 4-10 ng/mL became available. In this trial, two different cutoff levels for the ratio were used - 25% and 22%. If a ratio of >25% was used to decide whether biopsy was needed (those with ratio >25% did not undergo biopsy), 95% of prostate cancers were detected and 20% of unnecessary biopsies avoided. Using a cutoff of >22%, the cancer detection rate decreased to 90% but unnecessary biopsies were reduced by 29%. Based on these types of results, the Food and Drug Administration approved the use of the free:total PSA ratio in men with serum PSA levels between 4-10 ng/mL.

This test is also useful when deciding whether to rebiopsy men after an initial negative prostate biopsy. In these types of patients, it has been found to be superior to other PSA modifications. In one study of men with serum PSA levels between 4-10 ng/mL, 90% of prostate cancers were detected with rebiopsy if a cutoff value of 30% was used. Using this cutoff value, the number of unnecessary biopsies were reduced by 50%.

In summary, the three modifications to the PSA test described above (PSA density, age-adjusted PSA, free:total PSA ratio) have been clearly shown to improve the specificity of the serum PSA in the detection of prostate cancer. All three modifications decrease the number of prostate biopsies performed in men who do not have prostate cancer. The reduction in the number of prostate biopsies performed, however, is associated with reduced test sensitivity. Therefore, at the current time, there is no consensus regarding the optimal use of PSA density, age-adjusted PSA testing, and free:total PSA ratio.

Use of PSA for Prostate Cancer Staging

Many studies have shown that the serum PSA directly correlates with advancing disease and pathologic stage. However, there is too much overlap in PSA levels between the stages to allow for its use in staging patients with prostate cancer. As a general rule, approximately 75% of prostate cancer patients with a serum PSA <4.0 ng/mL have organ-confined prostate cancer. Over 50% of patients with a serum PSA >10 ng/mL have prostate cancer characterized by capsular penetration. Approximately 75% of patients with a serum PSA >50 ng/mL have malignant involvement of pelvic lymph nodes.

While the serum PSA level alone is not used for staging of prostate cancer, the degree of elevation can help determine which of the following tests or procedures is necessary for the proper staging of the patient with prostate cancer:

- Bone scan
- CT scan
- MRI
- Surgical staging with pelvic lymph node dissection

PRETREATMENT STAGING OF PROSTATE CANCER

Determine tumor grade (based on the Gleason grading system)

Gleason score 2-4: Lower biologic aggressiveness
Gleason score 5-6: Intermediate biologic aggressiveness
Gleason score >7: Biologically aggressive tumor

Additional tests, based on preliminary staging include:

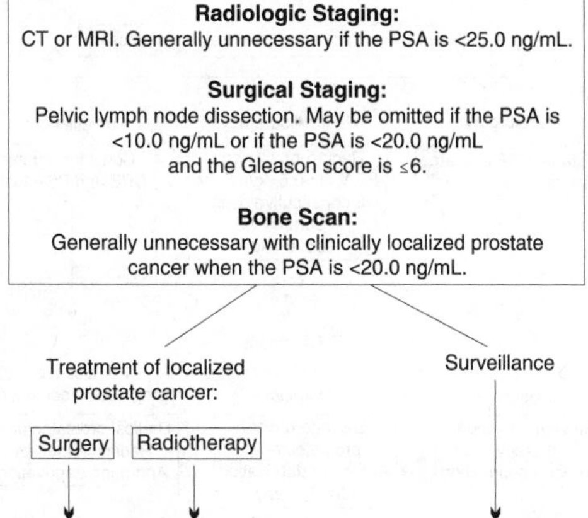
Radiologic Staging:
CT or MRI. Generally unnecessary if the PSA is <25.0 ng/mL.
Surgical Staging:
Pelvic lymph node dissection. May be omitted if the PSA is <10.0 ng/mL or if the PSA is <20.0 ng/mL and the Gleason score is ≤6.
Bone Scan:
Generally unnecessary with clinically localized prostate cancer when the PSA is <20.0 ng/mL.
Treatment of localized prostate cancer:
Surveillance
Surgery
Radiotherapy

Adapted from Carroll P, Coley C, McLeod D, et al, "Prostate-Specific Antigen Best Practice Policy - Part II: Prostate Cancer Staging and Post-Treatment Follow-up," *Urology*, 2001, 57:226.

Use of PSA Following Radical Prostatectomy

Undetectable serum PSA levels following radical prostatectomy suggest that the patient has been cured of the prostate cancer. Undetectable serum PSA levels are expected within 1 month of surgery. If levels do not become undetectable within 1 month of surgery, the clinician should suspect residual disease. If serum PSA becomes detectable during the follow-up of a patient who had initially undetectable levels, the clinician should be concerned about disease recurrence.

Use of PSA Following Radiotherapy

There is no general consensus regarding an acceptable serum PSA level after radiotherapy. One of two approaches are usually taken in the serial evaluation of serum PSA levels following radiotherapy.

- Assessment of serum PSA nadir

  After radiotherapy, serum PSA levels fall slowly, reaching a nadir at about 17 months (median value). When nadir PSA values are quite low (<0.5 ng/mL) or undetectable, relapse is not likely.

- Rise in serum PSA above nadir

  The American Society for Therapeutic Radiology and Oncology defines recurrence of disease based upon three consecutive rises in serum PSA above the nadir. Proponents of this method advocate serial testing of serum PSA levels every 3-6 months.

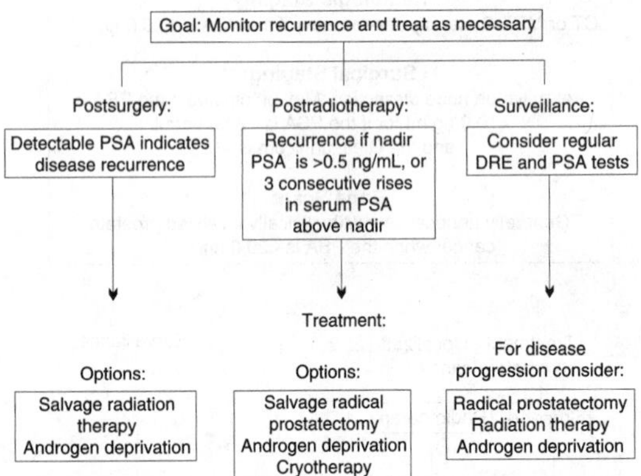

Adapted from Carroll P, Coley C, McLeod D, et al, "Prostate-Specific Antigen Best Practice Policy - Part II: Prostate Cancer Staging and Post-treatment Follow-up," *Urology*, 2001, 57:226.

References

Anderson C, "Casebook: PSA Dilemmas," *Practitioner*, 2000, 244(1614):739-41, 744, 748.

Barry MJ, "Clinical Practice. Prostate-Specific-Antigen Testing for Early Diagnosis of Prostate Cancer," *N Engl J Med*, 2001, 344(18):1373-7.

Brawer MK, "Prostate-Specific Antigen: Current Status," *CA Cancer J Clin*, 1999, 49(5):264-81.

Caplan A and Kratz A, "Prostate-Specific Antigen and the Early Diagnosis of Prostate Cancer," *Am J Clin Pathol*, 2002, 117(Suppl):S104-8.

Carroll P, Coley C, McLeod D, et al, "Prostate-Specific Antigen Best Practice Policy - Part II: Prostate Cancer Staging and Post-treatment Follow-up".

Egawa S, "Detection of Prostate Cancer by Prostate-Specific Antigen," *Biomed Pharmacother*, 2001, 55(3):130-4.

Gambert SR, "Prostate Cancer. When to Offer Screening in the Primary Care Setting," *Geriatrics*, 2001, 56(1):22-6, 29-31.

Gretzer MB and Partin AW, "PSA Markers in Prostate Cancer Detection," *Urol Clin North Am*, 2003, 30(4):677-86.

Ornstein DK and Pruthi RS, "Prostate-Specific Antigen," *Expert Opin Pharmacother*, 2000, 1(7):1399-411.

Pruthi RS, "The Dynamics of Prostate-Specific Antigen in Benign and Malignant Diseases of the Prostate," *BJU Int*, 2000, 86(6):652-8.

Van Der Cruijsen-Koeter IW, Wildhagen MF, De Koning HJ, et al, "The Value of Current Diagnostic Tests in Prostate Cancer Screening," *BJU Int*, 2001, 88(5):458-66.

URINALYSIS

Chemical analysis of urine is performed by using reagent strips. The following may be determined using these strips.

URINALYSIS INFORMATION OBTAINED WITH REAGENT STRIPS
pH
PROTEIN
GLUCOSE
KETONES
BILIRUBIN
UROBILINOGEN
BLOOD
NITRITES
LEUKOCYTE ESTERASE
SPECIFIC GRAVITY

When reagent strips are wetted by urine, a chemical reaction takes place which results in a change of color. The color obtained may be compared to a color chart that is distributed by the manufacturer to give qualitative results of the above. Results are reported as one of the following, depending on which reagent strips are used:

- Concentration (mg/dL)
- Small / moderate / large
- 1+ / 2+ / 3+ / 4+
- + / - / normal

Exceptions to this are specific gravity and pH which are always given a numerical value.

GROSS APPEARANCE / ODOR

Gross examination of the urine can be quite informative. The elements to be cognizant of include the following.

1. Color

   Urine is normally clear or yellow. The color of urine is determined by the concentration of urochrome pigment. Therefore, colorless urine may be the result of large fluid intake. Darker urine can be seen with poor fluid intake. A change in urine color is not synonymous with disease. For example, there are many foods and medications that can cause a variety of changes in urine color.

2. Turbidity / clarity

   It is important to recognize that in the majority of patients, cloudiness does not imply disease. However, a microscopic exam of the urine is necessary in every turbid, uncentrifuged urine specimen.

   The most common cause of cloudy urine is phosphaturia, which involves the precipitation of phosphate crystals in alkaline urine. This is completely benign and is often found after a meal high in protein. Another common cause of cloudy urine is pyuria. One can differentiate between the two by the fact that infected urine has a pungent odor and its microscopic examination reveals white blood cells.

The causes of cloudy urine are listed in the following box.

CLOUDY URINE DIFFERENTIAL DIAGNOSIS
PHOSPHATURIA PYURIA CHYLURIA LIPIDURIA HYPEROXALURIA HYPERURICOSURIA

What Information Can Be Gained by Examining Urine Odor?

In general, urine odor is not a helpful discriminating factor; nevertheless, the following are described in the literature.

Urine Odor and Associated Diseases

Disease	Odor
Ketones	Sweet or fruity
Maple syrup urine disease	Maple syrup
Phenylketonuria	Musty
Hypermethioninemia	Rancid
Tyrosinemia	Rancid
Isovaleric or glutaric acidemia	Sweaty feet
Excess butyric or hexanoic acid	Sweaty feet
Urea-splitting bacterial infection	Ammonia

URINE OSMOLALITY / SPECIFIC GRAVITY

What Information Can Be Gained by Measuring Osmolality?

The concentration of solutes in urine can be quantified by measuring either specific gravity or osmolality. Urine osmolality varies with hydration status. A maximally dilute urine has an osmolality of 50 mOsm/kg, whereas a maximally concentrated urine approaches 1400 mOsm/kg. A normal adult with normal fluid intake produces urine with an osmolality between 500 and 850 mOsm/kg. In the absence of renal disease, urine osmolality and specific gravity can be used interchangeably. However, with renal disease, specific gravity and osmolality do not correspond because of the greater contribution of high molecular weight substances, such as glucose and protein, to specific gravity. Therefore, in the patient with renal disease, the measurement of urine osmolality is preferred.

What Information Can Be Gained by Measuring Specific Gravity?

Specific gravity (SG) is a ratio of the weight of a volume of urine with the same volume of water. It reflects the state of hydration, varying between 1.001 and 1.035. Urine with a specific gravity <1.008 is dilute while that >1.020 is considered concentrated. When the ultrafiltrate of plasma enters Bowman's capsule, it has a specific gravity of 1.010. As ultrafiltrate passes through renal tubules, water and solutes are absorbed and secreted. If tubular function is impaired, the specific gravity of urine will be the same as that of the initial ultrafiltrate. This fixed specific gravity (1.010) is known as isothenuria, a finding that suggests significant tubular dysfunction.

Causes of decreased specific gravity are listed in the following box.

DECREASED SPECIFIC GRAVITY DIFFERENTIAL DIAGNOSIS
INCREASED FLUID INTAKE
DIURETICS
DECREASED RENAL CONCENTRATING ABILITY
DIABETES INSIPIDUS

The following can result in an increase in specific gravity.

INCREASED SPECIFIC GRAVITY DIFFERENTIAL DIAGNOSIS
DECREASED FLUID INTAKE
DEHYDRATION
DIABETES MELLITUS WITH GLUCOSURIA
SIADH
INTRAVENOUS CONTRAST

Further evaluation is required when urine SG falls above 1.035 or below 1.001, because such values are physiologically impossible. In cases where urine SG falls below 1.001, the clinician should ensure that the specimen being analyzed is truly urine. This can be done by measuring creatinine or urea concentration in the specimen. When urine SG is >1.035, the clinician should consider the presence of either radiographic contrast or mannitol.

Urine osmolality is a better measure of renal function than specific gravity. For example, if there are substances present in the urine with a higher molecular weight than normal urinary constituents, then there may be a relatively higher rise in specific gravity as compared to osmolality.

URINE pH

The normal range of urine pH is shown in the following table.

	Urine pH
Normal	4.5-8
Acidic	4.5-5.5
Alkaline	6.5-8

A pH that is >8 or <4 is physiologically impossible. When the pH is >8, the clinician should strongly suspect the urine was not processed expeditiously, resulting in the growth of urease-producing bacteria. In general, urine pH parallels serum pH.

What Are the Causes of Alkaline Urine?

In patients with urinary tract infection, the finding of alkaline urine with a pH >7.5 warrants consideration of a urea splitting organism such as *Proteus*. In these cases, ammonia is converted to the ammonium ion with precipitation of calcium magnesium aluminum phosphate crystals.

It is important to determine pH promptly because urine standing at room temperature will become alkalotic secondary to bacterial overgrowth. An alkaline urine may be appreciated in the following.

ALKALINE URINE DIFFERENTIAL DIAGNOSIS
UREA SPLITTING ORGANISM STANDING URINE VEGETARIANS CONSIDERABLE INTAKE OF CITRUS FRUIT METABOLIC ALKALOSIS RESPIRATORY ALKALOSIS MEDICATION-INDUCED Sodium bicarbonate Potassium citrate Acetazolamide

What Happens to Urine pH After a Meal?

The average person excretes urine with a pH between 5 and 6 because of endogenous acid production. However, after a meal, urine may be less acidic because of the so called "alkaline tide". Parietal cells secrete HCl into the stomach lumen leaving bicarbonate behind in the serum. This bicarbonate is filtered by the kidney resulting in an alkaline urine pH after a meal.

What Are the Causes of Acidic Urine?

The causes of acidic urine are listed in the following box.

ACIDIC URINE DIFFERENTIAL DIAGNOSIS
LARGE INTAKE OF MEAT CERTAIN FRUITS (cranberries) METABOLIC ACIDOSIS RESPIRATORY ACIDOSIS MEDICATION-INDUCED Ammonium chloride

What Is the Urine pH in Patients With Renal Tubular Acidosis (RTA)?

Urine pH can help establish a diagnosis of RTA. Urine pH is typically >5.5 in these patients. Urine pH that does not fall to <5.5 after an acid load is diagnostic of RTA.

URINE PROTEIN

What Information Can Be Gained From Dipstick Testing of Urine for Protein?

Normally, there is <150 mg of protein excreted in the urine over a 24-hour period. Excretion exceeding this amount may be the first indication of disease. In clinical practice, proteinuria is usually first detected by urine dipstick testing.

What Are the Normal Protein Constituents Excreted in the Urine?

Excreted protein comes from plasma and the urinary tract. Plasma proteins include both albumin and a globulin fraction. The major constituent of protein derived from the urinary tract is the Tamm-Horsfall protein, which is secreted by cells of the ascending limb of the loop of Henle and the distal tubule.

CONSTITUENTS OF PROTEIN IN NORMAL URINE
ALBUMIN 30%
GLOBULINS 30%
TAMM-HORSFALL 40%

Why Is It Important to Know the Specific Gravity When Interpreting the Results of Urinary Protein Determined by Dipstick?

Urine dipstick for protein should always be evaluated in relation to urine specific gravity. In a patient with dilute urine, significant proteinuria may not be detected by dipstick, giving a false-negative reading. Trace urine protein has a different implication, depending on urine specific gravity. While a trace amount of protein in concentrated urine may not carry much significance, such an amount in dilute urine may be the first indication of pathologic disease.

What Are the Causes of a False-Positive Urine Dipstick Test for Protein?

CAUSES OF A FALSE-POSITIVE URINE DIPSTICK TEST FOR PROTEIN
HIGHLY ALKALINE URINE
HEMATURIA
HIGH SPECIFIC GRAVITY
PYRIDIUM

Is Dipstick Testing for Protein Sensitive for All the Different Types of Protein?

Urine dipstick is most sensitive for albumin. It may be negative when low molecular weight proteins are present in urine. There are two situations where this becomes important.

1. Renal tubular disease

   One of the functions of the proximal tubules is the catabolism of low-molecular-weight protein that is filtered at the glomerulus. In certain tubular diseases, this catabolic function may be impaired, leading to the presence of significant low-molecular-weight proteinuria.

2. Immunoglobulin light chains

   A false-negative result with other proteins, especially immunoglobulin light chains (Bence Jones proteins in patients with multiple myeloma), may occur as well. Bence Jones proteinuria can be demonstrated in up to 75% of patients with multiple myeloma. Although immunoglobulin light chains can be detected by the sulfosalicylic acid test, the diagnostic method of choice is urine protein electrophoresis (UPEP).

What Is Microalbuminuria?

In the past few years, attention has focused on microalbuminuria in the setting of diabetes mellitus. Microalbuminuria refers to the daily urinary excretion of albumin that is clearly abnormal, but is below the detection capability of urine dipstick testing. Microalbuminuria is important because it is an early indicator of nephropathy in patients with diabetes. Screening diabetic patients for microalbuminuria on a regular basis can help identify patients at increased risk for developing diabetic nephropathy, allowing the clinician to intervene. For more information, please see the chapter, ***Microalbuminuria*** *on page 581.*

Why Should a 24-Hour Urine Collection for Protein Be Performed if the Urine Dipstick Result Is Readily Available?

It needs to be recognized that a urine dipstick for protein is not a quantitative measure. In the patient with a positive urine dipstick for protein, a 24-hour urine collection for protein is needed for quantitation. Creatinine from this sample can be measured as well, to ensure adequacy of the collection. Some investigators recommend calculating a protein:creatinine ratio in random samples of urine as a surrogate to 24-hour testing.

Protein:Creatinine Ratio in Determining the Severity of Proteinuria

Protein:Creatinine Ratio	Severity of Proteinuria
<0.1-0.2	Normal
1.0	1 g/day
>3.5	>3.5 g/day (nephrotic range)

URINE GLUCOSE

Glucose in blood is normally filtered at the glomerulus with almost complete reabsorption taking place in the proximal tubule. The appearance of glucose in urine signifies that the filtered load exceeded the absorptive capability of the proximal tubule. The blood level at which glucose appears in the urine varies from individual to individual, but usually occurs at >180 mg/dL. This is the renal threshold for glucose. However, because there is variation among individuals, some may spill glucose into the urine at lower levels. Two conditions characterized by a positive urine dipstick test for glucose in the absence of hyperglycemia are renal glucosuria and pregnancy.

Hyperglycemic conditions associated with glycosuria are listed in the following box.

HYPERGLYCEMIC CONDITIONS ASSOCIATED WITH GLUCOSURIA
DIABETES MELLITUS
ALIMENTARY GLUCOSURIA (transient)
INCREASED INTRACRANIAL PRESSURE
OTHER ENDOCRINE DISORDERS
Cushing's syndrome
Pheochromocytoma
Acromegaly
Chronic liver disease
Chronic pancreatitis
MEDICATIONS
Steroids
Thiazide diuretics

Glucose detected by dipstick is not synonymous with diabetes, but is a feature of the disease and warrants a search for undiagnosed diabetes mellitus.

What Are the Causes of a False-Negative Urine Dipstick Test for Glucose?

The causes of a false-negative urine dipstick test for glucose are listed in the following box.

CAUSES OF A FALSE-NEGATIVE URINE DIPSTICK TEST FOR GLUCOSE
ASCORBIC ACID
ASPIRIN

URINE KETONES

The three types of ketones include β-hydroxybutrate, acetoacetate, and acetic acid. When body stores of carbohydrates are diminished and breakdown of fat takes place, ketones are produced. Although small amounts of ketones are normally present in serum and urine, they are not detected by conventional testing. Therefore, a positive test for ketones in serum or urine indicates considerable excess. In diabetes, an increase in ketones should raise concern about the possibility of diabetic ketoacidosis (DKA). In the patient with DKA, urine may be negative for ketones if severe renal insufficiency exists, as the kidneys may be unable to filter ketones. Therefore, in a patient with severe renal insufficiency, even if the urine is negative for ketones, DKA may still be a consideration.

The utility of this test is also dependent on which ketone is predominant. The nitroprusside reaction that forms the basis of this test does not react with β-hydroxybutyrate, but reacts strongly with acetoacetic acid. In DKA and AKA (alcoholic ketoacidosis), most of the ketones present are in the form of β-hydroxybutyrate. Therefore, a negative or weakly positive urine ketone dipstick should not sway the clinician from the possibility of ketoacidosis if the clinical presentation is suggestive.

What Are Other Causes of Ketonuria?

Other causes of ketonuria include starvation, pregnancy, rapid weight reduction, fasting, and salicylate overdose.

Is There Anything That Might Cause a Falsely Elevated Urine Ketone Level?

A false-positive result may occur with certain dyes, metabolites of levodopa, α-methyldopa, captopril, MESNA, N-acetylcysteine, D-penicillamine, phenylketones, and phthaleins.

URINE BLOOD

What Is the Significance of a Urine Dipstick Positive for Blood?

A dipstick positive for blood always requires further evaluation. It indicates the presence of hematuria, hemoglobinuria, or myoglobinuria.

Microscopic examination of urine revealing a large amount of red blood cells (normal urine contains <3 RBCs/hpf) supports hematuria. If red blood cells are absent, one can differentiate between hemoglobinuria and myoglobinuria by obtaining a blood sample. In hemoglobinuria, centrifugation will result in a pink supernatant, whereas it will be clear in myoglobinuria. The reason for this is that free hemoglobin in serum binds to haptoglobin, a protein produced by the liver. This complex is water insoluble and therefore remains in the serum, imparting a pink color. Because myoglobin is water soluble, it is excreted immediately in the urine. It should be noted that hemolysis leading to true hemoglobinuria is uncommon. More often, RBCs enter the urine and are lysed. Since chemical methods detect both intact and lysed RBCs, the clinician should not misinterpret a positive dipstick as a reflection of true hemoglobinuria. Other laboratory tests should be ordered to exclude true hemoglobinuria (LDH, bilirubin, haptoglobin).

Comparison of Hematuria, Hemoglobinuria, and Myoglobinuria

	Urine Dipstick	Urine RBC	Serum Supernatant	LDH	Bilirubin	CPK
Hematuria	(+)	(+)	Clear	NL	NL	NL
Hemoglobinuria	(+)	(-)	Pink	↑	↑	NL
Myoglobinuria	(+)	(-)	Clear	NL	NL	↑

What Are the Causes of a False-Positive Urine Dipstick for Blood?

The sensitivity of dipstick in the detection of hematuria is >90%. However, specificity in comparison with microscopy is lower. A false-positive result may occur in the following.

FALSE-POSITIVE URINE DIPSTICK FOR BLOOD
MENSTRUAL / HEMORRHOIDAL BLOOD CONTAMINATION
INCREASED URINE SPECIFIC GRAVITY*
VITAMINS / FOODS HIGH IN OXIDANTS

*This occurs because of the increased concentration of RBCs.

What Are the Causes of a False-Negative Urine Dipstick for Blood?

False-negative results may occur with ascorbic acid and high nitrite concentrations.

How Can the Clinician Differentiate Between the Origins of Hematuria?

Documentation of hematuria raises concern about the possibility of either renal or urologic disease. Finding red blood cell casts or considerable protein in the urine argues for hematuria of renal origin. Even marked urologic hematuria will not raise the protein concentration to the +2 to +3 range.

Hematuria of glomerular etiology is characterized by dysmorphic erythrocytes. This refers to alterations in morphology of red blood cells. Dysmorphic red blood cells are not seen with tubulointerstitial disease or hematuria of urologic origin. Hematuria in these diseases is characterized by red blood cells uniformly having a round shape. It is best to use a phase contrast microscope to look for dysmorphic red blood cells but light microscopy may reveal changes as well.

	Erythrocyte Shape	Urine Protein	RBC Casts
Urologic	Round	Mild	(-)
Glomerular	Dysmorphic	Marked*	(+)*
Tubulointerstitial	Round	Mild to moderate	(-)

*Approximately 25% of patients proved to have glomerular origin by renal biopsy do not have evidence of red blood cell casts or proteinuria.

For more information, please refer to the chapter, ***Hematuria** on page 561.*

URINE LEUKOCYTE ESTERASE (LE) / NITRITE

WBCs may enter urine in response to a number of noninfectious and infectious conditions. The most common cause of pyuria, however, is a urinary tract infection (UTI). Traditionally, microscopy was used to establish the presence of WBCs in urine. Since LE is an enzyme that is present in WBCs, detection of LE by dipstick is consistent with the presence of WBCs in urine. Therefore, a positive result provides strong evidence for the diagnosis of UTI in the patient presenting with compatible signs and symptoms. In comparison with urine culture, it is 80% to 90% sensitive in the diagnosis of urinary tract infection. Sensitivity increases when a positive nitrite test is obtained as well.

A urine specimen that is positive for leukocyte esterase but negative for the presence of white blood cells on urine microscopy suggests the possibility of cell lysis. Cell lysis is not uncommon in alkaline or hypotonic urine. A urine specimen that contains primarily lymphocytes will have a negative LE test, as lymphocytes do not contain the enzyme. This might explain the situation in which white blood cells are present in urine but the leukocyte esterase test is negative.

What Information Can Be Gained From Urine Nitrite?

Certain bacteria can reduce nitrates to nitrites. A positive result for nitrites argues for the presence of bacteria in the urine. In order for the nitrite test to be positive, the following factors must be present:

- Bacteria present must be nitrite producers
- More than 4 hours must pass between voids
- There must be adequate intake of dietary nitrates

The sensitivity of this test is about 50%, considerably lower than that of leukocyte esterase in the diagnosis of urinary tract infections.

A false-positive result may be obtained with pyridium or if the specimen sits at room temperature for a prolonged period of time allowing for the growth of bacteria.

A false-negative result may occur with ascorbic acid.

URINE BILIRUBIN / UROBILINOGEN

Bilirubin is not normally detected in the urine. It is important to remember that only conjugated bilirubin can be found in urine because it is water soluble. Therefore, in disorders such as hepatobiliary disease, dipstick may reveal a positive result for bilirubin. Bilirubin in urine imparts a dark color. This change in color can actually be appreciated several days before the patient becomes icteric. A quick test to differentiate conjugated from unconjugated hyperbilirubinemia is the foam test. Yellow foam that develops after shaking is consistent with conjugated bilirubinemia.

False-positive results may occur with high nitrite concentrations and improper specimen storage, particularly when specimens are exposed to light.

What Is the Significance of Urine Urobilinogen?

In clinical practice, urobilinogen is not useful.

URINE MICROSCOPIC ANALYSIS

What Is the Significance of White Blood Cells in the Urine?

The normal range for white blood cells in urine is 0-5/hpf. The presence of an increased number of WBCs in the urine supports an inflammatory process. It is important to examine urine microscopically within 1 hour of collection because white blood cells can lyse in hypotonic or alkalotic urine. In women, care must be taken to prevent vaginal contamination which can result in pyuria as well. The presence of squamous epithelial cells supports vaginal contamination.

Pyuria of renal origin should be suspected if there is significant concomitant proteinuria. Although proteinuria may accompany nonrenal pyuria, it is usually of a milder degree. The presence of WBC casts supports a renal origin.

The presence of increased white blood cells in the urine may be consistent with a urinary tract infection. In such cases, pyuria is usually accompanied by bacteriuria. Tuberculosis is one exception in which pyuria is sterile (negative bacterial culture).

The causes of sterile pyuria are listed in the following box.

STERILE PYURIA DIFFERENTIAL DIAGNOSIS
FEVER
PREGNANCY
FOLLOWING ANTIBIOTIC TREATMENT
STEROID TREATMENT
RENAL TRANSPLANT REJECTION
PROSTATITIS
URETHRITIS
TUBULOINTERSTITIAL NEPHRITIS
CYCLOPHOSPHAMIDE THERAPY
INFECTION
Tuberculosis
Fungal infection
Atypical mycobacteria
Anaerobic bacteria
Fastidious bacteria

What Is the Significance of Red Blood Cells in the Urine?

The normal range for red blood cells is 0-5/hpf. As stated previously, hematuria may be of glomerular, tubulointerstitial, or urologic origin. The finding of red blood cell casts or dysmorphic red blood cells in the urine indicates a glomerular source. Dysmorphic red blood cells have a variety of morphologic alterations including spicules, blebs, and vesicles. Uniformly round red blood cells are characteristic of nonglomerular hematuria. When dipstick testing for blood is positive, but microscopy does not reveal RBCs in the urine, one of three possibilities exists:

1. True hemoglobinuria
2. Myoglobinuria
3. RBC lysis

To distinguish among these possibilities, refer to the section on urine dipstick testing for blood *on page 598*.

What Is the Significance of Bacteria in the Urine?

Bacteria in urine, or bacteriuria, is usually reported as few, moderate, or many per high power field. Recall that normal urine is sterile. Therefore, the presence of bacteria in urine either signifies infection or contamination. Bacteriuria accompanied by pyuria argues strongly for infection. When pyuria is absent, the clinician should suspect contamination as the cause of bacteriuria.

What Is the Significance of Renal Tubular Epithelial Cells in the Urine?

It is not uncommon to see a few tubular cells in normal urine. In patients with tubular or interstitial disease, increased numbers may be appreciated in the urine.

What Is the Significance of Squamous Epithelial Cells in the Urine?

In women and uncircumcised men, the presence of squamous epithelial cells suggests contamination. These cells are never pathologic.

What Is the Significance of Transitional Cells in the Urine?

It is not uncommon to see a few transitional cells in urine secondary to desquamation. There may be an increase in the number of transitional cells in patients with urinary tract infections. Urinary catheterization or other instrumentation may lead to transitional cells in clusters or sheets. However, sheets of transitional cells in a patient who has not recently been instrumented raises concern for possible transitional cell carcinoma, requiring further evaluation.

What Is the Significance of Casts in the Urine?

Casts refer to proteins that outline the shape of the renal tubules in which they were formed.

Type of Cast	Clinical Correlate
RBC cast	Nephritic syndrome
WBC cast	Pyelonephritis Tubulointerstitial disease
Hyaline cast	Nonspecific
Granular cast	Nonspecific
Muddy brown cast	Acute tubular necrosis
Renal tubular epithelial cell cast	Acute tubular necrosis
Fatty cast	Nephrotic syndrome Fat embolism
Broad cast	Chronic renal insufficiency
Waxy cast	Chronic renal insufficiency

What Is the Significance of Crystals in the Urine?

Crystals are a common finding in urine. Their clinical significance is limited. However, in a patient with nephrolithiasis, the type of crystal may provide information about the patient's kidney stones. In ethylene glycol intoxication, increased amounts of calcium oxalate may be appreciated. The finding of cystine, tyrosine, and leucine crystals in urine is always abnormal.

References

Fogazzi GB, Passerini P, Ponticelli C, et al, *The Urinary Sediment*, London: Chapman and Hall Medical, 1994.

Geyer SJ, "Urinalysis and Urinary Sediment in Patients With Renal Disease," *Clin Lab Med*, 1993, 13(1):13-20.

Handrigan MT, Thompson I, and Foster M, "Diagnostic Procedures for the Urogenital System," *Emerg Med Clin North Am*, 2001, 19(3):745-61.

King C, "Automated Methods in Urinalysis," *Clin Lab Sci*, 1998, 11(1):44-6.

Lorincz AE, Kelly DR, Dobbins GC, et al, "Urinalysis: Current Status and Prospects for the Future," *Ann Clin Lab Sci*, 1999, 29(3):169-75.

Misdraji J and Nguyen PL, "Urinalysis. When - and When Not - To Order," *Postgrad Med*, 1996, 100(1):173-176, 181-2, 185-8 passim.

Raymond JR and Yarger WE, "Abnormal Urine Color: Differential Diagnosis," *Southern Med J*, 1988, 81:837-41.

PART VII:

GASTROENTEROLOGY

LIVER FUNCTION TESTS

ASPARTATE AMINOTRANSFERASE / ALANINE AMINOTRANSFERASE (AST/ALT)

Aspartate aminotransferase (AST) and alanine aminotransferase (ALT), previously known as serum glutamic oxaloacetic transaminase (SGOT) and serum glutamic pyruvic transaminase (SGPT), respectively, are enzymes found in the liver cell. These enzymes are involved in the transfer of amino groups, as their name suggests, from aspartate and alanine to α-ketoglutarate, leading to the formation of oxaloacetic acid and pyruvic acid, respectively. With hepatocellular damage, AST and ALT levels may rise.

Sensitivity of AST and ALT in the Detection of Liver Disease

Normal transaminase levels do not exclude the presence of liver disease. In fact, it is not unusual for patients with cirrhosis to have normal transaminase levels because of the absence of continuing injury. In addition, many patients with chronic hepatitis C do not have an elevation in the transaminase levels. Studies have shown that 33% of patients with chronic hepatitis C (confirmed by liver biopsy) have persistently normal ALT levels. These examples highlight the fact that AST and ALT lack sensitivity in the diagnosis of chronic liver disease.

Uremia can lead to falsely low transaminase levels. The upper limit of normal in patients on hemodialysis is about 50% of that appreciated in healthy individuals. It is important to realize this because hemodialysis patients are at risk for certain types of liver disease including hepatitis C.

Specificity of AST and ALT in Detection of Liver Disease

It is important to realize that these enzymes are not entirely specific for the liver. In fact, both AST and ALT are found in many other organs. Organs or tissues with the highest AST content are listed in the following box (in descending order of frequency).

ORGANS OR TISSUES WITH HIGH AST CONTENT (descending order of frequency)		
1. LIVER	4. PANCREAS	7. LUNG
2. HEART	5. KIDNEY	8. WHITE BLOOD CELL
3. SKELETAL MUSCLE	6. BRAIN	9. RED BLOOD CELL

ALT content is highest in the liver and kidney. Lesser amounts are present in heart and skeletal muscle. Despite the fact that these enzymes are found in many other organs, elevations in transaminases can often be ascribed to liver disease if the clinical context is carefully considered. Of the two, an ALT elevation is more specific for liver disease. When AST and/or ALT elevation is due to nonhepatic disease, levels exceeding 300 IU/L are rare. An exception to this rule is in the patient with acute rhabdomyolysis, in which transaminase levels may rise to a range typically seen with acute hepatocellular disorders.

Factors, other than liver disease, affecting AST/ALT levels are listed in the following table.

Factors Affecting AST and ALT, Other Than Liver Injury

Factor	AST	ALT	Comments
Day-to-day	5% to 10% variation from one day to next	10% to 30% variation from one day to next	Similar in liver disease and health, and in elderly and young
Race / gender	15% higher in African-American men		No significant difference between African-American, other women
Body mass index (BMI)	40% to 50% higher with high BMI	40% to 50% higher with high BMI	Direct relationship between weight and AST, ALT
Exercise	Threefold increase with strenuous exercise	20% lower in those who exercise at usual levels than in those who do not exercise or exercise more strenuously than usual	Effect of exercise seen predominantly in men; minimal difference in women (<10%). Enzymes increase more with strength training.
Muscle Injury	Significant increase	Moderate increase	Related to amount of increase in CK
Hemolysis	Significant increase	Moderate increase attributable to release from red cell	Dependent on degree of hemolysis; usually severalfold lower than increases in LDH

Adapted from Dufour DR, Lott JA, Nolte FS, et al, "Diagnosis and Monitoring of Hepatic Injury, I. Performance Characteristics of Laboratory Tests," *Clin Chem*, 2000, 46(12):2031.

Degree of Transaminase Elevation

The degree of transaminase elevation can provides clues as to the etiology of the liver disease. As shown in the following table, transaminase elevation can be classified as mild, moderate, or severe.

Degree of Transaminase Elevation

Measurement	Normal (IU/L)*	Mild†	Moderate†	Severe†
AST	11-32	<2-3	2-3 to 20	>20
ALT	3-30	<2-3	2-3 to 20	>20

*Normal range varies with the assay used and should be obtained from the laboratory performing the test.

†Multiples of the upper limit of normal.

Conditions Associated With Marked Transaminase Elevation (>1000 units/L)

Conditions associated with markedly elevated AST and ALT are listed in the following box.

MARKEDLY ELEVATED TRANSAMINASE LEVELS (>1000 units/L) DIFFERENTIAL DIAGNOSIS	
ACUTE VIRAL HEPATITIS	ACUTE BILIARY OBSTRUCTION
DRUGS / TOXINS	AUTOIMMUNE HEPATITIS
ISCHEMIC HEPATITIS	

The differential diagnosis listed in the box above can be narrowed even further if the clinician considers the degree of transaminase elevation >1000 units/L. The highest transaminase elevations are seen in patients with acute ischemic hepatitis or acute toxic injury (>3000 units/L). In contrast, acute viral hepatitis and acute biliary obstruction are seldom associated with levels >3000 units/L.

The time course during which the transaminase levels return to normal is also helpful in differentiating among the causes of markedly elevated transaminases. For example, the patient with ischemic hepatitis develops liver injury after a period of hypotension during which there is poor liver perfusion. Shortly thereafter, there is an impressive rise in the transaminase levels. In most cases, the transaminases return to normal over a period of about a week. This is in contrast to the patient with viral hepatitis in which the liver injury is more sustained. In these cases, the transaminases may remain elevated for a prolonged period of time. The LDH level is also useful in distinguishing ischemic from viral hepatitis. In ischemic hepatitis, there may be a significant elevation in the LDH to a level that is not typically seen in acute viral hepatitis.

The classic biochemical profile of the patient with biliary obstruction is a rise in the alkaline phosphatase and bilirubin levels. However, acute biliary obstruction may be associated with a marked elevation in the transaminase levels, especially if the AST and ALT are assayed early in the course of the biliary obstruction. Transaminase elevation typically occurs within hours of the obstruction, peaking within the first 24-48 hours. Even without resolution of the obstruction, the levels fall over 1-3 days. Accompanying the fall in the transaminase levels are a rise in the alkaline phosphatase and bilirubin levels.

It seems intuitive to think that marked elevation in the transaminase levels would correlate well with the extent of liver cell necrosis. In reality, the degree of transaminase elevation does not correlate with the extent of hepatocellular damage. Therefore, the height of the transaminase elevation has no bearing on the patient's prognosis.

Conditions Associated With Mild to Moderate Transaminase Elevation

While the differential diagnosis of marked transaminase elevation is limited, lesser degrees of elevation are nonspecific and may be associated with many diseases. Of note, transaminase levels seldom climb to >400 units/L in patients with alcoholic liver disease. The clinician should suspect other causes of liver injury in alcoholic patients who present with transaminase levels >400 units/L.

AST:ALT Ratio >1

An AST:ALT ratio >1 should prompt consideration of alcoholic liver disease. A ratio >2 is particularly suggestive of alcoholic liver disease. In one study, >90% of patients who presented with a ratio >2 were found to have alcoholic liver disease on liver biopsy. This percentage increases to 96% if the AST:ALT ratio is >3.

An elevation in the AST:ALT ratio is not pathognomonic for alcoholic liver disease; certainly other types of liver disease can present with this pattern. Conversely, alcoholic liver disease is not always associated with a ratio >1. An AST:ALT ratio >1 is also frequently noted in patients with cirrhosis, irrespective of the etiology. Therefore in patients with cirrhosis, an AST:ALT ratio >1 is less useful in distinguishing alcoholic from nonalcoholic causes of liver disease.

AST:ALT Ratio <1

In most types of liver disease, ALT exceeds AST. Exceptions to this rule are patients with alcoholic liver disease and Reye's syndrome in which the AST:ALT ratio typically is >1. It is also important to realize that, while ALT usually exceeds AST in most types of liver disease, with progression to cirrhosis, it is not uncommon for the AST to rise above the ALT.

ALBUMIN

Albumin is synthesized exclusively by the liver. In the blood, albumin exerts a significant osmotic effect and is integral in the transport of both endogenous and exogenous substances. In fact, albumin constitutes approximately 60% of total protein in the blood.

Elevation in Serum Albumin Level

Causes of an elevated serum albumin level are listed in the following box.

CAUSES OF AN ELEVATED SERUM ALBUMIN LEVEL
DEHYDRATION*
PROLONGED TOURNIQUET USE DURING COLLECTION
SPECIMEN EVAPORATION

*Hemoglobin / hematocrit are often increased in these patients as well.

Causes of Hypoalbuminemia

The causes of hypoalbuminemia are listed in the following box.

CAUSES OF HYPOALBUMINEMIA	
MALNUTRITION	INTRAVENOUS FLUIDS
MALABSORPTION	RAPID HYDRATION
MALIGNANCY	OVERHYDRATION
INFLAMMATION (ACUTE OR CHRONIC)	CIRRHOSIS
INCREASED LOSS	CHRONIC LIVER DISEASE
Nephrotic syndrome	PREGNANCY
Protein-losing enteropathy	
Burns	
Exudative skin disease	

Sensitivity and Specificity of the Serum Albumin Level in the Diagnosis of Liver Disease

Although serum albumin levels are often obtained in patients suspected of having liver disease, it is important to realize that the use of the albumin level is neither sensitive nor specific for liver disease. The half-life of albumin is approximately 3 weeks. As such, the serum albumin level is a much better gauge of synthetic function in patients with chronic liver disease. In cases of acute hepatic necrosis, the serum albumin level may not accurately reflect the true derangement in liver function.

Although the serum albumin can serve as a gauge of the liver's synthetic capability, it is important to realize that the liver can increase albumin synthesis as much as twofold in response to any process that impairs its synthetic function. This may explain, to some extent, why 80% of outpatients with cirrhosis have normal serum albumin levels. In studies of patients presenting with severe decompensated liver disease, serum albumin levels are found to be normal in 15%.

There are also many nonhepatic conditions associated with hypoalbuminemia (see above box); therefore, hypoalbuminemia is not specific for liver disease. In general, a nonhepatic cause is more likely in patients who have no other liver function test abnormalities.

PROTHROMBIN TIME

Prothrombin time (PT) is a measure of the function of the extrinsic pathway. The factors integral to the determination of the PT are made in the liver.

Sensitivity of the PT in the Detection of Liver Disease

Although the PT is clearly a marker of the liver's synthetic function, it will remain normal until at least 80% of the liver's synthetic ability is compromised. For this reason, PT is normal in many patients with chronic liver disease and cirrhosis. Therefore, the PT is a relatively insensitive marker of liver disease.

Compared to albumin, the PT is a more useful gauge of synthetic function in patients with acute liver disease. This is because the coagulation factors integral to the determination of the PT have shorter half-lives (hours) than albumin (3 weeks).

Specificity of the PT in the Detection of Liver Disease

An elevated PT is not specific for liver disease as there are many other causes of an elevated PT. The major causes of an isolated elevation of the PT (normal PTT) are shown in the following box.

ISOLATED ELEVATION OF PT DIFFERENTIAL DIAGNOSIS
VITAMIN K DEFICIENCY*
WARFARIN†
LIVER DISEASE
FACTOR VII DEFICIENCY (inherited or acquired)
FALSE-POSITIVE TEST RESULT
Inadequate tube filling
High hematocrit

*Vitamin K is important in the gamma carboxylation of glutamic acid residues in factors II, VII, IX, X, and protein C and S. Gamma carboxylation is essential for the proper functioning of these coagulation factors. Any process which leads to vitamin K deficiency will lead to a prolongation of the PT. Vitamin K deficiency may result from malabsorption, malnutrition, or antibiotic use.

†Warfarin interferes with gamma carboxylation of glutamic acid residues on vitamin K-dependent coagulation factors.

It is usually not difficult to differentiate among the causes of an isolated elevation of the PT. Warfarin use can easily be excluded by knowledge of the patient's medication profile. Although reported, surreptitious ingestion of warfarin is rare. Factor VII deficiency, whether acquired or inherited, is very uncommon.

Therefore, in usual clinical practice, the clinician must differentiate between vitamin K deficiency and liver disease as the cause of an elevated PT. To differentiate between vitamin K deficiency and liver disease as the cause of an elevated PT, it is useful to administer parenteral vitamin K (10 mg subcutaneously). A decrease in PT by at least 30% within 24 hours of administration of vitamin K supports deficiency of this vitamin. Minimal to little decrease in the PT suggests that the elevation is due to liver disease. It is important to realize that, in some patients, the elevated PT may be due to both vitamin K deficiency and liver disease (ie, alcoholic patient with alcoholic liver disease and malnutrition.)

Using PT to Estimate Prognosis in Patients With Liver Disease

Prognostic scores have been developed for many types of liver disease. The PT is used in many of these prognostic scores. It plays a key role, for example, in estimating prognosis in patients with fulminant hepatic failure and acute alcoholic hepatitis. In general, there is good correlation between the degree of PT elevation and prognosis.

ALKALINE PHOSPHATASE

Alkaline phosphatase is an enzyme that catalyzes the hydrolysis of phosphate esters at an alkaline pH. Alkaline phosphatase is found in many organs, including the liver and biliary tree, bone, placenta, intestine, kidney, and white blood cells. Increases in alkaline phosphatase may be seen in tissues that are active in metabolism. Adolescence and pregnancy are, therefore, states when alkaline phosphatase may be elevated due to bone and placental growth, respectively. Clinically, elevations in alkaline phosphatase are usually of hepatobiliary or bone origin.

Factors Affecting Alkaline Phosphatase (Other Than Liver or Bone Disease)

Prior to considering liver or bone disease as the cause of an elevated alkaline phosphatase level, the clinician should be aware of other factors that can affect the alkaline phosphatase level. These factors are listed in the following table.

Factors Affecting Alkaline Phosphatase (Other Than Liver or Bone Disease)

Factor	Change	Comments
Food ingestion*	Increases as much as 30 units/L	In patients of blood groups B and O; remains increased for up to 12 hours; attributable to intestinal isoenzyme
Race / gender	15% higher in African-American men; 10% higher in African-American women	
Body mass index (BMI)	25% higher with increased BUN	
Hemolysis	Hemoglobin inhibits enzyme activity	
Pregnancy	Increase up to two- to threefold in third trimester	Attributable to placental isoenzyme
Smoking	10% higher	
Oral contraceptives	20% lower	

*If possible, alkaline phosphatase levels should be measured in the fasting state. A mildly elevated nonfasting value should be repeated after fasting. Further evaluation is necessary if the repeat fasting alkaline phosphatase level is elevated.

Adapted from Dufour DR, Lott JA, Nolte FS, et al, "Diagnosis and Monitoring of Hepatic Injury, I. Performance Characteristics of Laboratory Tests," *Clin Chem*, 2000, 46(12):2033.

Causes of an Elevated Alkaline Phosphatase Level

Causes of elevated alkaline phosphatase are listed in the following table.

CAUSES OF AN ELEVATED ALKALINE PHOSPHATASE
CHOLESTASIS
Intrahepatic
Medication-induced
Primary biliary cirrhosis
Benign recurrent intrahepatic cholestasis
Intrahepatic cholestasis of pregnancy
Total parenteral nutrition
Cholestasis of sepsis
Alcoholic hepatitis
Postoperative cholestasis
Systemic infection
Viral hepatitis
Extrahepatic
Stones
Biliary stricture
Malignancy (pancreatic, cholangiocarcinoma, ampullary carcinoma, lymphoma, duodenal carcinoma, metastases to portal lymph nodes)
Pancreatitis / pancreatic pseudocyst
Primary sclerosing cholangitis
Biliary malformation
AIDS cholangiopathy
INFILTRATIVE DISEASE (LIVER)
Granulomatous disease (tuberculosis, sarcoid, etc)
Amyloidosis
Leukemia
Lymphoma
MASS LESIONS (LIVER)
Malignancy (hepatoma, metastatic cancer)
Cyst
Abscess
PARENCHYMAL DISEASE (LIVER)
Viral hepatitis (acute or chronic)
Alcoholic liver disease
Hereditary liver disease (hemochromatosis, Wilson's disease, α_1-antitrypsin deficiency)
Cirrhosis
Congestive hepatopathy
Autoimmune hepatitis
Medication-induced
Ischemic hepatitis
Hepatic steatosis
BONE DISEASE
Fractures
Paget's disease
Rickets
Osteomalacia
Osteitis fibrosa cystica
Osteoblastic bone tumors (osteogenic sarcoma, metastatic tumors)
Bone growth (childhood and adolescence)

(continued)

CAUSES OF AN ELEVATED ALKALINE PHOSPHATASE *(continued)*
PREGNANCY
CHILDHOOD GROWTH
MISCELLANEOUS
Malignancy (renal cell carcinoma, lymphoma)
Hyperthyroidism
Acromegaly
Myelofibrosis
Mastocytosis
Hypervitaminosis D
Pulmonary infarct
Renal infarction
AIDS
C. difficile infection in AIDS patients

In most cases, differentiating among the above causes of an elevated alkaline phosphatase level is not difficult. The presence of other liver function test abnormalities suggests that the elevation is of hepatobiliary origin.

At times, however, an elevated alkaline phosphatase may occur in the setting of otherwise normal liver function tests. In these cases, it may be difficult to differentiate between hepatobiliary and bone disease as the etiology of the isolated elevation of the alkaline phosphatase. Measure of 5′ nucleotidase, which is specific for the hepatobiliary tree, is very helpful in discerning the source of an isolated elevation of alkaline phosphatase. If 5′ nucleotidase is not available, GGT (gamma-glutamyltranspeptidase) should be ordered. However, it is important to note that although GGT is very sensitive for biliary tract disease, it is not specific. Elevation of either the 5 nucleotidase or GGT indicates that the increased alkaline phosphatase level is at least, in part, caused by hepatobiliary disease. Normal levels, on the other hand, suggest that the origin of the alkaline phosphatase elevation is bone. The clinician should realize, however, that these enzymes do not always increase in parallel in patients with hepatobiliary disease. That is, some patients with an isolated elevation of the alkaline phosphatase due to hepatobiliary disease may present with normal 5 nucleotidase and GGT levels.

Degree of Alkaline Phosphatase Elevation

Although the degree of alkaline phosphatase elevation is not very reliable in differentiating among the causes of the elevation, markedly increased alkaline phosphatase levels should prompt the clinician to consider the following possibilities:

- Extrahepatic biliary obstruction
- Primary biliary cirrhosis
- Drug-induced cholestasis
- Primary sclerosing cholangitis
- Infiltrative processes

Of note, extrahepatic cholestasis cannot be differentiated from intrahepatic cholestasis based upon the degree of alkaline phosphatase elevation. Alkaline phosphatase levels >1000 units/L in the setting of a bilirubin level <1 mg/dL should prompt the clinician to consider granulomatous or infiltrative liver diseases.

Causes of a Low Alkaline Phosphatase

Causes of a low alkaline phosphatase level are listed in the following box.

CAUSES OF A LOW ALKALINE PHOSPHATASE	
WILSON'S DISEASE	MEDICATIONS
HYPOTHYROIDISM	Alendronate
PERNICIOUS ANEMIA	Clofibrate
ZINC DEFICIENCY	Estrogens in postmenopausal women
HYPOPHOSPHATASIA	Theophylline

BILIRUBIN

The evaluation of an elevated bilirubin level requires an understanding of bilirubin metabolism. Bilirubin is produced by the catabolism of senescent RBCs and other hemoproteins (ie, cytochrome P450).

Heme is initially converted to biliverdin by heme oxygenase. Biliverdin is then converted to bilirubin by biliverdin reductase. The resulting bilirubin is reversibly bound to albumin and transported into hepatocytes. Conjugation by the enzyme, UDP-glucuronyl transferase, is the next step. Conjugated bilirubin then undergoes canalicular secretion, which is the rate-limiting step. Conjugated bilirubin is then excreted from the biliary tree into the intestinal tract where it is reduced by bacteria to urobilinogen. Some of this urobilinogen is excreted in the feces, but a fair amount is reabsorbed. That which is reabsorbed is either excreted in urine (the urobilinogen that is reported in the urinalysis) or in bile (enterohepatic circulation).

Differentiating Conjugated From Unconjugated Hyperbilirubinemia

The evaluation of hyperbilirubinemia begins with the determination of whether the hyperbilirubinemia is conjugated or unconjugated. Patients with conjugated hyperbilirubinemia should be evaluated for hepatobiliary disease while patients with unconjugated hyperbilirubinemia do not always have hepatobiliary disease. There are several ways of making this distinction.

- Other liver function test abnormalities

  The causes of unconjugated hyperbilirubinemia are not typically associated with other liver function test abnormalities. In contrast, most cases of conjugated hyperbilirubinemia are accompanied by other liver function test abnormalities.

- Urine dipstick for bilirubin

  Of the two types of bilirubin, only conjugated bilirubin is water soluble. As a result, a positive urine dipstick for bilirubin signifies the presence of conjugated hyperbilirubinemia. When patients with hepatobiliary disease recover, urine bilirubin becomes negative well before normalization of the serum conjugated bilirubin level.

- Serum bilirubin fractionation

  A predominantly conjugated hyperbilirubinemia is said to exist when 30% or more of the serum bilirubin is in the conjugated form. In mild degrees of hyperbilirubinemia, the fractionation of the total serum bilirubin into direct (conjugated) and indirect (unconjugated) bilirubin levels is unreliable. In these cases, there may be an overestimation of the proportion of total bilirubin that is unconjugated. This is true when the standard diazo methods are used for bilirubin measurement. More precise techniques are now available and can be ordered in these types of cases.

Causes of Unconjugated Hyperbilirubinemia

Causes of unconjugated hyperbilirubinemia are listed in the following box.

UNCONJUGATED HYPERBILIRUBINEMIA DIFFERENTIAL DIAGNOSIS
HEMOLYSIS*
INEFFECTIVE ERYTHROPOIESIS†
RESORPTION OF LARGE HEMATOMA
DECREASE IN HEPATIC UPTAKE BY DRUGS (rifampin)
NEONATAL JAUNDICE
CRIGLER-NAJJAR SYNDROME‡
GILBERT'S SYNDROME§

*Chronic low level hemolysis rarely leads to bilirubin >5 mg/dL. Acute hemolysis or chronic hemolysis superimposed on underlying liver dysfunction can lead to more impressive elevations.

†A minor degree of ineffective erythropoiesis is present in normal bone marrow, but may be increased in conditions such as megaloblastic anemia, thalassemia, iron deficiency, sideroblastic anemia, and PCV.

‡There can be complete deficiency of UDP-glucuronyl transferase (type I) or partial deficiency (type 2).

§Gilbert's syndrome is characterized by unconjugated hyperbilirubinemia with bilirubin rarely >3 or 4 mg/dL. Investigators believe that the etiology may be multifactorial with increased hemolysis, decreased uptake, and decreased conjugation all playing a role. The syndrome typically presents with unconjugated hyperbilirubinemia in the absence of other liver function test abnormalities. It is typically precipitated by fasting, illness, stress, exercise, or lack of sleep. Gilbert's syndrome affects 7% of the population, but is clinically significant because it is often misdiagnosed as chronic hepatitis. However, as it is benign, recognition can obviate an expensive workup and alleviate the patient's concern.

Causes of Conjugated Hyperbilirubinemia

The causes of conjugated hyperbilirubinemia are listed in the following box.

CAUSES OF CONJUGATED HYPERBILIRUBINEMIA

HEPATOCELLULAR DISEASE

- Alcoholic hepatitis
- α_1-antitrypsin deficiency
- Autoimmune hepatitis
- Cirrhosis
- Drug-induced
- Dubin-Johnson syndrome
- Hemochromatosis
- Hepatotoxins
- Hepatic vein thrombosis
- Ischemia
- Rotor's syndrome
- Viral hepatitis
- Wilson's disease

CHOLESTASIS

- Extrahepatic
  - AIDS cholangiopathy
  - Biliary malformation
  - Choledocholithiasis
  - Malignancy
    - Ampullary
    - Cholangiocarcinoma
    - Duodenal
    - Lymphoma
    - Metastases to portal lymph nodes
    - Pancreatic
  - Pancreatic pseudocyst
  - Pancreatitis
  - Primary sclerosing cholangitis
- Intrahepatic
  - Alcoholic hepatitis
  - Benign recurrent intrahepatic cholestasis
  - Cholestasis of pregnancy
  - Drug-induced
  - Postoperative hyperbilirubinemia
  - Primary biliary cirrhosis
  - Systemic infection
  - Total parenteral nutrition
  - Viral hepatitis

Degree of Hyperbilirubinemia

Total serum bilirubin levels are usually not helpful in differentiating among the causes of conjugated hyperbilirubinemia because values overlap considerably. Bilirubin levels >15 mg/dL are rare in patients with common bile duct obstruction secondary to gallstones. As a general rule, extrahepatic cholestasis alone is unlikely in patients who have bilirubin levels >25-30 mg/dL. This degree of hyperbilirubinemia usually signifies hemolysis or renal insufficiency superimposed on hepatobiliary disease.

In some types of hepatobiliary disease, the degree of hyperbilirubinemia has been found to have prognostic significance. For example, mean survival is only 1.4 years in patients with primary biliary cirrhosis when bilirubin levels exceed 10 mg/dL. Bilirubin levels also provide prognostic information in patients with fulminant hepatic failure, primary biliary cirrhosis, and acute alcoholic hepatitis.

5′ NUCLEOTIDASE

An isolated increase in alkaline phosphatase is the only indication for the measurement of a 5′ nucleotidase. In these patients, an elevated 5′ nucleotidase supports a hepatobiliary origin of the increased alkaline phosphatase. 5′ nucleotidase has a higher predictive value than GGT and alkaline phosphatase in the detection of hepatobiliary disease. It also has a lower false positivity than GGT and alkaline phosphatase in the diagnosis of hepatobiliary disease. Alkaline phosphatase and 5′ nucleotidase usually increase and decrease in parallel in hepatobiliary disorders.

5′ nucleotidase is particularly helpful in detecting liver disease during childhood, adolescence, and pregnancy. These are times when alkaline phosphatase is physiologically elevated. When it is not clear whether an alkaline phosphatase elevation is physiologic, the clinician may wish to measure a 5′ nucleotidase level. An increased 5′ nucleotidase level should prompt the clinician to consider liver disease as the etiology of the alkaline phosphatase and 5′ nucleotidase elevations.

GAMMA GLUTAMYL TRANSFERASE (GGT)

Sensitivity of GGT in Detection of Liver Disease

GGT is found to be elevated in 80% to 95% of patients with acute hepatitis, irrespective of the cause. GGT levels increase in almost all types of liver disease; therefore, its use in differentiating among different types of liver disease is limited.

GGT does have a role in the patient presenting with an isolated elevation of the alkaline phosphatase. In these cases, it can be particularly difficult to differentiate between hepatobiliary and bone causes of an isolated alkaline phosphatase elevation. To make this distinction, a GGT level may be obtained. An elevated GGT level supports hepatobiliary disease as the etiology of the elevated alkaline phosphatase. A normal GGT level strongly argues against the presence of hepatobiliary disease.

Specificity of GGT in Detection of Liver Disease

GGT is present in many different tissues, as shown in the following box.

TISSUES WITH HIGH GGT CONTENT (in decreasing order of abundance)	
1. PROXIMAL RENAL TUBULE	3. PANCREAS
2. LIVER	4. INTESTINE

GGT is not specific for liver disease because an elevated GGT may reflect disease in other organs including the kidney, pancreas, and intestines. There are other factors that may affect GGT levels, as shown in the following table.

Factors Affecting GGT Level (nondisease factors)

Factor	Change	Comments
Race	Approximately double in African Americans	Similar differences in adult males, females
Body mass index (BMI)	25% higher with mild increase in BMI; 50% higher with BMI >30	Effect similar in adult males, females
Food ingestion	Decreases after meals; increases with increasing time after food ingestion	
Drugs*	Increased by carbamazepine, cimetidine, furosemide, heparin, isotretinoin, methotrexate, oral contraceptives, phenobarbital, phenytoin, valproic acid	Values up to 2 times reference limits are common, may be up to 5 times reference limits, especially with phenytoin
Smoking	10% higher with 1 pack/day; approximately double with heavier smoking	
Alcohol consumption†	Direct relationship between alcohol intake and GGT	May remain increased for weeks after cessation of chronic alcohol intake
Pregnancy	25% lower during early pregnancy	

*Because these medications induce GGT, GGT levels may not be helpful in assessing for hepatobiliary disease in patients taking these medications.

†GGT levels increase in the alcoholic patient because alcohol induces the enzyme. This can even occur in the absence of alcoholic liver disease. With cessation of alcohol use, GGT levels typically return to normal within 3-5 weeks. When GGT levels fail to return to normal, the clinician should suspect continued alcohol intake, the presence of liver damage, or another etiology.

Adapted from Dufour DR, Lott JA, Nolte FS, et al, "Diagnosis and Monitoring of Hepatic Injury, I. Performance Characteristics of Laboratory Tests," *Clin Chem*, 2000, 46(12):2034.

An isolated elevation of the GGT (other liver function tests are normal) requires no further evaluation, especially if the patient has no other evidence of liver disease.

AMMONIA

The final product of amino acid and nucleic acid metabolism is ammonia. The liver is the only organ that detoxifies ammonia by converting it into urea.

Sensitivity of Ammonia Level in the Detection of Hepatic Encephalopathy

The role of ammonia in the development of hepatic encephalopathy is unclear. Nonetheless, ammonia levels have been used to provide support for the diagnosis of hepatic encephalopathy. It is important to realize, however, that ammonia levels are not routinely recommended for the diagnosis of hepatic encephalopathy in patients with acute or chronic liver disease. This is because some patients with hepatic encephalopathy have normal ammonia levels. It must be emphasized that a normal ammonia level does not exclude the diagnosis of hepatic encephalopathy. It is a clinical diagnosis that is based upon the presence of neurological signs and symptoms consistent with hepatic encephalopathy in the setting of liver disease.

Specificity of Ammonia Level in the Detection of Hepatic Encephalopathy

The presence of an elevated ammonia level does not establish the diagnosis of hepatic encephalopathy. There are many other causes of an elevated ammonia level, as shown in the following box.

CAUSES OF ELEVATED AMMONIA LEVELS	
HEPATOCELLULAR DYSFUNCTION	BLOOD TRANSFUSION
EXCESSIVE BLEEDING (GI)	BONE MARROW TRANSPLANTATION
EXCESSIVE DIETARY PROTEIN	MEDICATIONS (valproic acid, glycine)
CONSTIPATION	NEUROGENIC BLADDER INFECTION
RENAL INSUFFICIENCY	HEMODIALYSIS
ALKALOSIS	URETEROSIGMOIDOSTOMY
PORTOSYSTEMIC VENOUS SHUNT	ASPARAGINASE THERAPY
HYPOKALEMIA	
ACUTE LEUKEMIA	

Other factors that affect ammonia levels are listed in the following table.

Factors Affecting Ammonia Level (nondisease factors)

Factor	Change	Comments
Specimen source	Arterial higher than venous	Arterial ammonia levels correlate better with change in liver function than venous ammonia levels; tourniquet use, clenching fist increase venous ammonia levels
Exercise	Increases up to threefold after exercise	Increase greater in males than in females
Smoking	Increases 10 µmol/L after 1 cigarette	
Delay in analysis	Ammonia levels increase because of metabolism by red blood cells: 20% in 1 hour and 100% by 2 hours	Use of ice water, rapid centrifugation, and separation of plasma minimize increase; rate of increase higher in liver disease

Adapted from Dufour DR, Lott JA, Nolte FS, et al, "Diagnosis and Monitoring of Hepatic Injury, I. Performance Characteristics of Laboratory Tests," *Clin Chem*, 2000, 46(12):2038.

In patients treated for hepatic encephalopathy, monitoring of ammonia levels is not recommended to assess response to therapy. Instead, the clinician should rely on the clinical evaluation to gauge the effectiveness of therapy.

ALPHA FETOPROTEIN (AFP)

The function of alpha fetoprotein is not clear. It is elevated in >90% of patients with hepatocellular cancer (50% to 80% have elevated AFP levels at the time of presentation), but it is not specific. It may also be elevated in other conditions including acute liver disease, chronic liver disease, cirrhosis, and hepatic metastasis.

However, these other conditions are usually characterized by mild increases in the AFP level. In contrast, there is a strong correlation between the presence of hepatocellular cancer and AFP levels >500 ng/mL, particularly in the presence of a liver mass. Unfortunately, at these levels, the tumor is usually not resectable.

In the patient with cirrhosis, serial measurements of the AFP level are useful. An increase should prompt the clinician to consider the possibility of hepatocellular cancer. AFP levels are also useful in monitoring response to treatment. With successful treatment of hepatocellular cancer, the levels will fall.

LACTATE DEHYDROGENASE (LDH)

Measurement of LDH is not routinely recommended in patients with liver disease. It typically provides no additional information than that already obtained from measurement of AST, ALT, albumin, bilirubin, and alkaline phosphatase levels. There are, however, several situations in which a LDH level may be helpful.

LDH levels may rise in acute viral hepatitis and ischemic hepatitis. In ischemic hepatitis, there may be an impressive elevation in the LDH level. This degree of LDH elevation is not seen in patients with acute viral hepatitis; when there is difficulty differentiating acute viral hepatitis from ischemic hepatitis, measurement of the LDH level may provide a clue to the diagnosis. Prolonged LDH elevation along with an increased alkaline phosphatase level may be seen in malignancy infiltrating the liver.

The ALT to LDH ratio may be useful in differentiating acute viral hepatitis (ratio >1.5) from shock liver and acetaminophen toxicity (ratio <1.5). The sensitivity and specificity of this ratio is 94% and 84%, respectively.

CHILD-TURCOTTE CLASSIFICATION

This is a useful classification that provides information about liver function and prognosis. A patient's particular Child's class can be calculated by considering the following.

Child-Turcotte Classification of Prognostic Factors in Liver Disease

	0 Points	1 Point	2 Points
Albumin (g/dL)	>3.5	2.8-3.5	<2.8
Bilirubin (mg/dL)	<2	2-3	>3
Prolongation of the PT (sec)	<4	4-6	>6
Ascites	None	Controlled	Refractory
Encephalopathy	None	Controlled	Refractory

The patient's class is calculated by totalling the points for each of the 5 categories:

- Class A: 0-1 point
- Class B: 2-4 points
- Class C: ≥5 points

Patients who are Class A have a good prognosis; in contrast, the prognosis for Class C is much more guarded. Patients who fall into Class B or C should be considered for liver transplantation because their life expectancy is limited.

References

Aranda-Michel J and Sherman KE, "Tests of the Liver: Use and Misuse," *Gastroenterologist*, 1998, 6(1):34-43.

Beckingham IJ and Ryder SD, "ABC of Diseases of Liver, Pancreas, and Biliary System. Investigation of Liver and Biliary Disease," *BMJ*, 2001, 322(7277):33-6.

Burke MD, "Liver Function: Test Selection and Interpretation of Results," *Clin Lab Med*, 2002, 22(2):377-90.

Dufour DR, Lott JA, Nolte FS, et al, "Diagnosis and Monitoring of Hepatic Injury. I. Performance Characteristics of Laboratory Tests," *Clin Chem*, 2000, 46(12):2027-49.

Dufour DR, Lott JA, Nolte FS, et al, "Diagnosis and Monitoring of Hepatic Injury. II. Recommendations for Use of Laboratory Tests in Screening, Diagnosis, and Monitoring," *Clin Chem*, 2000, 46(12):2050-68.

Gopal DV and Rosen HR, "Abnormal Findings on Liver Function Tests. Interpreting Results to Narrow the Diagnosis and Establish a Prognosis," *Postgrad Med*, 2000, 107(2):100-2, 105-9, 113-4.

Green RM and Flamm S, "AGA Technical Review on the Evaluation of Liver Chemistry Tests," *Gastroenterology*, 2002, 123(4):1367-84.

Johnston DE, "Special Considerations in Interpreting Liver Function Tests," *Am Fam Physician*, 1999, 15;59(8):2223-30.

Limdi JK and Hyde GM, "Evaluation of Abnormal Liver Function Tests," *Post Grad Med J*, 2003, 79(932):307-12.

Pratt DS and Kaplan MM "Evaluation of Abnormal Liver-Enzyme Results in Asymptomatic Patients," *N Engl J Med*, 2000, 342(17):1266-71.

APPROACH TO THE ASYMPTOMATIC PATIENT WITH MILD TRANSAMINASE ELEVATION

It is not uncommon to encounter an asymptomatic patient with mild AST and/or ALT elevation (<5 times the upper limit of normal). The first step in the evaluation of such a patient is to repeat the tests. Up to 50% of patients with an asymptomatic elevation of the AST and/or ALT will have normal values on repeat testing. In most of these cases, no further evaluation is warranted. The clinician should be aware of the fact that certain diseases of the liver are characterized by fluctuations in the transaminase levels (ie, chronic hepatitis C). In these cases, the clinician may be falsely reassured when repeat testing reveals normal transaminase levels. Studies have shown that 33% of patients with chronic hepatitis C (confirmed by liver biopsy) have persistently normal ALT levels. Therefore, if chronic hepatitis C is a concern, particularly in patients with risk factors for hepatitis C infection, further testing for hepatitis C is recommended even if repeat transaminase levels are normal.

If repeat testing confirms the elevation of the AST and/or ALT, further evaluation is warranted.

Since ALT is more specific for liver disease than AST, an elevated AST should always prompt the clinician to obtain an ALT level. A normal ALT level in the setting of an increased AST level should raise concern for nonhepatic disease. Even in patients who have elevations in both AST and ALT, nonhepatic disease remains a consideration.

These enzymes are found in many organs and may be released into the circulation when disease affects these organs. Levels approaching 2-3 times the upper limit of normal may be appreciated following strenuous physical exertion or after muscle injury, as in polymyositis and hypothyroidism. If there is any uncertainty as to the origin of the AST and ALT elevation, a CK level should be obtained to exclude muscle disease as the cause of the transaminase elevation.

If the clinician is certain that the origin of the transaminase elevation is the liver, then the next step involves consideration of the hepatic causes of mild transaminase elevation. These causes are listed in the following box.

HEPATIC CAUSES OF MILD TRANSAMINASE ELEVATION IN THE ASYMPTOMATIC PATIENT	
ALCOHOLIC LIVER DISEASE	HEMOCHROMATOSIS
CHRONIC HEPATITIS B	WILSON'S DISEASE
CHRONIC HEPATITIS C	$ALPHA_1$-ANTITRYPSIN DEFICIENCY
AUTOIMMUNE HEPATITIS	DRUG-INDUCED LIVER DISEASE
FATTY LIVER (hepatic steatosis)	CONGESTIVE HEPATOPATHY
NONALCOHOLIC STEATOHEPATITIS	ACUTE VIRAL HEPATITIS (A-E, EBV, CMV)
CIRRHOSIS	CELIAC DISEASE

APPROACH TO THE ASYMPTOMATIC PATIENT WITH MILD TRANSAMINASE ELEVATION

The history can provide clues to the etiology of the transaminase elevation, as shown in the following table.

Historical Clue	Condition Suggested
Heavy alcohol use	Alcoholic liver disease
Intravenous drug abuse Hemodialysis patients Sharing razor blades / toothbrushes Tattooing Body piercing Acupuncture Healthcare worker History of blood transfusion High-risk sexual activity	Chronic hepatitis B (risk factors) Chronic hepatitis C (risk factors)
Family history of liver disease	Wilson's disease Hemochromatosis Alpha$_1$-antitrypsin deficiency Autoimmune hepatitis
Medication history	Transaminase elevation following the start of a new medication suggests drug-induced liver disease
Onset of transaminase elevation after age 40	Argues against Wilson's disease
History of congestive heart failure	Congestive hepatopathy Hemochromatosis
History of diabetes mellitus	Hemochromatosis
Impotence	Hemochromatosis
History of arthritis	Hemochromatosis
Difficulty speaking (dysarthria) Tremor Writing difficulty Ataxia	Wilson's disease
Northern European ancestry	Hemochromatosis
History of COPD	Alpha$_1$-antitrypsin deficiency
History of other autoimmune disorders (thyroid disease, Sjögren's syndrome, ulcerative colitis, etc)	Autoimmune hepatitis

Physical examination findings that point to the etiology of the transaminase elevation are listed in the following table.

Physical Examination Finding	Condition Suggested
Hyperpigmentation	Hemochromatosis
Kayser-Fleischer rings on slit lamp examination	Wilson's disease
Hypertrophy of 2nd and 3rd metacarpophalangeal joints	Hemochromatosis
Spider angiomas Palmar erythema Gynecomastia Testicular atrophy Parotid gland enlargement	Stigmata of chronic liver disease

If clues are elicited during a thorough history and physical exam, appropriate laboratory testing should be pursued according to the condition suggested. If no clues are present in the history and physical examination, the following laboratory tests or interventions should be performed:

- Anti-HCV to assess for acute/chronic hepatitis C
- HB_sAg / HB_sAb / HB_cAb to assess for chronic hepatitis B
- IgM anti-HAV to assess for acute/chronic hepatitis A
- Serum iron, total iron binding capacity (TIBC), and ferritin to assess for hemochromatosis
- Ceruloplasmin (only if age <40 years) to assess for Wilson's disease
- Serum protein electrophoresis, antinuclear antibodies, and antismooth muscle antibodies to assess for autoimmune hepatitis
- Ultrasound of liver to assess for increased hepatic echogenicity suggestive of fatty infiltration
- Discontinuation of suspected drug(s) if drug-induced liver disease a possibility (since many patients, who take over-the-counter and herbal medications, do not think of them as medications, it is important to specifically ask about their use).

MEDICATIONS, HERBS, AND TOXINS THAT CAN CAUSE ELEVATIONS OF AMINOTRANSFERASES

MEDICATIONS AND DRUGS	*HERBS / ALTERNATIVE MEDICATIONS*
Acetaminophen	Chaparral leaf
Alpha-methyldopa	Ephedra
Amoxicillin-clavulanic acid	Gentian
Amiodarone	Germander
Carbamazepine	Jin Bu Huan
Dantrolene	Senna
Disulfiram	Kava kava
Etretinate	Scutellaria (skullcap)
Fluconazole	Shark cartilage
Glyburide	Vitamin A
Halothane	
Heparin	***ILLICIT DRUGS***
HMG-Co reductase inhibitors	Anabolic steroids
Isoniazid	Cocaine
Ketoconazole	Ecstasy (MDMA)
Labetalol	Phencyclidine (PCP)
Nicotinic acid	
Nitrofurantoin	***TOXINS***
NSAIDs	Carbon tetrachloride
Phenylbutazone	Chloroform
Phenytoin	Dimethylformamide
Propylthiouracil	Hydrazine
Protease inhibitors	Hydrochlorofluorocarbons
Sulfonamides	2-nitropropane
Trazodone	Trichloroethylene
Troglitazone	Toluene
Valproic acid	
Zafirlukast	

From Green RM and Flamm S, "AGA Technical Review on the Evaluation of Liver Chemistry Tests," *Gastroenterology*, 2002, 123(4):1367-84.

- Abstinence from alcohol
- Efforts to lose weight if clinical evaluation or imaging studies suggest that the patient may have fatty liver or nonalcoholic steatohepatitis

Abnormalities of any of the above laboratory tests should prompt the clinician to pursue further evaluation of the condition suggested by the abnormal lab tests. If the results of the above laboratory tests are normal, then the following tests should be obtained:

- Hepatitis C viral RNA
- Alpha$_1$-antitrypsin phenotyping
- Antigliadin, antitransglutaminase, and antiendomysial antibodies to assess for celiac sprue
- CK / aldolase to exclude muscle disease as the cause (if not already obtained)

When all laboratory testing is uneventful in the asymptomatic patient with mild transaminase elevation, the clinician should consider percutaneous liver biopsy, especially if the lab test abnormalities persist.

References

Aranda-Michel J and Sherman KE, "Tests of the Liver: Use and Misuse," *Gastroenterologist*, 1998, 6(1):34-43.

Beckingham IJ and Ryder SD, "ABC of Diseases of Liver, Pancreas, and Biliary System. Investigation of Liver and Biliary Disease," *BMJ*, 2001, 322(7277):33-6.

Burke MD, "Liver Function: Test Selection and Interpretation of Results," *Clin Lab Med*, 2002, 22(2):377-90.

Dufour DR, Lott JA, Nolte FS, et al, "Diagnosis and Monitoring of Hepatic Injury. I. Performance Characteristics of Laboratory Tests," *Clin Chem*, 2000, 46(12):2027-49.

Dufour DR, Lott JA, Nolte FS, et al, "Diagnosis and Monitoring of Hepatic Injury. II. Recommendations for Use of Laboratory Tests in Screening, Diagnosis, and Monitoring," *Clin Chem*, 2000, 46(12):2050-68.

Gopal DV and Rosen HR, "Abnormal Findings on Liver Function Tests. Interpreting Results to Narrow the Diagnosis and Establish a Prognosis," *Postgrad Med*, 2000, 107(2):100-2, 105-9, 113-4.

Green RM and Flamm S, "AGA Technical Review on the Evaluation of Liver Chemistry Tests," *Gastroenterology*, 2002, 123(4):1367-84.

Johnston DE, "Special Considerations in Interpreting Liver Function Tests," *Am Fam Physician*, 1999, 15;59(8):2223-30.

Limdi JK and Hyde GM, "Evaluation of Abnormal Liver Function Tests," *Post Grad Med J*, 2003, 79(932):307-12.

Pratt DS and Kaplan MM "Evaluation of Abnormal Liver-Enzyme Results in Asymptomatic Patients," *N Engl J Med*, 2000, 342(17):1266-71.

APPROACH TO THE ASYMPTOMATIC PATIENT WITH MILDLY ELEVATED TRANSAMINASE LEVELS

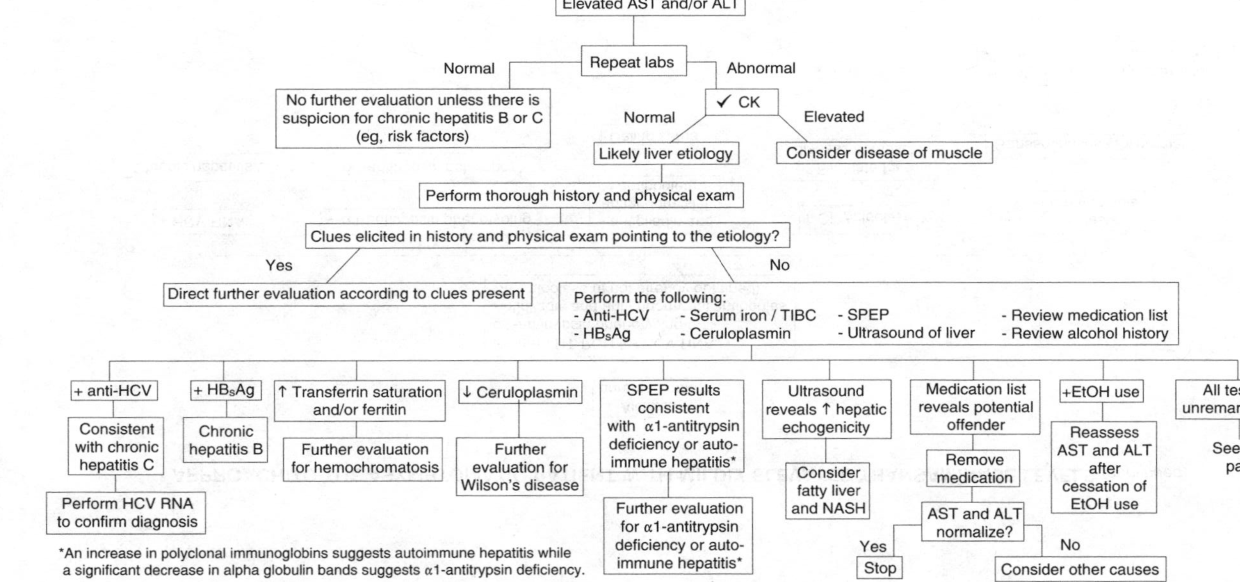
Elevated AST and/or ALT
Repeat labs
Normal
No further evaluation unless there is suspicion for chronic hepatitis B or C (eg, risk factors)
Abnormal
✓ CK
Normal
Elevated
Likely liver etiology
Consider disease of muscle
Perform thorough history and physical exam
Clues elicited in history and physical exam pointing to the etiology?
Yes
Direct further evaluation according to clues present
No
Perform the following:
- Anti-HCV
- HBsAg
- Serum iron / TIBC
- Ceruloplasmin
- SPEP
- Ultrasound of liver
- Review medication list
- Review alcohol history
+ anti-HCV
Consistent with chronic hepatitis C
Perform HCV RNA to confirm diagnosis
+ HBsAg
Chronic hepatitis B
↑ Transferrin saturation and/or ferritin
Further evaluation for hemochromatosis
↓ Ceruloplasmin
Further evaluation for Wilson's disease
SPEP results consistent with α1-antitrypsin deficiency or auto-immune hepatitis*
Further evaluation for α1-antitrypsin deficiency or auto-immune hepatitis*
Ultrasound reveals ↑ hepatic echogenicity
Consider fatty liver and NASH
Medication list reveals potential offender
Remove medication
AST and ALT normalize?
Yes
Stop
No
Consider other causes
+EtOH use
Reassess AST and ALT after cessation of EtOH use
All tests unremarkable
See next page
*An increase in polyclonal immunoglobins suggests autoimmune hepatitis while a significant decrease in alpha globulin bands suggests α1-antitrypsin deficiency.

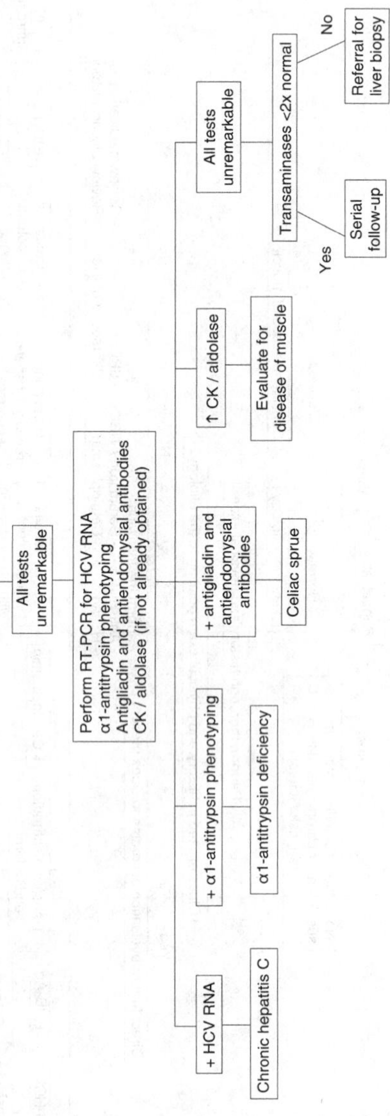
APPROACH TO THE ASYMPTOMATIC PATIENT WITH MILDLY ELEVATED TRANSAMINASE LEVELS (continued)
All tests unremarkable
Perform RT-PCR for HCV RNA
α1-antitrypsin phenotyping
Antigliadin and antiendomysial antibodies
CK / aldolase (if not already obtained)
+ HCV RNA
Chronic hepatitis C
+ α1-antitrypsin phenotyping
α1-antitrypsin deficiency
+ antigliadin and antiendomysial antibodies
Celiac sprue
↑ CK / aldolase
Evaluate for disease of muscle
All tests unremarkable
Transaminases <2x normal
Yes
Serial follow-up
No
Referral for liver biopsy

APPROACH TO THE PATIENT WITH AN ALKALINE PHOSPHATASE ELEVATION OUT OF PROPORTION TO THE TRANSAMINASE ELEVATION

Not uncommonly, patients are encountered who have elevations in both the transaminases and alkaline phosphatase. When the alkaline phosphatase level is much more elevated (>4x normal) than the transaminases (<300 units/L), the clinician should consider the presence of a cholestatic disorder. On the other hand, a disproportionate elevation in the transaminase levels should prompt the clinician to consider disorders characterized by hepatocellular injury. In this section, we will discuss the approach to the patient presenting with a disproportionate increase in the alkaline phosphatase level. As such, hepatocellular disorders will not be discussed here.

Cholestasis may be defined as an impairment in or lack of bile flow. Cholestasis may be divided into intrahepatic and extrahepatic forms. Extrahepatic cholestasis may be defined as the blockage of bile flow at the level of the larger bile ducts while intrahepatic cholestasis refers to a functional impairment of bile formation/flow at the level of the hepatocyte. As mentioned above, when the alkaline phosphatase level is much more elevated than the transaminases, cholestasis is the major consideration.

To differentiate between extrahepatic and intrahepatic causes of cholestasis, radiologic imaging is required. Either CT or US can be obtained. The finding of dilated bile ducts establishes the presence of a condition causing extrahepatic cholestasis. The causes of extrahepatic cholestasis are listed in the following box.

CAUSES OF EXTRAHEPATIC CHOLESTASIS
CHOLEDOCHOLITHIASIS
BILIARY STRICTURE
MALIGNANCY
Cholangiocarcinoma
Pancreatic carcinoma
Ampullary carcinoma
Duodenal carcinoma
Lymphoma
Metastases to portal lymph nodes
PANCREATITIS
PANCREATIC PSEUDOCYST
BILIARY MALFORMATION
PRIMARY SCLEROSING CHOLANGITIS
AIDS CHOLANGIOPATHY

When biliary dilatation is detected, the diagnosis of extrahepatic cholestasis is likely. In these cases, the clinician should pursue further evaluation to identify the cause of the extrahepatic cholestasis. Most often, the evaluation includes ERCP or PTC. The clinician should realize that the absence of biliary dilatation does not exclude the diagnosis of extrahepatic cholestasis. In early obstruction, enough time may not pass for the biliary ducts to dilate. As a result, even if radiologic findings are normal, further evaluation with ERCP or PTC (percutaneous transhepatic cholangiography) may be required if the clinician strongly suspects a condition causing extrahepatic cholestasis.

If no biliary dilatation is noted and suspicion for extrahepatic cholestasis is low, then intrahepatic cholestasis is likely. The causes of intrahepatic cholestasis are listed in the following box.

CAUSES OF INTRAHEPATIC CHOLESTASIS
ALCOHOLIC HEPATITIS
BENIGN RECURRENT INTRAHEPATIC CHOLESTASIS
DRUG-INDUCED CHOLESTASIS
INTRAHEPATIC CHOLESTASIS OF PREGNANCY
POSTOPERATIVE CHOLESTASIS
PRIMARY BILIARY CIRRHOSIS
SYSTEMIC INFECTION
TOTAL PARENTERAL NUTRITION
VIRAL HEPATITIS

Adapted from Desai SP, *Clinician's Guide to Diagnosis*, Hudson, OH: Lexi-Comp, Inc, 2001, 350.

A thorough history and physical examination will often provide clues to the cause of the intrahepatic cholestasis. When clues are present, appropriate testing should be obtained to confirm the diagnosis. This testing may include viral serology to exclude viral hepatitis as well as serology for antimitochondrial antibodies to assess for primary biliary cirrhosis. The detection of antimitochondrial antibodies supports the diagnosis of primary biliary cirrhosis; confirmation of the diagnosis requires liver biopsy.

If drug-induced cholestasis is a possibility, the suspect medication should be discontinued. Medications that can cause this type of liver function test pattern are listed in the following box.

MEDICATIONS THAT CAN CAUSE ELEVATION OF THE ALKALINE PHOSPHATASE	
Anabolic steroids	Gold salts
Allopurinol	Imipramine
Amoxicillin-clavulanic acid	Indinavir
Captopril	Iprindole
Carbamazepine	Nevirapine
Chlorpropamide	Methyltestosterone
Cyproheptadine	Oxaprozin
Diltiazem	Pizotyline
Erythromycin	Quinidine
Estrogens	Tolbutamide
Floxuridine	Total parenteral hyperalimentation
Flucloxacillin	Trimethoprim-sulfamethoxazole
Fluphenazine	

From Green RM and Flamm S, "AGA Technical Review on the Evaluation of Liver Chemistry Tests," *Gastroenterology*, 2002, 123(4):1367-84.

Normalization of the liver function tests after discontinuation of the suspect medication supports the diagnosis. The clinician should realize, however, that resolution of the liver function test abnormalities may take weeks to months after discontinuation of the offending medication.

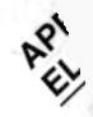

When the cause of the disproportionately elevated alk remains unexplained after consideration of the above caus should consider performing liver biopsy to establish the diagnos

References

Aranda-Michel J and Sherman KE, "Tests of the Liver: Use and Misuse," *Gastroenterologist*, 1998, 6(1):34-43.

Beckingham IJ and Ryder SD, "ABC of Diseases of Liver, Pancreas, and Biliary System. Investigation of Liver and Biliary Disease," *BMJ*, 2001, 322(7277):33-6.

Burke MD, "Liver Function: Test Selection and Interpretation of Results," *Clin Lab Med*, 2002, 22(2):377-90.

Dufour DR, Lott JA, Nolte FS, et al, "Diagnosis and Monitoring of Hepatic Injury. I. Performance Characteristics of Laboratory Tests," *Clin Chem*, 2000, 46(12):2027-49.

Dufour DR, Lott JA, Nolte FS, et al, "Diagnosis and Monitoring of Hepatic Injury. II. Recommendations for Use of Laboratory Tests in Screening, Diagnosis, and Monitoring," *Clin Chem*, 2000, 46(12):2050-68.

Gopal DV and Rosen HR, "Abnormal Findings on Liver Function Tests. Interpreting Results to Narrow the Diagnosis and Establish a Prognosis," *Postgrad Med*, 2000, 107(2):100-2, 105-9, 113-4.

Green RM and Flamm S, "AGA Technical Review on the Evaluation of Liver Chemistry Tests," *Gastroenterology*, 2002, 123(4):1367-84.

Johnston DE, "Special Considerations in Interpreting Liver Function Tests," *Am Fam Physician*, 1999, 15;59(8):2223-30.

Limdi JK and Hyde GM, "Evaluation of Abnormal Liver Function Tests," *Post Grad Med J*, 2003, 79(932):307-12.

Pratt DS and Kaplan MM "Evaluation of Abnormal Liver-Enzyme Results in Asymptomatic Patients," *N Engl J Med*, 2000, 342(17):1266-71.

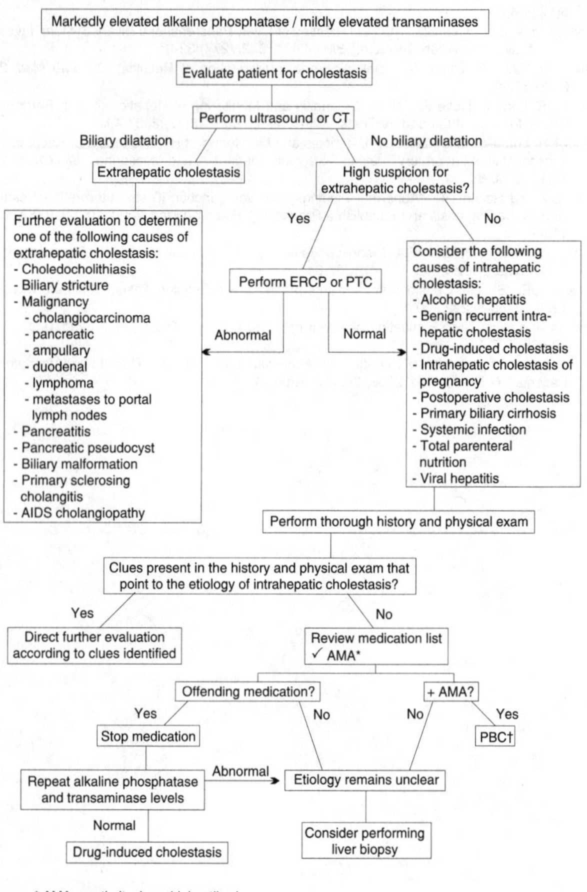
APPROACH TO THE PATIENT WITH AN ALKALINE PHOSPHATASE ELEVATION OUT OF PROPORTION TO THE TRANSAMINASE ELEVATION
Markedly elevated alkaline phosphatase / mildly elevated transaminases
Evaluate patient for cholestasis
Perform ultrasound or CT
Biliary dilatation
No biliary dilatation
Extrahepatic cholestasis
High suspicion for extrahepatic cholestasis?
Further evaluation to determine one of the following causes of extrahepatic cholestasis:
- Choledocholithiasis
- Biliary stricture
- Malignancy
- cholangiocarcinoma
- pancreatic
- ampullary
- duodenal
- lymphoma
- metastases to portal lymph nodes
- Pancreatitis
- Pancreatic pseudocyst
- Biliary malformation
- Primary sclerosing cholangitis
- AIDS cholangiopathy
Yes
No
Perform ERCP or PTC
Abnormal
Normal
Consider the following causes of intrahepatic cholestasis:
- Alcoholic hepatitis
- Benign recurrent intra-hepatic cholestasis
- Drug-induced cholestasis
- Intrahepatic cholestasis of pregnancy
- Postoperative cholestasis
- Primary biliary cirrhosis
- Systemic infection
- Total parenteral nutrition
- Viral hepatitis
Perform thorough history and physical exam
Clues present in the history and physical exam that point to the etiology of intrahepatic cholestasis?
Yes
No
Direct further evaluation according to clues identified
Review medication list
✓ AMA*
Offending medication?
+ AMA?
Yes
No
No
Yes
Stop medication
PBC†
Repeat alkaline phosphatase and transaminase levels
Abnormal
Etiology remains unclear
Normal
Drug-induced cholestasis
Consider performing liver biopsy
* AMA = antimitochrondrial antibody
† PBC = primary biliary cirrhosis

APPROACH TO THE PATIENT WITH ISOLATED ELEVATION OF ALKALINE PHOSPHATASE

The evaluation of the patient presenting with an isolated elevation of the alkaline phosphatase (other liver function tests normal) begins with a repeat test to confirm the elevation, particularly when the elevation is mild to moderate in degree. The clinician should ensure that the repeat test is done in a fasting state since the alkaline phosphatase level can increase after a meal, depending upon the patient's blood type. If the repeat fasting value remains elevated, further evaluation is necessary.

The clinician should realize that a physiologic increase in alkaline phosphatase does occur in pregnancy. In fact, alkaline phosphatase levels may increase up to two- to threefold in the third trimester of pregnancy due to the placental secretion of the enzyme. Physiologic increases in the alkaline phosphatase level may be also be appreciated in childhood and adolescence (up to two to three times the upper limit of normal). In these groups of patients (children, adolescents, pregnant women), separate reference intervals should be used for the interpretation of alkaline phosphatase levels.

If the alkaline phosphatase elevation is not physiologic, the next step involves the determination of the origin of the enzyme elevation. In usual clinical practice, a pathologic elevation of the alkaline phosphatase reflects either hepatobiliary or bone disease. To determine whether the alkaline phosphatase elevation is of hepatobiliary or bone origin, the clinician can obtain one of the following tests.

- High resolution electrophoresis and isoelectric focusing (most useful technique)

  Although the most sensitive and specific test, electrophoresis is not widely available. As a result, measurement of the 5′ nucleotidase or GGT level is much more commonly used to differentiate between hepatobiliary and bone causes of an isolated alkaline phosphatase elevation. Previously, heat and urea denaturation testing was performed to make this distinction; these techniques are not sufficiently sensitive and should no longer be used.

- 5′ nucleotidase or GGT

  It is not necessary to obtain both 5′ nucleotidase and GGT; measurement of one will suffice. An elevation of either the 5′ nucleotidase or GGT supports a hepatobiliary origin of the alkaline phosphatase elevation. Bone diseases presenting with an elevated alkaline phosphatase are not associated with increases in either of these enzymes. The clinician should realize, however, that an elevated GGT or 5′ nucleotidase does not exclude a coexisting bone disease (for example, malignancy with metastases to both liver and bone).

If the alkaline phosphatase elevation is found to be of bone origin, a thorough history and physical exam will usually provide clues as to the type of bone disease present. Bone diseases presenting with an isolated elevation of the alkaline phosphatase level will not be discussed further in the reminder of this section.

If the alkaline phosphatase elevation is found to be of hepatobiliary origin, the clinician should obtain a CT or ultrasound. CT or ultrasound may identify one or more of the following.

- Biliary dilatation

  The presence of biliary dilatation is consistent with extrahepatic cholestasis. Causes of extrahepatic cholestasis are listed in the following box.

CAUSES OF EXTRAHEPATIC CHOLESTASIS
CHOLEDOCHOLITHIASIS
BILIARY STRICTURE
MALIGNANCY
Cholangiocarcinoma
Pancreatic carcinoma
Ampullary carcinoma
Duodenal carcinoma
Lymphoma
Metastases to portal lymph nodes
PANCREATITIS
PANCREATIC PSEUDOCYST
BILIARY MALFORMATION
PRIMARY SCLEROSING CHOLANGITIS
AIDS CHOLANGIOPATHY

Further evaluation of extrahepatic cholestasis includes ERCP or PTC.

- Mass lesion

  The presence of a focal liver mass should prompt consideration of hepatocellular carcinoma, lymphoma, and liver metastases among other possibilities. Further evaluation may include aspiration of the mass under radiologic guidance.

When imaging of the liver and biliary tree reveals no biliary dilatation or focal liver mass, the clinician should consider intrahepatic cholestasis or infiltrative liver disease as the etiology of the isolated alkaline phosphatase elevation. Two major causes of intrahepatic cholestasis are drug-induced cholestasis and primary biliary cirrhosis. Medications are a common cause of intrahepatic cholestasis. Common offenders are listed in the following box.

MEDICATIONS COMMONLY ASSOCIATED WITH CHOLESTASIS
AMITRIPTYLINE
AMOXICILLIN AND CLAVULANIC ACID
ANDROGENIC STEROIDS
CAPTOPRIL
CYCLOSPORINE A
CYPROHEPTADINE
ERYTHROMYCIN
ESTROGENS
GLYBURIDE
H_2-BLOCKERS
IMIPRAMINE
NITROFURANTOIN
ORAL CONTRACEPTIVES
PENICILLIN DERIVATIVES
PHENOTHIAZINES
TAMOXIFEN

The list above only represents the common offenders and is, by no means, complete. Should the clinician suspect drug-induced cholestasis, the suspect medication should be discontinued. Normalization of the alkaline phosphatase level with discontinuation of the suspect medication supports the diagnosis. It is important to realize that normalization of the level may take weeks to months.

To assess for primary biliary cirrhosis, serologic tests for antimitochondrial antibodies should be obtained. Those with serum antimitochondrial antibodies should be referred for percutaneous liver biopsy to confirm the diagnosis of primary biliary cirrhosis.

If drug-induced cholestasis or primary biliary cirrhosis are not the cause of the isolated elevation of the alkaline phosphatase level, further evaluation is necessary. In patients who have an alkaline phosphatase level >50% above normal, liver biopsy and ERCP should be considered. Liver biopsy may reveal features consistent with drug-induced cholestasis or infiltrative liver disease. Infiltrative liver diseases include sarcoidosis, tuberculosis, atypical mycobacterial infection, brucellosis, coccidioidomycosis, histoplasmosis, candidiasis, Q fever, and syphilis.

The clinician may wish to observe the patient who has a lesser degree of alkaline phosphatase elevation, particularly if the patient is asymptomatic. This approach has been supported by recent studies.

References

Aranda-Michel J and Sherman KE, "Tests of the Liver: Use and Misuse," *Gastroenterologist*, 1998, 6(1):34-43.

Beckingham IJ and Ryder SD, "ABC of Diseases of Liver, Pancreas, and Biliary System. Investigation of Liver and Biliary Disease," *BMJ*, 2001, 322(7277):33-6.

Burke MD, "Liver Function: Test Selection and Interpretation of Results," *Clin Lab Med*, 2002, 22(2):377-90.

Dufour DR, Lott JA, Nolte FS, et al, "Diagnosis and Monitoring of Hepatic Injury. I. Performance Characteristics of Laboratory Tests," *Clin Chem*, 2000, 46(12):2027-49.

Dufour DR, Lott JA, Nolte FS, et al, "Diagnosis and Monitoring of Hepatic Injury. II. Recommendations for Use of Laboratory Tests in Screening, Diagnosis, and Monitoring," *Clin Chem*, 2000, 46(12):2050-68.

Gopal DV and Rosen HR, "Abnormal Findings on Liver Function Tests. Interpreting Results to Narrow the Diagnosis and Establish a Prognosis," *Postgrad Med*, 2000, 107(2):100-2, 105-9, 113-4.

Green RM and Flamm S, "AGA Technical Review on the Evaluation of Liver Chemistry Tests," *Gastroenterology*, 2002, 123(4):1367-84.

Johnston DE, "Special Considerations in Interpreting Liver Function Tests," *Am Fam Physician*, 1999, 59(8):2223-30.

Limdi JK and Hyde GM, "Evaluation of Abnormal Liver Function Tests," *Post Grad Med J*, 2003, 79(932):307-12.

Pratt DS and Kaplan MM "Evaluation of Abnormal Liver-Enzyme Results in Asymptomatic Patients," *N Engl J Med*, 2000, 342(17):1266-71.

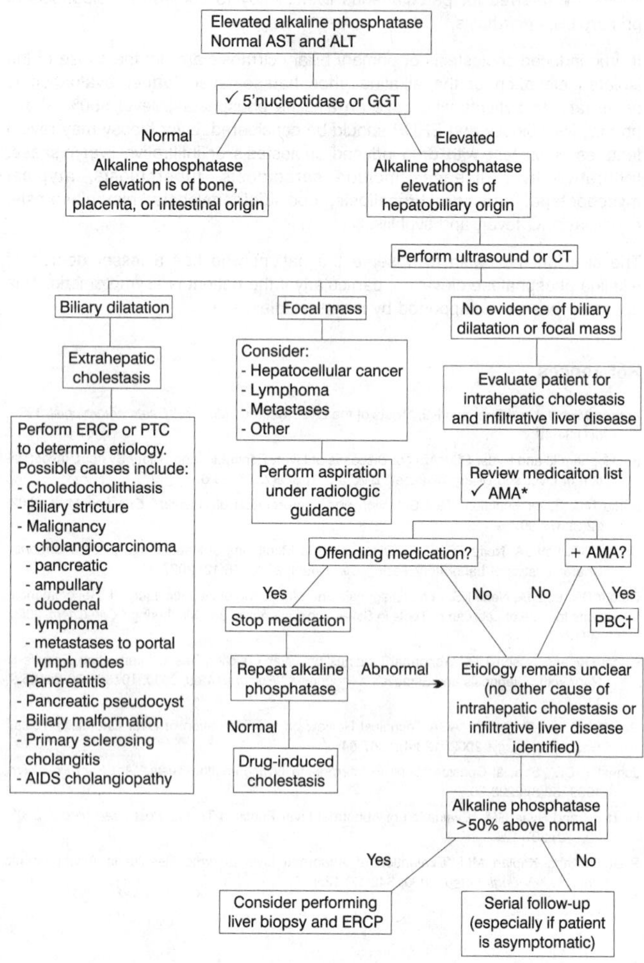

* AMA = antimitochondrial antibody
† PBC = primary biliary cirrhosis

JAUNDICE

STEP 1 – *What Are the Causes of Jaundice?*

Hyperbilirubinemia of sufficient magnitude may manifest as jaundice. Jaundice refers to a yellowing of the skin. Yellowing of the sclera is known as icterus. As a general rule, jaundice can be appreciated when the serum bilirubin exceeds 2.5 mg/dL. The causes of jaundice are listed in the following box.

CAUSES OF JAUNDICE

Unconjugated Hyperbilirubinemia	
Crigler-Najjar syndrome	Hemolysis
Drug-induced	Ineffective erythropoiesis
Gilbert's syndrome	Resorption of hematoma
Conjugated Hyperbilirubinemia	
Hepatocellular diseases	
Alcoholic hepatitis	Hepatotoxins
α_1-antitrypsin deficiency	Ischemia
Autoimmune hepatitis	Medications
Cirrhosis	Rotor's syndrome
Dubin-Johnson syndrome	Viral hepatitis (acute or chronic)
Hemochromatosis	Wilson's disease
Hepatic vein thrombosis	
Cholestatic diseases	
Intrahepatic	Extrahepatic
Alcoholic hepatitis	AIDS cholangiopathy
Benign recurrent intrahepatic cholestasis	Biliary malformation
	Choledocholithiasis
Cholestasis of pregnancy	Malignancy
Drug-induced	Ampullary
Postoperative jaundice	Cholangiocarcinoma
Primary biliary cirrhosis	Duodenal
Systemic infection	Lymphoma
Total parenteral nutrition	Metastases to portal lymph nodes
Viral hepatitis	Pancreatic
	Pancreatic pseudocyst
	Pancreatitis
	Primary sclerosing cholangitis

Proceed to Step 2.

STEP 2 – *Does the Patient Have Conjugated or Unconjugated Hyperbilirubinemia?*

The evaluation of jaundice begins with the determination of whether the hyperbilirubinemia is conjugated or unconjugated. The following lists several ways of making this distinction.

- Other liver function test abnormalities

  The causes of unconjugated hyperbilirubinemia are not typically associated with other liver function test abnormalities. In contrast, most cases of conjugated hyperbilirubinemia are accompanied by other liver function test abnormalities.

- Urine dipstick for bilirubin

  Of the two types of bilirubin, only conjugated bilirubin is water soluble. As a result, a positive urine dipstick for bilirubin signifies the presence of conjugated hyperbilirubinemia.

- Foam test

  When normal urine is shaken, the foam appears white. In the presence of bilirubinuria, however, the foam will be yellow. Because the yellow color characteristic of conjugated hyperbilirubinemia may be subtle, it is useful to compare the specimen with the white foam of a normal urine specimen.

- Serum bilirubin fractionation

  A predominantly conjugated hyperbilirubinemia is said to exist when 30% or more of the serum bilirubin is in the conjugated form.

If the patient has unconjugated hyperbilirubinemia, ***proceed to Step 3***.

If the patient has conjugated hyperbilirubinemia, ***proceed to Step 9***.

STEP 3 – *What Are the Causes of Unconjugated Hyperbilirubinemia?*

The approach to the patient presenting with unconjugated hyperbilirubinemia is more easily understood if one considers the steps involved in bilirubin metabolism. Close to 80% of the serum bilirubin originates from the breakdown of senescent red blood cells. The remainder is derived from the metabolism of other proteins containing heme as well as the destruction of red blood cell precursors in the bone marrow (ineffective erythropoiesis). The unconjugated bilirubin then travels to the liver. Uptake of bilirubin occurs at the liver cell followed by conjugation. Conjugation is catalyzed by the enzyme, UDP-glucuronyl transferase. Therefore, a process that leads to or affects any of the following steps in bilirubin metabolism can lead to unconjugated hyperbilirubinemia:

- Increased production of bilirubin
- Impaired hepatic uptake of bilirubin
- Impaired conjugation of bilirubin

The causes of unconjugated hyperbilirubinemia are listed in the box below.

CAUSES OF UNCONJUGATED HYPERBILIRUBINEMIA

INCREASED PRODUCTION	IMPAIRED HEPATIC UPTAKE
Hemolysis	Medications
Ineffective erythropoiesis	Gilbert's syndrome
Resorption of large hematoma	IMPAIRED CONJUGATION
	Crigler-Najjar syndrome
	Gilbert's syndrome

Proceed to Step 4.

STEP 4 – *Does the Patient Have Unconjugated Hyperbilirubinemia Secondary to Hemolysis?*

With hemolysis, the degradation of hemoglobin in large amounts overwhelms the liver's ability to excrete it. Because the liver has a remarkable capacity to excrete bilirubin, the hyperbilirubinemia that accompanies hemolysis is characteristically mild. The serum bilirubin is usually <5 mg/dL in patients with hemolysis. Only when the hemolysis is superimposed on underlying liver disease or the hemolytic disease involves the liver (eg, sickle cell anemia) will the bilirubin level rise above 5 mg/dL. Other laboratory test abnormalities that support the presence of hemolysis include the following:

- Anemia
- Reticulocytosis
- Increased LDH
- Decreased haptoglobin
- Urine hemosiderin

In many cases, the etiology of the hemolysis is known. In other cases, a thorough history, physical examination, and other laboratory testing will establish the diagnosis.

If the patient has unconjugated hyperbilirubinemia secondary to hemolysis, ***stop here***.

If the patient does not have unconjugated hyperbilirubinemia secondary to hemolysis, ***proceed to Step 5***.

STEP 5 – *Does the Patient Have Unconjugated Hyperbilirubinemia Secondary to Ineffective Erythropoiesis?*

Ineffective erythropoiesis refers to the increased destruction of red blood cells or red blood cell precursors in the bone marrow. Disorders associated with ineffective erythropoiesis are listed in the following box.

CAUSES OF INEFFECTIVE ERYTHROPOIESIS	
DYSERYTHROPOIETIC PORPHYRIA	SIDEROBLASTIC ANEMIA
FOLATE DEFICIENCY	THALASSEMIA
LEAD POISONING	VITAMIN B_{12} DEFICIENCY
SEVERE IRON DEFICIENCY ANEMIA	

The history and physical examination may direct the clinician to one of the above causes of ineffective erythropoiesis. As a general rule, the above conditions are not characterized by serum bilirubin levels in excess of 4 mg/dL unless there is concomitant liver disease.

If the patient has unconjugated hyperbilirubinemia secondary to ineffective erythropoiesis, ***stop here***.

If the patient does not have unconjugated hyperbilirubinemia secondary to ineffective erythropoiesis, ***proceed to Step 6***.

STEP 6 – *Does the Patient Have Unconjugated Hyperbilirubinemia Secondary to Decreased Hepatic Uptake of Bilirubin?*

This is an uncommon cause of unconjugated hyperbilirubinemia but may be noted with the use of certain medications. These medications include the following:

- Rifampin
- Probenecid
- Flavaspidic acid
- Some radiographic contrast agents (bunamiodyl)

Resolution of the unconjugated hyperbilirubinemia typically occurs within 48 hours of drug discontinuation. Another cause of impaired hepatic uptake of bilirubin is Gilbert's syndrome. However, since Gilbert's syndrome is a heterogeneous disorder characterized by defects of bilirubin conjugation as well, it will be discussed shortly.

If the patient has unconjugated hyperbilirubinemia secondary to decreased hepatic uptake of bilirubin, ***stop here***.

If the patient does not have unconjugated hyperbilirubinemia secondary to decreased hepatic uptake of bilirubin, ***proceed to Step 7***.

STEP 7 – *Does the Patient Have Unconjugated Hyperbilirubinemia Secondary to the Crigler-Najjar Syndrome?*

There are two types of Crigler-Najjar syndrome. Type I Crigler-Najjar syndrome is characterized by the absence of UDP-glucuronyltransferase activity. As a result, unconjugated hyperbilirubinemia develops immediately after birth. Infants often have impressive elevations in the serum bilirubin level. Left untreated, all affected patients will die of kernicterus. The only treatment is liver transplantation.

In type II Crigler-Najjar syndrome, also known as Arias disease, affected individuals have about 10% of the normal UDP-glucuronyltransferase activity. While most develop jaundice before the age of 1 year, some may not until later in life. It is unusual for affected individuals to present after the age of 10 years. The serum bilirubin levels typically range between 10-20 mg/dL. Therapy is usually not needed but, in those at risk for kernicterus, phenobarbital can decrease the bilirubin level.

If the patient has unconjugated hyperbilirubinemia secondary to the Crigler-Najjar syndrome, ***stop here***.

If the patient does not have unconjugated hyperbilirubinemia secondary to the Crigler-Najjar syndrome, ***proceed to Step 8***.

STEP 8 – *Does the Patient Have Gilbert's Syndrome?*

In outpatients, the most common cause of unconjugated hyperbilirubinemia is Gilbert's syndrome. Gilbert's syndrome is found in 3% to 8% of the Caucasian population. Inherited in an autosomal dominant pattern, this syndrome typically manifests during or after adolescence. Jaundice usually develops with the following precipitants.

- Intercurrent illness
- Exercise

- Stress
- Fatigue
- Alcohol use
- Fasting
- Nicotinic acid intake

The diagnosis should be suspected in younger patients who present with unconjugated hyperbilirubinemia but no other liver function test abnormalities. Defects in hepatic uptake and/or conjugation of bilirubin have been described in patients with Gilbert's syndrome.

A diagnosis of Gilbert's syndrome can be established in the patient who has the features listed in the following box.

FEATURES OF GILBERT'S SYNDROME	
NO BILIRUBINURIA	NORMAL MCV
NORMAL ALKALINE PHOSPHATASE	NORMAL PERIPHERAL BLOOD SMEAR
NORMAL AST/ALT	NORMAL RETICULOCYTE COUNT
NORMAL GGT	UNCONJUGATED HYPERBILIRUBINEMIA
NORMAL HEMOGLOBIN	

In most cases, the presence of the features listed above are sufficient to establish the diagnosis. If there is any uncertainty, the clinician can elect to perform either one of the following tests:

- Nicotinic acid stress test

  When nicotinic acid is given intravenously, an increase in serum bilirubin by more than >18 μmol/L has been found to have 100% sensitivity and specificity in the diagnosis of Gilbert's syndrome. One hour before the intravenous administration of nicotinic acid, 100 mg of indomethacin is recommended to prevent flushing.

- Caloric restriction test

  A rise in the serum bilirubin to greater than two times the upper limit of normal after two days of caloric restriction (400 kcal/day) is consistent with Gilbert's syndrome. Other causes of hyperbilirubinemia may be associated with a lesser rise in the serum bilirubin.

The following table offers a comparison between Gilbert's syndrome and the two types of Crigler-Najjar syndrome.

	Gilbert's Syndrome	Crigler-Najjar Syndrome (Type I)	Crigler-Najjar Syndrome (Type II)
Incidence	3% to 8%	Very rare	Uncommon
Inheritance Pattern	Autosomal dominant	Autosomal recessive	Autosomal recessive
Serum Bilirubin	<5 mg/dL	Usually >20 mg/dL	Usually <20 mg/dL
Response to Phenobarbital	Decrease in serum bilirubin	No response	Decrease in serum bilirubin
Prognosis	Normal	Death in infancy	Usually normal
Treatment	None needed	Liver transplantation	Phenobarbital if serum bilirubin markedly increased

Making the diagnosis of Gilbert's syndrome can obviate an unnecessary and expensive work-up. The patient can then be reassured that their illness is benign.

End of Section.

STEP 9 – *What Are the Causes of Conjugated Hyperbilirubinemia?*

The causes of conjugated hyperbilirubinemia are listed in the following box.

CAUSES OF CONJUGATED HYPERBILIRUBINEMIA

HEPATOCELLULAR DISEASE

- Alcoholic hepatitis
- α_1-antitrypsin deficiency
- Autoimmune hepatitis
- Cirrhosis
- Drug-induced
- Dubin-Johnson syndrome
- Hemochromatosis
- Hepatotoxins
- Hepatic vein thrombosis
- Ischemia
- Rotor's syndrome
- Viral hepatitis
- Wilson's disease

CHOLESTASIS

- Extrahepatic
  - AIDS cholangiopathy
  - Biliary malformation
  - Choledocholithiasis
  - Malignancy
    - Ampullary
    - Cholangiocarcinoma
    - Duodenal
    - Lymphoma
    - Metastases to portal lymph nodes
    - Pancreatic
  - Pancreatic pseudocyst
  - Pancreatitis
  - Primary sclerosing cholangitis
- Intrahepatic
  - Alcoholic hepatitis
  - Benign recurrent intrahepatic cholestasis
  - Cholestasis of pregnancy
  - Drug-induced
  - Postoperative hyperbilirubinemia
  - Primary biliary cirrhosis
  - Systemic infection
  - Total parenteral nutrition
  - Viral hepatitis

The initial step in elucidating the etiology of the conjugated hyperbilirubinemia is consideration of the other liver function tests.

If the conjugated hyperbilirubinemia is not accompanied by other liver function test abnormalities, ***proceed to Step 10***.

If the conjugated hyperbilirubinemia is accompanied by other liver function test abnormalities, ***proceed to Step 11***.

STEP 10 – *Does the Patient Have Conjugated Hyperbilirubinemia Secondary to Dubin-Johnson or Rotor's Syndrome?*

When the conjugated hyperbilirubinemia is not accompanied by other liver function test abnormalities, consideration should be given to the Dubin-Johnson and Rotor's syndrome. Both are inherited disorders that typically become apparent in childhood. Serum bilirubin levels typically range between 2-5 mg/

dL. The following table offers a comparison between these two congenital disorders.

	Dubin-Johnson Syndrome	Rotor's Syndrome
Incidence	Uncommon	Rare
Inheritance Pattern	Autosomal recessive	Autosomal recessive
Bilirubin	Usually between 2-5 mg/dL	Usually between 2-5 mg/dL
Plasma Sulfobromophthalein Disappearance	Slow initial disappearance with frequent secondary rise at 1.5-2 hours	Very slow disappearance without secondary rise
Oral Cholecystography	Faint or nonvisualization	Usually normal visualization
Liver Histology	Coarse pigment in centrilobular hepatocytes	Normal
Prognosis	Normal	Normal
Treatment	No specific treatment	No specific treatment

End of Section.

STEP 11 – *Are There Any Historical Clues That Point to the Etiology of the Conjugated Hyperbilirubinemia?*

When other liver function test abnormalities are present in the patient with conjugated hyperbilirubinemia, the clinician should consider the causes of hepatobiliary disease. Clues in the patient's history that may point to the etiology of the hepatobiliary disease are listed in the following table.

Historical Clue	Disease Suggested
Anorexia	Viral hepatitis Malignancy
Arthritis	Viral hepatitis Autoimmune hepatitis Primary sclerosing cholangitis Sarcoidosis Hemochromatosis
Pregnancy	Intrahepatic cholestasis of pregnancy Acute fatty liver of pregnancy Pre-eclampsia
Light stools	Cholestasis
Anorexia Myalgias Malaise	Viral hepatitis (prodrome)
History of COPD	α_1-antitrypsin deficiency
Right shoulder or subcapsular pain	Choledocholithiasis
Pruritus	Cholestasis
Aversion to cigarettes	Viral hepatitis
Weight loss	Malignancy Alcoholic hepatitis End stage liver disease or cirrhosis
Fever / chills	Cholangitis Viral hepatitis Amebic abscess Alcoholic hepatitis Drug-induced hepatitis
RUQ tenderness	Alcoholic hepatitis Viral hepatitis Amebic abscess Choledocholithiasis / cholangitis

(continued)

(continued)

Historical Clue	Disease Suggested
Pain in epigastric / RUQ region radiating to back Pain worsened by recumbency	Pancreatitis Pancreatic cancer
History of cholecystectomy	Retained common bile duct stone Biliary stricture
Receiving total parenteral nutrition	Cholestasis secondary to total parenteral nutrition
Alcohol use	Alcoholic hepatitis
History of inflammatory bowel disease	Primary sclerosing cholangitis
Recent surgery	Postoperative jaundice: Benign postoperative cholestasis Inhalational anesthetic Impaired hepatic perfusion Blood transfusion Occult sepsis
Family history of jaundice	Dubin-Johnson syndrome Rotor's syndrome Benign recurrent intrahepatic cholestasis
After transplantation Accompanied by rash and diarrhea	Graft-vs-host disease
Medications (including herbal and over-the-counter)	Drug-induced hepatitis or cholestasis
Daycare centers Institutions for the retarded Sharing drug paraphernalia Travel to endemic area Engaging in oral-anal sex Ingestion of raw shellfish	Hepatitis A (risk factors)
Intravenous drug abuse Hemodialysis patients Sharing razor blades / toothbrushes Tattooing Body piercing Acupuncture Healthcare worker History of blood transfusion High-risk sexual activity	Hepatitis B (risk factors)
Intravenous drug abuse Hemophilia History of blood transfusion Healthcare worker	Hepatitis C (risk factors)

Proceed to Step 12.

STEP 12 – *Are There Any Clues in the Physical Examination That Point to the Etiology of the Conjugated Hyperbilirubinemia?*

Clues in the physical examination that point to the etiology of the conjugated hyperbilirubinemia are listed in the following table.

Physical Examination Finding	Disease Suggested
Wasting	Advanced liver disease Malignancy
Needle track or skin popping	Intravenous drug abuse (risk factor for viral hepatitis)
Skin excoriations	Cholestasis
Generalized lymphadenopathy	Lymphoma
Supraclavicular lymphadenopathy	Gastric malignancy
Spider angiomas Gynecomastia Parotid enlargement Testicular atrophy Paucity of axillary and pubic hair Dupuytren's contracture	Chronic liver disease or cirrhosis
Palpable abdominal mass	Malignancy
Pulsatile liver	Tricuspid regurgitation (congestive hepatopathy)
Palpable gallbladder (Courvosier's sign)	Malignant biliary duct obstruction
Xanthomas	Primary biliary cirrhosis
Hyperpigmentation	Hemochromatosis Primary biliary cirrhosis
Abdominal scar in midline or right upper quadrant	Prior biliary surgery (suggestive of retained stone or biliary stricture)
Kayser-Fleischer ring	Wilson's disease
Fever	Acute cholangitis Alcoholic hepatitis Viral hepatitis Amebic abscess Pancreatitis

Proceed to Step 13.

STEP 13 – *Does the Patient Have Conjugated Hyperbilirubinemia Secondary to Hepatocellular Injury or Cholestasis?*

Consideration of the other liver function test abnormalities allows hepatocellular injury to be distinguished from cholestasis, which is defined as an impairment in bile flow. Specifically, the transaminase (AST and ALT) and alkaline phosphatase levels need to be obtained. The information in the table below allows the clinician to differentiate hepatocellular from cholestatic liver injury.

	Alkaline Phosphatase	Transaminases
Hepatocellular injury	Normal or <3 x normal	>400 units/L (acute) <300 units/L (chronic)
Cholestasis	>4 x normal	<300 units/L

At times, it can be difficult to make the distinction between hepatocellular injury and cholestasis because the laboratory test abnormalities described above may overlap.

If the patient has cholestasis, ***proceed to Step 14.***

If the patient has hepatocellular injury, ***proceed to Step 18.***

STEP 14 – *Does the Patient Have Extrahepatic or Intrahepatic Cholestasis?*

Cholestasis refers to an impairment in bile flow. As such, it may be intrahepatic or extrahepatic. It is important to make this distinction because prompt drainage is often necessary in patients with extrahepatic cholestasis. In contrast, drainage usually has no role in the management of intrahepatic cholestasis and, if performed, may result in increased morbidity and mortality.

The history and physical examination may provide clues as to whether the patient has extrahepatic (also known as obstructive jaundice) or intrahepatic cholestasis. These clues are described in the following table.

	Extrahepatic Cholestasis (Obstructive Jaundice)	Intrahepatic Cholestasis
Historical Clues	Abdominal pain Fever Shaking, chills Prior biliary surgery Older age	Anorexia, malaise, myalgias (suggestive of viral prodrome) Known infectious exposure Receipt of blood products Use of intravenous drugs Exposure to known hepatotoxin Family history of jaundice
Physical Examination Clues	High fever Abdominal tenderness Palpable abdominal mass Abdominal scar	Ascites Stigmata of chronic liver disease Prominent abdominal veins Gynecomastia Spider angiomas Asterixis Encephalopathy

Imaging with ultrasound or CT scan plays a prominent role in differentiating between extrahepatic and intrahepatic cholestasis. The demonstration of dilated bile ducts establishes the presence of extrahepatic cholestasis. Of note, mild dilatation of the common bile duct is commonly appreciated in postcholecystectomy patients. The advantages and disadvantages of these two radiologic tests in the evaluation of cholestasis are listed in the following table.

	Ultrasound	CT Scan
Noninvasive	Yes	Yes
Portable	Yes	Yes
Operator-Dependent	Yes	No
Expensive	No (relative to CT scan)	Yes
Sensitivity	55% to 91%	63% to 96%
Specificity	82% to 95%	93% to 100%
Contrast	No	Yes
Exposure to Radiation	No	Yes

If dilated bile ducts are demonstrated on ultrasound or CT, ***proceed to Step 15.***

If dilated bile ducts are not demonstrated on ultrasound or CT but high suspicion for extrahepatic cholestasis remains, ***proceed to Step 16.***

If bile ducts are not dilated on ultrasound or CT and suspicion for extrahepatic cholestasis is low, ***proceed to Step 17.***

STEP 15 – *What Are the Causes of Extrahepatic Cholestasis?*

The causes of extrahepatic cholestasis are listed in the following box.

CAUSES OF EXTRAHEPATIC CHOLESTASIS	
Choledocholithiasis	Pancreatitis
Biliary stricture	Pancreatic pseudocyst
Malignancy	Biliary malformation
Cholangiocarcinoma	Atresia
Pancreatic carcinoma	Choledochal cyst
Ampullary carcinoma	Primary sclerosing cholangitis
Duodenal carcinoma	AIDS cholangiopathy
Lymphoma	
Metastases to portal lymph nodes	

The presentation of the more common causes of extrahepatic cholestasis are considered below.

Choledocholithiasis

Patients with choledocholithiasis often present with signs and symptoms of biliary colic. The abdominal pain is steady, often lasting several hours in duration. Most patients complain of pain in the epigastrium and/or right upper quadrant.

Other patients with choledocholithiasis may seek medical care because of cholangitis, which results from infection in the setting of biliary obstruction. Charcot's triad of right upper quadrant pain, jaundice, and fever may be present in up to 75% of patients. Reynold's pentad includes this triad in combination with altered mental status and hypotension.

Soon after an attack of choledocholithiasis, the transaminases are markedly elevated. This is a transient finding, however, that is followed by a rise in the alkaline phosphatase. Rarely does the alkaline phosphatase exceed five times the upper limit of normal. Bilirubin rises in parallel, typically ranging between 2-14 mg/dL. Higher levels of alkaline phosphatase and/or bilirubin should prompt the clinician to consider malignancy. Ultrasound and CT have a sensitivity of about 20% and 50%, respectively, in the detection of common bile duct stones. In contrast, the sensitivity of ERCP is approximately 90%. It offers the clinician some therapeutic options as well including sphincterotomy and stone extraction.

Cholangiocarcinoma

Cholangiocarcinoma is a rare tumor that typically presents in middle age. There is a higher incidence of this malignancy in Southeast Asia, perhaps a reflection of an association with the liver fluke, *Clonorchis sinensis*. Cholangiocarcinoma is also associated with primary sclerosing cholangitis and biliary cysts. Nonspecific symptoms such as weight loss and fatigue are quite common while pain is uncommon. Cholangitis is unusual in these patients. The investigation of a patient suspected of having cholangiocarcinoma begins with either an ultrasound or CT scan. Of the two imaging modalities, CT scan usually provides more information. Confirmation of the diagnosis requires histologic analysis of cytologic brushings performed during an ERCP or PTC. While the sensitivity of the brushings is only 30%, a forceps biopsy in conjunction with brushings improves the sensitivity to 70%.

Pancreatic Cancer

Abdominal pain is a frequent complaint in patients with pancreatic cancer. Poor localization of the pain is not uncommon. The pain is typically constant with radiation from the upper abdomen to the back. There is usually a positional difference in the intensity of the pain; it is worse when supine but better when sitting up and leaning forward. Careful questioning of the patient usually reveals that the pain preceded the jaundice. Weight loss is almost invariably present. Diabetes mellitus is present in >60% of patients with pancreatic cancer. In a small percentage of patients, acute pancreatitis may be the initial presentation of the disease.

Physical examination typically reveals a jaundiced patient. Palpation of a mass argues for a lesion in the body or tail of the pancreas. In cases characterized by malignant biliary obstruction, the gallbladder may become distended and palpable (Courvosier's sign).

Abnormal laboratory tests are not uncommon at the time of presentation but, unfortunately, the abnormalities are often nonspecific. Mild elevations may be noted in the amylase and lipase concentrations. While both transaminases and alkaline phosphatase are often elevated, the alkaline phosphatase is often disproportionately so.

While ultrasound may detect a pancreatic cancer, more often, the utility of the test is poor because of overlying intraluminal gas. Even if the pancreas is not adequately visualized, ultrasound may provide important information such as the presence of biliary dilatation, which is suggestive of malignant biliary obstruction. CT scan can detect a pancreatic mass with an 80% sensitivity. ERCP is even better, exhibiting a 90% sensitivity in the diagnosis of pancreatic cancer. ERCP may demonstrate the double duct sign, which refers to a rather abrupt obstruction of both the common bile and pancreatic ducts. This finding is almost pathognomonic for pancreatic cancer. ERCP can also enable the clinician to obtain cytologic samples, yielding a sensitivity of nearly 40%. In recent years, endoscopic ultrasound has gained popularity because of its greater than 90% sensitivity in the diagnosis of pancreatic cancer. FNA of a mass can be performed with the guidance of endoscopic ultrasound.

Ampullary Tumor

Ampullary tumors are uncommon malignancies that can be benign (adenoma) or malignant (adenocarcinoma). While most malignant tumors originate from the mucosa of the ampulla of Vater, some ampullary tumors may arise from the pancreas, distal common bile duct, or duodenum. Jaundice, often cyclic, is the most common initial manifestation. Other symptoms include abdominal pain, nausea, vomiting, melena, and anorexia. The silver stool sign of Thomas, appreciated in <5% of patients, derives its appearance from acholic stools mixed with blood. Courvosier's sign may be appreciated in approximately 30% of patients.

Metastases to Portal Lymph Nodes (Porta Hepatis)

There are a number of malignancies that may metastasize to the periductal lymph nodes. With sufficient enlargement of the nodes in the porta hepatis, extrahepatic cholestasis may ensue. Tumors that have been reported to do so include colon cancer, breast cancer, gastric cancer, and melanoma. Lymphoma is also a consideration.

Primary Sclerosing Cholangitis (PSC)

Primary sclerosing cholangitis refers to bile duct injury in the absence of an apparent cause. It needs to be differentiated from secondary sclerosing cholangitis which occurs in the patient with a known predisposition. The injury to the bile ducts may take the form of inflammation, fibrosis, and strictures. PSC, a disease that has a predilection for young males, typically presents with pruritus, fatigue, and jaundice. Cholangitis is rare in these patients. A helpful clue is a history of inflammatory bowel disease since nearly 75% of patients have ulcerative colitis or Crohn's disease. Laboratory tests reveal elevations of the transaminases and alkaline phosphatase, with the latter being disproportionately elevated. ERCP can confirm the diagnosis.

Pancreatitis

Jaundice may be seen in alcoholic patients who present with both pancreatitis and hepatitis. Jaundice may also occur in pancreatitis that is secondary to gallstones. In these cases, the gallstones interrupt the flow of bile and pancreatic secretions in the distal common bile duct. Biliary obstruction may also occur if the pancreatitis is associated with extensive edema or is complicated by the development of a significant fluid collection.

Epigastric pain that typically radiates to the back is the hallmark of pancreatitis. The pain usually develops over a period of several hours but can last for days. There is a characteristic positional component to the pain. Most describe a worsening of the pain with recumbency and amelioration of the pain when leaning forward after assuming a sitting position. Nausea and vomiting frequently accompany the pain of pancreatitis. A low grade fever is also common.

Physical examination reveals epigastric tenderness with or without guarding. Tachycardia and decreased bowel sounds may also be appreciated. Less commonly observed are Cullen's and Grey Turner signs, which refer to periumbilical and flank ecchymoses, respectively. Laboratory testing reveals the characteristic rise in the amylase and lipase.

Pancreatic Pseudocyst

A pseudocyst may complicate either acute or chronic pancreatitis. Pseudocysts develop in approximately 10% of patients with acute pancreatitis. While patients with pancreatic pseudocysts may be asymptomatic, many complain of persistent abdominal pain. In some patients, physical examination may reveal an abdominal mass. Jaundice is one complication of pancreatic pseudocyst that typically occurs when a pseudocyst in the pancreatic head obstructs the common bile duct. Other complications include rupture, infection, compression of contiguous structures, erosion into nearby blood vessels, and fistula formation. Ultrasound and CT can readily establish the diagnosis.

AIDS Cholangiopathy

Pruritus and abdominal pain are common symptoms in patients with AIDS cholangiopathy, a disorder often associated with sclerosing cholangitis and/or papillary stenosis. Several organisms including *Microsporidia*, *Cryptosporidium*, *I. belli,* and CMV have been implicated in the pathogenesis. Ultrasound or CT may demonstrate the biliary dilatation that is characteristic of AIDS cholangiopathy. ERCP is required to confirm the diagnosis.

Biliary Stricture

Conditions associated with the development of biliary stricture are listed in the following box.

CONDITIONS ASSOCIATED WITH DEVELOPMENT OF BILIARY STRUCTURE	
AIDS CHOLANGIOPATHY	MALIGNANCY
BILE DUCT INJURY FROM SURGERY	Pancreatic
CHRONIC PANCREATITIS	Cholangiocarcinoma
MIRIZZI'S SYNDROME	Gallbladder
RADIATION	Ampullary
SCLEROSING CHOLANGITIS	Duodenal

Choledochal Cysts

More commonly seen in the Orient, extrahepatic biliary cysts, also known as choledochal cysts, tend to have a predilection for women. Although most cysts come to clinical attention in childhood with symptoms of obstructive jaundice, it is not unusual for the initial manifestations to appear in adulthood, usually in the form of pancreatitis or recurrent cholangitis. Intrahepatic biliary cysts (Caroli's syndrome) commonly present in young adulthood with fever. Abdominal pain and/or jaundice may be present. The diagnosis of both extrahepatic and intrahepatic biliary cysts requires imaging with ultrasound, CT, and cholangiography.

End of Section.

STEP 16 – *What Are the Results of ERCP or PTC?*

In patients strongly suspected of having extrahepatic cholestasis, the absence of biliary duct dilatation on ultrasound or CT should not prompt the clinician to discard this possibility. ERCP and PTC are invasive tests that should be considered when noninvasive testing (ultrasound or CT) is negative or equivocal in a patient likely to have extrahepatic cholestasis. ERCP and PTC have a sensitivity and specificity of 99% in the detection of ductal obstruction. In addition, the precise nature, extent, and location of the obstruction can be determined.

If the ERCP or PTC establishes the presence of extrahepatic cholestasis, ***proceed to Step 15.***

If the ERCP or PTC does not establish the presence of extrahepatic cholestasis, ***proceed to Step 17.***

STEP 17 – *What Is the Approach to the Patient With Intrahepatic Cholestasis?*

When imaging studies do not reveal biliary dilatation, intrahepatic cholestasis is likely. The causes of intrahepatic cholestasis are listed in the following box.

CAUSES OF INTRAHEPATIC CHOLESTASIS	
Alcoholic hepatitis	Postoperative cholestasis
Benign recurrent intrahepatic cholestasis	Primary biliary cirrhosis
Drug-induced	Systemic infection
Intrahepatic cholestasis of pregnancy	Total parenteral nutrition
	Viral hepatitis

Common causes of intrahepatic cholestasis are discussed below.

Primary Biliary Cirrhosis

Primary biliary cirrhosis, a disease of unknown etiology, is a chronic cholestatic illness. Nearly half of all patients are diagnosed at a time when they are asymptomatic. In these cases, the illness comes to clinical attention because of an elevated alkaline phosphatase level. Those who are symptomatic commonly complain of pruritus and fatigue. Approximately 25% of patients present with jaundice. Excoriations and hyperpigmentation of the skin may occur as a result of the frequent scratching.

The laboratory test abnormality that is the hallmark of the disease is the elevated alkaline phosphatase. While serum bilirubin levels are often normal at the time of presentation, hyperbilirubinemia develops in over 50% as the illness becomes more advanced. Antimitochondrial antibodies can be detected in 95% of patients. Serum protein electrophoresis may reveal IgM hypergammaglobulinemia. Imaging has a role in excluding extrahepatic causes of cholestasis in patients suspected of having primary biliary cirrhosis. The definitive diagnosis of primary biliary cirrhosis requires liver biopsy.

Viral Hepatitis

Cholestasis is not common in patients with viral hepatitis but may occur with any viral cause of hepatitis. It is more commonly appreciated in patients with hepatitis A. EBV and CMV are also considerations in the patient presenting with cholestasis thought to be secondary to a viral etiology.

In these patients, symptoms of acute viral hepatitis including fever, anorexia, and right upper quadrant pain are usually present. Jaundice and pruritus usually follow the onset of these symptoms. Early in the illness, the transaminase levels may exceed 1000 U/L but are usually less than 200 U/L by the time features of cholestasis manifest. During the cholestatic phase, the bilirubin and alkaline phosphatase levels are significantly elevated. Not uncommonly, cholestatic viral hepatitis persists for weeks to months.

Alcoholic Hepatitis

While alcoholic hepatitis usually presents with hepatocellular injury, some cases are characterized by cholestasis. In these cases, serum bilirubin and alkaline phosphatase levels are elevated out of proportion to the transaminase levels. Because patients with alcoholic hepatitis often present with fever and leukocytosis, it is necessary to exclude extrahepatic biliary obstruction.

Drug-Induced Cholestasis

Medications are a major cause of cholestasis. As such, drug-induced cholestasis should be considered in any patient with liver function test abnormalities consistent with cholestatic injury. Common offenders are listed in the following box.

MEDICATIONS COMMONLY ASSOCIATED WITH CHOLESTASIS	
Amoxicillin and clavulanic acid	Oral contraceptives
Androgenic steroids	Penicillin derivatives
Cyclosporine A	Phenothiazines
Estrogens	Tamoxifen
Glyburide	

Other medications may cause a mixed picture with features of both cholestasis and hepatocellular injury. These are listed in the following box.

MEDICATIONS CAUSING A MIXED PICTURE OF CHOLESTASIS AND HEPATOCELLULAR INJURY	
ACE inhibitors	Ketoconazole
Allopurinol	NSAIDs
Azathioprine	Oral hypoglycemic agents
Barbiturates	Penicillamine
Benzodiazepines	Phenothiazines
Clavulanic acid	Phenytoin
Erythromycin	Prochlorperazine
Fluoxetine	Propylthiouracil
H_2-blockers	Sulfonamides
Haloperidol	Tricyclic antidepressants

In most cases, cholestasis develops several weeks after starting the offending medication. In some cases, however, cholestasis has been described in patients several years after the institution of a medication. Most cases of drug-induced cholestasis come to clinical attention when abnormal liver function tests are found in an asymptomatic patient. Some patients may present with anorexia, abdominal pain, nausea, pruritus, or jaundice. Fever and rash are uncommon but, when present, should prompt the clinician to seriously consider drug-induced cholestasis.

Eosinophilia, although rare, lends support to the diagnosis. The diagnosis should be suspected in any patient who develops cholestatic liver injury within weeks to months after starting a new medication. Normalization of the liver function test abnormalities after cessation of the offending agent provides a strong argument for drug-induced cholestasis. While liver biopsy can demonstrate features consistent with drug-induced cholestasis, rarely is it diagnostic.

Total Parenteral Nutrition (TPN)

Not uncommonly, patients develop liver function test abnormalities 1-4 weeks after starting TPN. In most cases, these abnormalities resolve with time. While the most common hepatobiliary complication of TPN is steatohepatitis, cholestasis has also been reported.

Cholestatic liver disease tends to occur in patients receiving long-term TPN. Because these patients are also at risk for the development of biliary stones, it is important to exclude this possibility before attributing the cholestasis to TPN.

Systemic Infection

When jaundice develops in the febrile patient, the clinician should consider cholestasis secondary to systemic infection or sepsis. Affected patients are usually very ill. Jaundice is usually preceded by several days of symptoms and signs suggestive of infection. Both bilirubin and alkaline phosphatase levels are usually elevated.

Although cholestasis secondary to systemic infection has been well described in patients with Gram-negative enteric infections and toxic shock syndrome, it may also occur in Gram-positive infections. Extrahepatic biliary obstruction should be excluded in these patients.

Postoperative Jaundice

Jaundice occurs in approximately 1% of patients after an operative intervention requiring anesthesia. There are many causes of postoperative jaundice. In some cases, the etiology is multifactorial. Elucidating the precise etiology requires careful consideration of the temporal relationship between the onset of jaundice and the surgical procedure. Jaundice within the first few days suggests hepatic ischemia or hemolysis. In contrast, anesthetic related jaundice is unusual before the seventh postoperative day.

While postoperative jaundice may present with hepatocellular injury, in some cases, the injury is cholestatic. Bile duct injury may occur during abdominal surgery, resulting in jaundice. Such an injury should be suspected with certain surgeries such as laparoscopic cholecystectomy, other biliary tract surgery, and gastrectomy.

Cholestasis that occurs in the postoperative period is often multifactorial. Hypotension, hemorrhage, hypoxia, and sepsis are all factors that may play a role. This type of cholestatic syndrome manifesting after surgery has been referred to as benign postoperative jaundice.

Benign Recurrent Intrahepatic Cholestasis

Benign recurrent intrahepatic cholestasis is a rare condition that is characterized by recurrent episodes of acute cholestasis. Between exacerbations, patients are otherwise healthy. The onset of this illness is typically in childhood or adolescence. The episodes are characterized by symptoms of anorexia, pruritus, and jaundice. Liver function tests reveal a pattern consistent with cholestasis. After several weeks to months, the episode resolves, leaving the patient completely asymptomatic. With resolution of the illness, the liver function test abnormalities normalize. Although many have a family history of benign recurrent intrahepatic cholestasis, sporadic cases have been reported.

Intrahepatic Cholestasis of Pregnancy

Elevations in the alkaline phosphatase level are common during pregnancy because of the leakage of placental alkaline phosphatase into the serum. In the intrahepatic cholestasis of pregnancy, alkaline phosphatase elevation is accompanied by abnormalities of the GGT, transaminases, and bilirubin. This is an uncommon disorder that typically occurs late in pregnancy (70% during the 3rd trimester) and is characterized by pruritus. Jaundice occurs in about 25% of patients. Intrahepatic cholestasis of pregnancy is a benign condition that usually disappears after pregnancy. Affected individuals are at higher risk of developing a recurrence with subsequent pregnancies. A similar picture may develop when these individuals take oral contraceptives.

End of Section.

STEP 18 – *What Is the Etiology of the Hepatocellular Disease?*

Hepatocellular diseases associated with jaundice are listed in the following box.

HEPATOCELLULAR DISEASES ASSOCIATED WITH JAUNDICE	
Alcoholic hepatitis	Hepatic vein thrombosis
α_1-antitrypsin deficiency	Hepatotoxins
Autoimmune hepatitis	Ischemia
Cirrhosis	Viral hepatitis (acute or chronic)
Drug-induced	Wilson's disease
Hemochromatosis	

Some of the more common hepatocellular diseases are considered below.

Acute Viral Hepatitis

Acute viral hepatitis may manifest without any symptoms or signs. In these cases, the illness comes to clinical attention because of abnormal liver function tests along with serologic evidence of acute viral hepatitis. When symptomatic, patients with acute viral hepatitis often share some common features, irrespective of the viral etiology. Early in the course of the illness, patients may complain of malaise, fatigue, nausea, vomiting, anorexia, abdominal discomfort, and joint pain. On occasion, patients complain of losing the desire to drink alcohol or smoke cigarettes. Other complaints include low-grade fever and headache. These symptoms typically last 3-4 days but may linger for 2-3 weeks. This prodromal phase of the illness is followed by the icteric phase. During this phase, many patients note a darkening of the urine followed by stool discoloration and jaundice. It is important to realize that not all patients progress to the icteric phase (anicteric hepatitis).

Physical examination reveals a tender liver in up to 66% of patients. Fifteen percent of patients have mild splenomegaly.

At the time of clinical symptoms, patients with acute viral hepatitis usually have reached their peak AST and ALT levels. Levels may exceed 1000 U/L. Other findings include hyperbilirubinemia and a mild elevation in alkaline phosphatase. Identifying the specific viral etiology requires serologic testing. The following table lists the serologic tests (for the common causes of viral hepatitis) that should be obtained in the patient suspected of having acute viral hepatitis.

Viral Agent	Serologic Finding in Acute Viral Hepatitis
Hepatitis A	IgM anti-HAV
Hepatitis B	HB_sAg IgM anti-HB_c
Hepatitis C	Anti-HCV*

*Anti-HCV may not be detectable early in the course of acute hepatitis C. In these cases, it may be worthwhile to repeat the anti-HCV after a sufficient period of time has elapsed. Alternatively, the clinician may elect to obtain hepatitis C viral RNA to establish the diagnosis.

Chronic Viral Hepatitis

Jaundice is a cardinal manifestation of a number of chronic hepatocellular diseases. Chronic viral hepatitis is one such consideration. The major viral causes of chronic hepatitis are hepatitis B and C. Although patients with either chronic hepatitis B or C may recall a history of distant acute hepatitis, in many cases, no such history can be elicited. Most patients with chronic viral hepatitis are asymptomatic. Not uncommonly, chronic viral hepatitis comes to clinical attention only because of persistent liver function test abnormalities.

When symptoms are present, they are often nonspecific symptoms such as malaise, fatigue, and anorexia. Physical examination may reveal the stigmata of chronic liver disease such as prominent abdominal veins, spider angiomas, and gynecomastia. With advancing disease, patients with chronic viral hepatitis may present with jaundice and complications of portal hypertension. These complications include ascites, encephalopathy, and variceal hemorrhage. Viral serology for hepatitis B and C are necessary in patients suspected of having chronic viral hepatitis.

Alcoholic Hepatitis

Most patients with alcoholic hepatitis present with anorexia, malaise, fever, and abdominal pain. Physical examination often reveals scleral icterus, spider angiomas, and tender hepatomegaly. Portal hypertension may be evident in severe cases of alcoholic hepatitis. In these cases, the clinician may note splenomegaly, prominent abdominal veins, ascites, and encephalopathy.

Transaminase levels rarely exceed 300-400 U/L. Levels exceeding this should prompt the clinician to consider other causes of liver disease. In many cases, the AST to ALT ratio exceeds 2. Such a ratio in a patient with modest transaminase levels should always warrant consideration of alcoholic hepatitis. It is important to realize, however, that alcoholic hepatitis may present with an AST to ALT ratio <2.

Cirrhosis

The causes of cirrhosis are listed in the following box.

CAUSES OF CIRRHOSIS	
FAIRLY COMMON	**RARE**
Ethanol	α_1-antitrypsin deficiency
Viral	Cystic fibrosis
Hepatitis B (with or without D)	Drug-induced
Hepatitis C	Glycogen storage diseases
LESS COMMON	Jejunoileal bypass
Autoimmune hepatitis	Sarcoidosis
Cryptogenic cirrhosis	Wilson's disease
Hemochromatosis	
Primary biliary cirrhosis	
Primary sclerosing cholangitis	
Secondary biliary cirrhosis	

Many patients, particularly in the early stages of cirrhosis, are asymptomatic. With progression of the liver disease, nonspecific complaints of anorexia, malaise, fatigue, and weight loss may ensue. Complications of portal hypertension may occur in patients with advanced disease.

Although liver function tests may support the diagnosis, it is important to realize that they may be normal. A decreased serum albumin and an elevated prothrombin time are common in advanced disease, reflecting an impairment in hepatic synthetic function. Hypersplenism is a complication of portal hypertension and may result in anemia, thrombocytopenia, or leukopenia. Hyponatremia is a poor prognostic finding in patients with cirrhosis.

Elucidating the etiology of the cirrhosis often requires other laboratory testing. When the etiology is not clear, the clinician should consider obtaining the following tests:

Condition	Recommended Laboratory Tests
Hepatitis B	Hepatitis B surface antigen If positive, consider hepatitis D testing
Hepatitis C	Antibody to hepatitis C virus Hepatitis C viral RNA
Autoimmune hepatitis	Antinuclear antibodies Antismooth muscle antibodies Antiliver-kidney microsomal antibodies
Hemochromatosis	Ferritin Iron Total iron-binding capacity Transferrin
α_1-antitrypsin deficiency	Serum protein electrophoresis
Wilson's disease	Serum ceruloplasmin
Primary biliary cirrhosis	Antimichrondrial antibodies

Imaging studies are useful in providing evidence of cirrhosis or portal hypertension. In addition, complications of cirrhosis such as hepatocellular carcinoma may be detected.

Ultrasonographic findings that suggest the diagnosis of cirrhosis include the following:

- Dense reflective areas of irregular distribution and increased echogenicity

- Demonstration of a coarsely nodular liver surface
- Relatively enlarged caudate lobe
- Evidence of portal hypertension (portal vein diameter >1.4 cm, ascites, splenomegaly, portosystemic collaterals)

In addition, ultrasound may demonstrate a liver lesion, raising concern for hepatocellular carcinoma. Cirrhosis is a risk factor for the development of hepatocellular carcinoma.

CT findings may be normal in the early stages of cirrhosis. In advanced disease, the liver may be small with irregular edges and demonstrate inhomogeneous contrast enhancement. Not uncommonly, the caudate lobe is disproportionately larger than the other lobes of the liver. Findings of portal hypertension that may be demonstrated on CT include ascites, splenomegaly, and portosystemic collaterals.

Another imaging option available is 99mTc-sulfur colloid scintigraphy, which can assess liver size and blood flow. Heterogeneous uptake in the liver along with an increased uptake in the spleen and bone marrow are findings suggestive of cirrhosis. When these findings are present, a colloid shift is said to be present.

Taken together, the patient's clinical presentation, laboratory tests, and imaging studies can provide evidence that supports the diagnosis of cirrhosis. The definitive diagnosis, however, requires liver biopsy. In addition to confirming the presence of cirrhosis, the findings may point to a particular etiology, such as hemochromatosis.

Drug-Induced Liver Disease

Up to 5% of cases of jaundice in hospitalized patients are due to drug-induced liver disease. Drug-induced liver disease can take many forms including asymptomatic elevation in the transaminase levels, acute hepatitis, and fulminant hepatic failure. Most often, the clinician encounters the asymptomatic patient who has transaminase elevations secondary to a particular medication. The prevalence of hepatic enzyme elevation (in the asymptomatic patient) with various drugs is shown in the following table.

Prevalence (%)	Examples	Prevalence (%)	Examples
25-50	Tacrine	5-10	Chenodeoxycholate
20-25	Amiodarone		Disulfiram
	Chlorpromazine		Flucytosine
	Cisplatin		Penicillamine
	6-mercaptopurine	<5	Dantrolene
	Nicotinic acid		Ethionamide
	Papaverine		Gold salts
	Phenytoin		Quinidine
	Valproate		Salicylates
10-20	Androgens		Sulfonamides
	Erythromycin estolate		Sulfonylureas
	Etretinate		Ticarcillin
	Isoniazid		Tricyclic antidepressants
	Ketoconazole		

Adapted from *Clinical Practice of Gastroenterology*, Brandt LJ (ed), Philadelphia, PA: Current Medicine, Inc, 1999, 856.

Drug-induced liver disease can cause hepatocellular injury, cholestatic injury, or a mixed pattern. Medications that are predominantly associated with hepatocellular injury are listed in the following box.

MEDICATIONS CAUSING HEPATOCELLULAR INJURY	
ANESTHETICS	ANTIARRHYTHMICS
Enflurane	Amiodarone
Halothane	Procainamide
Methoxyflurane	Quinidine
ANTICONVULSANTS	LIPID-LOWERING AGENTS
Phenytoin	Nicotinic acid
Valproic acid	Statins
MAO INHIBITORS	ANTIBIOTICS
ANALGESIC	ANTIVIRAL AGENTS
Acetaminophen	AZT
NSAIDs	Didanosine
Salicylates	ANTINEOPLASTIC AGENTS
ANTITHYROID	MISCELLANEOUS
Propylthiouracil	Disulfiram
STEROIDS / HORMONAL AGENTS	Etretinate
Diethylstilbestrol	Loratadine
Tamoxifen	Pemoline
ANTIHYPERTENSIVES	Sulfasalazine
ACE-inhibitors	Tacrine
α-methyldopa	Tannic acid
β-blockers	Vitamin A
Hydralazine	
Verapamil	

The clinical presentation of drug-induced liver disease varies. The subclinical hepatic enzyme elevation that occurs with many different medications often does not lead to clinically significant liver disease despite continuing the offending medication. When a medication causes considerable hepatocellular necrosis, symptoms and signs resembling acute viral hepatitis may occur. In these cases, the degree of transaminase elevation may mimic that found in viral hepatitis.

A classic example is isoniazid hepatotoxicity. While subclinical hepatic enzyme elevation is more common, overt hepatitis occurs in 1% of patients receiving isoniazid. The risk of developing clinically significant hepatotoxicity increases with advancing age. The risk of hepatotoxicity is also increased when the medication is used in conjunction with rifampin or pyrazinamide.

Another example of drug-induced liver disease is acetaminophen hepatotoxicity, a major cause of fulminant hepatic failure. Characteristic of acetaminophen hepatotoxicity is a rise in the transaminase levels to >10,000 U/L.

Drug-induced liver disease should be suspected in any patient who presents with overt liver disease. Establishing the diagnosis begins with the exclusion of other causes of hepatocellular injury such as viral and alcoholic hepatitis. In drug-induced liver disease, resolution of the signs and symptoms along with normalization of the liver function test abnormalities following drug discontinuation provides a strong argument for the diagnosis. Rechallenging a patient with the suspect medication is not without risk. In patients who developed jaundice or other manifestations of liver disease, rechallenging the patient to confirm the diagnosis is not recommended. In those who had subclinical hepatic enzyme elevation, it is, however, possible to rechallenge the patient. Consultation with a hepatologist is recommended in these cases.

REFERENCES

Clinical Practice of Gastroenterology, Brandt LJ (ed), Philadelphia, PA: Current Medicine, Inc, 1999, 856.

Frank BB, "Clinical Evaluation of Jaundice. A Guideline of the Patient Care Committee of the American Gastroenterological Association," *JAMA*, 1989, 262(21):3031-4.

McGill JM and Kwiatkowski AP, "Cholestatic Liver Diseases in Adults," *Am J Gastroenterol*, 1998, 93(5):684-91.

Pasha TM and Lindor KD, "Diagnosis and Therapy of Cholestatic Liver Disease," *Med Clin North Am*, 1996, 80(5):995-1019.

Rossi RL, Traverso LW, and Pimentel F, "Malignant Obstructive Jaundice. Evaluation and Management," *Surg Clin North Am*, 1996, 76(1):63-70.

JAUNDICE

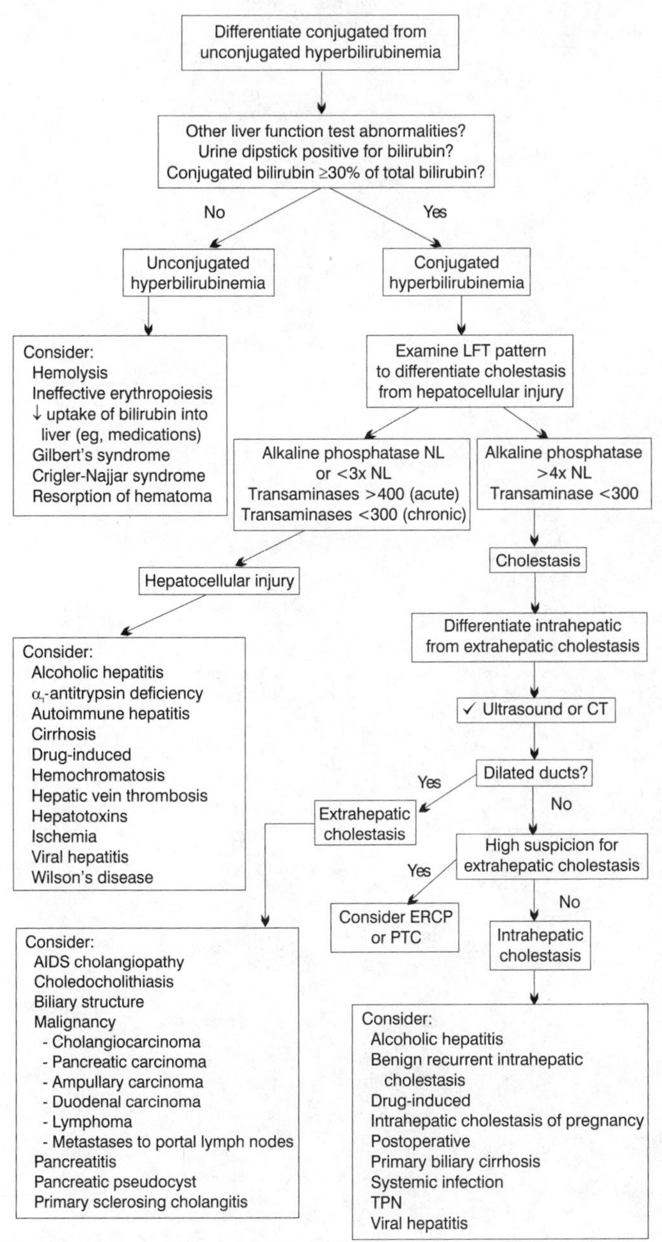
Differentiate conjugated from unconjugated hyperbilirubinemia
Other liver function test abnormalities? Urine dipstick positive for bilirubin? Conjugated bilirubin ≥30% of total bilirubin?
No
Yes
Unconjugated hyperbilirubinemia
Conjugated hyperbilirubinemia
Consider: Hemolysis; Ineffective erythropoiesis; ↓ uptake of bilirubin into liver (eg, medications); Gilbert's syndrome; Crigler-Najjar syndrome; Resorption of hematoma
Examine LFT pattern to differentiate cholestasis from hepatocellular injury
Alkaline phosphatase NL or <3x NL; Transaminases >400 (acute); Transaminases <300 (chronic)
Alkaline phosphatase >4x NL; Transaminase <300
Hepatocellular injury
Cholestasis
Consider: Alcoholic hepatitis; α1-antitrypsin deficiency; Autoimmune hepatitis; Cirrhosis; Drug-induced; Hemochromatosis; Hepatic vein thrombosis; Hepatotoxins; Ischemia; Viral hepatitis; Wilson's disease
Differentiate intrahepatic from extrahepatic cholestasis
✓ Ultrasound or CT
Dilated ducts?
Yes
No
Extrahepatic cholestasis
High suspicion for extrahepatic cholestasis
Yes
No
Consider ERCP or PTC
Intrahepatic cholestasis
Consider: AIDS cholangiopathy; Choledocholithiasis; Biliary structure; Malignancy - Cholangiocarcinoma - Pancreatic carcinoma - Ampullary carcinoma - Duodenal carcinoma - Lymphoma - Metastases to portal lymph nodes; Pancreatitis; Pancreatic pseudocyst; Primary sclerosing cholangitis
Consider: Alcoholic hepatitis; Benign recurrent intrahepatic cholestasis; Drug-induced; Intrahepatic cholestasis of pregnancy; Postoperative; Primary biliary cirrhosis; Systemic infection; TPN; Viral hepatitis

ACUTE VIRAL HEPATITIS

Acute viral hepatitis is characterized by hepatocellular necrosis. Elevated transaminases are the first laboratory abnormalities appreciated in patients with acute viral hepatitis and are often the last to resolve. The increase in transaminase levels begins in the late incubation period and usually peaks at the time jaundice is noted. There is no established diagnostic level for acute viral hepatitis as the peak transaminase level may vary from 3-100 times normal. Levels that exceed 100 times normal are very unusual in acute viral hepatitis and should prompt the clinician to consider other etiologies, particularly toxic and ischemic causes.

The ratio of AST to ALT is typically <1. In rare instances, the ratio may be >1 and even >2. This is likely to occur when viral hepatitis develops in the setting of preexisting alcoholic liver disease. In acute hepatitis due to coinfection with hepatitis B and D, there may be two transaminase peaks. The first peak corresponds to hepatitis B, followed later by a second peak from hepatitis D.

The bilirubin commonly rises, but rarely exceeds 20 mg/dL. Alkaline phosphatase also increases, but seldom climbs above three times the upper limit of normal. It may, however, be higher in the cholestatic variant of acute viral hepatitis. Hypoalbuminemia and increased PT are uncommon in most cases of acute viral hepatitis. Their presence should prompt consideration of severe, subfulminant, or fulminant disease.

These laboratory test findings are summarized in the following box.

ACUTE VIRAL HEPATITIS — LABORATORY FINDINGS

INCREASED TRANSAMINASES*
INCREASED BILIRUBIN†
NORMAL / INCREASED ALK PHOSPHATASE
PT / PTT NORMAL OR INCREASED (USUALLY)‡
NORMAL OR MILD DECREASE IN HEMOGLOBIN
NORMAL OR DECREASED WBC§
ATYPICAL LYMPHOCYTES
RELATIVE LYMPHOCYTOSIS
NORMAL OR DECREASED PLATELETS
NORMAL / SLIGHTLY DECREASED SERUM ALBUMIN
INCREASED FERRITIN
INCREASED SERUM IRON
INCREASED ESR
RARE COMPLICATIONS
- Pure red cell aplasia
- Aplastic anemia
- Membranous glomerulonephritis
- DIC
- Agranulocytosis
- Hemolytic anemia

*Transaminase levels peak near the onset of jaundice. Thereafter, there is a gradual fall in the transaminase levels. In acute viral hepatitis, the fall is typically slow, decreasing at an average of about 10% to 12% per day. AST and ALT levels remain elevated for 22±16 and 27±16 days, respectively. Once the transaminase levels have been noted to consistently decrease, there is no need to measure levels until the patient's signs and symptoms of acute viral hepatitis have resolved. The clinician should realize, however, that normalization of the transaminase level does not imply eradication of the hepatitis virus and recovery from infection. For example, patients with acute hepatitis B or C viral infection may go on to develop chronic infection which may be associated with normal transaminase levels. The clinician should also be aware of relapsing hepatitis, which most commonly occurs in acute hepatitis A viral infection. In relapsing hepatitis, signs, symptoms, and liver function test abnormalities recur weeks to months after the patient's condition has improved. With the relapse, the transaminases, which may have been normal or near-normal, rise again. Peak transaminase levels, at times, exceed the levels reached during the initial bout of the illness.

†In most cases, the serum bilirubin levels peaks about one week after the transaminase levels peak. Thereafter, there is a gradual decrease in the serum bilirubin level. Peak values exceeding 15-20 mg/dL are uncommon. Only 4% of patients with acute viral hepatitis have peak bilirubin levels exceeding 20 mg/dL (rarely does the level exceed 30 mg/dL). One study demonstrated that bilirubin levels are increased on average for 30± 20 days after peak levels are reached. On occasion, prolonged and marked hyperbilirubinemia may be noted, particularly in patients with hepatitis A viral infection. These patients are said to have cholestatic hepatitis. In this form of the disease, alkaline phosphatase levels are usually elevated but not to a striking degree.

‡More severe disease is suggested by a PT that is >4 seconds above reference limits.

§WBC >12,000 cells/mm^3 is rare unless fulminant hepatic failure develops.

Viral serology is indicated in all patients with acute viral hepatitis to not only confirm a viral etiology but also to determine the viral agent responsible for the illness. There are no clinical features that allow the clinician to discriminate reliably between the different causes of viral hepatitis. In patients with acute hepatic injury, testing for hepatitis A, B, and C should routinely be performed, as shown in the following table.

Essential Viral Serology in Acute Viral Hepatitis

Viral Agent	Recommended Testing
Hepatitis A*	IgM anti-HAV
Hepatitis B†	HB_sAg, IgM anti-HB_c
Hepatitis C‡	Anti-HCV

*On occasion, the IgM anti-HAV may be undetectable at the time of testing. In these patients, it is worthwhile to repeat testing in 1-2 weeks.

†Although HB_sAg usually precedes IgM anti-HB_c, both are typically present at the time of symptom onset. In patients who recover from acute hepatitis B viral infection, HB_sAg disappears several weeks to months after it appears. Loss of HB_sAg positivity occurs before disappearance of IgM anti-HBc. The clinician can rule out acute hepatitis B viral infection if both HB_sAg and IgM anti-HB_c are undetectable. Other hepatitis B viral markers and antibodies are not useful in the diagnosis of acute hepatitis B viral infection.

‡Anti-HCV testing has several limitations in the diagnosis of acute hepatitis C viral infection. When second-generation enzyme immunoassays (EIA-II) are used, 80% to 90% of patients with acute hepatitis C viral infection will be diagnosed by the presence of detectable anti-HCV. To detect the other 10% to 20% of patients with acute hepatitis C viral infection, the clinician has several choices. First, anti-HCV testing may be repeated 4-6 weeks later; conversion from negative to positive anti-HCV supports the diagnosis of acute hepatitis C viral infection. Alternatively, the clinician may wish to test for HCV RNA, which is the earliest marker of acute hepatitis C viral infection. HCV RNA appears just a few weeks after exposure.

Not all patients with acute viral hepatitis should be tested for hepatitis D viral infection. Patients who should be tested for antibodies to hepatitis D virus (anti-HDV) include the following.

- Patients with positive HB_sAg, especially if the patient has any of the following characteristics.
  - severe acute hepatitis
  - high risk for hepatitis D viral infection (ie, I.V. drug abuse)
  - biphasic pattern of illness
- Patients with history of chronic hepatitis B, who now present with severe acute hepatic injury or failure (suggestive of superinfection with hepatitis D viral infection)

As with hepatitis D, not all patients with acute hepatic injury require testing for hepatitis E. In the United States, hepatitis E is an unusual cause of acute viral hepatitis. It should be a consideration in patients who report a history of recent travel. It also deserves consideration in new immigrants with acute hepatic injury. For further information regarding the diagnosis of acute hepatitis D and E viral infection, see the chapters, ***Hepatitis D** on page 683* and ***Hepatitis E** on page 687*, respectively.

In patients who are diagnosed with acute hepatitis B viral infection, the clinician should repeat HB_sAg and anti-HB_s within 6-12 months. No further evaluation is necessary in patients who are negative for HB_sAg and positive for anti-HB_s. These patients have recovered from the hepatitis B viral infection and are not at risk for chronic hepatitis B. Persistence of HB_sAg for more than 6 months is indicative of chronic hepatitis B viral infection.

In patients who are diagnosed with acute hepatitis C viral infection, most will develop chronic hepatitis C. The diagnosis is based on the demonstration of persistent ALT elevation or HCV RNA in the serum for >6 months. Refer to the chapter, ***Chronic Viral Hepatitis** on page 663.*

References

Farrell GC, "Acute Viral Hepatitis," *Med J Aust*, 1998, 168(11):565-70.

Gill RQ and Sterling RK, "Acute Liver Failure," *J Clin Gastroenterol*, 2001, 33(3):191-8

Pappas SC, "Fulminant Viral Hepatitis," *Gastroenterol Clin North Am*, 1995, 24(1):161-73.

Regev A and Schiff ER, "Viral Hepatitis A, B, and C," *Clin Liver Dis*, 2000, 4(1):47-71, vi.

Ryder SD and Beckingham IJ, "ABC of Diseases of Liver, Pancreas, and Biliary System: Acute Hepatitis," *BMJ*, 2001, 322(7279):151-3.

Sheorey SH and Waters MJ, "Viral Hepatitis? Which Test Should I Order? " *Aust Fam Physician*, 2001, 30(5):433-7.

Weston SR and Martin P, "Serological and Molecular Testing in Viral Hepatitis: An Update," *Can J Gastroenterol*, 2001, 15(3):177-84.

CHRONIC VIRAL HEPATITIS

Although chronic viral hepatitis is just one cause of chronic hepatic injury, it is certainly the most common cause. Of the viral causes of hepatitis, hepatitis B and C are the major causes of chronic viral hepatitis. In the United States alone, approximately 2.5 million people have chronic hepatitis C viral infection. Another 1 to 1.25 million people are chronic carriers of hepatitis B.

In most cases, evaluation for chronic viral hepatitis begins when transaminases are found to be chronically elevated. The clinician should realize, however, that persistently normal ALT levels do not exclude the diagnosis of chronic hepatitis B or C viral infection. In fact, 15% to 30% of patients with chronic hepatitis C viral infection have persistently or intermittently normal ALT levels. Part of this may be due to the fact that these patients have fluctuations in the ALT level; that is, the ALT level fluctuates between normal and abnormal. The likelihood of persistently normal ALT levels decreases with multiple ALT measurements over time. In patients with chronic hepatitis C viral infection who have persistently normal ALT levels, liver biopsy usually reveals milder inflammation and lower rate of progression to cirrhosis than in their counterparts who have elevated ALT levels.

Viral serology for hepatitis B and C should certainly be obtained if ALT levels are increased on more than one occasion, particularly if another cause for the elevation is not present. If viral serology is only restricted to this group of patients, many individuals with chronic hepatitis B or C who have normal ALT levels will go undiagnosed. Therefore, in patients who have risk factors for chronic hepatitis B or C viral infection, viral serology for hepatitis B and C should be obtained, irrespective of the ALT level. Risk factors for chronic viral hepatitis are listed in the following box.

RISK FACTORS FOR CHRONIC VIRAL HEPATITIS
ESTABLISHED RISK FACTORS
Injection drug use
Chronic hemodialysis
Blood transfusion or transplantation prior to 1992
Receipt of blood (including needlestick) from a donor subsequently testing positive for hepatitis C viral infection
Receipt of clotting factor concentrates produced before 1987
Asian ancestry (endemic areas for hepatitis B viral infection)
Unvaccinated healthcare workers (hepatitis B viral infection)
Birth to mother with chronic hepatitis B or C viral infection
POSSIBLE RISK FACTORS
Body piercing or tattooing
Multiple sexual partners or sexually transmitted diseases
Healthcare workers (hepatitis C viral infection)
Contacts of hepatitis C viral infection positive persons

In patients suspected of having chronic viral hepatitis, the following tests of viral serology should be obtained.

- HB_sAg: Chronic hepatitis B viral infection is said to be present if persistence of HB_sAg is demonstrated for more than 6 months.
- Anti-HCV: While a positive anti-HCV test in the patient suspected of having chronic hepatitis C viral infection is suggestive of the diagnosis, the clinician should realize that the antibody is detectable in patients who have recovered from the infection as well. It is said that 15% to 25% of patients who become infected with the hepatitis C virus recover from the infection. To distinguish these patients who have recovered from others who have chronic hepatitis C viral infection, it is

necessary to obtain a qualitative HCV RNA test. The presence of HCV RNA confirms the diagnosis of chronic hepatitis C viral infection. A negative result should prompt the clinician to repeat the test, particularly in patients with an elevated ALT level.

Another cause of chronic viral hepatitis, chronic delta hepatitis, will not be discussed here. Please refer to the chapter, ***Hepatitis D*** *on page 683*.

References

Alexander G and Walsh K, "Chronic Viral Hepatitis," *Int J Clin Pract*, 2000, 54(7):450-6.

Farrell GC, "Chronic Viral Hepatitis," *Med J Aust*, 1998, 168(12):619-26.

O'Connor JA, "Acute and Chronic Viral Hepatitis," *Adolesc Med*, 2000, 11(2):279-92.

Ryder SD and Beckingham IJ, "ABC of Diseases of Liver, Pancreas, and Biliary System: Chronic Viral Hepatitis," *BMJ*, 2001, 322(7280):219-21.

Saab S and Martin P, "Tests for Acute and Chronic Viral Hepatitis. Finding Your Way Through the Alphabet Soup of Infection and Superinfection," *Postgrad Med*, 2000, 107(2):123-6, 129-30.

Walsh K and Alexander GJ, "Update on Chronic Viral Hepatitis," *Postgrad Med J*, 2001, 77(910):498-505.

Weston SR and Martin P, "Serological and Molecular Testing in Viral Hepatitis: An Update," *Can J Gastroenterol*, 2001, 15(3):177-84.

HEPATITIS A

In general, there are no particular signs and symptoms of acute hepatitis A viral infection that allow it to be distinguished from other viral causes of hepatitis. Laboratory diagnosis is essential in differentiating acute hepatitis A from other causes of acute viral hepatitis.

Liver Function Tests in Acute Hepatitis A Viral Infection

Liver function test abnormalities do not allow the clinician to distinguish acute hepatitis A viral infection from other causes of viral hepatitis. Liver function test abnormalities as well as other laboratory test findings in acute viral hepatitis have been discussed in the chapter, ***Acute Viral Hepatitis*** *on page 659*.

Establishing the Diagnosis of Acute Hepatitis A Viral Infection

The diagnosis of acute hepatitis A viral infection is based on the presence of IgM anti-HAV antibody, which appears 1-2 weeks after exposure. This antibody is indicative of a recent or current hepatitis A viral infection (within the past 6 months). The IgM component usually disappears by 4-6 months. However, persistence of this antibody for up to 1 year has been reported in a minority of patients. In one study, 86% of patients were IgM anti-HAV negative by 7 months after onset of symptoms.

The sensitivity and specificity of IgM anti-HAV measurement for the diagnosis of acute hepatitis A viral infection is 100% and 99%, respectively. On occasion, the test is negative at the time of clinical presentation. In these patients, a repeat test done 1-2 weeks later will usually reveal positivity.

Some patients with acute hepatitis A viral infection have relapsing infection. Studies have shown that up to 4% to 20% of patients with hepatitis A will suffer a relapse, usually 30-90 days after onset of icteric phase. In these patients, seemingly full recovery is followed by a flare characterized by signs and symptoms of hepatitis along with transaminase elevation. With a clinical relapse, there is usually a rise in the IgM anti-HAV. More than one relapse may occur and, in some patients, it may take up to 1 year for transaminase levels to return to normal. Eventually, full recovery does take place but, in these patients, IgM anti-HAV may be detectable for a prolonged period of time (1-2 years).

The IgG anti-HAV antibody, which is detectable 5-6 weeks after exposure, will remain positive indefinitely, imparting immunity against future infection with hepatitis A.

In summary, then, the diagnostic test of choice for the diagnosis of acute hepatitis A viral infection is the IgM anti-HAV. The IgM anti-HAV needs to be differentiated from the total anti-HAV. The latter includes measurement of both IgM anti-HAV and IgG anti-HAV. If the patient has a positive total anti-HAV but negative IgM anti-HAV, this is indicative of immunity consistent with either past infection or vaccination.

Serologic Pattern in the Diagnosis of Hepatitis A

Virus	Acute Illness	Convalescence
Hepatitis A	Total anti-HAV positive IgM anti-HAV positive	Total anti-HAV positive Appearance of IgG anti-HAV Disappearance of IgM anti-HAV

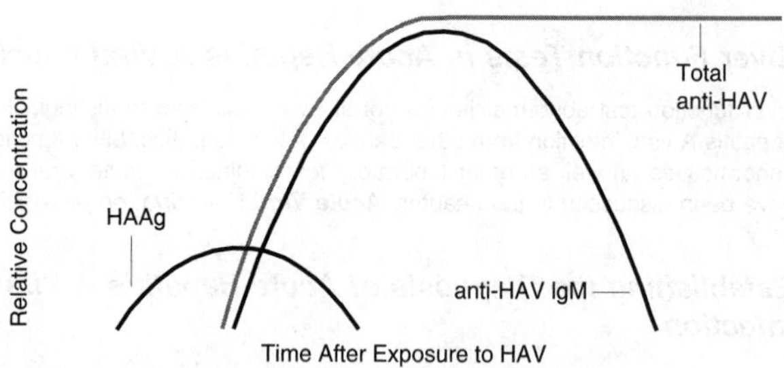

Reprinted from Abbott Diagnostics

References

Cuthbert JA, "Hepatitis A: Old and New," *Clin Microbiol Rev*, 2001, 14(1):38-58.

Farrell GC, "Acute Viral Hepatitis," *Med J Aust*, 1998, 168(11):565-70.

Kemmer NM and Miskovsky EP, "Hepatitis A," *Infect Dis Clin North Am*, 2000, 14(3):605-15.

Koff RS, "Hepatitis A," *Lancet*, 1998, 351(9116):1643-9.

Lemon SM, "Type A Viral Hepatitis: Epidemiology, Diagnosis, and Prevention," *Clin Chem*, 1997, 43(8 Pt 2):1494-9.

Regev A and Schiff ER, "Viral Hepatitis A, B, and C," *Clin Liver Dis*, 2000, 4(1):47-71, vi.

Ryder SD and Beckingham IJ, "ABC of Diseases of Liver, Pancreas, and Biliary System: Acute Hepatitis," *BMJ*, 2001, 322(7279):151-3.

Sacher RA, Peters SM, and Bryan JA, "Testing for Viral Hepatitis. A Practice Parameter," *Am J Clin Pathol*, 2000, 113(1):12-7.

Weston SR and Martin P, "Serological and Molecular Testing in Viral Hepatitis: An Update," *Can J Gastroenterol*, 2001, 15(3):177-84.

HEPATITIS B

VIRAL SEROLOGY

Hepatitis B Surface Antigen (HB_sAg)

In acute viral hepatitis B infection, HB_sAg is the first identified serologic marker, usually appearing 2-6 weeks before symptom onset (appears 1-10 weeks after exposure). HB_sAg positivity can be demonstrated before any rise in the transaminase levels. It disappears from the serum a few weeks to a few months after it is initially detected. In approximately 10% of patients, HB_sAg is not detectable at the time of presentation. In these patients, the clinician may miss the diagnosis of acute hepatitis B viral infection if an IgM anti-HB_c test is not obtained (see below).

It is important for the clinician to realize, however, that acute hepatitis associated with the presence of the HB_sAg is not synonymous with acute hepatitis B viral infection. There are many conditions which can cause acute hepatic injury in the patient with chronic hepatitis B viral infection, thus mimicking acute hepatitis B viral infection. These conditions include the exacerbation of chronic hepatitis B viral infection (HB_eAg seroconversion to anti-HB_e), hepatitis B virus reactivation, superinfection with other hepatotropic viruses (A, C, D, E, CMV, EBV), other infections (rickettsia, leptospirosis), alcohol, drugs, and ischemia.

In some patients, HB_sAg persists. Persistence of this antigen beyond 6 months suggests chronic hepatitis B viral infection.

Hepatitis E Antigen (HB_eAg)

In the setting of acute hepatitis B viral infection, HB_eAg usually appears in the serum shortly after HB_sAg is detected. This antigen is a measure of active viral replication, along with hepatitis B viral DNA (HBV DNA). It is a qualitative marker for infectivity. If infection resolves, the HB_eAg disappears from the serum shortly before the HB_sAg.

Hepatitis B Viral DNA (HBV DNA)

Like the HB_eAg, HBV DNA is a marker of active viral replication. In patients who recover from acute hepatitis B viral infection, it appears and disappears in the serum about the same time as HB_eAg. In patients with chronic hepatitis B infection, serum HBV DNA levels play a major role in the selection of candidates for antiviral therapy. Patients who have pretreatment serum HBV DNA levels exceeding 200 pg/mL are less likely to respond to interferon therapy. Serum HBV DNA levels are also measured after therapy to assess the patient's response to treatment.

Antibody to Hepatitis B Core Antigen (Anti-HB_c)

Anti-HB_c appears in the serum shortly after HB_sAg is first detected. It also appears prior to the detection of the antibody to HB_sAg (anti-HB_s). There are two types of anti-HB_c; IgM anti-HB_c and IgG anti-HB_c. In acute hepatitis B viral infection, it is the IgM anti-HB_c that is detectable. The IgM anti-HB_c is useful in the diagnosis of acute hepatitis B viral infection, particularly in the so-called "window period ". The window period is that period of time between the disappearance of HB_sAg and the appearance of anti-HB_s. IgM anti-HB_c needs to be measured in every patient suspected of acute hepatitis B viral infection. This ensures that the 10% of patients who have lost the HB_sAg, and are in the window period, will not be missed during serologic testing. After about 6-8 months, IgM anti-HB_c disappears from the serum of patients. Nevertheless, testing for anti-HB_c will remain positive in the form of IgG for many years.

Although patients with chronic hepatitis B typically have positive IgG anti-HB_c, with disease flares or exacerbations, there may be a rise in the IgM anti-HB_c

titer to detectable levels. This can lead to diagnostic confusion, especially when patients not previously known to have chronic hepatitis B present with a disease flare. In these cases, patients may erroneously be diagnosed as having acute hepatitis B viral infection rather than an exacerbation of chronic hepatitis B.

In some patients, hepatitis B serology is unremarkable except for the presence of anti-HB_c. These patients are said to be isolated anti-HB_c positive patients. When this situation is encountered, three possibilities should be considered as an explanation for this serologic pattern. These include the following:

- Window period of acute hepatitis B viral infection

  Approximately 10% of patients with acute hepatitis B viral infection present in the window period. During this time period, HB_sAg has fallen below the cut-off level for detection and anti-HB_s has not risen to detectable levels. In these cases, the diagnosis of acute hepatitis B viral infection is confirmed by the presence of IgM anti-HB_c.

- Recovery from hepatitis B viral infection

  Hepatitis B serology performed many years after recovery from hepatitis B viral infection may be negative for anti-HB_s. In these cases, anti-HB_s levels have fallen to undetectable levels and the only evidence of past infection is the presence of IgG anti-HB_c.

- Chronic hepatitis B viral infection

  Although most patients with chronic hepatitis B viral infection have detectable HB_sAg levels, after many years of infection, titers may decrease to undetectable levels. In these cases, the presence of isolated anti-HB_c may be an indication of chronic disease.

When a patient is encountered with an isolated anti-HB_c, serologic testing (anti-HB_c, HB_sAg, anti-HB_s) should be repeated to confirm the presence of the abnormality. If the patient continues to test positive for anti-HB_c, IgM anti-HB_c should be measured. If positive, the patient should be evaluated for recent acute hepatitis B viral infection. In patients who have a clinical presentation consistent with chronic liver disease, testing for HBV DNA should be performed to rule out chronic hepatitis B viral infection.

Antibody to Hepatitis B Surface Antigen (Anti-HB_s)

In patients who recover from acute hepatitis B viral infection, anti-HB_s is detected shortly after the disappearance of the HB_sAg. Anti-HB_s remains detectable for years to come. In a minority, however, there may be disappearance of anti-HB_s. Anti-HB_s is also the only antibody produced during vaccination.

ACUTE HEPATITIS B VIRAL INFECTION

The clinical presentation of acute viral hepatitis B infection is similar to that seen with other viral causes of hepatitis. Because there are no features in the clinical presentation that are discriminating enough to allow the clinician to make the distinction, diagnosis of acute hepatitis B viral infection is based upon the results of viral serologic testing.

Liver Function Tests in Acute Hepatitis B Viral Infection

Liver function test abnormalities do not allow the clinician to distinguish acute hepatitis B viral infection from other causes of viral hepatitis. Liver function test abnormalities as well as other laboratory test findings of acute viral hepatitis have been discussed in the chapter, ***Acute Viral Hepatitis** on page 659*.

Establishing the Diagnosis of Acute Hepatitis B Viral Infection

To confirm the diagnosis of acute hepatitis B viral infection, the following tests should be ordered:

- HB_sAg
- IgM anti-HB_c

Remember that most patients with acute hepatitis B will have the HB_sAg. Only 10% will present at a time in their illness when the HB_sAg is negative. A positive IgM anti-HB_c will establish diagnosis in these patients. Serologic findings in patients with acute hepatitis B viral infection are summarized in the following table.

Serologic Markers in Acute Hepatitis B Viral Infection

Phase of Acute Hepatitis B Viral Infection	Serologic Markers Present
Early phase of acute hepatitis B viral infection	HB_sAg
	IgM anti-HB_c
	HB_eAg*
	HBV DNA*
Window period	IgM anti-HB_c
Recovery	Anti-HB_s
	IgG anti-HB_c

*It is not necessary to order HBV DNA or HB_eAg. Although these are likely to be positive, they add very little in the way of useful information in the diagnosis of acute hepatitis.

CHRONIC HEPATITIS B VIRAL INFECTION

When HB_sAg persists for more than 6 months, a diagnosis of chronic hepatitis B has been established. The highest risk of developing chronic hepatitis B is among neonates born to mothers who are hepatitis B virus carriers. Overall, recovery from acute hepatitis B occurs in >95% of patients. In the remaining 5% of patients, hepatitis B persists either as chronic (replicative) hepatitis or as an asymptomatic chronic (nonreplicative) carrier state.

Liver Function Tests in Chronic Hepatitis B Viral Infection

Transaminase levels may be completely normal in patients with chronic hepatitis B, especially in those who are hepatitis B carriers or who have well-compensated cirrhosis. Most patients, however, have mild to moderate elevations, with ALT levels generally higher than AST levels. Occasionally, transaminase levels climb markedly with exacerbations (rise in ALT of up to 50 times the upper limit of normal). While a marked rise in the transaminase levels may merely reflect an exacerbation of chronic hepatitis B viral infection, the clinician should ensure that other causes of hepatic injury are not present (see below).

Progression of liver disease to cirrhosis should be considered when leukopenia or thrombocytopenia develops, suggesting the presence of splenomegaly. Also, the finding of hypoalbuminemia or a prolonged PT should raise the same concern.

Establishing the Diagnosis of Chronic Hepatitis B Viral Infection

Chronic hepatitis B viral infection is diagnosed when there is persistence of HB_sAg in the serum beyond 6 months. IgG anti-HB_c is usually present in these patients. Once the diagnosis of chronic hepatitis B viral infection has been established, the clinician should perform further testing. In particular, testing for HBV DNA and HB_eAg is useful in distinguishing replicative from nonreplicative

HEPATITIS B PROFILE

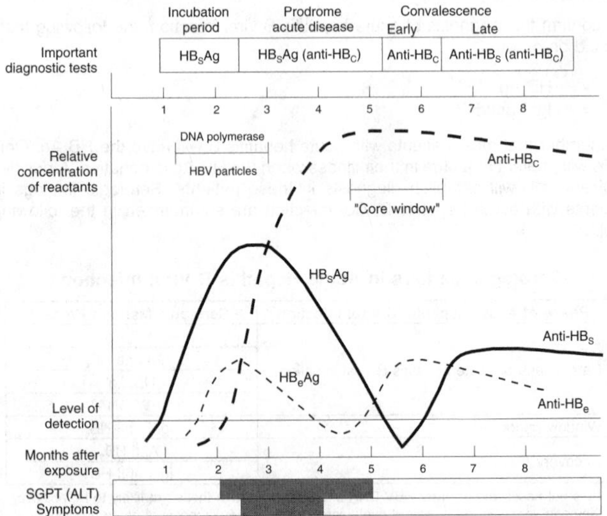

Serologic and clinical patterns observed during acute hepatitis B viral infection. From Hollinger FB and Dreesman GR, *Manual of Clinical Immunology*, 2nd ed, Rose NR and Friedman H, eds, Washington, DC: American Society for Microbiology, 1980, with permission.

infection (see below). In addition, the information obtained from these additional serologic tests will help guide decisions regarding the need for antiviral therapy.

Serologic patterns of chronic hepatitis B may vary depending on the replicative state of the virus. Active viral replication is likely if the following pattern is obtained on serologic testing.

Hepatitis B Chronic (Replicative) State

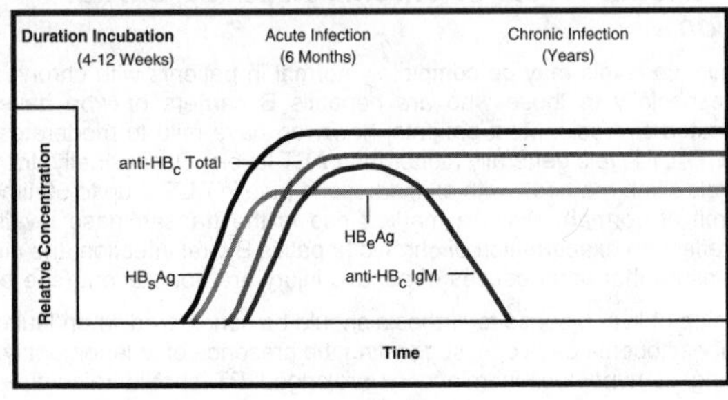

CHRONIC HEPATITIS B ACTIVE REPLICATION			
(+)	HBV DNA	(-)	Anti-HBs
(+)	HBeAg	(-)	Anti-HBe
(+)	HBsAg	(+)	Anti-HBc

The chronic (nonreplicative) carrier state is defined based on the following pattern.

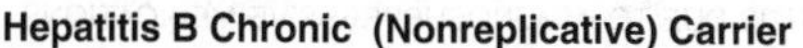

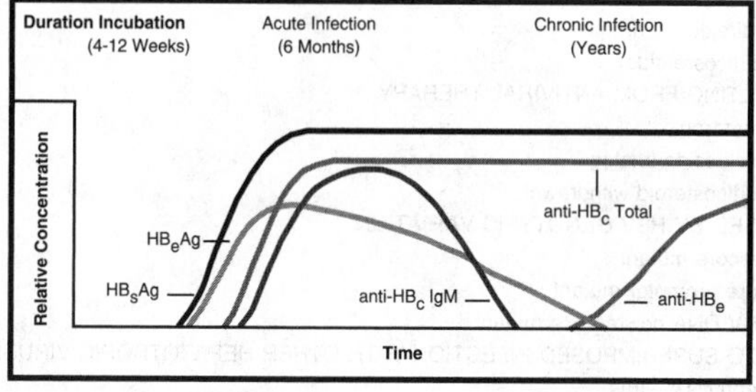

CHRONIC HEPATITIS B CARRIER STATE			
(-)	HBV DNA	(-)	Anti-HB_s
(-)	HB_eAg	(+)	Anti-HB_e
(+)	HB_sAg	(+)	Anti-HB_c

Chronic Hepatitis: A Comparison of the Replicative and Nonreplicative States

	HB_sAg	HBV DNA	HB_eAg	Anti-HB_s	Anti-HB_c	Anti-HB_e
Replicative state	(+)	(+)	(+)	(-)	(+)	(-)
Nonreplicative state	(+)	(-)	(-)	(-)	(+)	(+)

Many patients cycle back and forth between the replicative and nonreplicative states. With transformation of the replicative state into the nonreplicative state, HB_eAg is lost and anti-HB_e is detected in the serum. There is a 10% to 15% likelihood of spontaneous conversion from the replicative to the nonreplicative state of hepatitis B infection each year.

Flares or Exacerbations of Chronic Hepatitis B Viral Infection

Acute flares or exacerbations in chronic hepatitis B are common. Although these flares are often spontaneous, the clinician should realize that other factors may be involved. These other causes of flares or exacerbations of chronic hepatitis B are listed in the following box.

ETIOLOGIC CLASSIFICATION OF ACUTE FLARES IN CHRONIC HEPATITIS B
SPONTANEOUS REACTIVATION OF CHRONIC HEPATITIS B
REACTIVATED HEPATITIS DUE TO IMMUNOSUPPRESSIVE MEDICATIONS
Cancer chemotherapy
Antirejection drugs
Corticosteroids
RESULTING FROM ANTIVIRAL THERAPY
Interferon
Nucleoside analogs
Corticosteroid withdrawal
INDUCED BY HBV GENOTYPIC VARIATION
Precore mutant
Core promoter mutant
HBV DNA polymerase mutant
DUE TO SUPERIMPOSED INFECTION WITH OTHER HEPATOTROPIC VIRUSES
Hepatitis A virus
Hepatitis C virus
Hepatitis D virus
CMV
EBV
DUE TO OTHER TYPES OF INFECTION (NONVIRAL)
Leptospirosis
Rickettsia
DRUGS
ISCHEMIA
ALCOHOL
CAUSED BY INTERACTION WITH HIV INFECTION
Reactivated hepatitis
Effect of immune reconstitution therapy

Adapted from Perrillo R, "Acute Flares in Chronic Hepatitis B: The Natural and Unnatural History of an Immunologically Mediated Liver Disease," *Gastroenterology*, 2001, 120:1010.

The natural history of chronic hepatitis B is such that spontaneous flares of the disease occur. During these flares, a significant elevation in the transaminase levels may occur (2-5 times previous levels). These acute exacerbations often represent reactivated infection; that is, most clinically recognizable flares occur in patients who transform from a nonreplicative to replicative phase. During the flare, IgM anti-HB_c may become detectable. This is a marker that is traditionally associated with acute hepatitis B viral infection, disappearing with recovery from infection. It is now known that IgM anti-HB_c may accompany flares of chronic hepatitis B. If the patient is not known to have chronic hepatitis B, the presence of both HB_sAg and IgM anti-HB_c may prompt the clinician to erroneously diagnose the patient with acute hepatitis B.

While flares of chronic hepatitis B may be part of the natural history of the infection, the clinician should ensure that the flare does not represent superimposed infection with other hepatotropic viruses (hepatitis A, C, D, or E). Therefore, it is reasonable to obtain appropriate viral serology in patients with flares. Studies have shown that as many as 30% of flares may be caused by infection with other viral agents.

Spontaneous Resolution of Chronic Hepatitis B

In general, the patient who has developed chronic hepatitis B faces a lifelong disease. Among untreated patients, the average rate of spontaneous development of immunity, characterized by disappearance of HB_sAg and appearance of anti-HB_s, is about 1% to 2% per year.

Hepatitis B Vaccination

Patients receiving immunization for hepatitis B are immunized with HB_sAg. The antibody profile is positive only for anti-HB_s.

Serologic Results in Hepatitis B

	HB_sAg	HBV DNA	HB_eAg	Anti-HB_s	Anti-HB_c	Anti-HB_e
Hepatitis B immunization	(-)	(-)	(-)	(+)	(-)	(-)
Acute hepatitis B (early)	(+)	(+)	(+)	(-)	(-)	(-)
Hepatitis B window period	(-)	(-)	(-)	(-)	(+)	(+)
Chronic hepatitis B (replicative)	(+)	(+)	(+)	(-)	(+)	(-)
Chronic hepatitis B (nonreplicative)	(+)	(-)	(-)	(-)	(+)	(+)

Laboratory Testing Before and During Antiviral Treatment

In recent years, much attention has focused on antiviral treatment of chronic hepatitis B. The two major treatment options currently available are interferon and nucleoside analog therapy. Laboratory testing plays a role in deciding which patients with chronic hepatitis B should receive antiviral treatment. Candidates for interferon therapy typically have the following laboratory test profile:

- Abnormal transaminase levels
- Presence of HB_sAg in serum
- Presence of HB_eAg and/or HBV DNA in serum
- Chronic hepatitis demonstrated on liver biopsy

In patients who are to receive interferon therapy, laboratory testing also plays a role not only before but also during treatment, as shown in the following box.

ALGORITHM FOR THERAPY OF HEPATITIS B

INITIAL EVALUATION

SERIAL ALT LEVELS
PRESENCE OF HB_sAg, HB_eAg, HBV DNA
LIVER BIOPSY

MONITORING DURING THERAPY

EVERY 2-4 WEEKS
ALT, AST, bilirubin, albumin
CBC with differential
AT 2 AND 4 MONTHS
HB_eAg, HB_sAg, PT, TSH

(continued)

(continued)

ALGORITHM FOR THERAPY OF HEPATITIS B
FOLLOW-UP AFTER THERAPY
EVERY 2-3 MONTHS
ALT, AST, bilirubin, albumin
CBC
AT 6 MONTHS
HB_eAg, HB_sAg, PT, TSH*

*Testing for HB_sAg, HB_eAg, and HBV DNA should be performed at the completion of therapy as well as 6 months afterwards. A beneficial response is defined as the disappearance of HB_eAg and HBV DNA for at least 6 months after cessation of therapy. After completing therapy, not uncommonly, months to years pass before HB_sAg and HB_eAg disappear. Thyroid function tests are important because abnormalities of thyroid function are common with interferon therapy.

Bacon BR and DiBisceglie AM, *Liver Disease Diagnosis and Management*, Philadelphia, PA: Churchill Livingstone, 2000, 100.

References

Badur S and Akgun A, "Diagnosis of Hepatitis B Infections and Monitoring of Treatment," *J Clin Virol*, 2001, 21(3):229-37.

Dufour DR, Lott JA, Nolte FS, et al, "Diagnosis and Monitoring of Hepatic Injury. II. Recommendations for Use of Laboratory Tests in Screening, Diagnosis, and Monitoring," *Clin Chem*, 2000, 46(12):2050-68.

Lin KW and Kirchner JT, "Hepatitis B," *Am Fam Physician*, 2004, 69(1):75-82.

Lok AS, "Hepatitis B Infection: Pathogenesis and Management," *J Hepatol*, 2000, 32(1 Suppl):89-97.

Lok AS, Heathcote EJ, and Hoofnagle JH, "Management of Hepatitis B: 2000 - Summary of a Workshop," *Gastroenterology*, 2001, 120(7):1828-53.

Mahoney FJ, "Update on Diagnosis, Management, and Prevention of Hepatitis B Virus Infection," *Clin Microbiol Rev*, 1999, 12(2):351-66.

Perrillo RP, "Acute Flares in Chronic Hepatitis B: The Natural and Unnatural History of an Immunologically Mediated Liver Disease," *Gastroenterology*, 2001, 120(4):1009-22.

Regev A and Schiff ER, "Viral Hepatitis A, B, and C," *Clin Liver Dis*, 2000, 4(1):47-71, vi.

Ryder SD and Beckingham IJ, "ABC of Diseases of Liver, Pancreas, and Biliary System: Acute Hepatitis," *BMJ*, 2001, 20;322(7279):151-3.

Ryder SD and Beckingham IJ, "ABC of Diseases of Liver, Pancreas, and Biliary System: Chronic Viral Hepatitis," *BMJ*, 2001, 322(7280):219-21.

Walsh K and Alexander GJ, "Update on Chronic Viral Hepatitis," *Postgrad Med J*, 2001, 77(910):498-505.

Weston SR and Martin P, "Serological and Molecular Testing in Viral Hepatitis: An Update," *Can J Gastroenterol*, 2001, 15(3):177-84.

HEPATITIS C

VIRAL SEROLOGY

Enzyme Immunoassay (EIA)

The screening antibody test for hepatitis C is the enzyme immunoassay (EIA). There are now three versions of the EIA. EIA-1 was replaced by EIA-2 in 1992, because of its improved sensitivity (95% vs 80%) and specificity. Because of its increased sensitivity, EIA-2 allows for earlier identification of new infections (mean of 10 weeks for EIA-2 vs 16 weeks for EIA-1). With its use, the incidence of post-transfusion hepatitis C has decreased considerably. With the arrival of EIA-3, there was a further increase in sensitivity and specificity (sensitivity and specificity of the current third-generation tests are 99% in immunocompetent patients). Acute hepatitis C viral infection can be diagnosed earlier using EIA-3 assays (mean time of 2-3 weeks earlier).

It is important to realize, however, that EIA testing does not differentiate among acute, chronic, or resolved infection. Advantages and disadvantages of the EIA test for anti-HCV are listed in the following box.

ADVANTAGES AND DISADVANTAGES OF EIA TESTING FOR ANTI-HCV

ADVANTAGES

READILY AVAILABLE
EASE OF PERFORMANCE
REPRODUCIBILITY BETWEEN LABORATORIES
RELATIVE LOW COST (compared to other screening tests)

DISADVANTAGES

FALSE-NEGATIVE TESTS
- Immunocompromised
  - Organ transplant recipients
  - Hemodialysis
  - HIV
- Early acute hepatitis C viral infection
- Cryoglobulinemia

Recombinant Immunoblot Assay (RIBA)

Because the earlier EIA tests for anti-HCV were not as sensitive and specific, recombinant immunoblot assay tests for anti-HCV were developed to confirm the actual presence of hepatitis C virus. Over the years, three generations of RIBA testing have been developed (RIBA-1, RIBA-2, RIBA-3). With each successive generation, sensitivity of the RIBA test has increased. RIBA-3 is more specific than RIBA-2. Its use is also associated with fewer indeterminate results.

Not all patients found to have antibodies to hepatitis C virus by EIA require RIBA testing for confirmation of the diagnosis. RIBA testing is only required in patients who are deemed at low risk for hepatitis C infection. Low risk groups include those with normal transaminase levels, no evidence of chronic liver disease, and blood donors. RIBA testing should be considered in these groups as a confirmatory test only if the EIA test for anti-HCV is positive. In these groups, false-positive anti-HCV test results are more common than in groups who have a high prevalence of hepatitis C infection. In these cases, RIBA testing can be performed to determine which anti-HCV tests are false-positives. Further evaluation of EIA-positive patients is not required if RIBA testing is negative. These patients do not have ongoing infection. A positive or indeterminate RIBA test results needs to be followed by an HCV RNA test. In recent years, the use of RIBA testing has diminished with the advent of virologic testing (HCV RNA by PCR).

Hepatitis C Viral RNA (HCV RNA)

Also available are tests to detect the presence of hepatitis C viral RNA in the serum of affected individuals. These tests are now considered the gold standard in the diagnosis of hepatitis C viral infection. With HCV RNA tests, the presence of viremia can be established just a few days after exposure to the virus, well before antibody to the virus or transaminase elevations occur.

HCV RNA testing may be performed by polymerase chain reaction, transcription-mediated amplification, or branched DNA methodology. Testing is either quantitative or qualitative. Qualitative tests are read as either positive or negative (ie, virus is present or not). Quantitative tests will provide a measurement of the viral load, traditionally reported as HCV copies/mL but now more often reported in units of IU/mL.

The currently available PCR-based tests are highly sensitive. In fact, viral loads as low as 25 IU/mL can be detected. In patients with active HCV infection, circulating HCV levels are generally above 50,000 IU/mL. When performing HCV RNA testing for the diagnosis of HCV infection, many clinicians prefer to test with a quantitative assay. If the quantitative assay is negative, a qualitative test can be performed since this type of testing is a bit more sensitive, albeit not much more so.

In most cases, initial testing of the patient suspected of having HCV infection begins with anti-HCV (EIA). EIA testing, however, is subject to false-positive test results, especially in patients deemed to be at low risk for hepatitis C infection. To confirm that a positive test result is indeed a true positive, the clinician should obtain a confirmatory test. Traditionally, RIBA testing was the confirmatory test of choice. With the arrival of HCV RNA testing, however, clinicians are now turning to this type of testing to confirm the presence of hepatitis C infection in low risk populations. The clinician should realize that HCV viremia can fluctuate with levels being, at times, undetectable in patients with active HCV infection. Therefore, a negative test result does not exclude the diagnosis completely.

Quantitative testing for HCV RNA should be performed when a patient with HCV is being considered for antiviral therapy. There is good evidence to suggest that quantitative testing to determine the viral load can predict response to therapy. A lower viral load is considered to be a favorable factor.

Guide to the Interpretation of Hepatitis C Testing

Antibody to HCV	HCV RNA	Usual Interpretation	Other Possible Interpretation
Negative	Negative	No infection	—
Positive	Positive	HCV present	—
Positive	Negative	Resolved infection	1. False positive (<1%) 2. Treated, HCV below detectable limits (verify with qualitative HCV RNA PCR)
Negative	Positive	Infection present (usually in immuno-compromised patients or patients undergoing hemodialysis)	1. Early infection 2. False-positive or contaminated test system

Adapted from Carey W, "Tests and Screening Strategies for the Diagnosis of Hepatitis C," *Cleve Clin J Med*, 2003, 70(Suppl 4):S10.

Hepatitis C Virus Genotyping

Many different genotypes of HCV have been identified. Testing is available to differentiate among these genotypes. Knowledge of the patient's HCV genotype helps determine the likelihood of response to antiviral therapy. In addition, it provides information regarding the optimal treatment duration.

ACUTE HEPATITIS C VIRAL INFECTION

Patients with acute hepatitis C viral infection may present with signs and symptoms indistinguishable from those of other viral causes of hepatitis. In the United States, hepatitis C viral infection accounts for about 20% of acute hepatitis cases.

More often, they do not develop an illness that brings them to clinical attention. In these patients, the diagnosis of acute hepatitis C viral infection may go undiagnosed. Later, they may be found to have chronic hepatitis C viral infection.

Establishing the Diagnosis of Acute Hepatitis C Viral Infection

In patients with acute hepatitis C viral infection, the diagnosis may be confirmed by performing one or both of the following tests.

- Anti-HCV

  Although the measurement of anti-HCV is positive in many patients with acute hepatitis C viral infection, the antibody may not be measurable until after the onset of symptoms. On occasion, the antibody response may be undetectable for weeks or months after acquisition of the infection, as shown in the following table.

Using Anti-HCV in the Diagnosis of Acute Hepatitis C Viral Infection

Time Since Exposure to Hepatitis C	Percentage of Patients Who Have Detectable Anti-HCV
Within 15 weeks of exposure	80%
Within 5 months of exposure	>90%
Within 6 months of exposure	>97%

In these cases, the clinician may choose to repeat testing after a sufficient period of time. Conversion of the anti-HCV from negative to positive confirms the diagnosis of acute hepatitis C viral infection. Alternatively, the clinician may wish to obtain testing for HCV RNA.

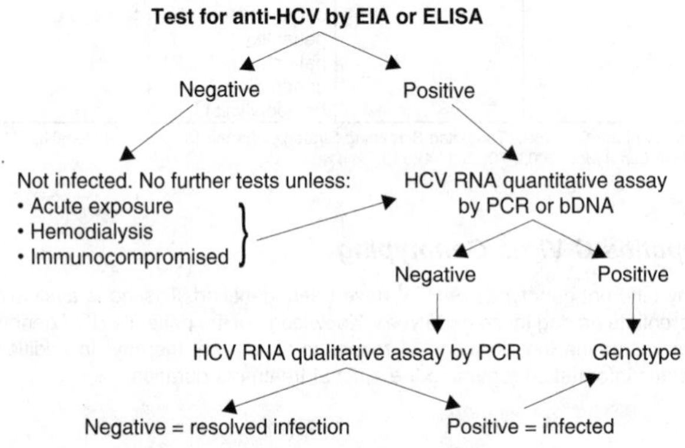

Anti-HCV = antibody to hepatitis C virus; EIA = enzyme immunoassy; ELISA = enzyme-lined immunosorbent assay; PCR = polymerase chain reaction; bDNA = branched DNA

- HCV RNA

  HCV RNA is usually detectable within 1-2 weeks of the acquisition of the virus.

Resolution of Acute Hepatitis C Viral Infection

Although normalization of serum transaminase levels would intuitively seem to suggest clearance of the virus, many of these patients have chronic hepatitis C viral infection. Chronic infection develops in 80% to 85% of patients who acquire hepatitis C.

In the 15% to 20% of patients who are fortunate enough to recover, recovery can be ascertained by testing for HCV RNA by PCR. Those who are found to be negative for HCV RNA have recovered from hepatitis C. Anti-HCV cannot be used to differentiate recovery from chronic hepatitis C viral infection because, once present, it remains positive for years.

CHRONIC HEPATITIS C VIRAL INFECTION

Although patients who acquire hepatitis C may become symptomatic with an illness that is indistinguishable from other causes of acute viral hepatitis, more often, patients are asymptomatic or develop a nonspecific illness for which they do not seek medical attention. Many of these affected patients are diagnosed with chronic hepatitis C viral infection years later when asymptomatic elevations of transaminases are noted on routine laboratory testing. This is consistent with the fact that 80% to 85% of patients who acquire hepatitis C go on to develop chronic hepatitis C.

Liver Function Tests in Chronic Hepatitis C Viral Infection

While many patients with chronic hepatitis C viral infection have mild to moderate transaminase elevation, some patients may present with normal AST and ALT levels. Therefore, normal transaminase levels do not exclude the diagnosis.

Chronic hepatitis C viral infection is a well known cause of fluctuations in AST and ALT levels; that is, transaminase levels fluctuate between normal and abnormal. Therefore, in patients with risk factors for hepatitis C, hepatitis C viral serology should be obtained, irrespective of the transaminase levels. See Figure 1.

Figure 1.
Time Course of Serologic Markers in Acute Hepatitis C Infection

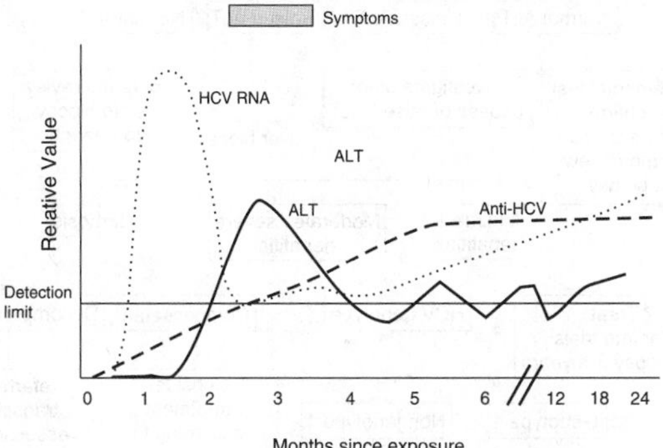

Adapted from Dufour DR, Lott JA, Nolte FS, et al, "Diagnosis and Monitoring of Hepatic Injury. I. Performance Characteristics of Laboratory Tests," *Clin Chem*, 2000, 46(12):2041.

Establishing the Diagnosis of Chronic Hepatitis C Viral Infection

While a positive anti-HCV test in the patient suspected of having chronic hepatitis C viral infection is suggestive of the diagnosis, the clinician should realize that the antibody is detectable in patients who have recovered from the infection as well. It is said that 15% to 25% of patients who become infected with the hepatitis C virus recover from the infection. To distinguish these patients who have recovered from others who have chronic hepatitis C viral infection, it is necessary to obtain a qualitative HCV RNA test. The presence of HCV RNA confirms the diagnosis of chronic hepatitis C viral infection. A negative result should prompt the clinician to repeat the test, particularly in patients with an elevated ALT level. To establish the diagnosis of chronic HCV, serology consistent with the diagnosis must be demonstrated on two occasions over a period of six months or more.

Laboratory Testing During Treatment of Chronic Hepatitis C Viral Infection

The following algorithm and table describe the recommended laboratory testing during treatment of chronic hepatitis C viral infection.

MANAGEMENT OF ANTI-HCV ANTIBODY-POSITIVE PATIENTS

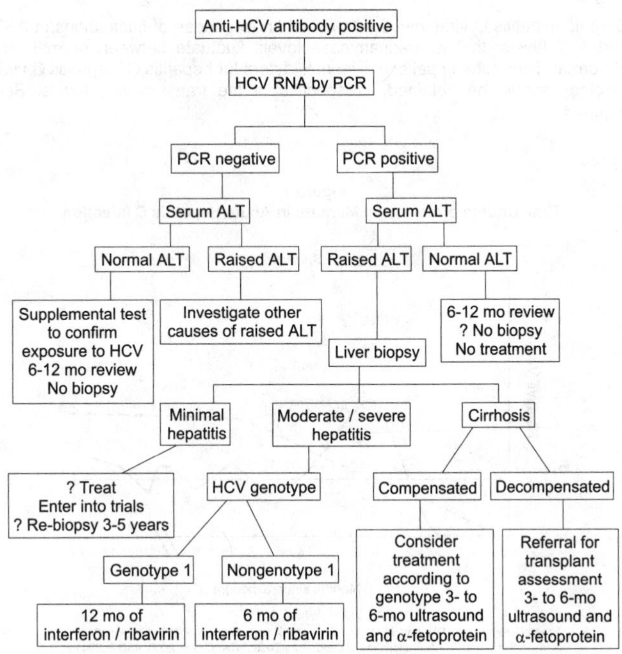

Adapted from *Comprehensive Clinical Hepatology,* O'Grady JG, Lake JR, and Howdle PD, eds, London, UK: Harcourt Publishers Ltd, 2000, 3:13.17.

RECOMMENDED LABORATORY TESTS DURING INTERFERON / RIBAVIRIN THERAPY*

	Baseline	Treatment				Monthly During Treatment	End of Treatment	Monthly for 6 Mo Post-Treatment	6 Mo After Completion of Therapy
		Week 1	Week 2	Week 4	Week 24				
Hemoglobin	X	X	X	X		X			
WBC	X	X	X	X		X			
Platelets	X	X	X	X		X			
HCV-RNA	X				X		X		X
Pregnancy*	X					X		X	
ALT / AST	X					†			
TSH	X					†			

WBC: White blood cell count; HCV-RNA: Hepatitis C virus RNA; ALT: Alanine transaminase; AST: Aspartate transaminase; TSH: Thyroid-stimulating hormone

* If applicable

†Should be individualized for each patient by the treating physician

Adapted from *Management of Chronic Viral Hepatitis*, Gordon SC, New York, NY: Marcel Dekker, 2002, 203.

References

Barrera JM, "Diagnostic Tests for Hepatitis C Virus Infection," *Nephrol Dial Transplant*, 2000, 15(Suppl 8):15-8.

Bonkovsky HL and Mehta S, "Hepatitis C: A Review and Update," *J Am Acad Dermatol*, 2001, 44(2):159-82.

Carey W, "Tests and Screening Strategies for the Diagnosis of Hepatitis C," *Cleve Clin J Med*, 2003, 70(Suppl 4):S7-13.

Carithers RL Jr, Marquardt A, and Gretch DR, "Diagnostic Testing for Hepatitis C," *Semin Liver Dis*, 2000, 20(2):159-71.

Cheney CP, Chopra S, and Graham C, "Hepatitis C," *Infect Dis Clin North Am*, 2000, 14(3):633-67.

Erensoy R, "Diagnosis of Hepatitis C Virus (HCV) Infection and Laboratory Monitoring of its Therapy," *J Clin Virol*, 2001, 21(3):271-81.

Krajden M, "Hepatitis C Virus Diagnosis and Testing," *Can J Public Health*, 2000, 91(Suppl 1):S34-9, S36-42.

Larson AM and Carithers RL, "Hepatitis C in Clinical Practice," *J Intern Med*, 2001, 249(2):111-20.

Lauer GM and Walker BD, "Hepatitis C Virus Infection," *N Engl J Med*, 2001, 345(1):41-52.

Orland JR, Wright TL, and Cooper S, "Acute Hepatitis C," *Hepatology*, 2001, 33(2):321-7.

Pawlotsky JM, "Use and Interpretation of Hepatitis C Virus Diagnostic Assays," *Clin Liver Dis*, 2003, 7(1):127-37.

Regev A and Schiff ER, "Viral Hepatitis A, B, and C," *Clin Liver Dis*, 2000, 4(1):47-71, vi.

Rodes J and Sanchez Tapias SM, "Hepatitis C," *Nephrol Dial Transplant*, 2000, 15(Suppl 8):2-11.

Rubinstein ML and Miele ME, "Hepatitis C Virus Infection: Detection and Treatment," *Clin Lab Sci*, 2003, 16(4):203-8.

Ryder SD and Beckingham IJ, "ABC of Diseases of Liver, Pancreas, and Biliary System: Chronic Viral Hepatitis," *BMJ*, 2001, 322(7280):219-21.

Ryder SD and Beckingham IJ, "ABC of Diseases of Liver, Pancreas, and Biliary System: Acute Hepatitis," *BMJ*, 2001, 322(7279):151-3.

Walsh K and Alexander GJ, "Update on Chronic Viral Hepatitis," *Postgrad Med J*, 2001, 77(910):498-505.

Weston SR and Martin P, "Serological and Molecular Testing in Viral Hepatitis: An Update," *Can J Gastroenterol*, 2001, 15(3):177-84.

HEPATITIS D

ACUTE DELTA HEPATITIS

Only patients with hepatitis B can acquire hepatitis D because hepatitis D is a defective RNA virus requiring the presence of hepatitis B for its replication. Coinfection may occur with hepatitis B and hepatitis D. Superinfection of a chronic hepatitis B infected patient with acute hepatitis D may occur as well.

Acute delta hepatitis must be differentiated from chronic delta hepatitis. Acute delta hepatitis may be the manifestation of either coinfection or superinfection. In either case, the infection may persist, in which case the patient is said to have chronic delta hepatitis.

Clinical Presentation

Signs and symptoms of acute hepatitis D viral infection are indistinguishable from other causes of viral hepatitis. Coinfection and superinfection are also clinically indistinguishable from one another. However, a biphasic course of illness separated by an interval of 2-5 weeks may be appreciated in some patients with coinfection.

Coinfection results in fulminant hepatitis much more often than hepatitis B viral infection alone. Most patients with coinfection do not develop a hepatitis B carrier state. In fact, <5% of patients with coinfection progress to chronicity. Of the patients who do become carriers, the progression to chronic liver disease is more rapid.

Biphasic illness is not a feature of superinfection. Superinfection should be considered in any patient with chronic hepatitis B who develops acute hepatitis. Similar to coinfection, fulminant hepatitis occurs more often in superinfection as compared to hepatitis B viral infection alone.

The development of chronic hepatitis D viral infection is much more common with superinfection than with coinfection.

Liver Function Tests in Acute Delta Hepatitis

Tests of liver function do not distinguish coinfection from superinfection, nor do they distinguish hepatitis D infection from other viral causes of hepatitis. Coinfection may be characterized in some patients by a biphasic transaminase elevation separated by weeks. The transaminase elevation in the first week corresponds to the hepatitis B infection.

Indications for Hepatitis D Serology in Acute Hepatic Injury

Acute delta hepatitis should be a consideration in patients who present with the following:

- Clinical presentation consistent with fulminant hepatitis
- Acute hepatic injury in the patient with chronic hepatitis B viral infection

It is in these groups of patients that testing for hepatitis D viral infection is warranted.

Establishing the Diagnosis of Coinfection

The diagnosis of coinfection can only be made when serology reveals the following markers of acute hepatitis B infection (in addition to HDV markers):

- HB_sAg
- IgM Anti-HB_c

Of note, although HB_sAg is usually present, on occasion, the patient may have cleared the HB_sAg at the time of presentation. In these cases, the IgM anti-HB_c will be positive, establishing the diagnosis of acute hepatitis B viral infection.

The concomitant presence of hepatitis D can then be established by obtaining appropriate hepatitis D viral serology. The earliest markers of hepatitis D viral infection are serum HDAg and HDV RNA (appearing within 1-10 days of symptom onset). It is important to realize that the sensitivity of the serum HDAg test is low because of its transient presence. For this reason, serial samples are recommended.

If these tests are not available, the clinician can obtain total anti-HD antibody levels. Total anti-HD antibody levels consist of both IgM and IgG fractions. IgM anti-HD becomes detectable approximately 2-3 weeks after symptom onset.

If these tests are negative in the patient thought to have coinfection, more sensitive testing is available. One such test is detection of intrahepatic HDAg by immunofluorescence or immunoperoxidase assays. These assays may be particularly useful in patients with fulminant hepatitis, in whom the serum markers of hepatitis D may be undetectable.

Figure 1. Schematic Diagram of the Typical Serologic Course in HDV-HBV Coinfection

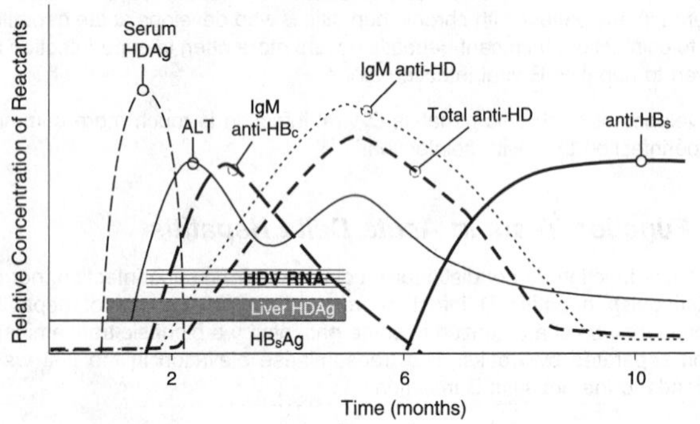

Establishing the Diagnosis of Superinfection

In patients with superinfection, IgM anti-HB_c is absent, but HB_sAg is detectable. HDV serology will typically reveal the presence of high total anti-HD. Chronicity of the hepatitis D viral infection, which is common in these patients, is suggested by the persistence of high titer IgM and IgG antibodies to the hepatitis D virus.

It is usually not necessary to obtain more sensitive tests to establish the diagnosis of chronicity because the demonstration of high titer anti-HD that persists suffices in the diagnosis. The clinician may wish, however, to obtain HDV RNA by PCR to determine the likelihood of progression to chronic hepatitis D viral infection. In patients who have detectable serum HDV RNA 4 weeks after onset of superinfection, chronic hepatitis D viral infection is very likely. Chronic hepatitis D viral infection is defined as HDV viremia lasting longer than 6 months.

Markers of Acute HBV and HBV / HDV Hepatitis

Marker	Acute HBV	Acute HBV / HDV Coinfection	Acute HBV / HDV Superinfection
Anti-HB_s	---	---	---
HB_sAg	±	±	±
IgM anti-HB_c	+	+	---
HBV DNA	+	±	±
Total anti-HD	---	+ (late, transient)	+
IgM anti-HD	---	+ (late, transient)	+
Liver HDAg	---	+	+
Serum HDAg	---	+ (early, transient)	+
Serum HDV RNA	---	+	+

Adapted from "Hepatitis Delta Virus: The Molecular Basis of Laboratory Diagnosis," *Crit Rev Clin Lab Sci*, 2000, 37(1):68.

Figure 2. Schematic Diagram of the Typical Serologic Course in HDV-HBV Superinfection

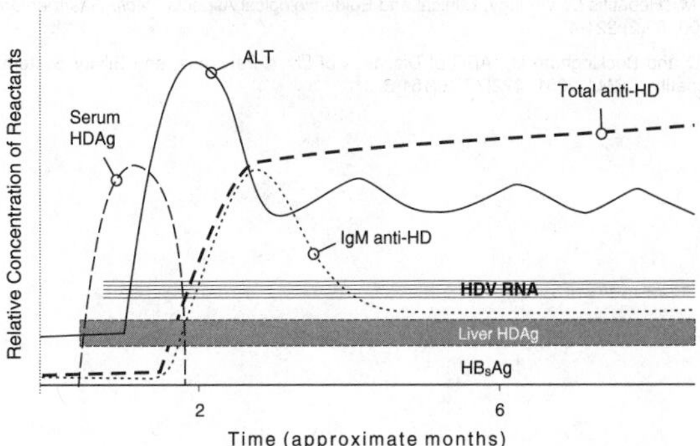

CHRONIC DELTA HEPATITIS

To establish the diagnosis of chronic delta hepatitis, the following hepatitis D viral markers may be assayed:

- Serum HDV RNA
- Serum HDAg
- Anti-HD (IgM and IgG)
- Intrahepatic HDAg

Of these tests, it seems that the detection of serum HDV RNA by dot blot is most accurate to detect chronic delta hepatitis infection. There is some evidence to suggest the sensitivity of this marker may be increased by using reverse transcriptase PCR assay.

Markers of Chronic HBV/HDV Hepatitis

Marker	Chronic HBV/HDV Hepatitis
Anti-HB_s	---
IgM anti-HB_c	---
Serum HB_sAg	+
Serum HBV DNA	+
Total anti-HD	+ (late, persistent)
IgM anti-HD	+ (late, persistent)
Liver HDAg	+
Serum HDAg	+ (early, transient)
Serum HDV RNA	+

Adapted from "Hepatitis Delta Virus: The Molecular Basis of Laboratory Diagnosis," *Crit Rev Clin Lab Sci*, 2000, 37(1):68.

References

Casey JL, "Hepatitis Delta Virus: Molecular Biology, Pathogenesis and Immunology," *Antivir Ther*, 1998, 3(Suppl 3):37-42.

Modahl LE and Lai MM, "Hepatitis Delta Virus: The Molecular Basis of Laboratory Diagnosis," *Crit Rev Clin Lab Sci*, 2000, 37(1):45-92.

Rizzetto M, "Hepatitis D: Virology, Clinical and Epidemiological Aspects," *Acta Gastroenterol Belg*, 2000, 63(2):221-4.

Ryder SD and Beckingham IJ, "ABC of Diseases of Liver, Pancreas, and Biliary System: Acute Hepatitis," *BMJ*, 2001, 322(7279):151-3.

HEPATITIS E

This virus is transmitted via the fecal-oral route and most commonly occurs with ingestion of contaminated water. The virus has mainly been found among patients in Asia, Africa, India, and Central America. It is an unusual cause of acute viral hepatitis in the United States. It should be a consideration, however, in patients who report a history of recent travel to developing countries as well as in those who are new immigrants.

Liver Function Tests in Acute Hepatitis E Viral Infection

Liver function test abnormalities in acute hepatitis E viral infection do not allow the clinician to distinguish this infection from other causes of viral hepatitis. Liver function test abnormalities as well as other laboratory test findings in acute viral hepatitis have been discussed in the chapter, ***Acute Viral Hepatitis*** *on page 659.*

Establishing the Diagnosis of Acute Hepatitis E Viral Infection

To establish the diagnosis of acute hepatitis E viral infection, it is necessary to perform serologic testing for the hepatitis E virus. This includes assays for both IgM and IgG anti-HEV. During acute hepatitis E viral infection, both IgG and IgM titers increase, with the IgM rise preceding the IgG rise. There is a rapid decrease in the IgM anti-HEV levels during convalescence. Detectable levels of IgG anti-HEV usually persist for a longer period of time, but, in most cases, antibody levels are undetectable 6-12 months after disease onset. In some patients, however, antibody levels may be detectable for at least several years. It is important to realize that serologic testing is not widely available. Although the testing can be performed in commercial laboratories, as of yet, the assays have not been approved by the FDA. In addition to antibody testing, PCR tests for the detection of HEV RNA in serum and stool specimens are available, but outside of research settings they are seldom used in the diagnosis. These PCR tests may need to be performed, however, when antibody testing is negative in the patient suspected of having acute hepatitis E viral infection. In fact, in 10% to 20% of acute hepatitis E cases confirmed by PCR testing, anti-HEV IgM testing is negative.

References

Aggarwal R and Krawczynski K, "Hepatitis E: An Overview and Recent Advances in Clinical and Laboratory Research," *J Gastroenterol Hepatol*, 2000, 15(1):9-20.

Harrison TJ, "Hepatitis E Virus – An Update," *Liver*, 1999, 19(3):171-6.

Krawczynski K, Aggarwal R, and Kamili S, "Hepatitis E," *Infect Dis Clin North Am*, 2000, 14(3):669-87.

Ryder SD and Beckingham IJ, "ABC of Diseases of Liver, Pancreas, and Biliary System: Acute Hepatitis," *BMJ*, 2001, 322(7279):151-3.

Weston SR and Martin P, "Serological and Molecular Testing in Viral Hepatitis: An Update," *Can J Gastroenterol*, 2001, 15(3):177-84.

Winn WC Jr, "Enterically Transmitted Hepatitis. Hepatitis A and E Viruses," *Clin Lab Med*, 1999, 19(3):661-73.

ALCOHOLIC LIVER DISEASE

Alcoholic liver disease should be considered in every patient with liver disease of unknown etiology. It should also be considered in patients who report significant amounts of alcohol intake. The clinician should realize, however, that many patients with alcoholic liver disease deny alcohol use.

The term "alcoholic liver disease" is a broad one. It is more useful to identify the type of alcoholic liver disease that is present. Patients may present with one of the following types of alcoholic liver disease:

- Fatty liver
- Alcoholic hepatitis
- Alcoholic cirrhosis

The clinician should realize, however, that one or more of the above types of alcoholic liver disease can be present at the same time. In order to make the diagnosis of alcoholic liver disease, the clinician must document both alcohol abuse and the presence of liver disease. In addition, other potential causes must be excluded.

Clinical Presentation

Alcoholic fatty liver can develop even after a short period of moderate to heavy alcohol use (3-4 weeks). Although most patients are asymptomatic, some may report nonspecific symptoms such as bloating, flatulence, fatigue, and pressure sensation in the right upper abdomen. The physical examination may reveal hepatomegaly but the absence of this finding does not exclude the diagnosis.

The clinical presentation of alcoholic hepatitis varies. While some patients may be asymptomatic, most report symptoms such as nausea, vomiting, anorexia, fatigue, fever, weight loss, jaundice, and right upper quadrant pain. Some patients may present with ascites, hepatic encephalopathy, or gastrointestinal bleeding due to esophageal varices. Although these are features classically seen in cirrhosis, the clinician should realize that many patients with a clinical diagnosis of alcoholic hepatitis are found to have significant fibrosis and cirrhosis when liver biopsy is performed. Physical examination may reveal fever, scleral icterus, jaundice, spider angiomata, parotid gland enlargement, splenomegaly, and tender hepatomegaly.

Patients with alcoholic cirrhosis are often asymptomatic. When symptomatic, these patients usually report the same complaints that patients with alcoholic hepatitis have. Not uncommonly, alcoholic cirrhosis patients present with complications of their liver disease. These complications include portal hypertension, edema, ascites, splenomegaly, coagulopathies, and esophageal varices.

Liver Function Test Abnormalities

AST levels are commonly elevated in patients with alcoholic liver disease. AST levels >500 IU/L are unusual and should prompt the clinician to consider other possibilities or a condition superimposed on alcoholic liver disease. ALT levels may be elevated as well but are typically increased to a lesser degree. In patients with fatty liver, transaminase levels are normal or mildly elevated. Alcoholic cirrhosis patients may also present with normal AST and ALT levels, especially if they have progressed to end-stage liver disease.

Classically, the AST to ALT ratio is >2 in patients with alcoholic liver disease but the clinician should realize that this is not entirely specific for alcoholic liver disease. Furthermore, 30% to 50% of patients with alcoholic liver disease will present with an AST to ALT ratio <2.

Alkaline phosphatase levels are normal or mildly elevated in patients with alcoholic fatty liver. Levels are also mildly elevated in alcoholic hepatitis but, at times, the disease may present with a cholestatic picture, characterized by significant elevations in the alkaline phosphatase and bilirubin levels. This cholestatic presentation, especially if accompanied by fever and leukocytosis, may mimic biliary tract disease.

Hyperbilirubinemia is unusual in patients with fatty liver. An increase in the serum bilirubin level is more commonly appreciated in patients with alcoholic hepatitis or more advanced liver disease. The serum bilirubin level in combination with the PT provides the best index of disease severity in patients with alcoholic hepatitis. The Maddrey discriminant function is most widely used in predicting prognosis in patients with alcoholic hepatitis. It can be calculated using the following formula:

Maddrey discriminant function = 4.6 x (PT - control) + bilirubin (mg/dL)

Values >32 signify an increased 30-day mortality in this group of patients.

The presence of hypoalbuminemia should prompt the clinician to consider the presence of alcoholic hepatitis or cirrhosis.

GGT is often used as a marker for alcoholic liver disease but it is not specific for alcoholic liver disease. It is often elevated in other hepatobiliary diseases as well as disease of other organs. GGT levels can be increased in patients who consume alcohol but have no significant alcoholic liver disease.

Other Laboratory Test Abnormalities

Frequent measurement of the serum ethanol level may be needed in patients suspected of having alcoholic liver disease who deny alcohol use.

Leukocytosis is not uncommon in patients with alcoholic hepatitis. Its presence, however, should prompt a search for infection or sepsis. The elevated white blood cell count should only be attributed to the alcoholic hepatitis if there is no evidence for infection.

In patients with alcoholic liver disease, anemia may be the result of iron deficiency from gastrointestinal blood loss, folate deficiency, hypersplenism, or anemia of liver disease. A hemolytic anemia may occur in patients who develop Zieve's syndrome. Zieve's syndrome is characterized by the triad of jaundice, hyperlipidemia, and hemolysis. It typically occurs after acute alcohol consumption, manifesting with anorexia, nausea, vomiting, and diarrhea. These patients often report severe abdominal pain. These manifestations usually resolve after several weeks of abstinence from alcohol.

Macrocytosis is commonly noted with heavy drinking regardless of whether or not the patient has alcoholic liver disease. Anemia is not always present. Other causes of macrocytosis such as vitamin B_{12} and folate deficiency should be considered in these patients. Because of the relatively long life span of red blood cells (120 days), macrocytosis that is due to alcohol abuse may take several months to resolve in the patient who ceases to drink alcohol.

Thrombocytopenia may be due to the direct effects of alcohol on the bone marrow. Alternatively, it may be a manifestation of hypersplenism in patients with advanced alcoholic liver disease. Patients with hypersplenism may also present with leukopenia and anemia. Folic acid deficiency is another cause of thrombocytopenia in patients who abuse alcohol.

Serum ferritin levels are often elevated in patients with alcoholic hepatitis, often to impressive degrees. Ferritin levels will return to normal within several months after the cessation of alcohol intake. The clinician should realize, however, that an elevated serum ferritin level is also a manifestation of hemochromatosis. If ferritin levels do not return to normal after cessation of alcohol intake or the patient has clinical manifestations of hemochromatosis, consideration should be given to evaluating the patient for this hereditary condition.

Metabolic acidosis may be noted due to alcoholic ketoacidosis. These patients present with nausea, vomiting, fruity odor on breath, dehydration, and hyperventilation. Ketonemia and ketonuria are key features of the illness while a modest degree of hyperglycemia may not always be present. The clinician should also realize that patients who abuse alcohol are at risk for other causes of metabolic acidosis.

The presence of hyponatremia is suggestive of alcoholic cirrhosis. Other electrolyte abnormalities commonly found in alcoholic liver disease include hypokalemia, hypomagnesemia, and hypophosphatemia.

Indications for Liver Biopsy

Liver biopsy is not necessary in all patients with alcoholic liver disease but may be useful in certain situations. Liver biopsy can confirm the diagnosis and exclude other causes of liver disease. Studies have shown that 20% of patients suspected of having alcoholic liver disease are diagnosed with another condition after liver biopsy. Liver biopsy may also be performed to determine the severity of the disease. The clinical and laboratory features of alcoholic liver disease are not reliable predictors of the severity of the liver disease. The treatment of alcoholic liver disease revolves around abstinence from alcohol use. In the patient who continues to have liver function test abnormalities despite cessation of alcohol use, liver biopsy may be necessary.

References

Chedid A, Mendenhall CL, Gartside P, et al, "Prognostic Factors in Alcoholic Liver Disease. VA Cooperative Study Group," *Am J Gastroenterol*, 1991, 86(2):210-6.

Diehl AM, "Alcoholic Liver Disease," *Med Clin North Am*, 1989, 73(4):815-30 (review).

Diehl AM, "Liver Disease in Alcohol Abusers: Clinical Perspective," *Alcohol*, 2002, 27(1):7-11.

Leevy CM and Leevy CB, "Liver Disease in the Alcoholic," *Gastroenterology*, 1993, 105(1):294-6.

Lieber CS, "Medical Disorders of Alcoholism," *N Engl J Med*, 333(16):1058-65 (review).

Menon KV, Gores GJ, and Shah VH, "Pathogenesis, Diagnosis, and Treatment of Alcoholic Liver Disease," *Mayo Clin Proc*, 2001, 76(10):1021-9.

Sherlock S, "Alcoholic Liver Disease," *Lancet*, 1995, 345(8944):227-9 (review).

Zetterman RK, "Alcoholic Liver Disease," *Curr Hepatol*, 1993, 13:159-77.

ISCHEMIC HEPATITIS

Ischemic hepatitis is characterized by a rapid and marked elevation of the serum transaminases due to an acute fall in liver perfusion. The causes of ischemic hepatitis may be divided into cardiac and noncardiac etiologies.

Clinical Presentation

Ischemic hepatitis can follow any condition that is complicated by hypotension or shock. Most often, it results from acute myocardial infarction or arrhythmia. Other conditions that may lead to ischemic hepatitis include sepsis, hemorrhage, dehydration, and burns.

The illness that resulted in poor perfusion to the liver typically dominates the clinical presentation. Most patients report symptoms of weakness and apathy. On occasion, the clinician may encounter ischemic hepatitis patients with mental status changes, flapping tremor, jaundice, and even coma.

Laboratory Testing

Laboratory testing typically reveals a rapid increase in serum transaminases, usually to levels between 10 and 20 times the upper limit of normal. Peak levels of up to 250 times the upper limit of normal have been described. Peak levels are typically reached within 1-3 days.

If the cause of the impaired perfusion to the liver is corrected or resolves, the transaminase levels will fall more than 50% within 72 hours of the insult. Near normal levels are reached within 10 days of the insult. This is one of the key features that differentiate ischemic hepatitis from other causes of marked transaminase elevation, such as viral, alcoholic, and drug-induced hepatitis. In these latter conditions, the transaminase elevation is sustained.

LDH levels are often markedly elevated to a degree that is not usually seen with other causes of marked transaminase elevation. Increased serum bilirubin and alkaline phosphatase levels are not uncommon but levels seldom rise above 4 and 2 times the upper limit of normal, respectively. On occasion, laboratory test abnormalities indicative of consumptive coagulopathy may be present, including prolonged PT / PTT, low fibrinogen levels, thrombocytopenia, and elevated fibrin-fibrinogen degradation products.

Studies of patients with ischemic hepatitis have revealed other laboratory test abnormalities. In one series of patients, elevation of the serum creatinine and BUN were consistent findings, reflecting damage from kidney hypoperfusion. In another series of patients, hyperglycemia was reported in 66% of patients, occurring within 48 hours of the insult. Hypoglycemia has also been reported to occur in ischemic hepatitis patients.

References

DeLeve LD, "Vascular Liver Disease," *Curr Gastroenterol Rep*, 2003, 5(1):63-70.

Gill RQ and Sterling RK, "Acute Liver Failure," *J Clin Gastroenterol*, 2001, 33(3):191-8.

Lee WM, "Acute Liver Failure," *Am J Med*, 1994, 96(1A):3S-9S.

Naschitz JE, Slobodin G, Lewis RJ, et al, "Heart Diseases Affecting the Liver and Liver Diseases Affecting the Heart," *Am Heart J*, 2000, 140(1):111-20.

α-1 ANTITRYPSIN DEFICIENCY

α-1 antitrypsin deficiency, the most common genetic metabolic disease of the liver, has a prevalence of about 1 in 2000 (United States). Occurring most often in Caucasians, it exhibits autosomal recessive inheritance.

α-1 antitrypsin, an antiprotease, functions to inactivate a number of proteases, including trypsin and elastase. Liver disease and cirrhosis occur in 15% to 30% of patients who have the PiZZ phenotype, which represents the homozygous form of the disease. Some evidence suggests that the heterozygous forms of the disease (PiZ, PiMZ, PiSZ) may also be complicated by liver disease.

Clinical Presentation

Some patients with α-1 antitrypsin deficiency will manifest in childhood. Others do not come to clinical attention until adulthood when abnormal liver function tests or signs and symptoms of cirrhosis are noted. It should be a consideration in any patient who presents with chronic hepatitis or cirrhosis, especially if the etiology is unclear.

Laboratory Testing

The tests available in the diagnosis of α-1 antitrypsin deficiency are listed in the following box.

LABORATORY TESTING FOR α-1 ANTITRYPSIN DEFICIENCY
SERUM α-1 ANTITRYPSIN LEVEL
SERUM PROTEIN ELECTROPHORESIS
IMMUNOFIXATION WITH PHENOTYPE ANALYSIS
PERCUTANEOUS LIVER BIOPSY

Serum α-1 antitrypsin level is a useful initial test. It should be obtained in any patient with chronic hepatitis or cirrhosis of unclear etiology. A strong argument can be made for the diagnosis when the serum level is 25% less than the lower limit of normal. The clinician should realize that the serum α-1 antitrypsin level may be falsely elevated in inflammatory conditions. Failure to recognize this may be falsely reassuring.

Serum protein electrophoresis is another test available in the diagnosis of α-1 antitrypsin deficiency. A significant reduction or absence of the α-1 globulin band is characteristic of α-1 antitrypsin deficiency.

If liver biopsy is performed, periodic acid-Schiff diastase stain can demonstrate abnormal deposits of α-1 antitrypsin within the liver cells. These deposits will appear as periodic acid-Schiff diastase resistant globules in the hepatocytes. The presence of these deposits is supportive of the diagnosis but, on occasion, these inclusions may be found in patients with other types of liver disease.

The gold standard for the diagnosis of α-1 antitrypsin deficiency is serum α-1 antitrypsin phenotyping (Pi typing). Phenotyping, which should be performed in all patients suspected of having the disease, may be done by isoelectric focusing or immunofixation.

References

Eriksson S, "Alpha-1 Antitrypsin Deficiency," *J Hepatol*, 1999, 30(Suppl 1):34-9 (review).

Morrison ED and Kowdley KV, "Genetic Liver Disease in Adults. Early Recognition of the Three Most Common Causes," *Postgrad Med*, 2000, 107(2):147-52, 155, 158-9.

Perlmutter DH, "Alpha-1 Antitrypsin Deficiency," *Semin Liver Dis*, 1998, 18(3):217-25.

Perlmutter DH, "Alpha-1 Antitrypsin Deficiency: Biochemistry and Clinical Manifestations," *Ann Med*, 1996, 28(5):385-94.

Perlmutter DH, "Clinical Manifestations of Alpha-1 Antitrypsin Deficiency," *Gastroenterol Clin North Am*, 1995, 24(1):27-43.

Qu D, Teckman JH, and Perlmutter DH, "Review: Alpha-1 Antitrypsin Deficiency Associated Liver Disease," *J Gastroenterol Hepatol*, 1997, 12(5):404-16.

Eriksson S, [illegible], 1996, 240 Suppl 1:[illegible].

Mahadeva R and Lomas DA, [illegible]

[illegible]

Perlmutter DH, [illegible]

Perlmutter DH, [illegible]

[illegible] Gastroenterology, [illegible]

HEREDITARY HEMOCHROMATOSIS

Hereditary hemochromatosis is a condition characterized by iron overload. It is a disorder of iron regulation that leads to the excessive gastrointestinal absorption of dietary iron. With the passage of time, the deposition of iron in various organs leads to iron overload, manifesting with cirrhosis, arthritis, cardiomyopathy, diabetes mellitus, hepatoma, or other chronic disorders.

Prevalence

Genetic hemochromatosis is characterized by autosomal recessive inheritance. The gene responsible for this disease has a prevalence of about 10% in populations of North-West European descent. Although the prevalence of hemochromatosis varies depending upon the screening tests used to establish the diagnosis as well as the population studied, the average prevalence is between 0.1% and 0.5%. In the United States, hemochromatosis is the most common genetic disorder among Caucasians (10% to 15% of U.S. population are thought to be heterozygous carriers).

Clinical Features

Despite the fact that it is the most common genetic disorder among Caucasians in the United States, the disease is often not recognized by clinicians. Much of this has to do with the fact the disease has a gradual onset, usually presenting with nonspecific symptoms. As a result, there is often a delay in diagnosis and treatment, which can lead to increased morbidity and mortality.

For these reasons, it behooves the clinician to become familiar with the clinical features of hemochromatosis, which are listed in the following box.

CLINICAL FEATURES OF HEREDITARY HEMOCHROMATOSIS

PITUITARY
- Hypogonadotropic hypogonadism

SKIN
- Pigmentation

LIVER
- Hepatomegaly
- ±cirrhosis
- ±hepatoma

HANDS
- Porphyria cutanea tarda
- Arthritis in 2nd and 3rd metacarpophalangeal joints

HEART
- Cardiomyopathy

SPLEEN
- Splenomegaly

PANCREAS
- Diabetes mellitus

KNEES
- Chondrocalcinosis

GENITOURINARY
- Loss of hair in axillae and pubis
- Testicular atrophy

The presence of any of the above clinical features should prompt consideration of hemochromatosis. The classic profile of the patient with hereditary hemochromatosis includes skin hyperpigmentation (bronzing), cirrhosis, and type 2 diabetes mellitus. In reality, this classic triad is rarely present. Instead, patients may present with a wide variety of other symptoms and signs. Some of the heterogeneity in the clinical presentation of these patients has to do with when patients present in the course of their disease, as shown in the following box.

EARLY AND LATE SIGNS AND SYMPTOMS OF HEREDITARY HEMOCHROMATOSIS
EARLY
ELEVATED LIVER ENZYMES (AST, ALT)
DEPRESSION
IRRITABILITY
FATIGUE
JOINT PAIN
IMPOTENCE
AMENORRHEA
LATE
GRAY OR BRONZE SKIN TONE
CIRRHOSIS
HEPATOMA
HEART DISEASE / FAILURE
DIABETES MELLITUS
HYPOPITUITARISM
HYPOGONADISM
CHRONIC ABDOMINAL PAIN
SEVERE FATIGUE
INCREASED INCIDENCE OF BACTERIAL INFECTION
SPLENOMEGALY

Adapted from Laudicina RJ and Legrys VA, "Hereditary Hemochromatosis: A Case Study and Review," *Clin Lab Sci*, 2001, 14(3):201.

In recent years, however, more and more patients are being evaluated for hemochromatosis when abnormal liver function tests or serum ferritin levels are encountered. Knowledge of the laboratory tests available in the diagnosis of hemochromatosis is essential in not only establishing the diagnosis but also in differentiating it from other causes of iron overload.

Laboratory Testing

The laboratory tests available for the diagnosis of hereditary hemochromatosis are listed in the following box.

LABORATORY TESTS AVAILABLE IN THE DIAGNOSIS OF HEREDITARY HEMOCHROMATOSIS
SERUM IRON
TOTAL IRON BINDING CAPACITY
TRANSFERRIN SATURATION
SERUM FERRITIN
DNA ANALYSIS FOR HFE MUTATIONS
HEPATIC IRON INDEX

Serum Iron

Although serum iron levels are elevated in hereditary hemochromatosis, levels may also be raised in other conditions such as acute hepatitis. There are a number of factors that can affect serum iron levels including diet, pregnancy, oral contraceptive use, and ingestion of oral iron supplements. Fasting levels are recommended because levels can be increased after a meal. It is preferable to measure serum rather than plasma iron levels. If plasma is used, the clinician must make sure to avoid the use of anticoagulants, such as EDTA and citrate, which chelate iron. Because of these factors, serum iron levels alone lack sensitivity and specificity for the diagnosis of hereditary hemochromatosis.

Total Iron Binding Capacity

Measurement of the serum iron and total iron binding capacity can be used to calculate the percentage of transferrin saturation (TS), as follows:

Transferrin saturation = (serum iron / TIBC) x 100

When compared to the serum iron level, the transferrin saturation is more sensitive and specific for the diagnosis. Fasting transferrin saturation >50% and 60% in women and men, respectively, is associated with a sensitivity of 92% and specificity of 93% for the diagnosis of hereditary hemochromatosis. Using these values, the positive predictive value is 86%. There are many who advocate the use of a lower cutoff TS. If 45% is used as the cutoff value, the sensitivity is certainly increased (98%) but the specificity and positive predictive value decrease. The American Association for the Study of Liver Diseases advocates the use of the transferrin saturation as the initial test of choice in patients suspected of having hereditary hemochromatosis.

Like the serum iron, transferrin saturation may be affected by many factors including diet and coexisting diseases. Falsely normal values have been obtained in hereditary hemochromatosis patients with chronic blood loss or inflammatory disease. Patients must discontinue vitamins containing iron or oral contraceptives several days before testing. A second transferrin saturation should be obtained if the initial value is increased.

Serum Ferritin

Although the upper limit of normal for serum ferritin varies from laboratory to laboratory, in general, upper limits for men and postmenopausal women are 300 ng/mL. For premenopausal women, 200 ng/mL should be considered the upper limit of normal. An elevated serum ferritin level is consistent with the diagnosis of hereditary hemochromatosis. A normal serum ferritin level, however, does not exclude the diagnosis, especially in children and women. It is important to realize that young homozygotes may have normal serum ferritin levels despite the presence of considerably increased total iron body stores.

An elevated serum ferritin level may also be found in other conditions, such as cancer, inflammation, or infection. This has to do with the fact that ferritin is an acute phase reactant, rising in patients who have inflammatory disease. In patients with inflammatory conditions, serum ferritin levels are not as useful in estimating iron status. The degree of hyperferritinemia can be used, to some extent, in differentiating between inflammatory states and hemochromatosis. Serum ferritin levels are rarely >700 μmol/L when the elevation is due to an inflammatory condition.

Therefore, serum ferritin lacks sensitivity and specificity as a screening test for the diagnosis of hereditary hemochromatosis. For these reasons, serum ferritin levels alone should never be used as a screening test for the diagnosis. Studies have shown that elevations in both the serum ferritin and transferrin saturation have a 90% sensitivity and specificity for the diagnosis of hereditary hemochromatosis, particularly when other medical illnesses are not present.

Because of limitations when used alone, serum iron, total iron binding capacity, and serum ferritin should be used together in the diagnosis of hereditary hemochromatosis, keeping in mind that a number of factors can affect the results of these tests. These factors are outlined in the following table.

Confounding Variables in Iron Testing

Variable	Iron	TIBC	Transferrin Saturation	Ferritin
Day to day variation	Large	Small	Follows iron	Small
Menstrual cycle	Lower with menses; higher premenstrually	Small	Follows iron	Unknown
Oral iron	Increases after each dose, as much as 100-300 mg/dL	No change	Increase after each dose	Increase after many days
Iron contamination of sample	Increase	No change	Increase	No change
Hepatitis (viral, alcoholic, other)	Increase	Increase in some methods	Increase	Increase
Inflammable/acute phase reaction	Decrease	Decrease	Decrease	Increase
Oral contraceptives	Increase	No change	Decrease	No change
Biological variation	Large (20%)	Small (5%)	Large (20%)	Small (10%)

Adapted from Witte DL, "Hereditary Hemochromatosis: Practice Guideline Development Task Force of the College of American Pathologists," *Clin Chim Acta*, 1996, 235:139-200.

Patients who have a normal serum ferritin level and a transferrin saturation <45% usually require no further testing for hereditary hemochromatosis. This combination of lab test results has a negative predictive value of 97%.

DNA Testing

DNA testing for hereditary hemochromatosis is available. Genotypic testing/mutation analysis can determine the presence of the *HFE* gene mutations C282Y and H63D. Patients with C282Y/C282Y genotype are said to be homozygous for the hereditary hemochromatosis disease. Those that are heterozygous for the disease have a C282Y/wild type genotype. Compound heterozygotes are defined as having the C282Y/H63D genotype. Over 90% of hereditary hemochromatosis patients have been found to have the C282Y/C282Y genotype while compound heterozygotes account for 3% to 5% of cases. The clinician should realize, however, that other gene mutations may also be responsible for the disease.

At the present time, however, genotypic testing is not recommended for routine screening, especially in asymptomatic patients. Currently, a study is underway to determine if routine population screening for hereditary hemochromatosis is warranted. Until the results become available, mutation analysis should be considered in the following situations:

- Confirming the diagnosis of hereditary hemochromatosis in patients with documented iron overload (high transferrin saturation and ferritin levels)
- Testing in presymptomatic individuals (high transferrin saturation, normal serum ferritin, normal liver function tests)
- Screening family members of patients with hereditary hemochromatosis

  All first-degree relatives (genetic testing of children is controversial) should undergo mutation analysis for the *HFE* gene mutation. It is important to assess for the presence of both the C282Y and H63D mutations. Understandably, hereditary hemochromatosis patients are concerned about the risk their children have of acquiring the disease. In these cases, the spouse should undergo genotypic testing. If mutation analysis reveals no mutations, there is no need for evaluation of the children. If the spouse has the C282Y or H63D mutation, then the children are at risk for either being a C282Y homozygote or compound heterozygote (C282Y/H63D). It is recommended that children of these parents have serum ferritin levels performed on a yearly basis.

Liver Biopsy

The gold standard for the diagnosis of hereditary hemochromatosis has traditionally been liver biopsy. Histologic examination can assess iron deposition in hepatocytes. In addition, the presence of fibrosis or cirrhosis can be determined. Because other conditions may also be characterized by iron overload, liver biopsy is also useful to distinguish these conditions from hereditary hemochromatosis.

Of key importance is the determination of the following.

- Grading of hemosiderin deposits in liver tissue

  Liver biopsy with Perls Prussian blue stain can be used to not only detect hemosiderin deposits in liver tissue but also to grade the siderosis. Grade III or IV siderosis is more suggestive of hereditary hemochromatosis.

- Hepatic iron index

  The hepatic iron index is calculated by dividing the hepatic iron content (micromoles/g dry weight of liver) by the age of the patient (in years). A hepatic iron index <1.1 is considered to be normal. Homozygotes of the hereditary hemochromatosis gene have an index >1.9 while heterozygotes have a value <1.9. Alcoholic liver disease, which is a cause of secondary iron overload, is characterized by a hepatic iron index <1.7.

Traditionally, liver biopsy was performed on all patients with hereditary hemochromatosis, but, in recent years, there is general consensus that it is not needed in all patients. In particular, C282Y homozygotes who have a low likelihood for significant hepatic fibrosis or cirrhosis may proceed directly to therapeutic phlebotomy without undergoing liver biopsy. In these patients, the following features suggest a low likelihood for significant hepatic fibrosis or cirrhosis:

- Age <40 years
- Normal ALT
- Serum ferritin level <1000 ng/mL
- No clinical evidence of liver disease

If the patient does not have all of the above features, however, liver biopsy is warranted to determine the degree of hepatic fibrosis.

Quantitative Phlebotomy

On occasion, liver biopsy may not be performed because of contraindications or patient refusal. In these cases as well as in cases where the liver biopsy results are equivocal, the clinician may wish to perform quantitative phlebotomy. The premise of this test is that the removal of significant amounts of blood on a weekly basis will not lead to anemia in hereditary hemochromatosis because of the excess amounts of iron present within the body. Most patients with hereditary hemochromatosis have 3-4 g body iron. If one considers that a unit of blood has 250 mg of iron, at least sixteen units of blood can be removed without the development of anemia. Removal of this amount of blood through successive phlebotomies without the development of anemia is diagnostic of iron overload.

Differentiating Hereditary Hemochromatosis From Other Causes of Iron Overload

It is essential to differentiate hereditary hemochromatosis from secondary causes of iron overload. There are many conditions that may be associated with secondary iron overload, as shown in the following box.

CAUSES OF SECONDARY IRON OVERLOAD
ANEMIA
Thalassemia
Sideroblastic anemia
Congenital dyserythropoietic anemia
Refractory hypoplastic anemia
Severe hemolytic anemia
Any recurrent anemia that requires repeated blood transfusion
ALCOHOLIC CIRRHOSIS*
NONALCOHOLIC CIRRHOSIS / STEATOHEPATITIS
CHRONIC VIRAL HEPATITIS (B or C)
DEFECTS OF IRON TRANSPORT
PORPHYRIA CUTANEA TARDA
AFTER PORTOCAVAL SHUNT
DIETARY IRON OVERLOAD
NEONATAL IRON OVERLOAD
IRON-DEXTRAN INJECTIONS
AFRICAN IRON OVERLOAD

*In 20% of patients with alcoholic liver disease, hemosiderin deposits may be noted in the liver (hepatic siderosis). Hyperferritinemia is also quite common in patients with alcoholic liver disease. For these reasons, the iron overload of alcoholic liver disease may be difficult to distinguish from that due to hereditary hemochromatosis. Although transferrin saturation or serum ferritin may be elevated in alcoholic liver disease, both are not usually elevated together. Even when one is elevated, the degree of elevation is usually less than that seen in patients with hereditary hemochromatosis. When hepatic siderosis due to alcoholic liver disease is demonstrated by Perls staining of liver biopsy tissue, grading of the hemosiderin deposits usually demonstrates grade 1 or 2 siderosis. Rarely are grade 3 or 4 siderosis demonstrated in patients with alcoholic liver disease. In equivocal cases, the hepatic iron index allows the clinician to distinguish between these two conditions. An index >1.9 is consistent with hereditary hemochromatosis. Alcoholic liver disease is characterized by an index <1.7.

Other Laboratory Test Abnormalities

Because one of the clinical features of hereditary hemochromatosis is diabetes mellitus, blood glucose levels should be checked in all patients. Although AST and/or ALT may be elevated in patients with hereditary hemochromatosis, in many cases, the levels are normal. Therefore, the absence of transaminase elevation should not exclude the diagnosis. Other liver function tests such as albumin, PT, and bilirubin are usually normal. Abnormalities of these tests in the patient suspected of having hereditary hemochromatosis should prompt the clinician to consider the presence of chronic liver disease or cirrhosis.

Laboratory Testing During Therapy of Hereditary Hemochromatosis

Removal of excess iron by weekly venesection is the preferred treatment for hereditary hemochromatosis. During the period of weekly venisections, laboratory testing with serum ferritin and hemoglobin levels is performed at 4- to 6-week intervals. The removal of excess stores of iron is the goal of therapy. To reach this objective, clinicians aim to bring the hemoglobin in men and women to 12 and 11 g/dL, respectively, or the serum ferritin level to <50 µg/L.

Once these target values have been reached, venesection no longer has to be performed on a weekly basis but still must be performed at longer intervals (3-6 months) to maintain low or normal iron stores. These patients should be monitored for evidence of iron accumulation. It is thought that transferrin saturation may be a more reliable test than serum ferritin in assessing patients for reaccumulation of iron stores.

References

Bacon BR, "Hemochromatosis: Diagnosis and Management," *Gastroenterology*, 2001, 120(3):718-25.

Harrison SA and Bacon BR, "Hereditary Hemochromatosis: Update for 2003," *J Hepatol*, 2003, 38(Suppl 1):S14-23.

Laudicina RJ and Legrys VA, "Hereditary Hemochromatosis: A Case Study and Review," *Clin Lab Sci* 2001, 14(3):196-208; quiz 220-2.

Pietrangelo A, "Haemochromatosis," *Gut*, 2003, 52(Suppl 2):ii23-30.

Powell LW and Yapp TR, "Hemochromatosis," *Clin Liver Dis*, 2000, 4(1):211-28, viii.

Powell LW, Subramaniam VN, and Yapp TR, "Haemochromatosis in the New Millennium," *J Hepatol*, 2000, 32(1 Suppl):48-62.

Ryder SD and Beckingham IJ, "ABC of Diseases of Liver, Pancreas, and Biliary System. Other Causes of Parenchymal Liver Disease," *BMJ*, 2001, 322(7281):290-2.

Worwood M, "What Is the Role of Genetic Testing in Diagnosis of Haemochromatosis?" *Ann Clin Biochem*, 2001, 38(Pt 1):3-19.

HEREDITARY HEMOCHROMATOSIS

Algorithm for Investigation of Iron Overload

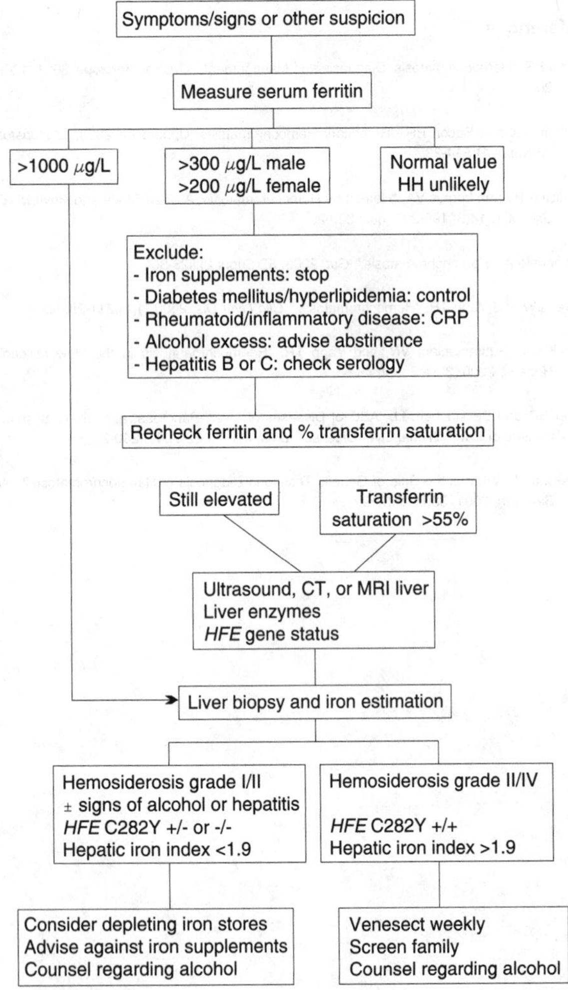

Adapted from O'Grady JG, Lake JR, and Houdle PD, *Comprehensive Clinical Hepatology*, Harcourt, 2000, 3.20.8.

HEREDITARY HEMOCHROMATOSIS

Algorithm for Screening Relatives

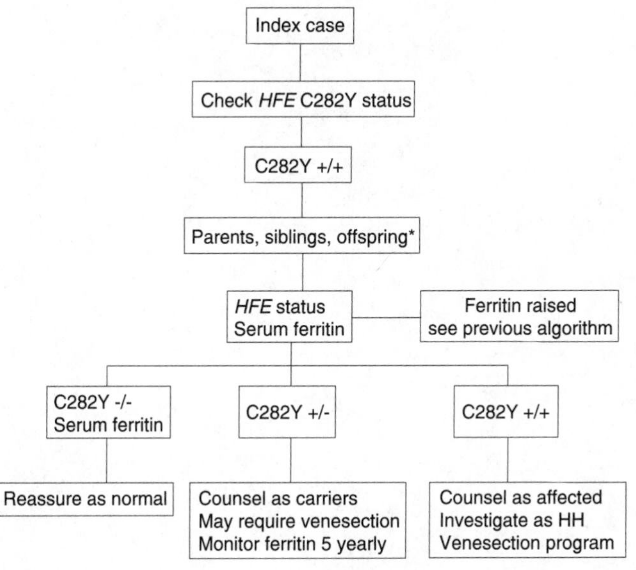

*When children are very young, the other parent may be tested, if C282Y -/- (90% cases), the children need not be tested until adulthood.

Adapted from O'Grady JG, Lake JR, and Houdle PD, *Comprehensive Clinical Hepatology*, Harcourt, 2000, 3.20.11.

WILSON'S DISEASE

Clinical Presentation

Wilson's disease is a genetic disorder of copper metabolism. The clinical presentation of Wilson's disease varies, but most patients present with liver disease and/or neuropsychiatric signs and symptoms. None of the clinical features of Wilson's disease is diagnostic. Because of greater awareness of the disease, patients are being diagnosed earlier, even before the development of classic features such as Kayser-Fleischer rings and severe neurologic symptoms.

Most patients with Wilson's disease have some manifestations of liver disease. In some cases, the liver disease precedes the neurologic manifestations by years. Studies have shown that liver disease alone may be the initial presentation of Wilson's disease in 20% to 46% of cases. In these patients, Wilson's disease may present with asymptomatic elevations in the liver function tests, acute hepatitis, chronic hepatitis, cirrhosis, and fulminant hepatic failure.

Although neurologic symptoms typically develop in adolescence or young adulthood, cases have been described in which the onset of symptoms was later in adulthood. Initially, it is not uncommon for patients to present with subtle symptoms including mild tremor, speech difficulty, and writing problems. With time, these patients may develop a progressive movement disorder.

Laboratory Testing

Liver function test abnormalities vary depending upon the hepatic presentation of the disease. Patients with Wilson's disease may present with acute liver failure, chronic hepatitis, acute hepatitis, asymptomatic elevations of the transaminases, or cirrhosis.

Renal tubular abnormalities are frequently noted in patients with Wilson's disease. These include glycosuria, aminoaciduria, hypophosphatemia, or renal tubular acidosis. These abnormalities may occur alone or together in what is known as the renal Fanconi syndrome.

Although the liver function test and/or renal tubular abnormalities may be suggestive of the diagnosis, the evaluation of patients suspected of having Wilson's disease begins with screening tests. The screening tests available in the diagnosis of Wilson's disease include the following:

- 24-hour urine collection for copper
- Kayser-Fleischer rings
- Serum ceruloplasmin level

24-Hour Urine Collection for Copper

Normal 24-hour urine copper excretion is 20-50 µg. A value >100 µg is indicative of Wilson's disease. When performing a 24-hour urine collection for copper, there are several important points of which to be aware.

- A complete 24-hour urine collection must be obtained. To ensure that the specimen submitted is a complete collection, it is necessary to measure the 24-hour urine creatinine. Males and females excrete 20-25 mg/kg and 15-20 mg/kg of creatinine over a 24-hour period, respectively. Creatinine levels that are below this range are suggestive of an incomplete 24-hour urine collection.
- Not every laboratory has the capability to perform accurate copper measurements of the urine. The specimen should be sent to a laboratory that has expertise in measuring copper.
- Elevated values are not synonymous with Wilson's disease. For example, levels >100 µg have been described in patients with long-

standing hepatic failure and hepatic obstruction (>1 year). Mildly elevated values may be noted in heterozygous carriers of Wilson's disease. Ten percent of these patients may have copper levels between 65 μg and 100 μg.

- The urine collecting material must not be contaminated with copper. In general, new plasticware is usually not contaminated with copper.
- Urine copper will be elevated during therapy with penicillamine or trientine (as well as for a few days after stopping these medications). For a few weeks after discontinuing the medications, a rebound lowering of copper levels may be appreciated.
- Presymptomatic Wilson's disease patients may not have urine copper levels >100 μg. In fact, only 75% of these patients will have levels this high. In the other 25%, levels will range from 65-100 μg.

In summary, the 24-hour urine copper is an excellent screening test for symptomatic patients with Wilson's disease. However, in presymptomatic patients, it is diagnostic in only 75% of cases. False-positive test results may occur in patients with chronic hepatic obstruction.

Kayser-Fleischer Rings

The deposition of copper around the outer portions of the cornea may be visualized as Kayser-Fleischer rings. These rings may be noted in many patients with Wilson's disease. In many cases, these rings are visible without any ophthalmological instrumentation. But much better for establishing or excluding their presence is ophthalmological evaluation with slit lamp examination.

Although Kayser-Fleischer rings are present in at least 99% of patients with the neuropsychiatric form of Wilson's disease, they are not always present in patients with the hepatic form of the disease. In addition, Kayser-Fleischer rings may be absent in presymptomatic patients.

The presence of these rings is not pathognomonic for Wilson's disease as they have been described, albeit rarely, in patients with long-standing hepatic failure or obstruction.

DIAGNOSTIC PITFALLS IN THE USE OF KAYSER-FLEISCHER RINGS IN THE DIAGNOSIS OF WILSON'S DISEASE
Not always present with hepatic presentation of the disease
At an early stage only detected by slit lamp exam
Difficult to see in brown or green eyes
Not pathognomonic - can occur in long-standing hepatic failure or obstruction

Serum Ceruloplasmin

Serum ceruloplasmin is a commonly used screening test for Wilson's disease. In most patients with Wilson's disease, the serum ceruloplasmin level is low. In 15% of patients, the levels may be normal or just below the lower limit of normal. It is also important to realize that heterozygous carriers of Wilson's disease may present with low ceruloplasmin levels as well.

In most laboratories, the reference interval for serum ceruloplasmin is 20-35 mg/dL. A strong argument can be made for Wilson's disease in patients who have levels <5 mg/dL. Rarely, heterozygous carriers may have levels this low. Levels ranging between 5-10 mg/dL are strongly suggestive of the disease.

Values between 10-20 mg/dL are found not only in Wilson's disease but also heterozygous carriers of Wilson's disease. While 20% of carriers have levels <20 mg/dL, the remainder have levels exceeding this. Other causes of low serum ceruloplasmin levels include malnutrition and familial hypoceruloplasminemia.

Values >30 mg/dL argue against the diagnosis of Wilson's disease. However, it is important to realize that false elevation of serum ceruloplasmin levels can occur, particularly in patients taking oral contraceptives, steroids, or estrogen.

DIAGNOSTIC PITFALLS IN THE USE OF SERUM CERULOPLASMIN IN THE DIAGNOSIS OF WILSON'S DISEASE
May be >20 mg/dL in 10% of cases, particularly in chronic hepatic inflammation
May be <20 mg/dL in 5% to 10% of heterozygous carriers
May be <20 mg/dL in acute liver failure or decompensated cirrhosis from other causes
May be low in malnutrition and familial hypoceruloplasminemia
May be falsely elevated in patients taking oral contraceptives, estrogens, or steroids

Establishing the Diagnosis

Since all of the screening tests for Wilson's disease have some limitations, the clinician should base the decision as to which one to perform on the signs and symptoms the patient with suspected Wilson's disease is presenting with. The following table describes the preferred screening test in the various forms of Wilson's disease.

Recommended Screening Tests for Wilson's Disease

Type of Wilson's Disease Presentation	Comment
Neurologic / psychiatric presentation	
24-hour urine copper	Generally unambiguous. Values >100 μg/24 hours indicate Wilson's disease, and are always present. Values significantly <100 rule out Wilson's disease.
Kayser-Fleischer ring	Generally unambiguous
Hepatic presentation	
24-hour urine copper	Generally quite reliable. Values >100 μg/24 hours indicates Wilson's disease. Interpret cautiously with long-standing hepatic failure or obstruction. Values significantly <100 rule out Wilson's disease.
Kayser-Fleischer ring	If present, very helpful. Interpret cautiously with long-standing hepatic failure or obstruction.
Serum ceruloplasmin	May be helpful (see above)
Presymptomatic patients	
24-hour urine copper	Over 100 μg/24 hours in about 75% of patients, and this indicates Wilson's disease. However, in about 25% of truly affected patients, it may not have reached 100.
Kayser-Fleischer ring	Present 30% to 40% of time. Essentially diagnostic when present.
Serum ceruloplasmin	May be helpful (see above)
Haplotype analysis	Applicable if a sibling has been diagnosed with the disease. Can be very useful, if the technique is available.

Adapted from Brewer GJ, *Wilson's Disease: A Clinician's Guide to Recognition, Diagnosis, and Management,* Kluwer Academic Publishers, 2001, 37.

The gold standard for the diagnosis of Wilson's disease is liver biopsy. A hepatic copper level >200 µg/g dry weight of tissue is diagnostic of Wilson's disease if the following criteria are met:

- Absence of long-standing hepatic failure (>1 year)
- Absence of long-standing hepatic obstruction (>1 year)

Normal hepatic copper levels are 20-50 µg/g dry weight. Heterozygous carriers of Wilson's disease may have elevated levels but rarely do these levels exceed 125 µg/g dry weight. A false-negative test result may occur because of sampling error.

Not all patients require liver biopsy, however, to establish the diagnosis. In many, the diagnosis can be established short of liver biopsy if the clinical presentation and biochemical testing is convincing for the diagnosis. The following table describes clinical scenarios in which liver biopsy is not indicated.

CLINICAL SCENARIOS IN WHICH LIVER BIOPSY IS NOT NEEDED FOR THE DIAGNOSIS OF WILSON'S DISEASE
Typical neurologic symptoms, Kayser-Fleischer rings, and urine copper >100 µg/24 hours
Sibling of affected patient, urine copper >100 µg/24 hours, and haplotype analysis identical to affected sibling
Kayser-Fleischer rings and urine copper >100 µg/24 hours
Hepatic presentation with urine copper >100 µg/24 hours (in the absence of long-standing hepatic failure or obstruction) and serum ceruloplasmin levels <10 mg/dL

Adapted from Brewer GJ, *Wilson's Disease: A Clinician's Guide to Recognition, Diagnosis, and Management,* Kluwer Academic Publishers, 2001, 43.

Long-standing hepatic failure or obstruction may also present with an increase in hepatic copper content to the levels seen in Wilson's disease. It can be quite challenging to differentiate these conditions from Wilson's disease because, in addition to increased hepatic copper content, increased urinary copper excretion and Kayser-Fleischer rings may also be noted in these patients.

In these cases, the serum ceruloplasmin levels may be helpful. Values <5 mg/dL are strongly suggestive of Wilson's disease. Values between 5-10 mg/dL are also suggestive of the diagnosis. Levels exceeding this are not reliable in differentiating Wilson's disease from long-standing hepatic failure or obstruction. In these difficult cases, a radiocopper test, DNA analysis, or therapeutic trial may need to be performed to establish the correct diagnosis.

References

El-Youssef M, "Wilson's Disease," *Mayo Clin Proc*, 2003, 78(9):1126-36.

Gaffney D, Fell GS, and O'Reilly DS "ACP Best Practice No 163. Wilson's Disease: Acute and Presymptomatic Laboratory Diagnosis and Monitoring," *J Clin Pathol*, 2000, 53(11):807-12.

Gitlin JD, "Wilson's Disease," *Semin Liver Dis*, 2000, 20(3):353-64.

Loudianos G and Gitlin JD, "Wilson's Disease," *Gastroenterology*, 2003, 125(6):1868-77.

Robertson WM, "Wilson's Disease," *Arch Neurol*, 2000, 57(2):276-7.

Ryder SD and Beckingham IJ, "ABC of Diseases of Liver, Pancreas, and Biliary System. Other Causes of Parenchymal Liver Disease," *BMJ*, 2001, 3;322(7281):290-2.

Sternlieb I, "Wilson's Disease," *Clin Liver Dis*, 2000, 4(1):229-39, viii-ix.

WILSON'S DISEASE

Algorithm for Establishing the Diagnosis of Asymptomatic or Hepatic Wilson's Disease

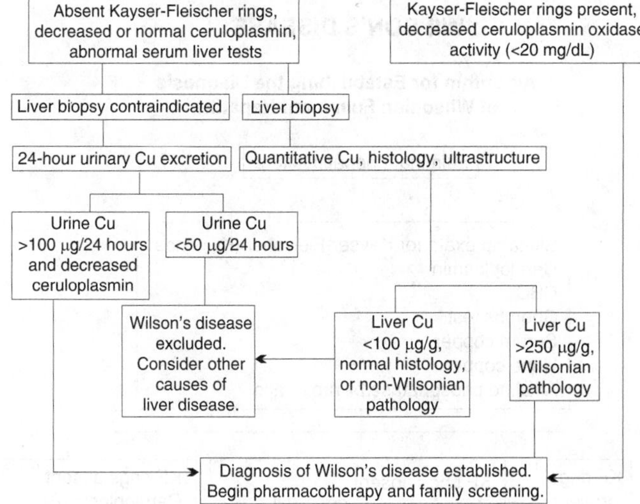

Algorithm for Establishing the Diagnosis of Wilson's Disease With Neuropsychiatric Presentation

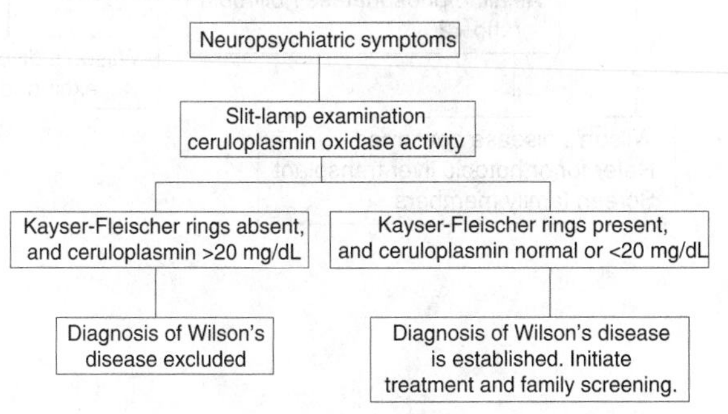

Adapted from Uv GY and Israel J, *Diseases of the Liver*, Humana Press, 1998.

WILSON'S DISEASE

Algorithm for Establishing the Diagnosis of Wilsonian Fulminant Hepatitis

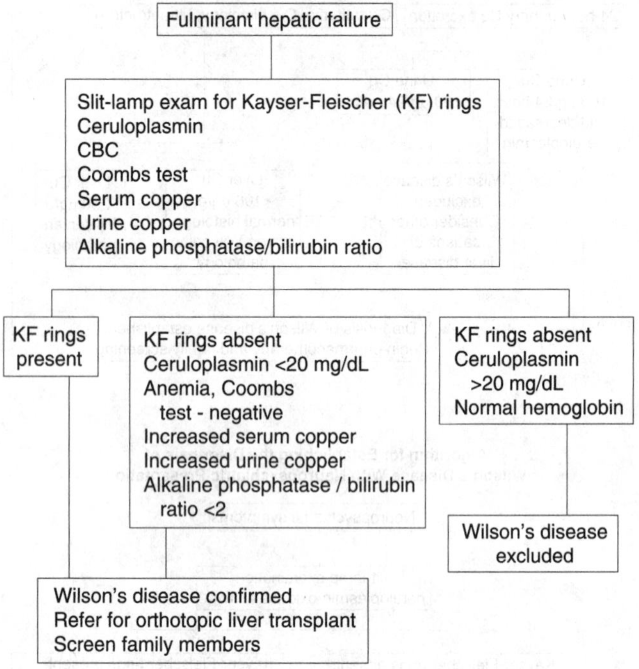

AUTOIMMUNE HEPATITIS

Autoimmune hepatitis is a chronic inflammatory liver disease that tends to have a predilection for women. In fact, it is four times more common in women. It is a type of chronic hepatitis characterized by the presence of hypergammaglobulinemia and serum autoantibodies.

Clinical Presentation

Although typically considered chronic, a considerable number of patients may present with an acute illness characterized by jaundice, mimicking the presentation of acute viral hepatitis. On occasion, it may present with acute liver failure.

More often, however, autoimmune hepatitis presents insidiously with nonspecific symptoms such as fatigue, malaise, and anorexia. In these patients, the diagnosis may not be made until the liver disease is advanced. Physical examination findings include jaundice, hepatomegaly, splenomegaly, and spider nevi.

Between 30% and 80% of patients may present with manifestations of cirrhosis. Decompensated cirrhosis with ascites or hepatic encephalopathy may be the initial presentation in up to 20% of patients.

A clue to the diagnosis of autoimmune hepatitis is its frequent association with other autoimmune diseases. These include thyroiditis, ulcerative colitis, rheumatoid arthritis, diabetes mellitus, alopecia, nail dystrophy, Sjögren's syndrome, and glomerulonephritis.

Laboratory Testing

Laboratory testing usually reveals elevated transaminase levels, typically ranging from two to ten times the upper limit of normal. Autoimmune hepatitis is also a consideration in patients who present with marked transaminase elevation (>1000 IU/L). The absence of transaminase elevation does not exclude the diagnosis. In fact, AST and ALT may be normal in autoimmune hepatitis patients who have progressed to cirrhosis.

Although serum bilirubin and alkaline phosphatase levels are often increased, mild increases are typically noted. Substantial increases should prompt consideration of alternative diagnoses. In a small percentage of autoimmune hepatitis cases, however, a cholestatic pattern characterized by marked increases of the alkaline phosphatase and bilirubin is noted. In these patients, a thorough evaluation should be performed to exclude other causes of cholestasis.

Prolonged PT and/or hypoalbuminemia are suggestive of progression to cirrhosis.

Serum immunoglobulins are elevated in the majority of autoimmune hepatitis patients. Hypergammaglobulinemia with polyclonal increase in IgG is most commonly noted but elevations in IgM and IgA may also be appreciated. In type II autoimmune hepatitis (see below), there may be a reduction in serum IgA levels.

The laboratory hallmark of autoimmune hepatitis is the presence of circulating autoantibodies. Antibody testing should include antinuclear antibodies (ANA), antismooth muscle antibodies (ASMA), antiliver-kidney microsomal antibodies (LKM-1), autoantibodies against soluble liver antigens (SLA), and antibodies against liver-pancreas antigen (LP). Using these antibodies, autoimmune hepatitis may be subdivided further, as shown in the following table.

Classification of Autoimmune Hepatitis

Autoimmune Hepatitis Type	Autoantibody Present
Type I	ANA/ASMA
Type II	LKM-1 (ANA and ASMA absent)
Type III	SLA/LP

Among the different types of autoimmune hepatitis, type I is much more common than types II and III.

ANA are found in 2/3 of autoimmune patients. It is important to realize that other hepatic conditions (primary biliary cirrhosis, primary sclerosing cholangitis, drug-induced hepatitis, alcoholic liver disease, nonalcoholic steatohepatitis, chronic viral hepatitis) may present with positive ANA. Of note, titers in autoimmune hepatitis are typically above 1:160. There is no correlation between the titer and the activity or prognosis of the disease.

ASMA are found not only in autoimmune hepatitis (87%) but may also be noted in other hepatic illnesses. Like the ANA, ASMA titers do not correlate with prognosis.

Anti-LKM testing is usually negative in autoimmune hepatitis patients in the United States. In Europe, however, up to 20% of adult patients are found to have anti-LKM. They are not specific for autoimmune hepatitis and may be found in patients with drug-induced hepatitis.

Establishing the Diagnosis

The abnormalities of the liver function tests do not allow the clinician to differentiate autoimmune hepatitis from other causes of liver disease. Although autoantibodies and serum immunoglobulin levels are helpful in the diagnosis of autoimmune hepatitis, the clinician should realize that other liver diseases, such as drug-induced hepatitis and chronic viral hepatitis, may also be associated with the presence of autoantibodies. To make the diagnosis of autoimmune hepatitis, the clinician should make every effort to exclude other possible causes of the patient's clinical presentation. Liver biopsy remains a key component in the evaluation of suspected autoimmune hepatitis. It also provides information about disease severity and can help exclude other types of liver disease.

Recently, a scoring system was devised by the International Autoimmune Hepatitis Group to aid in the diagnosis of this disease. The patient's score is based on the presence or absence of various biochemical, epidemiologic, and clinical markers. Although the scoring system was originally developed for research purposes, studies have shown that the use of this score has validity in the clinical setting as well. A sensitivity of the diagnosis of definite or probable autoimmune hepatitis is 97% to 100%. This scoring system is described in the following table.

Diagnostic Scoring System for Autoimmune Hepatitis in Adults

Category	Factor	Score
Sex	Female	+2
Ratio of alkaline phosphatase to AST or ALT	>3
<1.5	-2 +2
γ-globulin or immunoglobulin G level (three times above upper limit or normal)	>2.0 1.5-2.0 1.0-1.5
<1.0	+3 +2 +1 0
ANA, ASMA (anti-smooth muscle antibodies), or anti-LKM1 titers	>1:80 1:80 1:40
<1:40	+3 +2 +1 0
Antimitochondrial antibodies	Positive	-4

Diagnostic Scoring System for Autoimmune Hepatitis in Adults *(continued)*

Category	Factor	Score
Viral markers of active replication	Positive Negative	-3 +3
Hepatotoxic drugs	Yes No	-4 +1
Alcohol consumption	<25 g/day >60 g/day	+2 -2
Concurrent immune disease	Any nonhepatic disease or an immune nature	+2
Other autoantibodies	Anti-SLA/LP, actin, LC1, pANCA	+2
Histologic features	Interface hepatitis Plasma cells Rosettes None of the above Biliary changes Atypical features	+3 +1 +1 -5 -3 -3
Human leukocyte antigen	DR3 or DR4	+1
Treatment response	Remission alone Remission with relapse	+2 +3
Pretreatment score	Definite diagnosis >15	Probable diagnosis 10-15
Post-treatment score	Definite diagnosis >17	Probable diagnosis 12-17

From Luxon BA, "Autoimmune Hepatitis," *Postgraduate Medicine*, 2003, 114(1):81.

Also from Alvarez F, Berg PA, Bianchi FB, et al, "International Autoimmune Hepatitis Group Report: Review of Criteria for Diagnosis of Autoimmune Hepatitis," *J Hepatol*, 1999, 31(5):929-38.

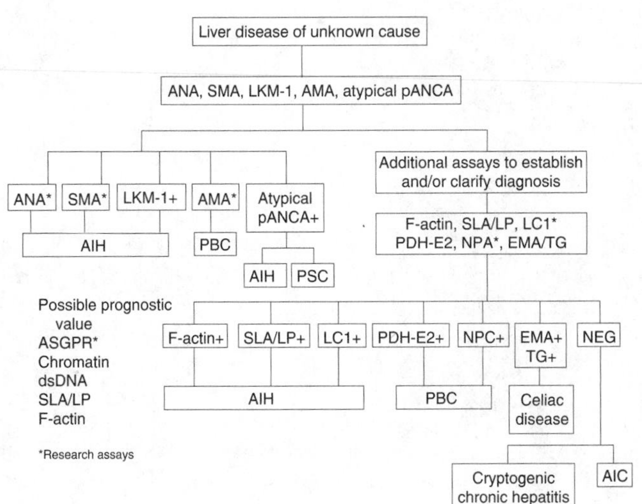

References

Gish RG and Mason A, "Autoimmune Liver Disease. Current Standards, Future Directions," *Clin Liver Dis*, 2000, 5(2):287-314.

Luxon BA, "Autoimmune Hepatitis. Making Sense of All Those Antibodies," *Postgrad Med*, 2003, 114(1):79-82, 85-8.

Mackay IR, "Antinuclear (Chromatin) Autoantibodies in Autoimmune Hepatitis," *J Gastroenterol Hepatol*, 2001, 16(3):245-7.

Manns MP and Strassburg CP, "Autoimmune Hepatitis: Clinical Challenges," *Gastroenterology*, 2001, 120(6):1502-17.

McFarlane IG, "Autoimmune Hepatitis: Clinical Manifestations and Diagnostic Criteria," *Can J Gastroenterol*, 2001, 15(2):107-13.

McFarlane IG, "Autoimmune Hepatitis: Diagnostic Criteria, Subclassifications, and Clinical Features," *Clin Liver Dis*, 2002, 6(3):317-33.

Obermayer-Straub P, Strassburg CP, and Manns MP, "Autoimmune Hepatitis," *J Hepatol*, 2000, 32(1 Suppl):181-97.

Ryder SD and Beckingham IJ, "ABC of Diseases of Liver, Pancreas, and Biliary System. Other Causes of Parenchymal Liver Disease," *BMJ*, 2001, 322(7281):290-2.

Strassburg CP and Manns MP, "Autoantibodies and Autoantigens in Autoimmune Hepatitis," *Semin Liver Dis*, 2002, 22(4):339-52.

FATTY LIVER

Fatty liver, also known as hepatic steatosis, is defined as the accumulation of lipid within liver cells. It is a common condition that is associated with a number of conditions. Most cases, however, are due to excessive amounts of alcohol intake. Other common causes of fatty liver include obesity, hyperlipidemia, diabetes mellitus, and medications. Although most cases are benign in nature, some causes of fatty liver may be associated with necroinflammatory changes. When these changes are demonstrated on histologic examination of liver tissue in the absence of alcohol intake, nonalcoholic steatohepatitis is said to be present. It is important to make the distinction between fatty liver and nonalcoholic steatohepatitis because only patients with the latter are at risk of progression to chronic liver disease and cirrhosis.

Clinical Presentation

Most patients with fatty liver are asymptomatic. Up to 20% of patients, however, may present with right upper quadrant pain.

Laboratory Testing

In usual clinical practice, most patients with fatty liver come to clinical attention with one or more of the following:

- Enlarged liver
- Abnormal liver function tests
- Findings consistent with fatty liver on imaging study

Mild elevations in the transaminases, alkaline phosphatase, and GGT may be present. Rarely do the levels of these liver function tests exceed three to four times the upper limit of normal. Serum albumin and bilirubin levels are usually normal.

It is important to realize that fatty liver does not always present with abnormal liver function tests. Therefore, the absence of liver function test abnormalities does not exclude the diagnosis.

Radiologic Imaging

In patients suspected of having fatty liver, an ultrasound or CT scan may provide evidence to support the diagnosis. Ultrasound findings consistent with fatty liver include increased echogenicity of the liver parenchyma. Low attenuation of the liver compared to the spleen is the CT scan finding that should prompt consideration of fatty liver. It is important to realize, however, that the absence of radiologic findings consistent with hepatic steatosis does not exclude the diagnosis.

Liver Biopsy

Liver biopsy is the gold standard for establishing the diagnosis of fatty liver. Liver biopsy, however, is usually not required. In patients who have radiologic findings consistent with fatty liver but have normal liver function tests, there is no need to proceed with liver biopsy. In other patients, the decision to perform liver biopsy should be based on whether or not the findings would change patient management. If the findings could alter the management of the patient, liver biopsy should be considered.

Causes

Causes of hepatic steatosis are listed in the following box.

CAUSES OF HEPATIC STEATOSIS	
MICROVESICULAR	***MACROVESICULAR***
INBORN ERRORS	CHRONIC ALCOHOL INGESTION*
ACUTE FATTY LIVER OF PREGNANCY	TYPE II DIABETES*
REYE'S SYNDROME	OBESITY*
MEDICATIONS / TOXINS	JEJUNOILEAL BYPASS*
Salicylate	HYPERALIMENTATION*
Tetracycline	PROTEIN-CALORIE MALNUTRITION
Valproic acid	LIMB LIPODYSTROPHY*
Amiodarone*	CORTICOSTEROIDS
Perhexiline maleate	ABETALIPOPROTEINEMIA*
Dideoxyinosine	WILSON'S DISEASE
ACUTE ALCOHOL INGESTION	AZT

*Indicates conditions commonly associated with either steatosis or steatohepatitis.

Adapted from O'Grady JG, Lake JR, and Howdle PD, *Comprehensive Clinical Hepatology*, London, England: Harcourt Publishers Ltd, 2000, 3.22.3.

As indicated in the above box, hepatic steatosis may be categorized as microvesicular or macrovesicular. These are histologic terms that refer to whether fat is present in small or large vacuoles in the hepatocyte.

Clinical Course

In most cases, fatty liver is a benign condition, carrying a good prognosis. There are, however, some causes of fatty liver which are associated with an increased risk of progression to hepatic fibrosis and cirrhosis. These include chronic alcohol ingestion, amiodarone therapy, and jejunoileal bypass.

When a cause can be identified, steps taken to correct the cause or remove the precipitant can lead to normalization of the liver function tests and improvement or even resolution of the radiologic findings of fatty liver.

References

Diehl AM, "Nonalcoholic Steatohepatitis," *Semin Liver Dis*, 1999, 19(2):221-9.

Kumar KS and Malet PF, "Nonalcoholic Steatohepatitis," *Mayo Clin Proc*, 2000, 75(7):733-9.

Lonardo A, "Fatty Liver and Nonalcoholic Steatohepatitis. Where Do We Stand and Where Are We Going?" *Dig Dis*, 1999, 17(2):80-9.

Marchesini G, McCullough AJ, Falck-Ytter Y, et al, "Clinical Features and Natural History of Nonalcoholic Steatosis Syndromes," *Semin Liver Dis*, 2001, 21(1):17-26.

Mullhall BP, Ong JP, and Younossi ZM, "Non-alcoholic Fatty Liver Disease: An Overview," *J Gastroenterol Hepatol*, 2002, 17(11):1136-43.

Reid AE, "Nonalcoholic Steatohepatitis," *Gastroenterology*, 2001, 121(3):710-23.

Sanyai AJ, "AGA Technical Review on Nonalcoholic Fatty Liver Disease," *Gastroenterology*, 2002, 123(5):1705-25.

Williams CN, "Nonalcoholic Steatohepatitis," *Can J Gastroenterol*, 1999, 13(8):639-40.

ACUTE PANCREATITIS

Clinical Presentation

Acute pancreatitis is classically characterized by the gradual onset of epigastric pain, which often radiates to the back. The pain is generally steady, taking some time to reach maximal intensity. The severity of the pain varies, with some patients describing the pain as the most severe they have ever experienced. Many patients report that leaning forward alleviates the pain. Nausea, vomiting, and anorexia commonly accompany the pain, so much so that it is said that their absence should prompt consideration of other etiologies.

Acute pancreatitis is fatal in up to 10% of patients. One factor thought to play a major role in the mortality of acute pancreatitis is suboptimal management due to either a delay in diagnosis or missing the diagnosis altogether. Recent studies have revealed that up to 42% of acute pancreatitis cases are not diagnosed until postmortem examination. Part of the difficulty in establishing the diagnosis lies with the fact that there is a wide variation in the clinical presentation of acute pancreatitis. Atypical clinical presentations are common, especially in the elderly. This coupled with the relative lack of sensitivity and specificity of the available confirmatory laboratory tests (serum amylase and lipase) make the diagnosis of acute pancreatitis a challenging one.

Sensitivity of Serum Amylase in the Detection of Acute Pancreatitis

The serum amylase is a widely used test for the diagnosis of acute pancreatitis. One of the major problems with the use of the test is that it is often not ordered because the diagnosis of acute pancreatitis is not suspected. As a general rule, most experts recommend obtaining serum amylase levels if there is clinical suspicion for acute pancreatitis. In addition, many support obtaining a serum amylase level in all patients who present with acute abdominal pain.

Even when the serum amylase is ordered, however, the interpretation of the serum amylase level is fraught with potential pitfalls. Eighty percent of patients with acute pancreatitis will have an elevated serum amylase if the test is obtained within 24 hours of the onset of abdominal pain. In the remaining 20% of patients, however, an amylase elevation will be lacking for a variety of reasons. Reasons why the serum amylase level may be normal in the patient with acute pancreatitis include the following.

- Sensitivity of the serum amylase level is lower in acute alcoholic pancreatitis (when compared to other etiologies).
- Acute exacerbations of chronic pancreatitis may not be associated with a rise in the serum amylase level.
- Serum amylase levels may not have risen if the patient presents early after the onset of abdominal pain (a rise in the serum amylase is first detected 2-12 hours after symptom onset).
- Serum amylase levels may have returned to normal if the patient presents too late in the course of the disease (serum amylase levels usually return to normal within 5 days of symptom onset, even if pancreatic inflammation persists).
- A significant increase in the lipid level (lipemic serum) can result in normal serum amylase levels in the face of acute pancreatitis. In these cases, the hyperlipidemia inhibits serum amylase activity. The elevation in the serum amylase level may be appreciated if the clinician instructs the lab to dilute the serum.

The precise sensitivity of the serum amylase level in the diagnosis of acute pancreatitis has been difficult to establish but most authorities state that the sensitivity is about 90% when blood specimens are obtained within 24-36 hours of symptom onset.

Specificity of the Serum Amylase in the Detection of Acute Pancreatitis

The limitations of the serum amylase level in the detection of acute pancreatitis are not confined to sensitivity alone. The serum amylase level also lacks specificity in the diagnosis of acute pancreatitis.

Although amylase can be found in a number of different tissues, the pancreas and the salivary gland are the two main sources of amylase. The serum amylase level is dependent upon the activity of these two isoenzymes (salivary and pancreatic) of amylase. Therefore, disease affecting nonpancreatic organs can result in an increase in the serum amylase level. Causes of serum amylase elevation are listed in the following box.

CAUSES OF INCREASED SERUM AMYLASE LEVELS

PANCREATIC DISEASE
- Pancreatitis
- Pseudocyst
- Abscess
- Carcinoma
- Ductal obstruction
- Trauma (including surgery and ERCP)
- Early cystic fibrosis

SALIVARY DISEASE
- Infection (mumps)
- Trauma (including surgery)
- Radiation
- Ductal obstruction
- Tumor

GASTROINTESTINAL DISEASE
- Perforated/penetrating peptic ulcer
- Mesenteric ischemia/infarction
- Intestinal obstruction
- Gut perforation (stomach, small intestine, large intestine)
- Acute appendicitis
- Acute cholecystitis
- Common bile duct obstruction
- Esophageal perforation
- Hepatitis
- Cirrhosis
- Abdominal trauma with hematoma formation
- Afferent loop obstruction
- Gastroenteritis (severe)

GYNECOLOGIC DISEASE
- Ruptured ectopic pregnancy
- Pelvic inflammatory disease
- Ovarian cysts
- Fallopian cysts

MALIGNANCY
- Solid tumors (ovary, lung, esophagus, prostate, breast, thymus)
- Multiple myeloma
- Pheochromocytoma

CAUSES OF INCREASED SERUM AMYLASE LEVELS *(continued)*
MISCELLANEOUS
Renal failure
Diabetic ketoacidosis
Anorexia nervosa
Macroamylasemia
Cerebral trauma
Burns
Postoperative
Pregnancy
Ruptured aortic aneurysm or dissection
Postictical
Alcohol use
AIDS
MEDICATIONS
Sphincter of Oddi spasm
Cholinergics
Bethanechol
Codeine
Morphine
Fentanyl
Meperidine
Pentazocine
Other narcotics
Parotitis
Phenylbutazone (causes parotitis)
Potassium iodide (causing parotitis)
Procyclidine
Drugs causing pancreatitis

In other cases, an elevation in serum amylase is not due to disease of nonpancreatic or pancreatic organs. In patients with renal insufficiency, impaired clearance of the enzyme can lead to an elevated serum amylase level. Levels are usually less than three times the upper limit of normal in patients with renal failure. Even less common is a serum amylase elevation secondary to macroamylasemia, a condition in which amylase binds to high molecular weight compounds. Macroamylasemia is reported to account for up to 5% of cases of hyperamylasemia.

Authorities have attempted to improve the specificity of the serum amylase level by increasing the amylase level at which acute pancreatitis is diagnosed. Instead of using the upper limit of normal, these investigators recommend using three times the upper limit of normal as the diagnostic threshold for acute pancreatitis. While a rise in the serum amylase level to above three times the upper limit of normal is almost diagnostic for the diagnosis of acute pancreatitis, the improved specificity comes at a price of reduced sensitivity.

More specific than total serum amylase levels is determination of pancreatic isoamylase. Unfortunately, measurement of pancreatic isoamylase is not readily available.

Sensitivity of the Serum Lipase Level in the Detection of Acute Pancreatitis

Most authorities feel that the sensitivity of the serum amylase and lipase are about the same during the first day after symptom onset. After the first day, the sensitivity of the serum lipase in the detection of acute pancreatitis is clearly higher. Much of this has to due with the time course of elevation and return to normal of these pancreatic enzymes.

Serum amylase levels first rise 2-12 hours after symptom onset, peak at 12-72 hours, and return to normal within 5 days. Serum lipase levels climb within 4-8 hours of symptom onset, peaking at 24 hours. In contrast to serum amylase, serum lipase levels return to normal more slowly, often taking 8-14 days.

Like the serum amylase level, serum lipase levels may be normal in patients with acute exacerbations of chronic pancreatitis. In these cases, so much acinar tissue may have been destroyed that a rise in either amylase or lipase is not possible despite the presence of pancreatic inflammation.

Specificity of the Serum Lipase in the Detection of Acute Pancreatitis

While serum lipase levels are considered to be more specific than serum amylase levels in the detection of acute pancreatitis, the serum lipase level may be increased in a number of nonpancreatic diseases. Most of these conditions are intestinal or hepatobiliary disorders in which there is a rise in nonpancreatic lipase. The causes of serum lipase elevation are listed in the following box.

CAUSES OF SERUM LIPASE ELEVATION

PANCREATIC DISEASE
- Acute pancreatitis
- Chronic pancreatitis
- Post-ERCP/trauma
- Calculus
- Carcinoma
- Abscess
- Pseudocyst

GASTROINTESTINAL / HEPATOBILIARY DISEASE
- Intestinal ischemia/infarction
- Intestinal obstruction
- Acute appendicitis
- Acute cholecystitis
- Common bile duct obstruction
- Gut perforation (stomach, small intestine, colon)
- Esophageal perforation

MEDICATIONS
- Drugs causing pancreatitis
- Sphincter of Oddi spasm
  - Meperidine
  - Codeine
  - Cholinergics
  - Bethanechol
  - Pentazocine
  - Methacholine
  - Morphine
  - Secretin
- Acetaminophen overdose
- Valproic acid

MISCELLANEOUS
- Renal failure
- Macrolipasemia
- Idiopathic
- Intracranial bleeding
- Malignancy
- Hemodialysis
- HIV

Despite this, the clinician should realize that lipase has significantly less tissue distribution than amylase; therefore, serum lipase levels are less commonly elevated in patients with nonpancreatic disease. Even when the serum lipase level rises in nonpancreatic disease, seldom does the level rise above three times the upper limit of normal. In fact, lipase elevations exceeding three times the upper limit of normal have been found to be 98% specific for the diagnosis of acute pancreatitis.

Like the serum amylase level, the serum lipase level may be elevated in patients with renal failure due to prolonged clearance. Levels exceeding three times the upper limit of normal, however, are unusual in patients with renal failure.

Use of Amylase and Lipase Together in the Detection of Acute Pancreatitis

While there continues to be some debate regarding the use of one or both enzymes in the detection of acute pancreatitis, most authorities recommend obtaining both serum amylase and lipase levels. They advocate the use of both enzymes together in an effort to maximize sensitivity and specificity.

In one study of 65 patients with acute pancreatitis who had a normal amylase level, approximately 66% were found to have a serum lipase elevation. In this study, the combined use of both amylase and lipase increased the sensitivity from 81% (amylase alone) to 94% (both enzymes together). Other experts do not believe that a combination of these two tests improves diagnostic accuracy.

The use of both tests together has led to situations in which one enzyme is elevated but the other is normal. Normal serum amylase levels may occur in the setting of hyperlipasemia in the following situations.

- Acute pancreatitis patients who present with a longer duration of symptoms

  Amylase levels rise within 2 -12 hours of symptom onset, peak at 12-72 hours, and return to normal within 5 days. Lipase levels rise within 4-8 hours, peak at 24 hours, and return to normal 8-14 days after symptom onset. Therefore, blood specimens drawn in patients with a longer duration of symptoms may be characterized by hyperlipasemia but normoamylasemia.

- Impaired renal function

  The clearance of lipase is prolonged in patients with renal failure. The serum amylase level may also be increased in patients with renal failure but, sometimes, only the serum lipase level is increased.

- Macrolipasemia

  Macrolipasemia, which is less common than macroamylasemia, is another explanation for an elevated serum lipase level in the setting of normoamylasemia. In this condition, lipase binds to high molecular weight compounds, which results in prolonged clearance.

- Nonpancreatic sources of lipase

  Lipase is found in a number of different organs. Most of the conditions characterized by hyperlipasemia are abdominal or hepatobiliary disorders. While some of these conditions may also be characterized by serum amylase elevation, not uncommonly, only the serum lipase level is found to be high. Serum lipase elevation that is due to nonpancreatic disease seldom exceeds three times the upper limit of normal.

Because of the problems with the sensitivity and specificity of serum amylase and lipase in the diagnosis of acute pancreatitis, the best use of these tests is to support rather than confirm the diagnosis of acute pancreatitis in patients with a compatible clinical presentation.

Relationship Between the Degree of Serum Amylase / Lipase Elevation and the Severity of Acute Pancreatitis

No correlation has been established between the degree of serum amylase / lipase elevation and the severity of the acute pancreatitis. Neither serum amylase or lipase are used in the severity scores commonly used in acute pancreatitis (ie, Ranson criteria). Therefore, the admission or peak amylase or lipase level has no bearing on the severity of the disease.

Persistently Elevated Serum Amylase / Lipase Levels in the Patient With Acute Pancreatitis

Persistently elevated serum amylase or lipase levels should prompt the clinician to consider a complication of acute pancreatitis. In particular, consideration should be given to the possibility of pancreatic abscess or pseudocyst. Imaging may be indicated in these cases. Remember that serum amylase levels should return to normal within 5 days of symptom onset.

Other Laboratory Test Abnormalities in Acute Pancreatitis

By no means are the serum amylase and lipase the only tests to be abnormal in patients with acute pancreatitis. Many other lab test abnormalities have been described, as shown in the following table. Of key importance is the fact that while these abnormalities have been noted in acute pancreatitis, the same lab test abnormalities have been described in patients with other acute abdominal emergencies.

Laboratory Test	Acute Pancreatitis (%)	Other (%)
Serum amylase (Somogyi units/dL)		
>500	59	1
200-500	36	4
<200	5	95
Hematocrit (%)		
>45	31	23
<45	69	77
White blood cell count (cells/mm^3)		
>12,000	41	53
<12,000	59	47
Blood glucose (mg/dL)		
>300	7	0
200-300	9	7
Diabetics excluded: <200	84	93
Serum calcium (mg/dL)		
>9	76	67
8-9	15	31
<8	9	2
Serum LDH (IU/L)		
>225	48	24
<225	52	76
SGOT (Sigma-Frankel units/dL)		
>100	37	8
<100	63	92

Adapted from "Diagnostic Standards for Acute Pancreatitis," *World J Surg*, Vol 21, Ranson JH, ed, 1997, 137.

Using Laboratory Tests to Estimate Prognosis in Acute Pancreatitis

Certain laboratory tests may be used to predict the severity of the acute pancreatitis attack. While a number of severity scores have been developed, one that is quite popular is Ranson's criteria, originally developed in 1974. Ranson's criteria are listed in the following box.

RANSON'S PROGNOSTIC FACTORS IN ACUTE PANCREATITIS
AT ADMISSION OR DIAGNOSIS
Age >55 years
White blood cell count >16,000/µL
Blood glucose level >200 mg/dL
Serum LDH concentration >350 IU/L
SGOT >250 IU/L
AFTER 48 HOURS
Hematocrit decrease >10%
Blood urea nitrogen increase >5 mg/dL
Serum calcium level <8 mg/dL
Arterial pO_2 <60 mm Hg
Base deficit >4 mEq/L
Estimated fluid sequestration >6 L

Calculation of the Ranson's prognostic score can be used to predict mortality in patients with acute pancreatitis, as shown in the following table.

Mortality of Acute Pancreatitis Based on Ranson's Prognostic Score

Ranson's Prognostic Score	Mortality
<2	<5%
3-5	10%
>5	≥60%

The major limitation of the Ranson's criteria is that 48 hours must pass before the severity score can be calculated. This is a limitation it shares with many of the other available scoring systems, with the exception of the APACHE II system.

Using Laboratory Tests to Assess Etiology of Acute Pancreatitis

The two major causes of acute pancreatitis include alcohol and gallstone disease, both accounting for approximately 80% to 90% of cases. Studies have been done to determine if laboratory test abnormalities can differentiate acute pancreatitis secondary to gallstone disease from other causes. One meta-analysis revealed that an ALT elevation >150 IU/L was 96% specific in the diagnosis of gallstone pancreatitis. When ALT levels exceed this value, one can make a fairly strong argument for the diagnosis. It is important to realize, however, that the sensitivity of this degree of ALT elevation is only 48%. Therefore, an ALT level <150 IU/L does not exclude the diagnosis of gallstone pancreatitis.

Several other causes of acute pancreatitis may be identified by laboratory testing. Hypertriglyceridemia is a well known cause of acute and chronic pancreatitis. An attack of acute pancreatitis may be precipitated by serum triglyceride levels exceeding 1000 mg/dL. One cannot make the diagnosis during or soon after an attack of acute pancreatitis because hyperlipidemia may be the result of the attack itself rather than the causative factor. For this reason, a lipid profile should be obtained weeks after the acute pancreatitis episode has resolved.

Hypercalcemia is also a cause of acute pancreatitis. At the time of an acute pancreatitis episode, however, an increased serum calcium level may be masked by the hypocalcemia that commonly accompanies acute pancreatitis. Therefore, it is reasonable to obtain a serum calcium level at some point after the episode has resolved.

References

Beckingham IJ and Borbman PC, "ABC of Diseases of Liver, Pancreas, and Biliary System. Acute Pancreatitis," *BMJ*, 2001, 322(7286):595-8.

Cartmell MT and Kingsnorth AN, "Acute Pancreatitis," *Hosp Med*, 2000, 61(6):382-5.

Frank B and Gottlieb K, "Amylase Normal, Lipase Elevated: Is It Pancreatitis? A Case Series and Review of the Literature," *Am J Gastroenterol*, 1999, 94(2):463-9.

Gates LK Jr, "Severity Scoring for Acute Pancreatitis: Where Do We Stand in 1999?" *Curr Gastroenterol Rep*, 1999, 1(2):134-8.

Kemppainen EA, Hedstrom JI, Puolakkainen PA, et al, "Advances in the Laboratory Diagnostics of Acute Pancreatitis," *Ann Med*, 1998, 30(2):169-75.

Kingsnorth A, "Diagnosing Acute Pancreatitis: Room for Improvement?" *Hosp Med*, 1998, 59(3):191-4.

Munoz AN and Katerndahl DA, "Diagnosis and Management of Acute Pancreatitis," *Am Fam Physician*, 2000, 62(1):164-74.

Ranson JH, "Diagnostic Standards for Acute Pancreatitis," *World J Surg*, 1997, 21(2):136-42.

Smotkin J and Tenner S, "Laboratory Diagnostic Tests in Acute Pancreatitis," *J Clin Gastroenterol*, 2002, 34(4):459-62.

Somogyi L, Martin SP, Venkatesan T, et al, "Recurrent Acute Pancreatitis: An Algorithmic Approach to Identification and Elimination of Inciting Factors," *Gastroenterology*, 2001, 120(3):708-17.

Vissers RJ, Abu-Laban RB, and McHugh DF, "Amylase and Lipase in the Emergency Department Evaluation of Acute Pancreatitis," *J Emerg Med*, 1999, 17(6):1027-37.

Yadav D, Agarwal N, and Pitchumoni CS, "A Critical Evaluation of Laboratory Tests in Acute Pancreatitis," *Am J Gastroenterol*, 2002, 97(6):1309-18.

BILIARY DISEASES

ACUTE CHOLECYSTITIS

Gallstone impaction of the cystic duct is the cause of acute cholecystitis in >90% of cases. In approximately 2% to 5% of cases, however, acalculous cholecystitis, characterized by the absence of gallstones, is present.

Clinical Presentation

Patients with acute cholecystitis complain of abdominal pain, which is classically located in the right upper quadrant. Less commonly, the pain may be located in the epigastrium, left upper quadrant, chest, or other parts of the abdomen. In a minority of patients, there is radiation of the pain to the right shoulder or tip of the scapula. Common accompanying symptoms include fever, nausea, and vomiting.

In addition to fever, physical examination typically reveals right upper quadrant abdominal tenderness. Signs of peritoneal irritation may also be present. Quite characteristic of acute cholecystitis is Murphy's sign, which is said to be present if inspiratory arrest upon palpation of the gallbladder is noted.

Laboratory Testing

There are no laboratory test abnormalities diagnostic of acute cholecystitis. A moderate leukocytosis (10,000-15,000 cells/mm^3) with or without a left shift is commonly noted. A white blood cell count >15,000 cells/mm^3 is uncommonly appreciated in patients with uncomplicated acute cholecystitis. If the white blood cell count exceeds this number, the clinician should consider the development of empyema or perforation, particularly when the patient continues to have high fever and/or significant pain.

Fifty percent of patients have a mild increase in the serum bilirubin level (2-4 mg/dL). AST and alkaline phosphatase levels are increased in 40% and 25% of patients, respectively. When these are elevated, the values are typically mildly increased. A disproportionate elevation of the alkaline phosphatase relative to the transaminases should prompt consideration for choledocholithiasis. Ten percent of patients present with a mild increase in the serum amylase level.

Serum bilirubin and amylase levels exceeding 4 mg/dL and 1000 units/dL should prompt consideration of common bile duct obstruction or acute pancreatitis, respectively.

Establishing the Diagnosis

In patients who present classically with fever, right upper quadrant tenderness, and leukocytosis, the clinician may be fairly certain of the diagnosis. In other cases, the presentation is not classic. Regardless of whether the presentation is classic or not, confirmation of the diagnosis requires radiologic testing with either ultrasound or nuclear medicine (HIDA-scintigraphy).

Ultrasound findings consistent with the diagnosis of acute cholecystitis include gallstones, gallbladder wall thickening, dilated lumen of the gallbladder, positive sonographic Murphy's sign, and pericholecystic fluid. Nonvisualization of the gallbladder despite common bile duct and small intestinal visualization are the hallmark findings of acute cholecystitis when HIDA-scintigraphy is performed.

ACUTE CHOLECYSTITIS

Adapted from Wu GY and Israel J, *Diseases of the Liver and Bile Ducts*, Humana Press, 1998.

ACUTE CHOLANGITIS

Acute cholangitis refers to an ascending infection of the biliary tree proximal to an area of obstruction. Most commonly, acute cholangitis develops in the setting of gallstone impaction of the common bile duct.

Clinical Presentation

Charçot's triad of right upper quadrant pain, jaundice, and fever is present in 70% of acute cholangitis cases. Reynold's pentad is said to be present if mental status changes and hypotension accompany Charçot's triad. Only 10% of patients, however, present will all five elements of the pentad.

Physical examination reveals fever in about 95% of cases. Right upper quadrant tenderness and jaundice are noted in about 90% and 80% of patients, respectively. Fifteen percent of patients present with peritoneal signs.

Laboratory Testing

Leukocytosis, often marked, is present in most patients (80%) with acute cholangitis. The leukocytosis may or may not be accompanied by a left shift. A left shift may also be noted in many of the patients who do not present with leukocytosis.

Serum bilirubin levels exceed 2 mg/dL in 80% of cases, with levels often exceeding 4 mg/dL. Alkaline phosphatase levels are also commonly elevated, usually to levels greater than those seen in acute cholecystitis. A moderate elevation in the serum AST may also be noted.

Acute cholecystitis must be differentiated from acute cholangitis. Features favoring a diagnosis of acute cholangitis include the following:

- Patient is more ill
- Serum bilirubin levels are >4 mg/dL
- Alkaline phosphatase is much more elevated
- Ultrasound reveals an obstructed biliary tree with dilated hepatic and common bile ducts

In contrast to acute cholecystitis, blood cultures in acute cholangitis are more often positive. When positive, *E. coli* is most commonly isolated (52%), followed by *B. fragilis* (22%) and *C. perfringens* (16%).

Ultrasound or CT scan is usually obtained to demonstrate the presence of common bile duct dilatation, which is present in 75% of patients. Therefore, the absence of common bile duct dilatation in the patient with a compatible clinical presentation does not exclude the diagnosis. Although most cases of acute cholangitis are due to stone impaction in the common bile duct, common bile duct stones are detected by ultrasound in only 50% of cases. ERCP is the gold standard test for the diagnosis of common bile duct stones.

PRIMARY BILIARY CIRRHOSIS

Primary biliary cirrhosis is a chronic disorder characterized by progressive cholestasis. The illness has a predilection for women, often presenting in middle age.

Clinical Presentation

The disease varies in its presentation. In fact, some patients are detected at an asymptomatic stage, coming to clinical attention because of abnormal laboratory tests. Others present with the characteristic symptoms of pruritus and lethargy. Occasionally, decompensated liver disease is the initial manifestation of primary biliary cirrhosis. These patients may present with bleeding esophageal varices or ascites.

Liver Function Tests

Prior to the onset of symptoms, patients may have normal liver function tests. More often, however, these patients are found to have an elevated alkaline phosphatase. Elevation of the alkaline phosphatase and GGT levels are the earliest liver function test abnormalities. These enzymes remain elevated throughout the course of the illness but the degree of elevation has not been shown to have any prognostic importance.

Serum transaminases may also be elevated but rarely do the levels exceed five times the upper limit of normal. The degree of elevation has little, if any, prognostic importance.

With progression of the disease (ie, cirrhosis), other liver function test abnormalities including hypoalbuminemia, hyperbilirubinemia, and PT prolongation may be noted, as shown in the following table.

Liver Function Tests in Primary Biliary Cirrhosis

	Early	Late
Albumin	Normal	Decreased
Bilirubin	Normal	Increased
Alkaline phosphatase	Elevated	Increased
AST/ALT	Normal or increased	Normal or increased
Prothrombin time	Normal	Increased

Adapted from O'Grady JG, Lake JR, and Howdle PD, *Comprehensive Clinical Hepatology*, Harcourt Publishers Ltd, 2000, 3.17.5.

Antimitochondrial Antibodies (AMA)

Approximately 95% of patients have antimitochondrial antibodies. There are many different types of antimitochondrial antibodies, some of which can be detected in other diseases such as systemic lupus erythematosus, tuberculosis, syphilis, and hepatitis C viral infection. Ten percent of patients with autoimmune hepatitis are found to have antimitochondrial antibodies.

Standard immunofluorescent techniques do not reveal the presence of antimitochondrial antibodies in a minority of patients with primary biliary cirrhosis. In some of these patients, antimitochondrial antibody testing using immunoblotting may reveal the presence of these antibodies. In others, the test may become positive with disease progression. There remains a subset of patients, however, who remain negative for antimitochondrial antibodies. In these patients, liver biopsy is essential to confirm the diagnosis as is ERCP to assess and exclude other biliary diseases. Patients who have AMA-negative PBC often have high-titer antinuclear or antismooth muscle antibodies.

Of note, survival is not affected by the presence or absence of AMA in PBC patients. The AMA titer also has no bearing on survival.

Other Laboratory Test Abnormalities

Lipid profile often reveals hypercholesterolemia. Early in the disease course, HDL levels are elevated, but with progression of the disease, HDL levels fall.

Measurement of serum immunoglobulins often reveals increases in serum IgM and IgG. IgA levels are usually normal.

CBC is typically unremarkable. However, examination of the differential cell count may reveal the presence of eosinophilia. Thrombocytopenia is usually indicative of portal hypertension.

There are many diseases associated with primary biliary cirrhosis, the diagnosis of which depends upon appropriate laboratory testing. Thyroid antibodies are present in up to 25% of patients. Although biochemical and clinical hypothyroidism is rare, it is important to screen primary biliary cirrhosis patients with thyroid function tests. Rheumatoid factor positivity is noted in up to 25% of patients, many of whom do not have signs and symptoms of rheumatoid arthritis.

Renal tubular acidosis is commonly found in patients with primary biliary cirrhosis.

Circulating antibodies that may be found include antinuclear, antithyroid, lymphocytotoxic, antiplatelet, antiribonucleoprotein antigen Ro, antiacetylcholine receptor, antihistone, and anticentromere antibodies.

Liver Biopsy

Liver biopsy provides confirmation of the diagnosis. It is also useful in estimating prognosis and plays a major role in evaluating the response to therapy. Histologic features of primary biliary cirrhosis include granulomatous and nonsuppurative destructive cholangitis.

PRIMARY BILIARY CIRRHOSIS (PBC)

Symptoms compatible with PBC:
- Lethargy
- Pruritus

↑ alkaline phosphatase of unclear etiology

✓ alkaline phosphatase

Perform ultrasound or CT of liver and biliary tree

NL → Consider other causes of the patient's symptoms

↑ → ✓ antimitochondrial antibody

Dilated ducts?

No → Consider PBC as well as other causes of ↑ alkaline phosphatase

Yes → Perform further evaluation (ie, ERCP, PTC)

✓ antimitochondrial antibody

+ → PBC*

- → No other cause for ↑ alkaline phosphatase found → Consider liver biopsy

*There is some debate as to whether liver biopsy is needed to confirm the diagnosis of PBC in patients with positive antimitochondrial antibodies.

PRIMARY SCLEROSING CHOLANGITIS

Primary sclerosing cholangitis is a chronic cholestatic disease characterized by diffuse inflammation and fibrosis affecting the intrahepatic and extrahepatic bile ducts. If left untreated, patients develop biliary cirrhosis, portal hypertension, and liver failure.

Clinical Presentation

Primary sclerosing cholangitis can affect individuals of all ages. It does tend to have a predilection for young Caucasian males. In one study, the mean age at the time of diagnosis was about 40 years. It varies in its presentation ranging from asymptomatic elevation of liver function tests to decompensated liver disease (ascites, variceal bleeding, hepatic encephalopathy).

There is an association between primary sclerosing cholangitis and inflammatory bowel disease that is well recognized. The diagnosis of primary sclerosing cholangitis is being made with increasing frequency in inflammatory bowel disease patients who present with abnormal liver function tests.

Laboratory Testing

No liver function test abnormalities are specific for the diagnosis of primary sclerosing cholangitis. Most often, patients present with an elevated alkaline phosphatase, usually to levels exceeding two times the upper limit of normal. Levels approaching 20 times the upper limit of normal have been reported. The clinician should realize, however, that cases of primary sclerosing cholangitis have been diagnosed in the setting of normal alkaline phosphatase levels.

Serum transaminase levels are increased in 92% of patients. Rarely do levels exceed five times the upper limit of normal.

Serum bilirubin levels may be normal (elevated in 65% of patients at the time of diagnosis) in early primary sclerosing cholangitis. With progression to advanced disease, hyperbilirubinemia becomes quite common. Hypoalbuminemia and prolonged PT have been described at the time of diagnosis (20% and 10%, respectively). In these patients, advanced disease is more likely.

Hypergammaglobulinemia has been reported in up to 30% of patients. Antinuclear, antismooth muscle, and antimitochondrial antibodies have been noted in primary sclerosing cholangitis patients. One study revealed that 35% and 55% of patients had antismooth muscle and antinuclear antibodies, respectively. Although antimitochondrial antibodies are present in <2% of patients, more sophisticated testing usually reveals that the type of antimitochondrial antibodies present in primary sclerosing cholangitis differs from that seen in primary biliary cirrhosis.

Perinuclear ANCA (pANCA) have been described in 65% to 85% of primary sclerosing cholangitis patients. Since these antibodies may be found in other conditions, this is a nonspecific finding.

Although the clinical presentation and laboratory features may be supportive of the diagnosis, ERCP is essential in establishing the diagnosis and may reveal multiple strictures of the extrahepatic and intrahepatic bile ducts. Histologic examination of liver tissue showing periportal fibrosis and obliteration of interlobular bile ducts is supportive of the diagnosis.

Laboratory test abnormalities due to associated diseases may also be present in these patients. Diseases associated with primary sclerosing cholangitis include inflammatory bowel disease, chronic pancreatitis, sarcoidosis, thyroiditis, celiac sprue, autoimmune hepatitis, systemic lupus erythematosus, rheumatoid arthritis, systemic sclerosis, Sjögren's syndrome, membranous nephropathy, bronchiectasis, histiocytosis X, cystic fibrosis, autoimmune hemolytic anemia, idiopathic thrombocytopenic purpura, and vasculitis.

References

Angulo P and Lindor KD, "Primary Biliary Cirrhosis and Primary Sclerosing Cholangitis," *Clin Liver Dis*, 1999, 3(3):529-70.

Heathcote J, "Update on Primary Biliary Cirrhosis" *Can J Gastroenterol*, 2000, 14(1):43-8.

Indar AA and Beckingham IJ, "Acute Cholecystitis," *BMJ*, 2002, 325(7365):639-43.

Nishio A, Keeffe EB, Ishibashi H, et al, "Diagnosis and Treatment of Primary Biliary Cirrhosis," *Med Sci Monit*, 2000, 6(1):181-93.

Prince MI and Jones DE, "Primary Biliary Cirrhosis: New Perspectives in Diagnosis and Treatment," *Postgrad Med J*, 2000, 76(894):199-206.

Ryder SD and Beckingham IJ, "ABC of Diseases of Liver, Pancreas, and Biliary System. Other Causes of Parenchymal Liver Disease," *BMJ*, 2001, 322(7281):290-2.

Sherlock S, "Primary Biliary Cirrhosis, Primary Sclerosing Cholangitis, and Autoimmune Cholangitis," *Clin Liver Dis*, 2000, 4(1):97-113.

Stiehl A, Benz C, and Sauer P, "Primary Sclerosing Cholangitis," *Can J Gastroenterol*, 2000, 14(4):311-5.

Strassburg CP, Jaeckel E, and Manns MP, "Anti-Mitochondrial Antibodies and Other Immunological Tests in Primary Biliary Cirrhosis," *Gastroenterol Hepatol Eur J*, 1999, 11(6):595-601.

Talwalkar JA and Lindor KD, "Primary Biliary Cirrhosis," *Lancet*, 2003, 362(9377):53-61.

Trowbridge RL, Rutkowski NK, and Shojania KG, "Does This Patient Have Acute Cholecystitis?" *JAMA*, 2003, 289(1):80-6.

Zein CO and Lindor KD, "Primary Sclerosing Cholangitis," *Semin Gastrointest Dis*, 2001, 12(2):103-12.

APPROACH TO THE PATIENT WITH IRON DEFICIENCY ANEMIA

STEP 1 – *How Common Is Iron Deficiency Anemia?*

Iron deficiency anemia is the most common type of anemia. In fact, 2% and 5% of women and men in the United States, respectively, have iron deficiency anemia.

In women, iron deficiency anemia is quite common, especially during the reproductive years. During this time in a woman's life, menstrual and pregnancy-related losses of iron may lead to iron deficiency anemia.

In postmenopausal women and men, the presence of iron deficiency anemia raises concern about the possibility of occult gastrointestinal bleeding. Although there are many causes of occult gastrointestinal bleeding, of major concern is the possibility of gastrointestinal malignancy.

Proceed to Step 2.

STEP 2 – *Does the Patient Truly Have Iron Deficiency Anemia?*

Evaluation to elucidate the etiology of iron deficiency anemia can be quite expensive. For this reason, the clinician should ensure that iron deficiency anemia is truly present prior to pursuing a workup that, at times, can be quite extensive.

The gold standard for the diagnosis of iron deficiency anemia is bone marrow biopsy with Prussian blue staining. In most cases, however, bone marrow biopsy is not needed because the results of the iron studies (serum iron, ferritin, TIBC) allow the clinician to make a secure diagnosis of iron deficiency anemia. There are, however, pitfalls in the interpretation of iron studies which, at times, make it difficult for the clinician to not only establish the diagnosis of iron deficiency anemia but also to differentiate it from other causes of anemia. For further information regarding the diagnosis of iron deficiency anemia, the clinician should refer to the chapter, ***Approach to the Patient With Anemia*** *on page 21*.

The remainder of this approach assumes that the diagnosis of iron deficiency anemia has been established with confidence.

If the patient is a male, ***proceed to Step 4***.

If the patient is a postmenopausal female, ***proceed to Step 4***.

If the patient is a premenopausal female, ***proceed to Step 3***.

STEP 3 – *Should Premenopausal Women With Iron Deficiency Anemia Have a Gastrointestinal Evaluation?*

Iron deficiency anemia is quite common among premenopausal women. Traditionally, the iron deficiency anemia has been attributed to menstrual blood loss. In recent years, however, there is some evidence to suggest that it is unwise to assume that iron deficiency anemia in premenopausal women is due to menstrual loss of blood.

In one study, a serious gastrointestinal condition was identified in 12% of premenopausal women with iron deficiency anemia. Gastric and colorectal carcinoma were two of the serious conditions identified. This study raised concern that gastrointestinal disease causing iron deficiency anemia may be more common in premenopausal women than previously thought.

At the current time, there is no general consensus regarding which premenopausal women with iron deficiency anemia should undergo gastrointestinal evaluation. Despite this, many clinicians pursue gastrointestinal evaluation if the patient meets any of the following criteria:

- Presence of abdominal symptoms
- Positive fecal occult blood test
- Hemoglobin <10 g/dL
- Failure to respond to trial of iron replacement therapy

If the patient meets any of the above criteria, gastrointestinal evaluation should be considered. ***Proceed to Step 4***.

If the patient does not meet any of the above criteria, the iron deficiency anemia is likely to be pregnancy-related or due to menstrual blood loss. ***Stop here.***

STEP 4 – *Should the Upper or Lower Gastrointestinal Tract Be Evaluated?*

Once the presence of iron deficiency anemia has been established, the clinician should consider the causes of iron deficiency anemia. While there are a number of causes, most cases are due to gastrointestinal blood loss (if the patient's clinical presentation is consistent with a nongastrointestinal source of blood loss, proceed to step 10). While patients may provide a history of frank gastrointestinal bleeding, in most cases, iron deficiency anemia is the manifestation of occult gastrointestinal bleeding.

Since iron deficiency anemia may result from a lesion in either the upper or lower gastrointestinal tract, a common dilemma that clinicians encounter is whether to begin the evaluation with a test to evaluate the upper or lower gastrointestinal tract.

Most clinicians base their decision on the presence or absence of symptoms. Therefore, an upper gastrointestinal tract lesion is suggested if the patient reports one or more of the following symptoms:

- Dysphagia
- Heartburn
- Nausea
- Vomiting
- Upper abdominal pain

A lower gastrointestinal tract lesion should be considered in patients who present with one or more of the following symptoms:

- Altered bowel habits
- Diarrhea
- Constipation
- Hematochezia
- Lower abdominal pain

Although decision-making is often based upon the type of symptoms present, studies that have examined the correlation between the type of gastrointestinal symptoms present and the location of the lesions have yielded mixed results. Nonetheless, because some studies have shown a positive correlation, most clinicians continue to base the decision of whether to evaluate the upper or lower gastrointestinal tract upon the type of gastrointestinal symptoms present.

If no symptoms are present, the clinician should begin the evaluation by performing testing to identify a lower gastrointestinal lesion.

If the patient has symptoms suggestive of an upper gastrointestinal lesion, ***proceed to Step 5***.

If the patient has symptoms suggestive of a lower gastrointestinal lesion, ***proceed to Step 7***.

If the patient has no symptoms suggestive of an upper or lower gastrointestinal lesion, ***proceed to Step 7***.

STEP 5 – *What Test Should Be Performed in Patients With Iron Deficiency Anemia Who Have Symptoms Suggestive of an Upper Gastrointestinal Lesion?*

When the decision has been made to begin the evaluation of iron deficiency anemia with testing to identify an upper gastrointestinal lesion, the clinician must choose between radiologic imaging (upper GI series) and upper endoscopy. While radiologic imaging is useful in detecting mass and large ulcerating lesions, upper endoscopy can do the same. In addition, upper endoscopy is more sensitive in the diagnosis of mucosal lesions (eg, esophagitis) and vascular ectasia, both of which can present with iron deficiency anemia. For these reasons, upper endoscopy is favored over radiologic imaging in the evaluation of iron deficiency anemia patients suspected of having an upper gastrointestinal lesion.

If upper endoscopy identifies a significant lesion (eg, large ulceration, mass, severe inflammation), no further evaluation is necessary. Not uncommonly, however, a trivial lesion (eg, mild inflammation) may be identified. Since trivial lesions do not bleed significantly, the clinician should be wary in attributing the iron deficiency anemia to the trivial lesion. In these cases, evaluation of the lower gastrointestinal tract should be highly considered.

If a significant lesion that could account for the iron deficiency anemia is identified by upper endoscopy, the clinician should direct further workup according to the lesion identified.

If a trivial lesion is identified by upper endoscopy, ***proceed to Step 6***.

If no lesion is identified by upper endoscopy, ***proceed to Step 6***.

STEP 6 – *What Are the Results of the Lower Gastrointestinal Tract Evaluation?*

When a trivial lesion is encountered during upper endoscopy, the clinician should not assume that the lesion is the cause of the iron deficiency anemia. These patients should have a lower gastrointestinal tract evaluation. Likewise, patients who have no abnormality identified during upper endoscopy should also have a lower gastrointestinal tract evaluation.

Colonoscopy is preferred over air-contrast barium enema in the evaluation of patients suspected of having a lower gastrointestinal tract lesion. Although air-contrast barium enema is useful in the diagnosis of large masses or ulcerating lesions, mucosal lesions (eg, colitis) and vascular ectasia may not be detected. All of these lesions will be evident during colonoscopy.

If the colonoscopy reveals a significant lesion (ie, large mass or severe inflammation), the clinician can feel comfortable in linking the iron deficiency anemia to the lesion discovered. When a trivial lesion (ie, mild inflammation or small adenoma) is encountered, however, the clinician should be wary in assuming that the trivial lesion is the etiology of the iron deficiency anemia.

If a significant lesion that could account for the iron deficiency anemia is identified by colonoscopy, the clinician should direct further workup according to the lesion identified.

If a trivial lesion is identified by colonoscopy, ***proceed to Step 9***.

If no lesion is identified by colonoscopy, ***proceed to Step 9***.

STEP 7 – *What Test Should Be Performed in Patients With Iron Deficiency Anemia Who Have Symptoms Suggestive of a Lower Gastrointestinal Lesion?*

When the decision has been made to begin the evaluation of iron deficiency anemia with testing to identify a lower gastrointestinal lesion, the clinician must choose between radiologic imaging (air-contrast barium enema) and colonoscopy. While radiologic imaging is useful in detecting mass and large ulcerating lesions, colonoscopy can do the same. In addition, colonoscopy is more sensitive in the diagnosis of mucosal lesions (eg, colitis) and vascular ectasia, both of which can present with iron deficiency anemia. For these reasons, colonoscopy is favored over radiologic imaging in the evaluation of iron deficiency anemia patients suspected of having a lower gastrointestinal lesion.

If colonoscopy identifies a significant lesion (eg, large ulceration, mass, severe inflammation), no further evaluation is necessary. Not uncommonly, however, a trivial lesion (eg, mild inflammation or small adenoma) may be identified. Since trivial lesions do not bleed significantly, the clinician should be wary in attributing the iron deficiency anemia to the trivial lesion. In these cases, evaluation of the upper gastrointestinal tract should be highly considered.

The upper gastrointestinal tract should also be evaluated in patients who have no abnormality identified during colonoscopy.

If a significant lesion that could account for the iron deficiency anemia is identified by colonoscopy, the clinician should direct further workup according to the lesion identified.

If a trivial lesion is identified by colonoscopy, ***proceed to Step 8***.

If no lesion is identified by colonoscopy, ***proceed to Step 8***.

STEP 8 – *What Are the Results of the Upper Gastrointestinal Tract Evaluation?*

When a trivial lesion is encountered during colonoscopy, the clinician should not assume that the lesion is the cause of the iron deficiency anemia. These patients should have an upper gastrointestinal tract evaluation. Likewise, patients who have no abnormality identified during colonoscopy should also have an upper gastrointestinal tract evaluation.

Upper endoscopy is preferred over radiologic imaging (eg, upper GI series) in the evaluation of patients suspected of having an upper gastrointestinal tract lesion. Although the upper GI series is useful in the diagnosis of large masses or ulcerating lesions, mucosal lesions (eg, esophagitis) and vascular ectasia, both of which may lead to iron deficiency anemia, may not be detected. All of these lesions will be evident during upper endoscopy.

If the upper endoscopy (ie, large mass or severe inflammation) reveals a significant lesion, the clinician can feel comfortable in linking the iron deficiency anemia to the lesion discovered. When a trivial lesion (ie, mild inflammation) is encountered, however, the clinician should be wary in assuming that the trivial lesion is the etiology of the iron deficiency anemia.

If a significant lesion that could account for the iron deficiency anemia is identified by upper endoscopy, the clinician should direct further workup according to the lesion identified.

If a trivial lesion is identified by upper endoscopy, ***proceed to Step 9***.

If no lesion is identified by upper endoscopy, ***proceed to Step 9***.

STEP 9 – *What Testing Should Be Performed in Patients Who Have an Unremarkable Upper Endoscopy and Colonoscopy?*

Unremarkable upper endoscopy and colonoscopy studies are not uncommon in patients with iron deficiency anemia. In fact, even after upper endoscopy and colonoscopy, the etiology of iron deficiency anemia remains unexplained in up to 52% of cases. These patients should be started on iron replacement therapy.

If the iron deficiency anemia is recurrent or persistent, then further evaluation is warranted. These patients are said to have obscure bleeding, which is defined by the American Gastroenterological Association as bleeding of unknown origin (iron deficiency anemia) that persists or recurs after negative colonoscopy and/ or upper endoscopy.

It is in these patients that the clinician should consider one or more of the following tests:

- Repeat upper endoscopy
- Repeat colonoscopy
- Enteroscopy
- Small bowel follow-through
- Enteroclysis
- Small bowel biopsy

These tests will be discussed in further detail in the remainder of this step.

Repeat Upper Endoscopy

Several studies have shown that the use of repeat upper endoscopy in patients with obscure bleeding has a diagnostic yield of nearly 30%. The lesions may have simply been missed at the time of initial upper endoscopy. Alternatively, less common causes of occult upper gastrointestinal bleeding may not have been recognized by the endoscopist because of their unusual nature.

Repeat Colonoscopy

Repeat colonoscopy should also be considered in patients with obscure bleeding. As with upper endoscopy, the endoscopist may simply have missed the causative lesion.

Enteroscopy

Endoscopy of the small intestine, also known as enteroscopy, has been found to be more sensitive than radiologic imaging for detecting small intestinal lesions, particularly mucosal and vascular lesions.

Despite this, at the current time, the data does not support the routine use of enteroscopy in all patients with iron deficiency anemia who have unremarkable upper endoscopy and colonoscopy unless they meet criteria for obscure bleeding, as defined by the American Gastroenterological Association.

Small Bowel Follow-Through / Enteroclysis

Studies have shown that the radiologic evaluation of the small intestine (enteroclysis or small bowel follow through) is not very useful in elucidating a small intestinal etiology of iron deficiency anemia. These studies have demonstrated that radiologic imaging has a low diagnostic yield. Although radiologic imaging is effective in identifying small intestinal tumors or prominent lesions of the small intestinal mucosa, vascular malformations are difficult to detect by radiologic imaging.

For these reasons, enteroscopy is favored over radiologic imaging in the evaluation of the small intestine. The clinician may consider performing enteroclysis, however, as a follow-up to enteroscopy in patients with obscure bleeding.

Small Bowel Biopsy

Iron deficiency anemia is quite commonly encountered in patients with celiac sprue. In these cases, the iron deficiency anemia is thought to be due to the malabsorption of iron. Small bowel biopsy is required to confirm the diagnosis of celiac sprue.

If the cause of the iron deficiency anemia is identified, ***stop here***.

If the cause of the iron deficiency anemia is not identified, ***proceed to Step 10***.

STEP 10 – *What Should Be Done in the Patient With Unexplained Iron Deficiency Anemia?*

In patients with unexplained iron deficiency anemia (normal endoscopy, normal colonoscopy, normal small intestinal evaluation), the clinician should consider the following questions.

- Does the patient truly have iron deficiency anemia or has the patient been misdiagnosed?

  As described in Step 2, the diagnosis of iron deficiency anemia can, at times, be difficult. Although serum iron studies are fairly reliable in establishing the presence of iron deficiency anemia, at times, the results may be such that it is difficult to differentiate iron deficiency anemia from other causes of anemia. A negative gastrointestinal evaluation should, at least, prompt the clinician to ascertain whether the diagnosis of iron deficiency anemia is secure.

- Does the patient have a nongastrointestinal source of blood loss?

  A negative gastrointestinal evaluation should also prompt the clinician to consider other causes of iron deficiency anemia, such as nongastrointestinal blood loss, nutritional deficiency, or increased requirements. The causes of iron deficiency anemia are listed in the following box.

CAUSES OF IRON DEFICIENCY ANEMIA
BLOOD LOSS
Gastrointestinal
Uterine
Urinary
Intrapulmonary hemorrhage
Hemolysis (hemoglobinuria)
Self-inflicted blood loss
Postoperative
Blood donation
Iatrogenic (repeated blood draws)
DECREASED DIETARY INTAKE
IMPAIRED ABSORPTION
Gastrectomy
Malabsorption (gluten-induced enteropathy)
INCREASED REQUIREMENTS
Pregnancy
Growth

References

Baker WF Jr, "Iron Deficiency in Pregnancy, Obstetrics, and Gynecology," *Hematol Oncol Clin North Am*, 2000, 14(5):1061-77.

Chamberlain SA and Soybel DI, "Occult and Obscure Sources of Gastrointestinal Bleeding," *Curr Probl Surg*, 2000, 37(12):861-916.

De Bossett V, Gonvers JJ, Burnand B, et al, "Appropriateness of Colonoscopy: Iron-Deficiency Anemia," *Endoscopy*, 1999, 31(8):627-30.

Dugdale M, "Anemia," *Obstet Gynecol Clin North Am*, 2001, 28(2):363-81.

Jolobe OM, "Does This Elderly Patient Have Iron Deficiency Anaemia, and What Is The Underlying Cause?" *Postgrad Med J*, 2000, 76(894):195-8.

Rockey DC, "Gastrointestinal Tract Evaluation in Patients With Iron Deficiency Anemia," *Semin Gastrointest Dis*, 1999, 10(2):53-64.

Rockey DC, " Occult Gastrointestinal Bleeding," *N Engl J Med*, 1999, 341(1):38-46.

Zuckerman GR, Prakash C, Askin MP, et al, "AGA Technical Review on the Evaluation and Management of Occult and Obscure Gastrointestinal Bleeding," *Gastroenterology*, 2000, 118(1):201-21.

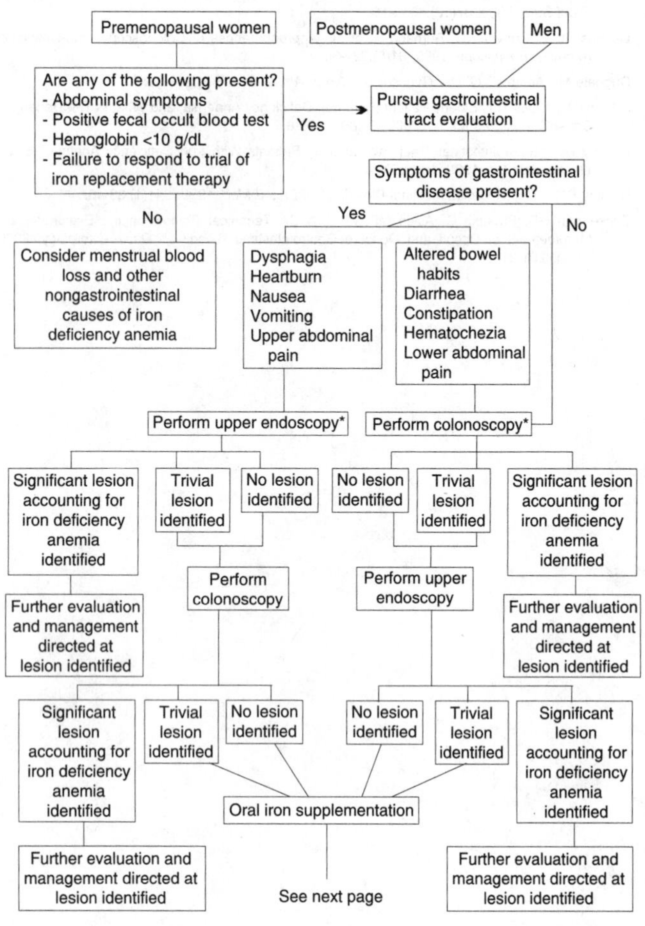
IRON DEFICIENCY ANEMIA
Premenopausal women
Postmenopausal women
Men
Are any of the following present?
- Abdominal symptoms
- Positive fecal occult blood test
- Hemoglobin <10 g/dL
- Failure to respond to trial of iron replacement therapy
Yes
Pursue gastrointestinal tract evaluation
Symptoms of gastrointestinal disease present?
No
Yes
No
Consider menstrual blood loss and other nongastrointestinal causes of iron deficiency anemia
Dysphagia
Heartburn
Nausea
Vomiting
Upper abdominal pain
Altered bowel habits
Diarrhea
Constipation
Hematochezia
Lower abdominal pain
Perform upper endoscopy*
Perform colonoscopy*
Significant lesion accounting for iron deficiency anemia identified
Trivial lesion identified
No lesion identified
No lesion identified
Trivial lesion identified
Significant lesion accounting for iron deficiency anemia identified
Further evaluation and management directed at lesion identified
Perform colonoscopy
Perform upper endoscopy
Further evaluation and management directed at lesion identified
Significant lesion accounting for iron deficiency anemia identified
Trivial lesion identified
No lesion identified
No lesion identified
Trivial lesion identified
Significant lesion accounting for iron deficiency anemia identified
Oral iron supplementation
Further evaluation and management directed at lesion identified
See next page
Further evaluation and management directed at lesion identified

IRON DEFICIENCY ANEMIA *(continued)*

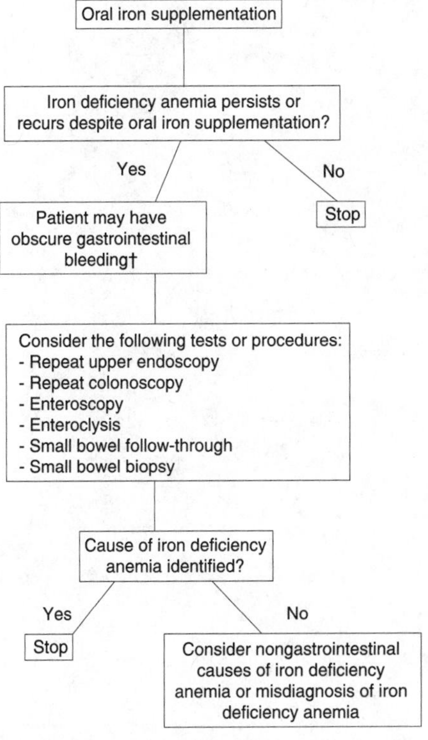

*UGI series and barium enema may be substituted for upper endoscopy and colonoscopy, respectively, if contraindicaitons to endoscopy are present.

†The American Gastroenterological Association defines obscure bleeding as bleeding of unknown origin (iron deficiency anemia) that persists or recurs after negative colonoscopy and/or upper endoscopy.

IRON DEFICIENCY ANEMIA (continued)

[illegible] iron supplementation)

Iron deficiency anemia [illegible] iron supplementation?

Yes — No

No: Stop

Yes: [illegible] have [illegible] bleeding?

Consider the following tests or procedures:
- Repeat upper endoscopy
- Repeat colonoscopy
- Enteroscopy
- Enteroclysis
- Small bowel follow-through
- Small bowel biopsy

Cause of iron deficiency anemia identified?

Yes: Stop

No: Consider [illegible] causes of iron deficiency anemia [illegible] iron deficiency anemia

[illegible]

FECAL OCCULT BLOOD TESTING

STEP 1 – *When Is Fecal Occult Blood Testing Indicated?*

Fecal occult blood testing was developed to screen asymptomatic patients for colon cancer. With screening, colorectal cancer can be diagnosed at an earlier stage. Treatment of colorectal cancer is more likely to be successful when the malignancy is detected at an earlier stage.

Although colorectal cancer screening using fecal occult blood testing has been practiced for many years, only recently did a study reveal that annual fecal occult blood testing reduces mortality from colorectal cancer. With this knowledge in mind, annual fecal occult blood testing has been advocated by the American Cancer Society and World Health Organization as an appropriate screening test for the detection of colorectal cancer in those over the age of 50 years.

Proceed to Step 2.

STEP 2 – *What Are the Different Types of Fecal Occult Blood Tests Available for Use as Screening Tests for Colorectal Cancer?*

A number of different fecal occult blood tests are available. These tests employ one of three techniques for the detection of fecal occult blood.

- Guaiac-based

  Commonly used guaiac-based tests include the Hemoccult II and Hemoccult II Sensa.

- Immunochemical

  Commonly used immunochemical tests include Heme Select and FlexSure OBT.

- Heme-porphyrin

  The HemoQuant is the most commonly used heme-porphyrin test.

Of the three methods, guaiac-based testing is the most commonly used fecal occult blood test. Compounds that have peroxidase activity or oxidants are able to turn guaiac from colorless to blue. A positive guaiac test is said to be present when this color change occurs. When the amount of blood lost in the gastrointestinal tract is of sufficient degree, guaiac testing of the stool will be positive. This is because the heme moiety of hemoglobin is able to induce this color change through its pseudoperoxidase activity.

The following table compares the characteristics of these three methods.

Comparison of Fecal Occult Blood Test Methods

	Guaiac-Based	Immunochemical*	Heme-porphyrin†
Qualitative or quantitative	Qualitative	Qualitative	Quantitative
Office based or laboratory processed	Office based	Office based or laboratory processed	Laboratory processed
Cost	Inexpensive	Moderate	More expensive
Time to develop	1 minute	5 minutes to 24 hours	1 hour

*Immunochemical fecal occult blood tests employ antibodies directed against intact human hemoglobin and its epitopes. Because small amounts of blood loss from the upper gastrointestinal tract are not detected by this technique, immunochemical fecal occult blood testing seems to be better at localizing bleeding to the large intestine. Limitations of this technique include greater expense, need for laboratory processing, and loss of globin antigenicity at room temperature.

†Heme-porphyrin fecal occult blood testing relies on spectrofluorometric techniques to detect the presence of hemoglobin. Although this type of fecal occult blood test allows exact measurement of the amount of hemoglobin present in stools, it is not widely used because of its greater expense and need for laboratory processing.

Adapted from Rockey DC, "Occult Gastrointestinal Bleeding," *N Engl J Med*, 1999, 341(1):39.

Also adapted from "Gastrointestinal Bleeding," *Curr Probl Surg*, 2000, 875.

Proceed to Step 3.

STEP 3 – *What Are Causes of False-Positive and False-Negative Fecal Occult Blood Test Results?*

All types of fecal occult blood tests are subject to false-positive and negative test results. Reasons for false-positive and negative test results are listed in the following table.

Reasons for False-Positive and Negative Fecal Occult Blood Tests

Characteristic	Guaiac-Based	Heme-porphyrin	Immuno-chemical
Reasons for false-positive results			
Nonhuman hemoglobin	++++	++++	0
Dietary peroxidases	+++	0	0
Rehydration	+++	0	0
Iron	0	0	0
Reasons for false-negative results			
Hemoglobin degradation	+++	0	+++
Storage	++	0	++
Vitamin C	++	0	0

*Relative comparisons are shown on a scale of 0 to ++++, with ++++ indicating highly likely and 0 highly unlikely.

Adapted from Rockey DC, "Occult Gastrointestinal Bleeding," *N Engl J Med*, 1999, 341(1):39.

If the heme-porphyrin or immunochemical fecal occult blood test is positive, ***proceed to Step 5.***

If the heme-porphyrin or immunochemical fecal occult blood test is negative, repeat testing should be based upon current guidelines.

If guaiac testing is to be performed, ***proceed to Step 4.***

STEP 4 – *What Instructions Should Be Given to the Patient Before Performing Guaiac-Based Fecal Occult Blood Testing?*

The instructions that need to be given to patients prior to performing guaiac-based tests focus on efforts to avoid false-positive and negative test results. In this regard, the main issues that need to be addressed revolve around the following:

- Interaction of diet and medications with guaiac-based fecal occult blood tests
- Sample collection technique

These issues will be discussed in further detail in the remainder of this step.

Interaction of Diet and Medications With Guaiac-Based Fecal Occult Blood Testing

There are many dietary and medication-related factors that can affect the results of guaiac-based testing. Many foods, including a number of different fruits and vegetables, contain peroxidases. The ingestion of dietary peroxidases can lead to false-positive test results. Medications such as aspirin and NSAIDs, which can cause gastrointestinal blood loss from gastric mucosal inflammation, should be avoided before testing. These as well as other factors that can impact upon the results of guaiac-based testing are listed in the following box.

FACTORS THAT AFFECT GUAIAC TESTING
CAUSES OF FALSE-POSITIVE TEST RESULTS
Uncooked fruits and vegetables (contain dietary peroxidases)
Radishes
Turnips
Cantaloupes
Bean sprouts
Cauliflower
Broccoli
Grapes
Hemoglobin from red meat
Aspirin
NSAIDs
Rehydration of test cards
CAUSES OF FALSE-NEGATIVE TEST RESULTS
Bacterial degradation of heme in the colon
Vitamin C (ascorbic acid)
Delayed development of testing cards (more than 4 days)
Improper sampling/developing
Degradation of hemoglobin by colonic bacteria

To avoid false-positive and false-negative guaiac-based test results, patients should be counseled about adhering to the recommendations listed in the following box.

GUAIAC TESTING RECOMMENDATIONS
AVOID THE FOLLOWING FOR 3 DAYS BEFORE AND DURING TESTING:
Radishes
Turnips
Cantaloupes
Bean sprouts
Broccoli
Grapes
Red meat
DISCONTINUE THESE MEDICATIONS 1 WEEK BEFORE AND DURING TESTING:
Aspirin
NSAIDs
Vitamin C
DEVELOP CARDS WITHIN 3 DAYS OF SAMPLE COLLECTION*
DEVELOP CARDS WITHOUT REHYDRATION†

*Some positive guaiac-based tests may become negative if 4 or more days are allowed to pass before testing of the sample.

†Rehydration of the stool specimen is not recommended. Although the sensitivity of the test may increase with rehydration, the specificity and positive predictive value decrease.

Sample Collection Technique

While it is certainly important to discuss the above recommendations with the patient prior to performing guaiac-based testing, equally important is a discussion about sample collection technique. Because colorectal cancers bleed intermittently, patients are told to sample three consecutive stools. Quite often, patients are given a disposable stool collection device. This is done to discourage collecting stool from toilet water. Collection from toilet water can lead to a false-positive test result from the presence of toilet sanitizer.

In addition, patients are instructed to sample two different areas of each stool. This is because blood loss from a cancer is not always evenly distributed throughout the stool. In total, six small samples should be submitted for analysis.

In recent years, there has been considerable controversy regarding the collection of samples by clinicians during digital rectal examination. The concern is that false-positive test results could be induced by trauma inflicted during the rectal examination. In addition, when samples are collected by a clinician, it is unlikely that the patient has followed recommendations to minimize false-positive and false-negative test results, as indicated in the preceding box.

Recently, a study was performed assessing the diagnostic yield of colonoscopy in patients found to have positive fecal occult blood tests detected either by the spontaneous passage of stools or during a digital rectal examination. No difference was noted in the number of adenomas and carcinomas found during colonoscopy in these two patient groups. Thus, a positive fecal occult blood test noted during digital rectal examination warrants further evaluation.

Interaction of Oral Iron With Guaiac-Based Fecal Occult Blood Testing

It is widely held that oral iron therapy can cause positive guaiac-based test results. In reality, oral iron supplements do not cause a positive test result. With iron therapy, however, the color of the stool may change to dark-green or black. It is this change in stool color that may cause confusion with the blue color of a positive guaiac. Other medications, including antacids and bismuth-containing antidiarrheal agents, can also cause a darkening of the stool. This darkening of the stool does not result in a positive guaiac-based test but does make the interpretation of the test more difficult.

If the guaiac-based fecal occult blood test is positive, ***proceed to Step 5.***

If the guaiac-based fecal occult blood test is negative, repeat testing should be based upon current screening guidelines.

STEP 5 – *What Are the Causes of a Positive Fecal Occult Blood Test?*

Although many factors can influence the results of fecal occult blood testing, once a positive result is obtained, it must be evaluated as a true positive test result. In these patients, there is concern that the positive result may be a manifestation of a potentially serious gastrointestinal disorder, such as colorectal cancer.

While fecal occult blood testing is often considered to play a key role in screening patients for colorectal cancer, a positive test result is not specific for colorectal cancer. A wide variety of upper and lower gastrointestinal lesions, both benign and malignant, may present with a positive fecal occult blood test. The causes of occult gastrointestinal bleeding are listed in the following box.

CAUSES OF OCCULT GASTROINTESTINAL BLEEDING

MASS LESIONS
- Carcinoma (any size)*
- Large (>1.5 cm) adenoma (any site)

INFLAMMATION
- Erosive esophagitis*
- Ulcer (any site)*
- Cameron lesions
- Erosive gastritis
- Celiac disease
- Ulcerative colitis
- Crohn's disease
- Colitis (nonspecific)
- Idiopathic cecal ulcer

VASCULAR DISORDERS
- Vascular ectasia (any site)*
- Dieulafoy's vascular malformation
- Watermelon stomach
- Varices (any site)
- Hemangioma
- Portal hypertensive gastropathy or colopathy

INFECTIOUS DISEASES
- Hookworm
- Whipworm
- Strongyloidiasis
- Ascariasis
- Tuberculous enterocolitis
- Amebiasis

SURREPTITIOUS BLEEDING
- Hemoptysis
- Oropharyngeal bleeding (including epistaxis)

OTHER CAUSES
- Hemosuccus pancreaticus
- Hemobilia
- Long-distance running
- Factitious cause

*These abnormalities are the most common.

Adapted from Rockey DC, "Occult Gastrointestinal Bleeding," *N Engl J Med*, 1999, 341(1):39.

Proceed to Step 6.

STEP 6 – *Should Endoscopy or Radiologic Imaging (eg, barium enema) Be Performed?*

When evaluating the patient with a positive fecal occult blood test, the clinician needs to decide between endoscopy and radiologic imaging (eg, barium enema). There is some controversy regarding which modality is preferred in the evaluation of these patients.

Most clinicians, however, favor endoscopy over radiologic imaging. When comparing colonoscopy with air-contrast barium enema in the evaluation of the large intestine in patients with a positive fecal occult blood test, for example, most studies have shown that colonoscopy is more accurate than the air-contrast barium enema study. With that being said, air-contrast barium enema may be an alternative to colonoscopy depending upon factors such as cost, acceptance by patient, risk of conscious sedation, general condition of the patient, and comorbid diseases. When air-contrast barium enema is performed *in lieu of* colonoscopy, flexible sigmoidoscopy must also be performed since the barium enema study does not allow adequate visualization of the rectosigmoid region.

Since most patients will have endoscopy rather than radiologic imaging, the remainder of this approach will focus on the endoscopic evaluation of patients who present with a positive fecal occult blood test.

Proceed to Step 7.

STEP 7 – *Should the Patient Have an Upper or Lower Gastrointestinal Tract Evaluation?*

Because a positive fecal occult blood test provides no information on whether the responsible lesion is in the upper or lower gastrointestinal tract, the clinician must decide between upper endoscopy and colonoscopy as the initial test for the evaluation of these patients.

There is no consensus regarding which endoscopic procedure should be performed first. While studies have clearly demonstrated the usefulness of upper endoscopy and colonoscopy in the evaluation of a positive fecal occult blood test, most of these studies have not commented on the order in which the bidirectional endoscopy was performed.

Many clinicians decide to perform one or the other depending upon the presence of upper or lower gastrointestinal symptoms. Studies assessing whether or not symptoms correlate with the presence of a lesion have yielded mixed results. Because some studies have suggested a positive correlation, however, many clinicians guide their decision based upon the presence of symptoms. In patients with upper gastrointestinal symptoms, upper endoscopy is the initial test that is performed. On the other hand, colonoscopy is preferred when patients present with lower gastrointestinal symptoms.

When symptoms are not present, colonoscopy is the preferred initial test.

If upper endoscopy is performed as the initial test, ***proceed to Step 8.***

If colonoscopy is performed as the initial test, ***proceed to Step 9.***

STEP 8 – *What Are the Results of Upper Endoscopy?*

In some patients, upper endoscopy may reveal the presence of a malignant lesion. In these cases, no further evaluation (eg, colonoscopy) is indicated and the evaluation should proceed according to the malignancy noted.

If a malignancy is not found but another lesion is discovered, then colonoscopy is still indicated. This is because the prevalence of combined upper and lower gastrointestinal lesions may be as high as 17%.

If no abnormal findings are noted during upper endoscopy, the clinician should proceed with colonoscopy.

If an upper or lower gastrointestinal lesion is identified, ***stop here.***

If an upper or lower gastrointestinal lesion is not identified, ***proceed to Step 10.***

STEP 9 – *What Are the Results of the Colonoscopy?*

In some patients, colonoscopy may reveal the presence of a malignant lesion. In these cases, no further evaluation (eg, upper endoscopy) is indicated and the evaluation should proceed according to the malignancy noted.

If a malignancy is not found but another lesion is discovered, then upper endoscopy is still indicated. This is because the prevalence of combined upper and lower gastrointestinal lesions may be as high as 17%.

If no abnormal findings are noted during colonoscopy, the clinician should proceed with upper endoscopy.

If an upper or lower gastrointestinal lesion is identified, ***stop here.***

If an upper or lower gastrointestinal lesion is not identified, ***proceed to Step 10.***

STEP 10 – *What Should Be Done in Patients Who Have Negative Colonoscopic and Upper Endoscopic Studies?*

The etiology of positive fecal occult blood tests may remain unclear even after bidirectional endoscopy in as many as 52% of cases. In most of these cases, future fecal occult blood testing is negative. Prognosis of patients with positive fecal occult blood tests but no identifiable lesion in the gastrointestinal tract is generally good. Therefore, most patients will not require testing other than colonoscopy and/or upper endoscopy, even if the results are unremarkable.

If future fecal occult blood tests are positive (recurrent or persistent), then the patient is said to have obscure-occult bleeding. Obscure bleeding is defined as bleeding of unknown origin that persists after a negative upper endoscopy and/or colonoscopy. In these patients, further evaluation should be considered.

Further evaluation usually begins with repeat upper endoscopy and/or colonoscopy. This is because repeat studies will often identify lesions that were missed at the time of initial endoscopic studies. The clinician may wish to discuss management of this type of patient with specialists such as gastroenterologists who can advise the clinician on the usefulness of repeat endoscopy as well as studies to investigate the small bowel (eg, enteroclysis, small bowel follow through, enteroscopy).

References

Bond JH, "Fecal Occult Blood Test Screening for Colorectal Cancer," *Gastrointest Endosc Clin N Am*, 2002, 12(1):11-21.

Bond JH, "Fecal Occult Blood Tests in Occult Gastrointestinal Bleeding," *Semin Gastrointest Dis*, 1999, 10(2):48-52.

Harewood GC and Ahlquist DA, "Fecal Occult Blood Testing for Iron Deficiency: A Reappraisal," *Dig Dis*, 2000, 18(2):75-82.

Lang CA and Ransohoff DF, "On the Sensitivity of Fecal Occult Blood Test Screening for Colorectal Cancer," *J Natl Cancer Inst*, 1997, 89(19):1392-3.

Simon JB, "Fecal Occult Blood Testing: Clinical Value and Limitations," *Gastroenterologist*, 1998, 6(1):66-78.

Van Dam J, Bond JH, and Sivak MV Jr, "Fecal Occult Blood Screening for Colorectal Cancer," *Arch Intern Med.*, 1995, 155(22):2389-402.

FECAL OCCULT BLOOD TESTING (FOBT)

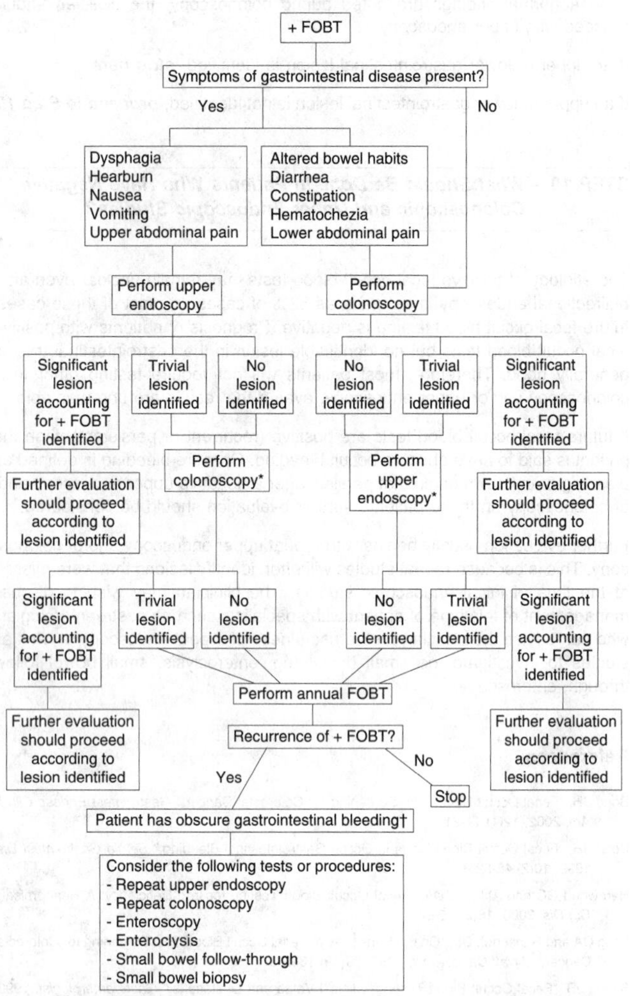

*UGI series and barium enema may be substituted for upper endoscopy and colonoscopy, respectively, if contraindications to endoscopy are present.
†The American Gastroenterological Association defines obscure bleeding as bleeding of unknown origin (+ FOBT) that persists or recurs after negative colonoscopy and/or upper endoscopy.

DIARRHEA (ACUTE)

STEP 1 – *What Is Acute Diarrhea?*

A diarrheal illness of less than 2 weeks duration is considered to be the definition of acute diarrhea. Chronic diarrhea is defined as diarrhea that lasts at least 1 month. That which falls between acute and chronic diarrhea is considered to be persistent diarrhea. This chapter will focus on the approach to the patient presenting with acute diarrhea.

Worldwide, diarrheal illnesses are the second leading cause of death. Even in developed countries such as the United States, diarrhea accounts for significant morbidity and mortality. In fact, in the United States alone, diarrhea is responsible for 1.5 million outpatient visits a year. Although most cases of acute diarrhea can be treated on an outpatient basis, over 450,000 patients are hospitalized every year with gastroenteritis, the most common cause of acute diarrhea. This accounts for 1.5% of all adult hospitalizations.

Proceed to Step 2.

STEP 2 – *What Are the Causes of Acute Diarrhea?*

The causes of acute diarrhea are listed in the following box.

CAUSES OF ACUTE DIARRHEA

INFECTION

- Bacterial
  - *Aeromonas*
  - *Bacillus cereus*
  - *Campylobacter*
  - *Chlamydia*
  - *Clostridium difficile*
  - *Clostridium perfringens*
  - *Escherichia coli*
  - *Neisseria gonorrhoeae*
  - *Plesiomonas*
  - *Salmonella*
  - *Shigella*
  - *Staphylococcus aureus*
  - *Treponema pallidum*
  - *Vibrio*
  - *Yersinia*
- Viral
  - Adenovirus
  - Astrovirus
  - Calicivirus
  - Coronavirus
  - Cytomegalovirus
  - Herpes simplex virus
  - Norwalk
  - Rotavirus
- Parasitic
  - *Cryptosporidium*
  - *Cyclospora*
  - *Entamoeba histolytica*
  - *Giardia lamblia*
  - *Isospora belli*
  - *Microsporidium*
  - Others

NONINFECTIOUS

- Acute radiation sickness
- Appendicitis
- Chemical poisons
  - Arsenic
  - Cadmium
  - Lead
  - Mercury
- Diverticulitis
- Fecal impaction
- Inflammatory bowel disease
- Ischemic bowel disease
- Medications
- Mushroom intoxication

Proceed to Step 3.

STEP 3 – *Are There Any Clues in the Patient's History That Point to the Etiology of Acute Diarrhea?*

Clues in the patient's history that point to the etiology of acute diarrhea are listed in the following table.

Historical Clue	Condition Suggested
Recent antibiotic use	*C. difficile* infection Other causes of antibiotic-associated diarrhea
Recently started new medication*	Medication-related diarrhea
Recent ingestion of undercooked ground beef or unpasteurized apple cider	Enterohemorrhagic *E. coli* (EHEC)
Diarrhea developing at least 72 hours after hospitalization	*C. difficile* infection Noninfectious causes Medication-related diarrhea Tube feedings Others Argues strongly against parasitic cause
Light-headedness or dizziness with standing Decreased urine output Weakness Thirst	Symptoms of dehydration
Male homosexual practicing anal intercourse†	*Neisseria gonorrhoeae* Herpes simplex virus *Chlamydia trachomatis* *Treponema pallidum*
Recent travel to developing countries	Traveler's diarrhea
Sore throat	*Yersinia enterocolitica* *Neisseria gonorrhoeae*
Recent excessive ingestion of chewing gum or sodas	Medication-related diarrhea (sorbitol)
History of prolonged bed rest, analgesic use, or recent constipation	Fecal impaction
History of peripheral vascular disease History of coronary artery disease Oral contraceptive use Bacterial endocarditis Prosthetic valve	Risk factors for ischemic bowel disease
Predominantly vomiting	Food poisoning Viral gastroenteritis
Manifestations of dysentery: Passage of bloody stools Small volume stools Passage of mucus Tenesmus	*Shigella* *C. jejuni* *Salmonella* *Aeromonas* *Vibrio parahaemolyticus* *Yersinia enterocolitica* *E. coli* (enteroinvasive or enterohemorrhagic) *Entamoeba histolytica*
History of inflammatory bowel disease	Relapse of inflammatory bowel disease
Acute diarrhea affecting two or more persons who have shared a meal	Food poisoning

(continued)

(continued)

Historical Clue	Condition Suggested
Neurologic symptoms and signs in patient with acute diarrhea	Ciguatera fish poisoning Neurotoxic shellfish poisoning Paralytic shellfish poisoning
Tenesmus	Proctocolitis

*Although any medication can cause diarrhea, the medications more commonly associated with acute diarrhea include antacids, antibiotics, antihypertensives, antineoplastic agents, diuretics, lactulose, metoclopramide, quinidine, sorbitol, and theophylline.

†Male homosexuals are also at risk for acute diarrhea due to any agent that is spread by fecal-oral transmission. In addition, those who have AIDS are also susceptible to pathogens not commonly encountered in immunocompetent hosts.

Epidemiologic clues to the etiology of infectious diarrhea are listed in the following table.

Vehicle	Classic Pathogen
Water (including foods washed in such water)	*Cryptosporidium* *Giardia* Norwalk virus *Vibrio cholerae*
Poultry	*Campylobacter* *Salmonella* *Shigella*
Beef, unpasteurized fruit juice	Enterohemorrhagic *E. coli*
Seafood and shellfish*	Hepatitis A, B, and C *Salmonella* species *Vibrio cholerae* *Vibrio parahaemolyticus* *Vibrio vulnificus*
Cheese, milk	*Listeria* species
Eggs	*Salmonella* species
Mayonnaise-containing food and cream pies	Staphylococcal and clostridial food poisonings
Fried rice	*Bacillus cereus*
Fresh berries	*Cyclospora* species
Canned vegetables or fruits	*Clostridium* species
Animal-to-person (pets and livestock)	*Campylobacter* *Cryptosporidium* *Giardia* *Salmonella*
Daycare center	*Campylobacter* *C. difficile* *Cryptosporidium* *Giardia* *Shigella* Viruses
Hospital, antibiotics, or chemotherapy	*C. difficile*
Swimming pool	*Cryptosporidium* *Giardia*

*Also includes fish poisonings such as scombroid, ciguatera, paralytic, diarrhetic, and neurotoxic disease

Adapted from Park SI and Giannella RA, "Approach to the Adult Patient With Acute Diarrhea," *Gastroenterol Clin North Am*, 1993, 22(3):482-97 (review); also from Yamada T, Alpers DH, Owyang C, et al (eds), *Textbook of Gastroenterology*, 3rd ed, Philadelphia, PA: Lippincott-Raven, 1999.

Proceed to Step 4.

STEP 4 – *Are There Any Clues in the Patient's Physical Examination That Point to the Etiology of Acute Diarrhea?*

Clues in the patient's physical examination that point to the etiology of the acute diarrhea are listed in the following table.

Physical Examination Finding	Condition Suggested
Absence of axillary sweat Diminished skin turgor Dry mucous membranes Postural hypotension Tachycardia	Volume depletion/dehydration
Fever*	Suggests invasive pathogen
Distention Hypoactive bowel sounds	Consider toxic megacolon (due to invasive pathogen or noninfectious condition)
Peritoneal signs or rigidity	Toxic megacolon or perforation
Anal fissure or fistula	Crohn's disease
Jaundice	Malaria
Skin rash	Rocky Mountain spotted fever *Salmonella typhi* (rose spots) Toxic shock syndrome *Vibrio vulnificus* (hemorrhagic bullae) Viral gastroenteritis
Bradycardia	Typhoid fever
Constricted pupils	Cholinesterase inhibitor poisoning

**Shigella*, *Salmonella*, *C. jejuni*, *C. difficile*, *Aeromonas*, and viruses are the major causes of febrile diarrhea.

After a thorough history and physical examination, the clinician may be able to elicit features in the clinical presentation that suggest infection of either the small or large intestine, as shown in the following table.

	Small Intestinal Pathogen	Large Intestinal Pathogen
Abdominal pain	Midabdominal	Lower abdominal or rectal
Stool volume	Large	Small
Stool consistency	Usually watery (rare blood)	Often mucoid or bloody
Stool for occult blood	Rarely positive	Often positive
Tenesmus	Absent	Often present

Determining the location of the enteric infection is a useful way of narrowing the differential diagnosis of acute infectious diarrhea. The predilection of pathogens for the large or small intestine is described in the following box.

PREDILECTION OF PATHOGENS FOR LARGE OR SMALL INTESTINE	
SMALL INTESTINE	**LARGE INTESTINE**
Cryptosporidium	*Aeromonas*
Cyclospora	*Campylobacter*
E. coli (enteropathogenic)	*C. difficile*
E. coli (enterotoxigenic)	Cytomegalovirus
Giardia lamblia	*E. coli* (enterohemorrhagic)
Isospora belli	*E. coli* (enteroinvasive)
Microsporidia	*E. histolytica*
Norwalk	*Plesiomonas*
Rotavirus	*Shigella*
Vibrio cholerae	

There are, however, certain pathogens that can involve both the lower small intestine and colon. These organisms include *Salmonella* and *Yersinia*. In most of these cases, the diarrheal illness is characterized by watery stools. Bloody diarrhea, however, does occur in some cases.

Proceed to Step 5.

STEP 5 – *Should Laboratory Tests Be Obtained in the Patient Presenting With Acute Diarrhea?*

Although there are many causes of acute diarrhea, infection is the leading etiology. Over 90% of patients with acute infectious diarrhea have a mild illness that readily improves with time. In fact, most patients have improved or recovered within 5 days. In these patients, laboratory evaluation to determine the etiologic organism is not recommended for the following reasons:

- Laboratory testing is expensive
- Test results are often unrevealing
- Testing does not affect treatment
- Testing does not affect outcome

The clinician's goal is to identify features in the patient's clinical presentation that suggest severe illness. Those patients having a severe acute diarrheal illness require further testing. In these patients, it is reasonable to send blood for determination of BUN, creatinine, electrolytes, CBC, and liver function tests. Blood cultures should be performed in clinically septic patients. The indications for fecal leukocyte testing, stool cultures for bacteria, ova and parasite examination, and proctosigmoidoscopy are discussed in the steps that follow.

Proceed to Step 6.

STEP 6 – *Should Testing for Fecal Leukocytes Be Performed?*

Since most cases of acute diarrhea due to infection are self-limited illnesses, fecal leukocyte testing should only be performed in certain situations. Indications for fecal leukocyte testing are listed in the following box.

INDICATIONS FOR FECAL LEUKOCYTE TESTING
Moderate or severe diarrhea*
Profuse watery diarrhea with dehydration
Passage of very small volume stools containing blood or mucus
Temperature >38.5°C or 101.3°F
≥6 unformed stools/24 hours
Duration >48 hours
Severe abdominal pain in patient >50 years of age
Diarrhea in elderly patient ≥70 years of age
Immunocompromised patient

*A diarrheal illness that forces a change in a patient's normal activities is referred to as moderate diarrhea. Severe diarrhea is said to be present when the illness confines the patient to bed.

The clinician should consider inflammatory causes of acute diarrhea when numerous fecal leukocytes are noted. Although the presence of fecal leukocytes is not specific for infection, this finding in the patient having clinical manifestations consistent with infectious diarrhea should prompt the clinician to consider invasive pathogens. These pathogens, as well as other causes of acute diarrhea associated with fecal leukocytes in the stool, are listed in the following box.

CAUSES OF ACUTE DIARRHEA ASSOCIATED WITH FECAL LEUKOCYTES IN THE STOOL
INFECTION
Aeromonas
Campylobacter
Clostridium difficile
E. coli
Enterohemorrhagic (EHEC)
Enteroinvasive (EIEC)
Salmonella
Shigella
Vibrio (noncholera species)
Yersinia enterocolitica
INFLAMMATORY BOWEL DISEASE

Significant numbers of fecal leukocytes are not found in patients with viral gastroenteritis, parasitic diarrhea, and enterotoxigenic diarrhea (eg, enterotoxigenic *E. coli*, cholera). The clinician must ensure that there is no delay in the processing of the stool specimen for fecal leukocytes as the cells may lyse readily.

Proceed to Step 7.

STEP 7 – *Should Stool Cultures Be Performed?*

It is not cost-effective to obtain a stool culture in every patient presenting with acute diarrhea, especially since the isolation rate of a pathogenic organism is about 3% to 20% in an unselected population. The diagnostic yield of stool culture is improved if the clinician takes the time to elicit certain features in the patient's clinical presentation. The features that should prompt the clinician to obtain stool cultures are listed in the following box.

INDICATIONS FOR STOOL CULTURE IN PATIENTS WITH ACUTE DIARRHEA	
AIDS-RELATED DIARRHEA	PERSISTENT DIARRHEA
BLOODY STOOLS	SEVERE DIARRHEA
+ FECAL LEUKOCYTES	TEMPERATURE >38.5°C or 101.3°F (oral)
+ OCCULT BLOOD IN STOOL	INFLAMMATORY BOWEL DISEASE*

*Stool culture may be useful in patients with inflammatory bowel disease who present with acute diarrhea. In these patients, testing may help to differentiate disease flare from superimposed infection.

There is no need to obtain stool cultures in hospitalized patients who develop diarrhea 72 hours or more after hospitalization. Although both infectious and noninfectious causes of acute diarrhea need to be considered in these patients, when infection is present, it is almost always due to *C. difficile* infection. The test of choice for establishing the diagnosis of *C. difficile* infection is not stool culture but toxin assay (see below).

Laboratories differ as to the pathogens that are tested when stool cultures are requested. In fact, most laboratories will routinely process stool specimens for *Shigella*, *Salmonella*, and *Campylobacter.* If other organisms are possibilities, it behooves the clinician to communicate these concerns with the laboratory. When the stool culture reveals the growth of a known gastrointestinal pathogen in a patient presenting with acute diarrhea, the clinician can be reasonably confident that the organism identified is the etiologic agent.

A history of recent antibiotic therapy should raise concern for the possibility of *C. difficile* infection. Other risk factors include recent hospitalization, daycare exposure, and recent chemotherapy. The most widely used test in the diagnosis of *C. difficile* diarrhea is detection of *C. difficile* toxin in stool specimens. Toxin assays, as well as other laboratory tests available in the diagnosis of *C. difficile* infection, are described in the following table.

Test	Sensitivity (%)	Specificity (%)	Clinical Utility
Endoscopy	51	100	Diagnostic of pseudomembranous colitis
Culture for *C. difficile**	89-100	84-99	Highly sensitive; confirmation of organism toxicity optimal
Cell culture cytotoxin test	67-100	85-100	With clinical data, diagnostic of CDAD†
EIA toxin test	63-99	75-100	With clinical data, diagnostic of CDAD†

(continued)

(continued)

Test	Sensitivity (%)	Specificity (%)	Clinical Utility
Latex test for *C. difficile* antigen	58-92	80-96	Less sensitive and specific than other tests; rapid results
PCR toxin gene detection	Undetermined	Undetermined	Research test

*Although *C. difficile* culture is a fairly sensitive test in the diagnosis of *C. difficile* infection, most laboratories are unable to differentiate between toxigenic and nonpathogenic strains of the organism. As a result, false-positive test results occur in up to 25% of cases.

†CDAD is an abbreviation for *Clostridium difficile*-associated disease.

Adapted from Gerding DN, Johnson S, Peterson LR, et al, "*Clostridium difficile*-Associated Diarrhea and Colitis," *Infect Control Hosp Epidemiol*, 1995, 16(8):459-77 (review); also from Mandell GL, Bennett JE, and Dolin R, *Principles and Practice of Infectious Disease*, 5th ed, New York, NY: Churchill Livingstone, 2000, 1117.

Proceed to Step 8.

STEP 8 – *Should an Ova and Parasite Examination Be Performed?*

Not all patients with acute diarrhea require stool examination for ova and parasites. In fact, the yield of the ova and parasite examination is low (<10%) in the absence of certain clinical or epidemiologic features. When indicated, three specimens should be sent on consecutive days. Indications for ova and parasite examination are listed in the following box.

INDICATIONS FOR STOOL OVA AND PARASITE EXAMINATION IN PATIENTS WITH ACUTE DIARRHEA
Community waterborne outbreak
Exposure to daycare center
HIV / AIDS
Homosexual males
Persistent diarrhea (>2 weeks)
Recent travel to developing countries, Russia, Nepal, or Rocky Mountains
Stools bloody but few fecal leukocytes noted

The clinician should not examine the stool for ova and parasites in the patient who develops diarrhea while in the hospital because a parasitic cause of the diarrhea is very unlikely in this setting. The clinician should be aware of substances that can negatively impact upon the yield of stool examination for ova and parasites. These substances include bismuth, antibiotic therapy (eg, tetracycline, erythromycin), barium, laxatives, antacids, and hypertonic enemas. If possible, these substances should be avoided.

Intestinal Amebiasis

The identification of cysts and trophozoites in stool specimens establishes the diagnosis of intestinal amebiasis. The yield of the stool examination is increased if the laboratory concentrates the fecal specimens. The clinician should realize that the organism will be identified in just 33% of cases if only one stool specimen is submitted for analysis. Hence, the recommendation for ova and parasite examination of three stool specimens when parasitic causes of acute diarrhea are a consideration.

The endoscopic appearance of amebiasis does not distinguish this infection from other infectious causes of acute diarrhea. However, biopsy or scrapings of lesions (wet preparation of ulcer aspirates or biopsy specimens) noted during endoscopy may reveal findings consistent with amebiasis. In recent years, serum antiamebic antibody tests have become available. These are probably the most useful tests in the diagnosis of amebiasis. One particular antibody test, the indirect hemagglutination test, yields positive results in almost 90% of intestinal amebiasis cases.

Giardiasis

Three separate stool specimens should be examined for the trophozoites and cysts of *Giardia lamblia.* If unrevealing, the clinician may choose to perform ELISA or immunofluorescence testing of the stool for *Giardia* antigens. Unremarkable stool studies should prompt consideration of duodenal aspiration, duodenal biopsy, or the Entero-Test string to establish the diagnosis.

Other Parasitic Causes of Diarrhea

Many of the other parasitic causes of acute diarrhea require acid-fast staining of the stool to identify the organism. Modified Kinyoun's acid-fast stain and trichrome staining of the stool, especially if the stool is concentrated, can demonstrate findings consistent with *Cryptosporidium*, *Isospora belli*, and microsporidiosis. Microsporidiosis may also be detected by light microscopy of properly stained stool specimens. At times, however, identification of these parasitic causes of acute diarrhea may require small intestinal aspirates or, even, jejunal biopsy. Recently, monoclonal-based tests (ELISA and immunofluorescence stains) have been developed for the detection of many of these parasites. The clinician should inform the laboratory if these parasitic causes of acute diarrhea are considerations, especially since routine ova and parasite examination does not always include screening for these protozoal organisms.

Proceed to Step 9.

STEP 9 – *Should Proctosigmoidoscopy Be Performed?*

It is uncommon for patients with acute diarrhea to require endoscopic evaluation. Indications for proctosigmoidoscopy in patients with acute diarrhea are listed in the following box.

INDICATIONS FOR PROCTOSIGMOIDOSCOPY IN ACUTE DIARRHEA
Amebiasis*
Chronic diarrhea
History of anal manipulation
HIV-positive with large bowel diarrhea or acute proctitis
Idiopathic inflammatory bowel disease
Ischemic colitis†
Severe antibiotic-associated diarrhea with equivocal test for *C. difficile* toxin†‡

*Indications for endoscopy in patients suspected of having amebiasis include the following:
- Stool ova and parasite exam is negative but serum antiamebic antibody test is positive.
- Stool ova and parasite exam is negative and immediate diagnosis is needed.
- High suspicion for amebiasis but stool ova and parasite examination and serum antiamebic antibody test are negative.

†Endoscopic evaluation should be considered when clinical and radiologic testing does not confirm a diagnosis of ischemic colitis in patients having a clinical presentation consistent with this condition.

‡The American College of Gastroenterology has developed guidelines for the role of endoscopy in patients suspected of having *C. difficile* infection. Their recommendations for endoscopy include the following:
- Rapid diagnosis is necessary but test results are either delayed or insensitive tests were performed.
- Patient has ileus and stool is not available.

Adapted from Fekety R, "Guidelines for the Diagnosis and Management of *Clostridium difficile*-Associated Diarrhea and Colitis. American College of Gastroenterology, Practice Parameters Committee," *Am J Gastroenterol*, 1997, 92(5):739-50 (review); also from "Intestinal Disease Caused by *Entamoeba histolytica*," *Amebiasis: Human Infection By Entamoeba histolytica*, Ravin JI (ed), New York, NY: Wiley, 1988, 495-510.

Proceed to Step 10.

STEP 10 – *Has the Diarrhea Resolved?*

Most cases of acute diarrhea resolve within 2 weeks. Even with extensive laboratory testing, an etiologic agent is not identified in up to 40% of cases. When a diarrheal illness persists after 2 weeks, the patient is said to have persistent diarrhea. Common causes of persistent diarrhea are listed in the following box.

COMMON CAUSES OF PERSISTENT DIARRHEA	
BACTERIAL DIARRHEA	INFLAMMATORY BOWEL DISEASE
Campylobacter	LACTASE DEFICIENCY
E. coli (enteropathogenic)	PARASITIC
Salmonella	*Cryptosporidium parvum*
Shigella	*Giardia lamblia*
Yersinia	*Isospora belli*
BRAINERD DIARRHEA	*Microsporidia*
HOST DEFICIENCY (ie, AIDS)	SMALL INTESTINAL BACTERIAL OVERGROWTH

References

Aranda-Michel J and Giannella RA, "Acute Diarrhea: A Practical Review," *Am J Med*, 1999, 106(6):670-6.

Cheney CP and Wong RK, "Acute Infectious Diarrhea," *Med Clin North Am*, 1993, 77(5):1169-96.

DuPont HL, "Guidelines on Acute Infectious Diarrhea in Adults. The Practice Parameters Committee of the American College of Gastroenterology," *Am J Gastroenterol*, 1997, 92(11):1962-75.

Farthing MJ, "Giardiasis," *Gastroenterol Clin North Am*, 1996, 25(3):493-515.

Fekety R, "Guidelines for the Diagnosis and Management of *Clostridium difficile*-Associated Diarrhea and Colitis. American College of Gastroenterology, Practice Parameters Committee," *Am J Gastroenterol*, 1997, 92(5):739-50 (review).

Gerding DN, Johnson S, Peterson LR, et al, "*Clostridium difficile*-Associated Diarrhea and Colitis," *Infect Control Hosp Epidemiol*, 1995, 16(8):459-77 (review).

Mandell GL, Bennett JE, and Dolin RA, *Principles and Practice of Infectious Disease*, 5th ed, New York, NY: Churchill Livingstone, 2000, 1117.

Park SI and Giannella R, "Approach to the Adult Patient With Acute Diarrhea," *Gastroenterol Clin North Am*, 1993, 22(3):483-97 (review).

Plevris JN and Hayes PC, "Investigation and Management of Acute Diarrhoea," *Br J Hosp Med*, 1996, 56(11):569-73.

Ravdin JI, "Intestinal Disease Caused by *Entamoeba histolytica*," *Amebiasis: Human Infection By Entamoeba histolytica*, New York, NY: Wiley, 1988, 495-510.

Talal AH and Murray JA, "Acute and Chronic Diarrhea. How to Keep Laboratory Testing to a Minimum," *Postgrad Med*, 1994, 96(3):30-2, 35-8, 43.

Textbook of Gastroenterology, 3rd ed, Yamada T, Alpers DH, Owyang C, et al (eds), Philadelphia, PA: Lippincott-Raven, 1999.

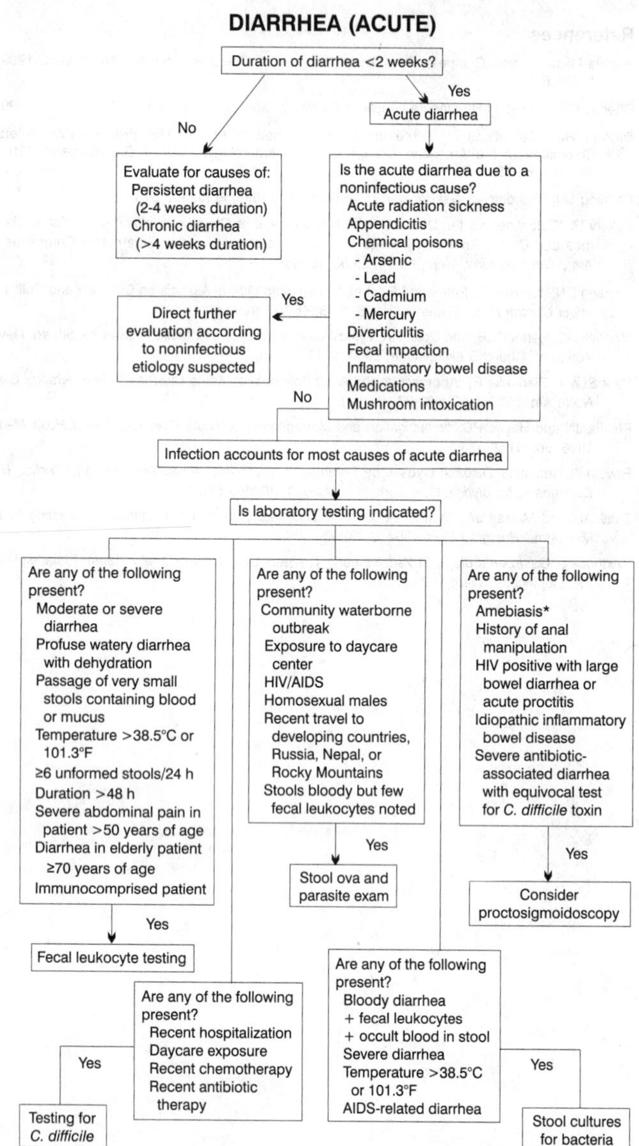
DIARRHEA (ACUTE)
Duration of diarrhea <2 weeks?
Yes
Acute diarrhea
No
Evaluate for causes of: Persistent diarrhea (2-4 weeks duration) Chronic diarrhea (>4 weeks duration)
Is the acute diarrhea due to a noninfectious cause? Acute radiation sickness Appendicitis Chemical poisons - Arsenic - Lead - Cadmium - Mercury Diverticulitis Fecal impaction Inflammatory bowel disease Medications Mushroom intoxication
Yes
Direct further evaluation according to noninfectious etiology suspected
No
Infection accounts for most causes of acute diarrhea
Is laboratory testing indicated?
Are any of the following present? Moderate or severe diarrhea Profuse watery diarrhea with dehydration Passage of very small stools containing blood or mucus Temperature >38.5°C or 101.3°F ≥6 unformed stools/24 h Duration >48 h Severe abdominal pain in patient >50 years of age Diarrhea in elderly patient ≥70 years of age Immunocomprised patient
Yes
Fecal leukocyte testing
Are any of the following present? Community waterborne outbreak Exposure to daycare center HIV/AIDS Homosexual males Recent travel to developing countries, Russia, Nepal, or Rocky Mountains Stools bloody but few fecal leukocytes noted
Yes
Stool ova and parasite exam
Are any of the following present? Amebiasis* History of anal manipulation HIV positive with large bowel diarrhea or acute proctitis Idiopathic inflammatory bowel disease Severe antibiotic-associated diarrhea with equivocal test for C. difficile toxin
Yes
Consider proctosigmoidoscopy
Are any of the following present? Recent hospitalization Daycare exposure Recent chemotherapy Recent antibiotic therapy
Yes
Testing for C. difficile
Are any of the following present? Bloody diarrhea + fecal leukocytes + occult blood in stool Severe diarrhea Temperature >38.5°C or 101.3°F AIDS-related diarrhea
Yes
Stool cultures for bacteria

*Indications for proctosigmoidoscopy in acute diarrhea patients suspected of having amebiasis include:
- Stool ova and parasite exam is nevative but serum antiamebic antibody test is positive
- Stool ova and parasite exam is negative and immediate diagnosis is needed
- High suspicion for amebiasis but stool ova and parasite examination and serum antiamebic antibody test are negative

ASCITIC FLUID ANALYSIS

Indications for Paracentesis

A paracentesis should be performed on all patients with the development of new onset ascites to help establish the etiology. In patients with ascites, an argument can also be made to sample ascitic fluid at the time of each hospital admission. Studies have shown that the prevalence of ascitic fluid infection at the time of admission varies between 10% and 27%. It is not always easy to clinically predict infected ascites, as manifestations may be very subtle. For these reasons, authorities recommend paracentesis in patients who meet one or more of the following criteria:

- All inpatients and outpatients with new-onset ascites
- All patients admitted to the hospital with ascites
- Whenever signs, symptoms, or laboratory features are consistent with infected ascites (abdominal pain or tenderness, fever, encephalopathy, renal failure, acidosis, hypotension, leukocytosis)

Contraindications for Paracentesis

Not uncommonly, the question that arises is whether it is safe to do a paracentesis in a patient with a coagulopathy. Only in the event of disseminated intravascular coagulation or clinically apparent fibrinolysis should a paracentesis not be performed. There is no level of PT or PTT above which the risk of paracentesis should preclude the procedure. There is also no data to support the routine administration of blood products (fresh frozen plasma or platelets) to minimize the risk of complications.

Gross Appearance

It is always important to comment on the gross appearance of ascitic fluid, which can be quite instructive in elucidating the cause of ascites. Normal ascitic fluid is transparent. Cloudiness of a specimen is most often caused by increased neutrophils. A bloody specimen may be either the result of a traumatic tap or from nontraumatic causes. There are several clues which help to differentiate between the two. These include the following.

- Often a bloody specimen from a traumatic tap will clot if it is not transferred to an anticoagulated tube. Nontraumatic bloody ascitic fluid will not clot.
- Blood associated with a traumatic tap tends to clear with ongoing paracentesis.
- Specimens that show blood streaking are indicative of a traumatic tap.

As for nontraumatic taps, it is not uncommon for patients with hepatocellular cancer to have a bloody tap. In contrast, in patients having peritoneal carcinomatosis or tuberculous peritonitis, only 10% and 5% of taps, respectively, are bloody.

A specimen that is milky and fails to clear after centrifugation raises the possibility of either chylous or pseudochylous ascites. Chylous ascites is not common but may be the result of a number of diseases including malignancy, tuberculosis, trauma, and cirrhosis.

A dark brown specimen raises concern about biliary perforation or upper gut perforation, particularly if the ascitic fluid bilirubin level is greater than the serum bilirubin concentration.

Black ascites is associated with both hemorrhagic pancreatitis and malignant melanoma.

Tests of the Ascitic Fluid

A number of tests of the ascitic fluid are available in establishing the etiology of the ascites. Too often, though, unnecessary ascitic fluid tests are obtained without careful consideration of the patient's clinical presentation. This practice of extensive ascitic fluid testing should be avoided for several reasons which include the following.

- Ordering every ascitic fluid test available can be quite expensive (and certainly not cost-effective).
- When tests that are not indicated are ordered, it is not unusual to encounter unexpectedly abnormal test results which can lead to diagnostic confusion.

The following box provides guidance regarding when to order ascitic fluid tests.

ASCITIC FLUID TESTS
ROUTINE
Albumin
Cell count
Culture (in blood culture bottles)
OTHER TESTS (if indicated, based on patient's clinical presentation)
Total protein
LDH
Glucose
Amylase
Gram stain
Tuberculosis smear/culture
Bilirubin
Triglyceride
Cytology
TESTS THAT ARE NOT USEFUL
pH
Lactate
Cholesterol

Classification

Years ago, clinicians relied on the total protein concentration of the ascitic fluid to determine if the patient had a transudate (<2.5 g/dL) or exudate (>2.5 g/dL). Separating ascitic fluid into transudates and exudates has now fallen out of favor and has given way to more sensitive tests. A more appropriate test for the classification of ascitic fluid is the serum-to-ascites albumin gradient (SAAG), which is really a subtraction, not a ratio. The formula for this calculation is as follows:

Serum - ascites albumin gradient (SAAG)

$$SAAG = albumin_{serum} - albumin_{ascitic\ fluid}$$

Conditions leading to ascites through portal hypertension characteristically have a gradient >1.1 g/dL. If the calculated gradient is <1.1 g/dL, one should consider those conditions that cause ascites in the absence of portal hypertension. There is 97% accuracy using this cutoff in the classification of ascites.

Classification of Ascites Based on the SAAG

Pathophysiology	SAAG
Portal hypertension	>1.1 g/dL
No portal hypertension	<1.1 g/dL

Differential Diagnosis of Ascitic Fluid Based on the SAAG

High Gradient (>1.1 g/dL)	Low Gradient (<1.1 g/dL)
Cirrhosis	Peritoneal carcinomatosis
Cardiac ascites	Tuberculous peritonitis (without cirrhosis)
Alcoholic hepatitis	Pancreatic ascites (without cirrhosis)
Massive liver metastasis	Biliary ascites
Fulminant hepatic failure	Nephrotic syndrome
Budd-Chiari syndrome	Serositis (connective tissue disease)
Portal vein thrombosis	Bowel obstruction
Hepatic veno-occlusive disease	Bowel infarction
Myxedema	Postoperative lymphatic leak
Acute fatty liver of pregnancy	
Mixed ascites	

Adapted from Runyon B, "Care of Patients With Ascites," *N Engl J Med*, 1999, 330(5):339.

Limitations of the SAAG in the Classification of Ascites

There are some limitations in the use of the SAAG for the classification of ascites. These include the following.

- In the patient with mixed ascites due to hepatic cirrhosis and peritoneal tuberculosis, for example, the gradient will be >1.1 g/dL, as the portal pressure remains elevated.
- If the serum albumin in a cirrhotic patient is <1.1 g/dL, the gradient may be misleadingly low.
- The clinician should ensure that the albumin assay that is performed is accurate at low albumin concentrations. Many patients with ascites have ascitic fluid albumin levels <1 g/dL. If the assay is not accurate at these levels, the SAAG can be affected, potentially leading to misclassification of the patient's ascites.
- The assay for albumin may be affected by lipids. Chylous ascites may have a falsely high albumin gradient.
- The hypotensive patient may have a decrease in the gradient because of a fall in portal pressure.
- An increase in the serum globulin fraction leads to a corresponding increase in the ascitic fluid globulin fraction. If significant enough, this may contribute to the oncotic forces in the ascitic fluid leading to a smaller gradient. The clinician should be aware of a correction factor for the SAAG in patients with peripheral hyperglobulinemia (>5 g/dL). The equation for correcting the SAAG is as follows:

  Corrected SAAG = uncorrected SAAG x 0.16 x [serum globulin (g/dL) + 2.5]
- It is important to obtain the ascites albumin and the serum albumin on the same day to avoid inaccurate comparisons.

Cell Count

Laboratories vary in how the cell count is reported. Some laboratories include mesothelial cells as part of the total white blood cell count, often reporting the sum (mesothelial cells + white blood cells) under the term "nucleated cells". The clinical significance of mesothelial cells in the ascitic fluid remains unclear.

The white blood cell count is probably the most useful test in the analysis of ascitic fluid. On occasion, the clinician may encounter difficulty obtaining ascitic fluid. In some cases, only a small amount of fluid may be available for analysis and the clinician may be faced with a dilemma as far as which test or tests should be ordered. In these situations, the cell count should most certainly be ordered since it is of utmost importance that infected ascites be excluded. The cell count will help support or argue against the diagnosis of infected ascites.

The WBC count in uncomplicated cirrhotic ascites is <500 cells/mm^3. The cell count, however, can climb to >1000 cells/mm^3 in cirrhotic patients undergoing diuresis. It is not wise to attribute this elevation solely to diuresis if a prediuresis count is not available for comparison, as patients with cirrhotic ascites are prone to infection. A predominance of lymphocytes and the lack of symptoms consistent with infected ascites support diuresis as the etiology. Additionally, the PMN cell count remains unaffected by diuresis and, therefore, if elevated, is highly suggestive of infection. The upper limit of a normal neutrophil count in uncomplicated cirrhotic ascites is 250 cells/mm^3.

Additionally, an increased WBC count may result from any inflammatory process, with spontaneous bacterial peritonitis being the most common. Approximately 90% of patients with spontaneous bacterial peritonitis (SBP) have a WBC count >500 cells/mm^3, at least 50% of which are neutrophils. An elevated leukocyte count may also be seen in both tuberculous peritonitis and peritoneal carcinomatosis, usually with a lymphocyte predominance.

The presence of blood in ascitic fluid can also raise the leukocyte count. A useful calculation to remember is that the corrected neutrophil count can be obtained by subtracting one neutrophil from the total neutrophil count for every 250 red blood cells present in the ascitic fluid. If the corrected count is >250 cells/mm^3, then infection is likely.

CAUSES OF INCREASED WBC COUNT IN ASCITIC FLUID
DIURESIS SPONTANEOUS BACTERIAL PERITONITIS TUBERCULOSIS PERITONITIS PERITONEAL CARCINOMATOSIS BLOODY ASCITES CHYLOUS ASCITES

Gram Stain

Gram stain is seldom positive. It requires the presence of substantial numbers of bacteria per mL of ascitic fluid. In spontaneous bacterial peritonitis, the number of bacteria causing infection is much lower, explaining the 10% sensitivity of this test. It is more useful with very serious infections or in the case of gut perforation.

Culture

In the past, it was thought that most infections of ascitic fluid were polymicrobial with high colony counts. It is now recognized that ascitic fluid infection is most often monomicrobial with low colony counts. With this in mind, there has been a shift in culture technique with plating falling out of favor. The inoculation of blood culture bottles at the bedside is now preferred as a more sensitive means. With bedside inoculation, microbial growth has been demonstrated in close to 80% of specimens.

AFB Smear and Culture

The AFB smear, like the Gram stain, is rarely positive. Culture of ascitic fluid for mycobacteria has a sensitivity of 50%; however, the sensitivity of histology and culture of a peritoneal biopsy is close to 100%.

Cytology

The overall sensitivity of cytology for all types of malignant ascites has been reported to be between 40% and 60%. However, there is great discrepancy between the sensitivity of cytology in the patient with peritoneal carcinomatosis (where the sensitivity approaches 97%) and the patient with hepatocellular carcinoma (where the sensitivity is reported as approximately 10%). This is easily understood if consideration is given to the differing pathophysiology of ascites formation in these two forms of malignancy. In peritoneal carcinomatosis, tumor cells lining the peritoneal cavity exfoliate directly in ascitic fluid. Contrast this with either hepatocellular cancer or extensive liver metastasis, where ascites is secondary to portal hypertension and a positive cytology would not be expected. Lymphatic obstruction leading to ascites in patients with lymphoma would present similarly.

Amylase

An amylase level in normal peritoneal fluid approximates the level in blood. Ascitic fluid amylase that is greater than three times the upper limits of normal argues for a pancreatic process leading to ascites (eg, acute pancreatitis, pseudocyst). However, there are other GI causes of ascitic fluid amylase elevation including, for example, gut perforation.

Triglyceride Level

Triglyceride levels are indicated when paracentesis reveals ascitic fluid that is opalescent or milky, which raises the possibility of chylous ascites. Chylous ascites refers to the presence of lymph in the ascitic fluid. Lymphatic obstruction is usually the cause and may result from trauma, tumor, tuberculosis, filariasis, and even congenital disorders. The triglyceride level is usually >200 mg/dL and, not uncommonly, >1000 mg/dL.

A turbid fluid may also be the result of inflammatory or tumor cells (so-called pseudochylous ascites) and may initially lead to confusion when the specimen is obtained at the bedside. However, a triglyceride level <200 mg/dL supports the diagnosis of pseudochylous ascites.

Bilirubin

A bilirubin level should be obtained on ascitic fluid that is brown. An ascitic fluid bilirubin level >6 mg/dL and one that exceeds the serum bilirubin level should raise concern for biliary or upper gut perforation.

Other Tests of the Ascitic Fluid

Investigators have found that the combination of total protein, LDH, and glucose in ascitic fluid are helpful in differentiating spontaneous bacterial peritonitis from gut perforation. If two of the three following criteria are met, strong consideration of surgical peritonitis is warranted.

CRITERIA FOR CONSIDERATION OF SURGICAL PERITONITIS
PROTEIN >1 g/dL GLUCOSE <50 mg/dL LDH > UPPER LIMIT OF NORMAL

References

Aalami OO, Allen DB, and Organ CH Jr "Chylous Ascites: A Collective Review," *Surgery*, 2000, 128(5):761-78.

Ahmad M and Ahmed A, "Tuberculous Peritonitis: Fatality Associated With Delayed Diagnosis," *South Med J*, 1999, 92(4):406-8.

Dugurnier T, Laterre PF, and Reynaert MS, "Ascites Fluid in Severe Acute Pancreatitis: From Pathophysiology to Therapy," *Acta Gastroenterol Belg*, 2000, 63(3):264-8.

Fernandez J, Bauer TM, Navasa M, et al, "Diagnosis, Treatment and Prevention of Spontaneous Bacterial Peritonitis," *Baillieres Best Pract Res Clin Gastroenterol*, 2000, 14(6):975-90.

Guarner C and Soriano G, "Spontaneous Bacterial Peritonitis," *Semin Liver Dis*, 1997, 17(3):203-17.

Han SH, Reynolds TB, and Fong TL, "Nephrogenic Ascites. Analysis of 16 Cases and Review of the Literature," *Medicine (Baltimore)*, 1998, 77(4):233-45.

Johst P, Tsiotos GG, and Sarr MG, "Pancreatic Ascites: A Rare Complication of Necrotizing Pancreatitis. A Case Report and Review of the Literature," *Int J Pancreatol*, 1997, 22(2):151-4.

Laroche M and Harding G, "Primary and Secondary Peritonitis: An Update," *Eur J Clin Microbiol Infect Dis*, 1998, 17(8):542-50.

Laterre PF, Dugurnier T, and Reynaert MS, "Chylous Ascites: Diagnosis, Causes and Treatment," *Acta Gastroenterol Belg*, 2000, 63(3):260-3.

McGuire BM and Bloomer JR, "Complications of Cirrhosis. Why They Occur and What to Do About Them," *Postgrad Med*, 1998, 103(2):209-12, 217-8, 223-4.

Parsons SL, Watson SA, and Steele RJ, "Malignant Ascites," *Br J Surg*, 1996, 83(1):6-14.

Rebuffoni G, Guadagni S, Somers DC, et al, "Peritoneal Carcinomatosis: Feature of Dissemination. A Review," *Tumori*, 1999, 85(1):1-5.

Rimola A, Garcia-Tsao G, Navasa M, et al, "Diagnosis, Treatment and Prophylaxis of Spontaneous Bacterial Peritonitis: A Consensus Document. International Ascites Club," *J Hepatol*, 2000, 32(1):142-53.

Saravanan R and Cramp ME, "Investigation and Treatment of Ascites," *Clin Med*, 2002, 2(4):310-3.

Uriz J, Cardenas A, and Arroyo V, "Pathophysiology, Diagnosis and Treatment of Ascites in Cirrhosis," *Baillieres Best Pract Res Clin Gastroenterol*, 2000, 14(6):927-43.

SELECTED CAUSES OF ASCITES

Causes of Ascites

The causes of ascites have already been classified according to the serum ascites to albumin gradient (SAAG) in the chapter, ***Ascitic Fluid Analysis** on page 763*. In the following table, the common causes of ascites in the United States are listed.

Causes of Ascites in the United States

Cause	Percentage of Total %*
Chronic parenchymal liver disease (includes cirrhosis and alcoholic hepatitis)	81.4
Malignancy	10.0
Congestive heart failure	3.0
Tuberculous	1.7
Nephrogenous (dialysis ascites)	1.0
Pancreatic	0.9
Miscellaneous (includes fulminant hepatic failure, biliary, lymphatic tear, *Chlamydia*, and nephrotic syndrome)	Each <1.0

*Mixed ascites (ie, more than one cause of ascites) found in 4.3% of patients.

Adapted from *Clinical Practice of Gastroenterology*, Brandt LJ, ed, Philadelphia, PA: Current Medicine, Inc, 1999, 988.

In the remainder of this chapter, the major causes of ascites will be discussed in further detail.

Cirrhotic Ascites

Although ascites due to liver disease can be a complication of alcoholic hepatitis or fulminant hepatic failure, most patients have cirrhotic ascites. Cirrhotic ascites is the major cause of ascites, accounting for >80% of cases. In some patients, ascites may be the first manifestation of cirrhosis. In these cases, the clinician should perform a thorough history and physical exam looking for features consistent with cirrhosis. Physical examination may reveal the stigmata of chronic liver disease including palmar erythema, spider angiomas, abdominal wall collateral veins, splenomegaly, and jaundice.

Laboratory studies that reveal abnormal levels of transaminases, alkaline phosphatase, and bilirubin support the diagnosis of cirrhotic ascites. PT prolongation and hypoalbuminemia are also consistent with cirrhosis, reflecting an impairment in the liver's synthetic capability. The clinician should realize, however, that there are other causes of ascites and hypoalbuminemia such as the nephrotic syndrome.

Ultimately, the diagnosis of cirrhotic ascites rests upon the analysis of the ascitic fluid. All patients suspected of having cirrhotic ascites require paracentesis. In addition, because these patients are at risk for spontaneous bacterial peritonitis, abdominal paracentesis should be performed in the following situation on patients with known cirrhotic ascites:

- At the time of hospital admission to rule out spontaneous bacterial peritonitis, irrespective of whether there are signs and symptoms of infection
- Whenever symptoms or signs of spontaneous bacterial peritonitis develop

Paracentesis usually reveals yellow, clear ascitic fluid in patients with uncomplicated cirrhosis. The clinician should suspect spontaneous bacterial peritonitis if a cloudy specimen is obtained. Although a serum to ascites albumin gradient >1.1 g/dL is consistent with cirrhotic ascites, there are other causes of an elevated gradient. Other causes can usually be excluded by history, physical examination, and laboratory testing. If the ascitic fluid PMN count is >250/mm^3, the clinician should consider the possibility of spontaneous bacterial peritonitis. This complication of cirrhotic ascites is discussed later in this chapter.

Malignancy-Related Ascites

Malignancy-related ascites accounts for <10% of cases. Not all cases of malignancy-related ascites are due to peritoneal carcinomatosis. The different types of malignancy-related ascites are listed in the following box.

CLASSIFICATION OF MALIGNANCY-RELATED ASCITES
PERITONEAL CARCINOMATOSIS MASSIVE LIVER METASTASES PERITONEAL CARCINOMATOSIS WITH MASSIVE LIVER METASTASES HEPATOCELLULAR CARCINOMA MALIGNANT LYMPH NODE OBSTRUCTION MALIGNANT BUDD-CHIARI SYNDROME CHYLOUS ASCITES

In patients with malignancy-related ascites, the results of ascitic fluid analysis will differ depending upon the mechanism of the ascites. Cytology will not be positive in all cases of malignancy-related ascites. Only in peritoneal carcinomatosis, in which tumor cells line the peritoneal cavity and exfoliate into the ascitic fluid, will cytology be positive. If another mechanism for ascites formation is present, cytology is unlikely to be revealing.

Therefore, cytology will be positive in 100% of patients with peritoneal carcinomatosis. When all patients with malignancy-related ascites are examined, however, cytology will only be positive in 60% to 70% since 33% of malignancy-related ascites is due to mechanisms of ascites formation other than peritoneal carcinomatosis.

Different types of malignancy-related ascites are compared in the following table.

Ascitic Fluid Test Results in Malignancy-Related Ascites

Type of Malignancy-Related Ascites	WBC Count	RBC Count	Cytology (% Positive Neoplastic Cells)	Biochemistry	SAAG
Peritoneal carcinomatosis	75% with >500	Few or none	100	Protein >2.5 g/dL	<1.1
Massive hepatic metastases	Usually <500	Few or none	0	Protein variable	>1.1
Peritoneal carcinomatosis + massive hepatic metastases	Variable, usually elevated	Few or none	80	Protein variable	>1.1
Malignant chylous	Often >300	Few or none	0	Triglyceride >200 mg/dL	Usually <1.1
Hepatoma	Often >500	Commonly increased	0	—	>1.1

Cardiac Ascites

Cardiac ascites is an uncommon cause of ascites, accounting for only 5% of cases. From time to time, it may be difficult to differentiate cardiac ascites from cirrhotic ascites. It is important to make the distinction between these two causes of ascites because some patients with cardiac ascites (ie, constrictive pericarditis) can potentially be cured of their ascites with proper treatment. The following table highlights the differences between cardiac and cirrhotic ascites.

Comparison of Parameters Between Cardiac and Cirrhotic Ascites*

Laboratory Test	Cardiac Ascites	Cirrhotic Ascites	P Value
Ascitic fluid total protein (g/dL)	3.9 ±1.1	1.0 ±0.72	<0.01
Ascitic fluid LDH (mU/mL)	110 ±44	54 ±95	<0.02
Ascitic fluid WBC count (cells/mm^3)	481 ±492	288 ±312	NS
Ascitic fluid neutrophil count (cells/mm^3)	42 ±57	29 ±43	NS
Ascitic fluid red blood cell count (cells/mm^3)	2066 ±1653	498 ±832	<0.01
Serum total protein (g/dL)	7.2 ±1.3	6.3 ±1.1	<0.05
Serum-ascites albumin gradient (g/dL)	1.41 ±0.28	1.65 ±0.34	<0.02
Peripheral hematocrit (%)	42.4 ±5.2	32.0 ±8.6	<0.001

*Values are mean ±SD. NS = not significant.

Adapted from Runyon BA, "Cardiac Ascites," *J Clin Gastroenterol*, 1988, 10(4):411.

To summarize the above findings, cardiac ascites like cirrhotic ascites is characterized by a serum to ascites albumin gradient >1.1 g/dL. When compared to cirrhotic ascites, cardiac ascites has significantly higher levels of the following:

- Ascitic fluid total protein concentration
- Ascitic fluid LDH level
- Ascitic fluid red blood cell count
- Peripheral hematocrit

Tuberculous Peritonitis

Tuberculous peritonitis is usually an insidious disease. Most patients have symptoms for several weeks or months before they seek medical attention. The symptoms and signs of tuberculous peritonitis are listed in the following box.

TUBERCULOUS PERITONITIS SYMPTOMS AND SIGNS

SYMPTOMS
- Ascites (65% to 100%)
- Fever (54% to 100%)
- Abdominal pain (36% to 93%)
- Weight loss (37% to 87%)
- Diarrhea (9% to 27%)

SIGNS
- Ascites (51% to 100%)
- Abdominal tenderness (65% to 87%)

Routine testing of the ascitic fluid can provide support for the diagnosis of tuberculous ascites, as shown in the following box.

ASCITIC FLUID TEST RESULTS IN TUBERCULOUS PERITONITIS

SAAG
- Often <1.1 g/dL
- May be >1.1 g/dL with mixed ascites (eg, tuberculosis and cirrhosis together)

PROTEIN CONCENTRATION
- Usually >2.5-3.0 g/dL

WBC COUNT
- Usually 1.5-4.0 x 1000 /mm^3

WBC DIFFERENTIAL
- Usually lymphocytic predominance
- PMN predominance in early tuberculous peritonitis

Although the above test results provide support for the diagnosis of tuberculous peritonitis, the definitive diagnosis usually requires one or more of the following tests.

- Ascitic fluid acid-fast smear

  The acid-fast smear does not have a high yield in establishing the diagnosis of peritoneal tuberculosis. In one study, <3% of tuberculous peritonitis cases were diagnosed by acid-fast smear of the ascitic fluid.

- Ascitic fluid culture for *M. tuberculosis*

  Ascitic fluid culture has been found to have higher yield than ascitic fluid acid-fast smear. In several studies, culture allowed for the diagnosis of tuberculous peritonitis in nearly 20% of cases. One study reported a higher yield of about 66%. Nonetheless, a significant number of cases will escape detection if the clinician relies only on the ascitic fluid culture. Another drawback to the use of the culture is that results are not available for as long as 4-8 weeks.

- Adenosine deaminase (ADA) level

  An ADA level >33 units/L in the ascitic fluid has a sensitivity of 100% and a specificity of 95% in the diagnosis of tuberculous peritonitis. The major drawback with this test is its lack of availability in the United States.

- Laparoscopy with directed biopsy

  A presumptive diagnosis of tuberculous peritonitis can be made in 85% to 95% of patients using laparoscopy with directed biopsy. Antituberculous therapy can be started if the peritoneum has the classic "millet seed" or "violin string" appearance. Histology and cultures of the peritoneal biopsy should be performed. Histology can demonstrate caseating granulomas in approximately 90% of patients. Currently, laparoscopy with directed biopsy is the technique of choice in establishing the diagnosis of tuberculous peritonitis.

Ascitic Fluid Infection

The following box categorizes five major types of ascitic fluid infection.

CLASSIFICATION OF ASCITIC FLUID INFECTION
SPONTANEOUS BACTERIAL PERITONITIS* MONOMICROBIAL NON-NEUTROCYTIC BACTERASCITES† CULTURE-NEGATIVE NEUTROCYTIC ASCITES‡ SECONDARY BACTERIAL PERITONITIS# POLYMICROBIAL BACTERASCITES§

*The diagnosis of spontaneous bacterial peritonitis (SBP) can be established if the following criteria are met: Ascitic fluid PMN count >250 cells/mm^3; positive ascitic fluid culture; No evidence for intra-abdominal surgically treatable source of infection.

†Monomicrobial non-neutrocytic bacterascites is said to be present if the following criteria are met: Positive ascitic fluid culture for one organism; ascitic fluid PMN count <250 cells/mm^3; No evidence for intra-abdominal surgically treatable source of infection.

‡The diagnosis of culture-negative neutrocytic ascites is established if the following criteria are met: Ascitic fluid PMN count >250 cells/mm^3; ascitic fluid culture reveals no growth of a bacterial organism; no antibiotics have been administered; No other cause of an elevated PMN count can be identified.

#Criteria for diagnosis of secondary bacterial peritonitis include: Ascitic fluid PMN count >250 cells/mm^3; ascitic fluid culture is positive (often reveals growth of multiple organisms); an intra-abdominal surgically treatable source of infection has been identified (ie, perforated gut).

§To establish the diagnosis of polymicrobial bacterascites, the following criteria must be met: Ascitic fluid PMN count <250 cells/mm^3; multiple bacterial organisms are noted on ascitic fluid Gram stain or culture.

The presence of polymicrobial bacterascites is consistent with gut perforation caused by the paracentesis needle. It should be a consideration when the paracentesis procedure was traumatic, particularly difficult, or associated with the aspiration of stool or air into the paracentesis syringe.

SBP, monomicrobial non-neutrocytic bacterascites, and culture-negative neutrocytic ascites usually occur in the setting of chronic liver disease. While commonly associated with chronic liver disease, such as cirrhosis, these types of infected ascites may also occur in acute or subacute liver disease. They are rare causes of infected ascites in patients with noncirrhotic ascites.

These causes of infected ascites need to be differentiated from secondary bacterial peritonitis. In secondary bacterial peritonitis, there is an intra-abdominal source of infection. Although SBP is clearly a more common cause of infected ascites than secondary bacterial peritonitis, secondary bacterial peritonitis needs to be considered in every patient who presents with neutrocytic ascites. This is because the treatment of secondary bacterial peritonitis, in contrast to SBP, is surgical. Failure to make this diagnosis can have grave consequences for the patient.

It may seem intuitive to think that SBP and secondary bacterial peritonitis are easily distinguished from one another (ie, presence of peritoneal signs supports diagnosis of secondary bacterial peritonitis). In reality, studies have shown that the signs and symptoms of these two conditions are not sufficiently distinctive to allow for their discrimination. The signs and symptoms of SBP and secondary bacterial peritonitis are described in the following table.

Symptom or Sign	SBP	Secondary Bacterial Peritonitis
Fever	68	33
Abdominal pain	49	67
Tender abdomen	39	50
Rebound	10	17
Mental status	54	33

Adapted from *Sleisinger and Fordtran's Gastrointestinal and Liver Disease*, 6th ed, Feldman M, Scharschmidt BF, and Sleisinger MH, eds, Philadelphia, PA: WB Saunders Co, 1998, 1323.

Secondary bacterial peritonitis should be suspected in any patient with neutrocytic ascites who has two or more of the following criteria:

- Ascitic fluid total protein concentration >1 g/dL
- Ascitic fluid glucose level <50 mg/dL
- Ascitic fluid LDH > upper limit of normal for serum LDH

In addition, growth of multiple bacterial organisms should also prompt consideration of secondary bacterial peritonitis. Patients thought to have secondary bacterial peritonitis need urgent radiological investigation to confirm the diagnosis followed by surgical intervention. In contrast, patients with SBP are managed medically with antibiotic therapy alone.

In patients with SBP, the results of the culture are often not available at a time when antibiotic therapy needs to be started. In most cases, the decision to start antibiotic therapy is based upon the PMN count of the ascitic fluid. In general, patients who have an ascitic fluid PMN count ≥250/mm^3 should be assumed to have an ascitic fluid infection until proven otherwise. In these cases, it behooves the clinician to begin empirical antibiotic therapy.

Selection of a particular antibiotic should be based upon knowledge of the flora involved in ascitic fluid infection. The following table lists the bacterial organisms most commonly found in patients with SBP.

Flora of Spontaneous Bacterial Peritonitis (SBP)

Organism	SBP
E. coli	37
K. pneumoniae	17
Miscellaneous gram-positive	14
S. pneumococcus	12
Miscellaneous gram-negative	10
S. viridans	9
Polymicrobial	1

Adapted from *Sleisinger and Fordtran's Gastrointestinal and Liver Disease*, 6th ed, Feldman M, Scharschmidt BF, and Sleisinger MH, eds, Philadelphia, PA: WB Saunders Co, 1998, 1323.

Pancreatic Ascites

Pancreatic ascites may develop as a complication of one of the following:

- Severe acute pancreatitis
- Rupture of pancreatic duct in acute or chronic pancreatitis
- Leakage from pancreatic pseudocyst

An elevated ascitic fluid amylase level is consistent with pancreatic ascites. In some cases, levels may even exceed 2000 IU/L.

Nephrotic Syndrome

Nephrotic syndrome is an uncommon cause of ascites in adults. In studies examining these patients, investigators found that coexisting liver disease or congestive heart failure was frequently present. Therefore, in patients thought to have ascites secondary to nephrotic syndrome, every effort should be undertaken to search for these coexisting conditions.

Nephrogenous Ascites

Nephrogenous ascites develops in patients with end-stage renal disease on hemodialysis. Information regarding this cause of ascites is limited and the etiology remains unclear.

Chylous Ascites

Obstruction or damage to the lymphatic vessels can lead to the accumulation of chyle within the peritoneal cavity. It should be suspected when milky fluid is aspirated during paracentesis. Although there are a number of causes, the major causes of chylous ascites include cirrhosis, malignancy (lymphoma, solid tumors), infection, and surgery. Ascitic fluid triglyceride levels exceed 200 mg/dL in patients with chylous ascites.

References

Aalami OO, Allen DB, and Organ CH Jr "Chylous Ascites: A Collective Review," *Surgery*, 2000, 128(5):761-78.

Ahmad M and Ahmed A, "Tuberculous Peritonitis: Fatality Associated With Delayed Diagnosis," *South Med J*, 1999, 92(4):406-8.

Cardenas A and Chopra S, "Chylous Ascites," *Am J Gastroenterol*, 2002, 97(8):1896-900.

Dugurnier T, Laterre PF, and Reynaert MS, "Ascites Fluid in Severe Acute Pancreatitis: From Pathophysiology to Therapy," *Acta Gastroenterol Belg*, 2000, 63(3):264-8.

Fernandez J, Bauer TM, Navasa M, et al, "Diagnosis, Treatment and Prevention of Spontaneous Bacterial Peritonitis," *Baillieres Best Pract Res Clin Gastroenterol*, 2000, 14(6):975-90.

Guarner C and Soriano G, "Spontaneous Bacterial Peritonitis," *Semin Liver Dis*, 1997, 17(3):203-17.

Han SH, Reynolds TB, and Fong TL, "Nephrogenic Ascites. Analysis of 16 Cases and Review of the Literature," *Medicine (Baltimore)*, 1998, 77(4):233-45.

Johst P, Tsiotos GG, and Sarr MG, "Pancreatic Ascites: A Rare Complication of Necrotizing Pancreatitis. A Case Report and Review of the Literature," *Int J Pancreatol*, 1997, 22(2):151-4.

Laroche M and Harding G, "Primary and Secondary Peritonitis: An Update," *Eur J Clin Microbiol Infect Dis.*, 1998, 17(8):542-50.

Laterre PF, Dugurnier T, and Reynaert MS, "Chylous Ascites: Diagnosis, Causes and Treatment," *Acta Gastroenterol Belg*, 2000, 63(3):260-3.

McGuire BM and Bloomer JR, "Complications of Cirrhosis. Why They Occur and What to Do About Them," *Postgrad Med*, 1998, 103(2):209-12, 217-8, 223-4.

Parsons SL, Watson SA, and Steele RJ, "Malignant Ascites," *Br J Surg*, 1996, 83(1):6-14.

Rebuffoni G, Guadagni S, Somers DC, et al, "Peritoneal Carcinomatosis: Feature of Dissemination. A Review," *Tumori*, 1999, 85(1):1-5.

Rimola A, Garcia-Tsao G, Navasa M, et al, "Diagnosis, Treatment and Prophylaxis of Spontaneous Bacterial Peritonitis: A Consensus Document. International Ascites Club," *J Hepatol*, 2000, 32(1):142-53.

Uriz J, Cardenas A, and Arroyo V, "Pathophysiology, Diagnosis and Treatment of Ascites in Cirrhosis," *Baillieres Best Pract Res Clin Gastroenterol*, 2000, 14(6):927-43.

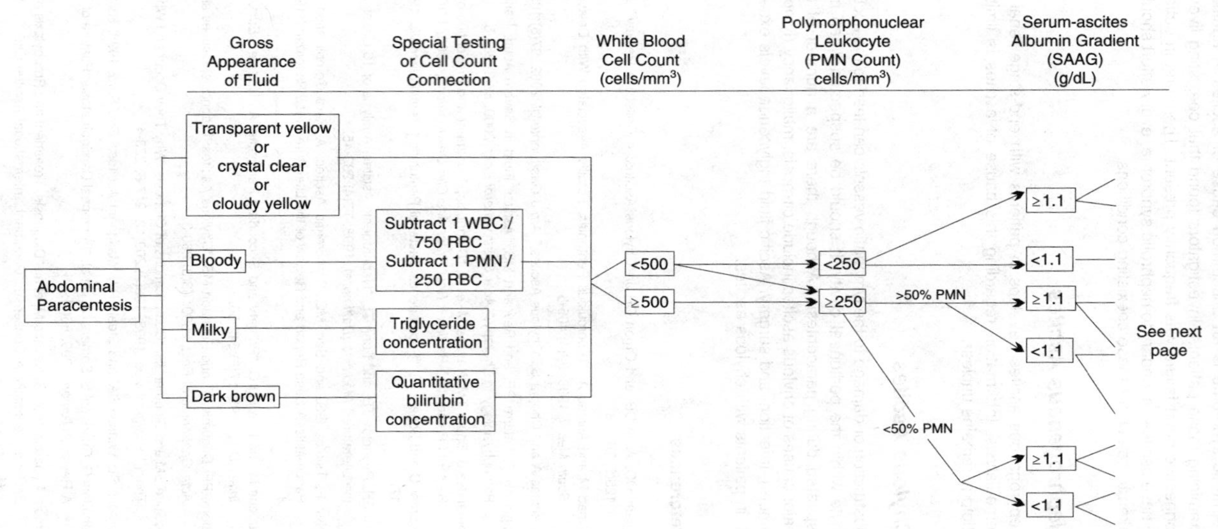
ASCITIC FLUID ANALYSIS
Gross Appearance of Fluid
Special Testing or Cell Count Connection
White Blood Cell Count (cells/mm³)
Polymorphonuclear Leukocyte (PMN Count) cells/mm³)
Serum-ascites Albumin Gradient (SAAG) (g/dL)
Abdominal Paracentesis
Transparent yellow or crystal clear or cloudy yellow
Bloody
Milky
Dark brown
Subtract 1 WBC / 750 RBC Subtract 1 PMN / 250 RBC
Triglyceride concentration
Quantitative bilirubin concentration
<500
≥500
<250
≥250
>50% PMN
<50% PMN
≥1.1
<1.1
≥1.1
<1.1
≥1.1
<1.1
See next page

ASCITIC FLUID ANALYSIS, *continued*

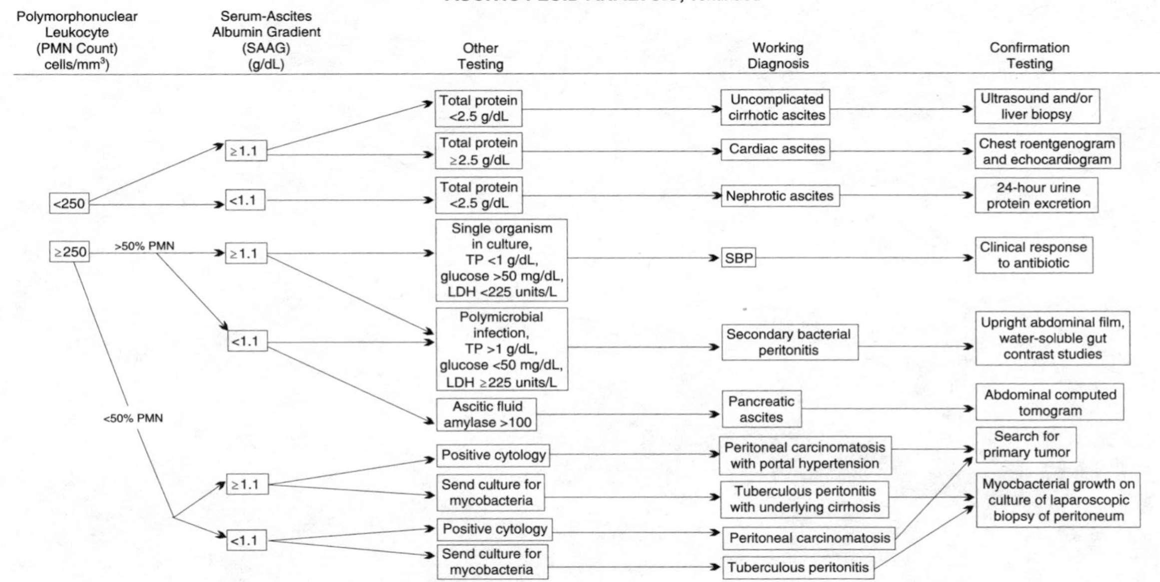

Adapted from Sleisenger and Fordtrans, *Gastrointesitnal and Liver Disease*, 6th ed, WB Saunders Co, 1998, 1314.

PART VIII:

RHEUMATOLOGY

ANTINUCLEAR ANTIBODIES (ANA)

Antinuclear antibodies, also known as ANAs, are commonly found in patients with connective tissue disease. When used together with the patient's clinical presentation, ANA testing is useful in the diagnosis and exclusion of connective tissue disease.

Reporting of the Test Results

Antinuclear antibodies are detected using indirect immunofluorescence testing. When human epithelial cells (Hep-2 cell line) are incubated with the patient's serum, antibody that is present in the serum will bind to cell nuclei. The antibody that binds can then be detected by the addition of fluorescent antihuman IgG. A positive test result may yield a number of different staining patterns. The four most common patterns are the homogenous, nucleolar, speckled, and centromere patterns. In the past, the type of fluorescence pattern present was thought to be indicative of a certain type of disease. In recent years, however, the use of the staining pattern has decreased in importance because it is now known that the fluorescent pattern is less sensitive and specific than autoantibody testing.

In addition to the fluorescent pattern, the titer (dilution at which nuclear fluorescence is no longer present) of the ANA will also be reported. In general, titers <1:40 are considered negative but some laboratories may report titers of 1:20 or 1:40 as being positive. Nevertheless, it is important to realize that patients with connective tissue disease rarely present with titers this low.

Although not recommended, at times, the ANA test is obtained in a patient with no signs and symptoms of connective tissue disease. If a positive test result is obtained, it can be difficult to determine the significance of the finding. It should be kept in mind that a positive ANA test result can be found in normal healthy individuals. In these cases, the titer can provide some guidance. Although higher titer values (>1:320), by itself, is not diagnostic of any autoimmune condition, such a finding should prompt a thorough evaluation to determine if the patient has an autoimmune disease. If the patient's clinical presentation is not compatible with an autoimmune disorder, then the patient should be assessed periodically for the development of one. Although a lower titer ANA (<1:80) is not as concerning in an asymptomatic patient, periodic follow-up is still necessary, but can be done less frequently.

Sensitivity of ANA Test for SLE

A positive ANA is present in almost all SLE patients (sensitivity approaches 100%). A negative test result should prompt consideration of other diseases that could account for the patient's clinical presentation.

Conditions Associated With Positive ANA Test

SLE is not the only condition that presents with a positive ANA test result. Other conditions associated with a positive ANA test result are listed in the following box.

CONDITIONS ASSOCIATED WITH A POSITIVE ANA TEST	
CONNECTIVE TISSUE DISEASE	
SLE	Scleroderma
Drug-induced lupus	Mixed connective tissue disease
Discoid lupus	Sjögren's syndrome
Rheumatoid arthritis	Polymyositis / dermatomyositis

(continued)

CONDITIONS ASSOCIATED WITH A POSITIVE ANA TEST *(continued)*	
INFECTION	DIABETES MELLITUS (type I)
Subacute bacterial endocarditis	MULTIPLE SCLEROSIS
HIV	HEALTHY INDIVIDUALS*
Infectious mononucleosis	ADVANCING AGE*
Hepatitis C	PREGNANCY
PULMONARY DISEASE	SILICONE GEL IMPLANTS
Pulmonary fibrosis	MEDICATIONS
Primary pulmonary hypertension	THYROID DISEASE
MALIGNANCY	Hashimoto's thyroiditis
LIVER DISEASE	Graves' disease
Autoimmune hepatitis	
Primary biliary cirrhosis	

*A positive ANA test result can occur in normal healthy individuals. The prevalence of a positive test result increases with advancing age. Women more commonly have positive results as well. In contrast to patients with connective tissue disease, ANAs in normal healthy persons are usually of low titer. In a study of 125 normal healthy individuals, only 3% had an ANA titer above 1:320. However, an ANA titer > 1:40 was noted in 32%.

The specificity of a positive ANA for SLE or a related condition increases with rising titers. In fact, a titer of 1:320 has a specificity of about 97% of the diagnosis of SLE or a related condition.

ANA Profile

A positive ANA test result should be followed with ANA profile, which will determine the type of antibodies present. The clinical significance of some of the more common autoantibodies is listed in the following table.

Clinical Significance of Specific Autoantibodies

Autoantibody	Clinical Significance
Antibodies to double-stranded DNA	Highly specific for SLE 40% to 60% prevalence Titers fluctuate with disease activity Correlation with renal disease recognized
Antibody to Smith antigen	Highly specific for SLE Positive in only 25% Not useful for management of SLE
Antibodies to histones	Found in 70% of SLE patients Positive in drug-induced lupus Can also be found in patients with other connective tissue diseases
Antibodies to U1-RNP	Present in mixed connective tissue disease
Antibodies to ribosomal P	Associated with psychosis and depression in SLE
Antibodies to Scl-70 (topoisomerase I)	Common in systemic sclerosis
Anticentromere antibodies	Commonly found in CREST syndrome
Antibodies to Ro (SSA)	Associated with Sjögren's syndrome, subacute cutaneous lupus, neonatal lupus, photosensitivity, and complement deficiencies
Antibodies to La (SSB)	Associated with Sjögren's syndrome, subacute cutaneous lupus, and neonatal lupus
Antibodies to single-stranded DNA	Frequently detected in SLE but not specific for SLE Can be found in other connective tissue disease

References

Kavanaugh A, Tomar R, Reveille J, et al, "Guidelines for Clinical Use of the Antinuclear Antibody Test and Tests for Specific Autoantibodies to Nuclear Antigens. American College of Pathologists," *Arch Pathol Lab Med*, 2000, 124(1):71-81.

Keren DF, "Antinuclear Antibody Testing," *Clin Lab Med*, 2002, 22(2):447-74.

Tozzoli R, Bizzaro N, Tonutti E, et al, "Guidelines for the Laboratory Use of Autoantibody Tests in the Diagnosis and Monitoring of Autoimmune Rheumatic Diseases," *Am J Clin Pathol*, 2002, 117(2):316-24.

Wanchu A, "Antinuclear Antibodies Clinical Applications," *J Postgrad Med*, 2000, 46(2):144-8.

RHEUMATOID FACTOR

Rheumatoid factor is an IgM antibody that is directed against the Fc portion of IgG. It is often obtained in the evaluation of patients suspected of having rheumatoid arthritis. In fact, a positive rheumatoid factor test is one of the criteria for the diagnosis of rheumatoid arthritis.

Sensitivity of Rheumatoid Factor for Rheumatoid Arthritis

Approximately 80% of rheumatoid arthritis patients are found to have a positive rheumatoid factor test result. It is important to realize that a negative test result does not exclude the diagnosis since about 20% of patients are seronegative. Seronegativity is more common early in the disease course (up to 40%). Herein lies the importance of understanding that a positive rheumatoid factor test result is just one of seven criteria established by the American College of Rheumatology for the diagnosis of rheumatoid arthritis. To establish the diagnosis, at least 4 of the seven criteria must be present. It is apparent that a diagnosis can be made even when the test is negative.

Specificity of Rheumatoid Factor for Rheumatoid Arthritis

The rheumatoid factor test may be positive in patients with other types of connective tissue disease. In addition, there are many other illnesses (nonrheumatic) in which a positive rheumatoid factor may be found. Conditions associated with a positive rheumatoid factor test result are listed in the following box.

DISEASES ASSOCIATED WITH A POSITIVE RHEUMATOID FACTOR TEST RESULT

CONNECTIVE TISSUE DISEASE
- Rheumatoid arthritis
- SLE
- Scleroderma
- Sjögren's syndrome
- Mixed connective tissue disease
- Cryoglobulinemia

INFECTION
- Bacterial endocarditis
- Syphilis
- Tuberculosis
- Viral (mumps, rubella, influenza)
- Parasitic

PULMONARY DISEASE
- Sarcoidosis
- Asbestosis
- Parasites
- Silicosis
- Interstitial pulmonary fibrosis

ADVANCING AGE*

MALIGNANCY (hematologic and solid)

PRIMARY BILIARY CIRRHOSIS

LIVER DISEASE (chronic)

*Low titers of rheumatoid factor are found in 3% of the general population. The prevalence of rheumatoid factor positivity increases with age. In fact, up to 20% of patients over the age of 65 years have a positive test result. In healthy elderly patients who have a positive test result, the titer is typically ≤1:40.

The specificity of a positive rheumatoid factor test result for the diagnosis of rheumatoid arthritis increases with higher titers.

Use of Rheumatoid Factor to Monitor Disease Activity

The rheumatoid factor cannot be used to monitor disease activity in rheumatoid arthritis patients. It is not useful for following disease progression. However, the disease tends to be more severe when patients are seropositive. Higher titers are associated with an increased risk of developing extra-articular manifestations of the disease. Once a patient with rheumatoid arthritis is known to be positive for rheumatoid factor, there is no use in repeating the test.

References

Newkirk MM , "Rheumatoid Factors: What Do They Tell Us?" *J Rheumatol*, 2002, 29(10):2034-40 (review).

ANTINEUTROPHIL CYTOPLASMIC ANTIBODIES (ANCA)

It can be challenging to distinguish vasculitis from other conditions that present similarly. In addition, differentiating among the various types of vasculitis can be equally daunting. In the 1980s, testing for antineutrophil cytoplasmic antibodies, or ANCA, became available and has proven to be useful in the diagnosis of vasculitis.

Types of ANCA

Using indirect immunofluorescence, two types of ANCA can be identified based upon the staining pattern. When the staining pattern is cytoplasmic, c-ANCA is said to be present. These antibodies are directed against the antigen, proteinase 3 (PR3). Perinuclear staining is consistent with the presence of p-ANCA, an autoantibody directed against myeloperoxidase (MPO). In recent years, antigen-specific immunochemical assays have begun to supplant indirect immunofluorescence ANCA testing. Using these assays, the terms, c-ANCA and p-ANCA, are replaced by proteinase 3-ANCA (PR3-ANCA) and myeloperoxidase-ANCA (MPO-ANCA), respectively.

Clinical Significance of ANCA

ANCA positivity, in and of itself, is not diagnostic for any type of vasculitis. However, a positive test result in the proper clinical context can help support the diagnosis. Further workup can then be pursued to confirm the suspected diagnosis.

C-ANCA testing is very sensitive for the diagnosis of Wegener's granulomatosis. The sensitivity, however, does vary depending upon the activity of the disease. In active, systemic disease, the sensitivity is reported to be 90% to 95%. This percentage falls to 60% to 65% in patients with organ-limited disease. The sensitivity is even less in those who are in remission (40%). The specificity of c-ANCA is about 90%. Some cases of microscopic polyangiitis and Churg-Strauss syndrome may be associated with the presence of c-ANCA but these diseases more commonly present with p-ANCA positivity. Despite the fact that c-ANCA may be positive in other diseases, a positive c-ANCA, in a patient who is presenting with classic symptoms and signs of Wegener's granulomatosis, may obviate biopsy.

Although p-ANCA is present in 66% and 75% of Churg-Strauss syndrome and microscopic polyangiitis patients, respectively, the test is neither sensitive nor specific enough to establish the diagnosis with confidence. At best, a positive test result can be considered supportive of the diagnosis if the patient has a clinical presentation consistent with one of these diseases. Confirmation of the diagnosis is recommended, often with biopsy. The test may also be positive in Wegener's granulomatosis, pauci-immune glomerulonephritis, rheumatoid arthritis, SLE, Goodpasture's syndrome, ulcerative colitis, autoimmune hepatitis, and other diseases.

Using ANCA to Assess Disease Activity

Although some patients with Wegener's granulomatosis patients have a rise in ANCA titer corresponding to a disease exacerbation or relapse, there are many others in whom a correlation between titer and disease activity cannot be found. At times, a rise in the titer may precede the onset of disease exacerbation. In these cases, experts would agree that treatment should not be started simply because the ANCA titer increases. Instead, this finding should prompt the clinician to assess the patient carefully for any signs and symptoms of active disease. In addition, most would agree that frequent monitoring would be indicated in such a patient.

With treatment that is successful, the ANCA titer often decreases. However, this is not true for every patient. It is recommended that a titer be obtained before starting therapy and then measured again periodically to determine if the patient is one in whom titers decrease with treatment. If so, then serial titer monitoring may be of use in the management of future exacerbations.

References

Bartunkova J, Tesar V, and Sediva A, "Diagnostic and Pathogenetic Role of Antineutrophil Cytoplasmic Autoantibodies," *Clin Immunol*, 2003, 106(2):73-82.

Kamesh L, Harper L, and Savage CO, "ANCA-Positive Vasculitis," *J Am Soc Nephrol*, 2002, 13(7):1953-60.

Langford CA, "Vasculitis," *J Allergy Clin Immunol*, 2003, 111(2 Suppl):S602-12.

Wilk A, "Rational Use of ANCA in the Diagnosis of Vasculitis," *Rheumatology (Oxford)*, 2002, 41(5):481-3.

ERYTHROCYTE SEDIMENTATION RATE (ESR)

The erythrocyte sedimentation rate or ESR is an acute phase reactant. Acute phase reactants are a group of proteins whose synthesis increases considerably in response to acute or chronic inflammation. The ESR is a measure of the distance in millimeters red blood cells settle within a specified tube over 1 hour. The Westergren tube is most often used.

Reference Range

For men and women <50 years of age, the upper limit of normal is 15 mm/hour and 20 mm/hour, respectively. The upper limit of normal increases to 20 mm/hour and 30 mm/hour in men and women, respectively, over the age of 50.

Factors That May Increase the ESR

Factors that may increase the ESR are listed in the following box.

FACTORS THAT MAY INCREASE THE ESR	
OLD AGE	MACROCYTOSIS
FEMALE GENDER	INCREASED PLASMA PROTEINS*
ANEMIA	TECHNICAL PROBLEMS
PREGNANCY	

*Seen with infection, inflammation, and malignancy

Although an elevated ESR is never diagnostic of a particular disease, it is often used in the evaluation and detection of inflammatory illnesses. It has an important role in the diagnosis of temporal arteritis and polymyalgia rheumatica. Patients with these disorders commonly have a significantly elevated ESR. In fact, the sensitivity of an elevated ESR is 80% and 95% for the diagnoses of polymyalgia rheumatica and temporal arteritis, respectively. Normal ESR levels should prompt consideration of alternative diagnoses. However, it is important to realize that some patients with these conditions may present with normal values. Therefore, a normal ESR does not exclude the presence of an inflammatory illness.

Factors That May Decrease the ESR

Factors that may decrease the ESR are listed in the following box.

FACTORS THAT MAY DECREASE THE ESR
POLYCYTHEMIA
MEDICATIONS (steroids, other anti-inflammatory drugs)
MICROCYTOSIS
SICKLE CELL DISEASE
SPHEROCYTOSIS
ACANTHOCYTOSIS
DECREASED PLASMA PROTEINS
Hypogammaglobulinemia
Hypofibrinogenemia
DYSPROTEINEMIA WITH HYPERVISCOSITY STATE
TECHNICAL PROBLEMS

Using the ESR to Monitor Clinical Activity of Disease

The ESR is also widely used in monitoring the clinical activity of connective tissue disease, especially rheumatoid arthritis. It also has a role in the management of temporal arteritis and polymyalgia rheumatica. In these conditions, it is used along with the patient's signs and symptoms to assess response to therapy.

References

Ng T, "Erythrocyte Sedimentation Rate, Plasma Viscosity and C-Reactive Protein in Clinical Practice," *Br J Hosp Med*, 1997, 58(10):521-3.

Saadeh C, "The Erythrocyte Sedimentation Rate: Old and New Clinical Applications," *South Med J*, 1998, 91(3):220-5.

Smith EM and Samadian S, "Use of the Erythrocyte Sedimentation Rate in the Elderly," *Br J Hosp Med*, 1994, 51(8):394-7.

SYNOVIAL FLUID ANALYSIS

Indications for Arthrocentesis

There are many clinicians who are advocates of arthrocentesis in all patients with joint disease. Although synovial fluid analysis is only diagnostic of a few conditions, it often provides important information that is impossible to know otherwise. Synovial fluid analysis, for example, can differentiate between inflammatory and noninflammatory types of arthritis. In some patients, more than one type of arthritis may be present. Quite often, these diagnoses cannot be made without analysis of the joint fluid. In joints that are significantly inflamed, especially if the clinical presentation is acute, there is concern that the patient may have septic arthritis. To make a definitive diagnosis, arthrocentesis is required. The same holds true for crystal-induced arthritis such as gout or pseudogout. In general, synovial fluid analysis is indicated when the etiology of joint symptoms is unclear.

There are also therapeutic reasons to perform arthrocentesis. For example, in patients with septic arthritis, treatment often includes removal of the inflammatory mediators present in the joint fluid. Patients may be very symptomatic with joint effusions that are tense and relief of pressure with arthrocentesis can result in amelioration of symptoms.

Routine Testing of the Synovial Fluid

While a number of synovial fluid tests may be obtained, tests that should be routinely ordered are listed in the following box.

ROUTINE LABORATORY TESTING OF THE SYNOVIAL FLUID	
WHITE BLOOD CELL COUNT	BACTERIAL CULTURE
WHITE BLOOD CELL COUNT DIFFERENTIAL	POLARIZED MICROSCOPY FOR CRYSTALS
GRAM STAIN	

Gross Appearance

Normally, synovial fluid is colorless and clear. Not uncommonly, it is yellow, especially in patients with arthritis. The yellow color is due to the presence of xanthochromia. The aspiration of bloody fluid may be due to trauma (previous joint trauma, traumatic tap) or to a number of different pathologic disorders.

DIFFERENTIAL DIAGNOSIS OF BLOODY SYNOVIAL FLUID	
TRAUMA	SICKLE CELL DISEASE
TRAUMATIC TAP	SCURVY
HEMANGIOMA OR AV MALFORMATIONS	PSEUDOXANTHOMA ELASTICUM
	EHLERS-DANLOS SYNDROME
MALIGNANCY (primary or metastatic)	TUBERCULOSIS
PIGMENTED VILLONODULAR SYNOVITIS	COAGULATION DISORDERS
	Hemophilia
CHARCOT'S JOINT	von Willebrand's Disease
THROMBOCYTOPENIA	Others
ESSENTIAL THROMBOCYTOSIS	ANTICOAGULATION THERAPY

Traumatic aspiration is likely when the aspiration of the blood is not homogenous.

Clarity

The clarity of the synovial fluid is a reflection of the amount of particles in the fluid (ie, density). Being able to read newsprint through a tube of synovial fluid is a characteristic of normal synovial fluid. With opacification of the fluid, it may be difficult to impossible to read newsprint in the manner described. Although a number of substances (lipids, debris commonly present in destructive forms of arthritis, crystals) can opacify synovial fluid, opacification is more commonly caused by the presence of increased numbers of white blood cells.

White Blood Cell Count and Differential

The synovial fluid white blood cell count and differential are two very useful tests to obtain. Because the cells can degenerate as early as one hour after arthrocentesis, it is recommended that testing be performed expeditiously. The upper limit of normal for the synovial fluid white blood cell count is 200 cells/mm^3. The synovial fluid can be categorized into different groups based on the degree of white blood cell elevation (see below). For example, the count can be used to distinguish between inflammatory and noninflammatory arthritis. Synovial fluid white blood cell counts between 200-2000/mm^3 are consistent with a noninflammatory process. It should be understood, however, that some systemic inflammatory conditions, such as SLE, often fall into the noninflammatory category.

Noninfectious inflammatory processes typically present with a synovial fluid white blood cell count between 2000-100,000 cells/mm^3. Crystal-induced arthritis is usually characterized by counts exceeding 30,000 cells/mm^3. As the synovial fluid white blood cell count approaches 100,000 cells/mm^3, the chance of an infectious etiology increases. With counts >100,000 cells/mm^3, a bacterial infection (ie, septic arthritis) should be considered to be present until proven otherwise. The finding of crystals by polarized microscopy should not eliminate the consideration of bacterial infection because the two can coexist. In this group of patients, empiric antibiotic therapy should be started while waiting for the results of microbiology studies. Rarely, this degree of elevation may be encountered in patients with crystal-induced arthritis or rheumatoid arthritis. A count <100,000 cells/mm^3 does not exclude the possibility of septic arthritis. This is particularly true in patients who are immunocompromised by their underlying disease or because of therapy with immunosuppressive or cytotoxic agents (ie, methotrexate, cyclosporine, cyclophosphamide). Partially treated infections may also present with lower synovial fluid white blood cell counts. It is important to realize that nonbacterial infections (viral, fungal, mycobacterial) often present with counts <100,000 cell/mm^3.

The white blood cell count differential is also useful in patients suspected of having septic arthritis. The PMN percentage typically exceeds 95%. However, other acute inflammatory processes may also be characterized by a PMN predominance.

Categorization of Synovial Fluid Based on Synovial Fluid Characteristics

	Class I (Noninflammatory)	Class II (Inflammatory)	Class III (Septic Arthritis)	Class IV (Hemorrhagic)
Color	Clear/yellow	Yellow/white	Yellow/white	Red
Clarity	Transparent	Translucent/ opaque	Opaque	Opaque
Viscosity	High	Variable	Low	Not applicable
Mucin clot	Firm	Variable	Friable	Not applicable
WBC count	200-2000/mm^3	2000-100,000/ mm^3	>100,000/mm^3	Not applicable

Categorization of Synovial Fluid
Based on Synovial Fluid Characteristics *(continued)*

	Class I (Noninflammatory)	Class II (Inflammatory)	Class III (Septic Arthritis)	Class IV (Hemorrhagic)
WBC differential	<25% PMN	>50% PMN	>95% PMN	Not applicable
Culture	Negative	Negative	Positive	Variable

Adapted from Klippel JH, Crofford LJ, and Stone JH, *Primer on Rheumatic Diseases*, National Book Network, Edition 12, 2001, 142.

Types of Synovial Fluid and Associated Conditions

Class I	Class II	Class III	Class IV
Osteoarthritis Osteonecrosis Traumatic arthritis Charcot's joint Pigmented villonodular synovitis Ochronosis Acromegaly Hyperparathyroidism	Rheumatoid arthritis Polymyositis Dermatomyositis Scleroderma SLE Vasculitis Seronegative spondyloarthropathies Psoriatic arthritis Reactive arthritis Juvenile rheumatoid arthritis Hydroxyapatite disease Gout Calcium pyrophosphate dihydrate disease Sarcoidosis Rheumatic fever Infection Viral Fungal Tuberculosis Lyme disease Whipple's disease Polychondritis Inflammatory bowel disease	Bacterial infection	See causes of bloody synovial fluid in the table above

Crystals

A diagnosis of crystal-induced arthritis can be made when characteristic intracellular crystals are noted with polarized microscopy.

Disease	Crystal	Description
Gout	Monosodium urate	Needle shaped Strongly negative birefringence
Pseudogout	Calcium pyrophosphate dihydrate	Rhomboid-shaped Weakly positive birefringence
Hydroxyapatite arthropathy*	Hydroxyapatite	Very small Not birefringent

*Hydroxyapatite crystals are usually too small to be appreciated under polarized light and can only be seen by electron microscopy.

Although patients with crystal-induced arthritis may have impressive elevations of the synovial fluid white blood cell count, infection must be excluded, even if crystals are demonstrated by polarized microscopy. It is not uncommon for the two diseases to coexist. It is also common for two different crystal-induced arthritides to be present in the same patient. In fact, 15% of gout patients also have calcium pyrophosphate deposition disease.

Culture

In patients with a clinical presentation consistent with septic arthritis, Gram stain and bacterial culture are clearly indicated. Because septic arthritis can lead to rapid destruction of joints, empiric antibiotic therapy should not be delayed while waiting for culture results. A negative Gram stain and culture do not exclude the presence of bacterial infection. Result may be negative if treatment was started before synovial fluid aspiration. Culture positivity also depends on the type of bacteria that is causing the infection. For example, cultures are negative in over 66% of patients with gonococcal arthritis. In these patients, it is important to culture other sites of infection such as the genitourinary tract. Other common bacterial causes of joint infection include staphylococcal and streptococcal species. Gram-negative organisms are less common but deserve consideration in immunocompromised or hospitalized patients as well as those who use intravenous drugs.

If the clinical presentation is consistent with tuberculous arthritis, an acid-fast stain and mycobacterial culture are indicated. The clinician should realize that the sensitivity of the acid-fast stain is only 20%. Cultures have a higher yield but it often takes considerable time for results to return. Not uncommonly, a synovial biopsy is necessary to establish the diagnosis. If tuberculosis is a consideration, then fungal arthritis needs to be considered in the differential diagnosis. Fungal cultures should be obtained but again, the diagnosis is often established only by histology and cultures of synovial tissue obtained at the time of biopsy.

Chemistry

In the past, glucose and protein were routinely ordered but are no longer recommended.

Synovial Fluid Biopsy

Synovial fluid biopsy may be needed to establish the diagnosis of certain types of infection, such as tuberculosis or fungal infection. Although special stains and cultures should be obtained if suspected, quite often, the results are unrevealing and the diagnosis is made only after tissue is obtained for histology and microbiology studies. A biopsy is also necessary in patients suspected of having malignancy (primary or metastatic). In these patients, the diagnosis is confirmed if malignant cells are noted in the synovial tissue. Other conditions that may be diagnosed with biopsy include amyloid arthropathy (apple-green birefringence in Congo-red stained synovial tissue), Whipple's disease (foamy macrophages containing PAS-positive material), and pigmented villonodular synovitis.

References

Dougados M, "Synovial Fluid Cell Analysis," *Baillieres Clin Rheumatol*, 1996, 10(3):519-34.

Joseph J and McGrath H, "Gout or Pseudogout: How to Differentiate Crystal-Induced Arthropathies," *Geriatrics.*, 1995, 50(4):33-9.

Ma DT and Carroll GJ, "Monoarthropathy, Could This Be Infection?" *Aust Fam Physician*, 1998, 27(1-2):28-31.

Sack K, "Monoarthritis: Differential Diagnosis," *Am J Med*, 1997, 102(1A):30S-34S.

Shmerling RH, "Synovial Fluid Analysis. A Critical Reappraisal," *Rheum Dis Clin North Am*, 1994, 20(2):503-12.

Shmerling RH, Delbanco TL, Tosteson AN, et al, "Synovial Fluid Tests. What Should Be Ordered?" *JAMA*, 1990, 264(8):1009-14.

Siva C, Velazquez C, Mody A, et al, "Diagnosing Acute Monoarthritis in Adults: A Practical Approach for the Family Physician," *Am Fam Physician*, 2003, 68(10:83-90.

Swan A, Amer H, and Dieppe P, "The Value of Synovial Fluid Assays in the Diagnosis of Joint Disease: A Literature Survey," *Ann Rheum Dis*, 2002, 61(6):493-8.

SYSTEMIC LUPUS ERYTHEMATOSUS (SLE)

The diagnosis of SLE is a clinical one. To aid clinicians in establishing the diagnosis, the American College of Rheumatology has proposed diagnostic criteria. A diagnosis of SLE is established if the patient has four or more of the eleven criteria listed in the box below. The sensitivity and specificity of the criteria are 96%.

DIAGNOSTIC CRITERIA FOR SLE
MALAR RASH
DISCOID RASH
PHOTOSENSITIVITY
ORAL ULCERS
ARTHRITIS
SEROSITIS
RENAL DISEASE
>0.5 g/dL of protein or >3 + dipstick proteinuria or cellular casts (red cell, granular, tubular, mixed)
NEUROLOGIC DISEASE
Seizures or psychosis*
HEMATOLOGIC DISORDER
Hemolytic anemia or decreased WBC count (<4000 cells/mm^3) or decreased lymphocytes (<1500 cells/mm^3)† or decreased platelets (<100,000 cells/mm^3)‡
IMMUNOLOGIC ABNORMALITY
Positive LE cell preparation or elevated anti-ds-DNA or elevated anti-Sm or false-positive serologic test for syphilis§
POSITIVE ANTINUCLEAR ANTIBODY#

*Seizures or psychosis cannot be drug-induced or due to a metabolic abnormality.

†On 2 or more occasions.

‡In the absence of offending drugs.

§Test must be positive for at least 6 months and must be confirmed by performing the *Treponema pallidum* immobilization or fluorescent treponemal antibody absorption test (FTA-ABS).

#In the absence of drugs known to be associated with drug-induced lupus.

Adapted from Tan EM, Cohen AS, Fries JF, et al, "The 1982 Revised Criteria for the Classification of Systemic Lupus Erythematosus," *Arthritis Rheum*, 1982, 25(11):1271-7.

These criteria were first developed to differentiate SLE from other autoimmune diseases. As a result, many of the signs and symptoms of SLE shared in common with other autoimmune diseases are not included. In addition, the criteria were developed in 1982 and while the LE cell preparation was not uncommon then, it is rarely performed today. Finally, because the sensitivity and specificity are just above 95%, there are some patients with SLE who will not have four or more criteria. Conversely, there are some patients who fulfill the criteria for SLE, but actually have another disease.

Antinuclear Antibodies (ANA) in SLE

More than 99% of patients with SLE have positive antinuclear antibodies. However, it is important to recognize that antinuclear antibodies may be present in other disease states, as well as in normal patients. Therefore, a positive ANA test is very sensitive, but not specific for the diagnosis of SLE. In fact, positive antinuclear antibodies have been found in 68%, 40% to 75%, and 25% to 50% of patients with Sjögren's syndrome, scleroderma, and rheumatoid arthritis, respectively. It is said that a fluorescent ANA test is so sensitive for the diagnosis of SLE that a negative test result essentially excludes the diagnosis.

Higher ANA titers lend more support to the diagnosis of SLE. Titers > 1:160 are considered to be significant and almost all SLE patients will present with such a titer. There is no need to repeat a positive ANA test, because the ANA titer does not change with disease activity.

A positive ANA test in a patient suspected of having SLE should be followed with an ANA profile. The ANA profile will identify the particular autoantibodies that are present. Although many different autoantibodies have been appreciated in SLE patients, autoantibodies that are most specific for the diagnosis include antidouble-stranded DNA (anti-ds-DNA) and anti-Smith antibodies (anti-Sm). Although the specificity of anti-ds-DNA for SLE is 95%, these antibodies have been found in patients with Sjögren's syndrome, rheumatoid arthritis, mixed connective tissue disease, scleroderma, Grave's disease, discoid lupus, autoimmune hepatitis, and Raynaud's phenomenon. Medications that have been associated with anti-ds-DNA include penicillamine, etanercept, and minocycline. The absence of anti-ds-DNA antibodies does not exclude the diagnosis of SLE since 50% of patients do not have these antibodies. Anti-Sm antibodies, which are also highly specific for SLE, are present in 10% to 40% of SLE patients.

There are associations between certain autoantibodies and specific SLE manifestations, as shown in the table below.

Autoantibodies Associated With Certain SLE Manifestations

Type of Autoantibody	Associated SLE Manifestation
Anti-ds-DNA	Lupus nephritis
Anti-Smith	Lupus nephritis CNS disease
Anti-RNP	Raynaud's phenomenon Myositis Less severe form of SLE
Anti-RA 33	Erosive arthritis
Anti-ribosomal P protein	Psychosis
Anti-La (SSB)	Sjögren's syndrome Neonatal lupus
Anti-Ro (SSA)	Sjögren's syndrome Lymphopenia Photosensitivity Subacute cutaneous lupus Neonatal lupus

Hematologic Disease in SLE

Leukopenia has been reported in >50% of patients with SLE and may be characterized by lymphopenia or granulocytopenia. The white blood cell count usually ranges between 2500-4000 cells/mm^3. Rarely does it fall to <1500 cells/mm^3. Patients are not usually symptomatic unless the counts are severely depressed. Although leukopenia is the classic finding, leukocytosis can also occur due to a disease flare, infection, or corticosteroid therapy. A left shift should prompt a search for infection.

Approximately 70% of SLE patients have the anemia of chronic disease. In these patients, the anemia is typically mild in severity. Less than 10% have autoimmune hemolytic anemia, despite the fact that the percentage of SLE patients with a positive direct Coombs' test is between 20% and 60%. Therefore, merely discovering a positive direct Coombs' test in this population does not confirm the diagnosis of hemolytic anemia. Anemia in SLE may also occur due to renal insufficiency (lupus nephritis). These patients are also prone to the development of iron deficiency anemia (gastrointestinal blood loss) secondary to chronic NSAID use. A thrombotic microangiopathic hemolytic anemia can occur in SLE patients. It may present with the manifestations of TTP or the hemolytic-uremic syndrome.

Although thrombocytopenia is appreciated in about 40% of patients, only 10% of patients have platelet counts <10,000/microliter. The decrease in the platelet count may be secondary to antiplatelet antibodies or because of antiphospholipid antibodies. Other causes include bone marrow suppression due to the use of immunosuppressive medications and thrombotic microangiopathy.

Pulmonary Disease in SLE

Pulmonary manifestations of SLE include acute pneumonitis, chronic pneumonitis, pulmonary hypertension, vanishing lung syndrome, pulmonary hemorrhage, bronchiolitis obliterans with organizing pneumonia, and lupus pleuritis. The pleural effusion of lupus pleuritis is exudative and is characterized by the presence of low complement levels. Low complement levels may also be seen with rheumatoid arthritis effusions. Traditionally, an increased pleural fluid ANA titer has been said to be very supportive of the diagnosis. Recently, however, it has been realized that the ANA is not sensitive or specific for the diagnosis of lupus pleuritis. Therefore, the diagnosis is now based on a compatible clinical presentation and supported by serum ANA testing.

Renal Disease in SLE

Renal disease due to SLE, or lupus nephritis, occurs in approximately 40% of SLE patients. The World Health Organization has established a classification system for patients with lupus nephritis based on histologic findings.

WHO CLASSIFICATION SYSTEM FOR LUPUS NEPHRITIS
Class I - Normal biopsy Class II - Mesangial lupus nephritis Class III - Focal proliferative lupus nephritis Class IV - Diffuse proliferative lupus nephritis Class V - Membranous lupus nephritis Class VI - Sclerosing

Many patients with lupus nephritis are asymptomatic at the time of diagnosis. In these patients, abnormalities detected on a urinalysis may bring the disease to clinical attention. In fact, once a diagnosis of SLE has been established, a urinalysis should be obtained periodically to assess for the development of lupus nephritis. At the time of SLE diagnosis, 50% of patients have urinalysis abnormalities (proteinuria, hematuria, pyuria). Symptoms and signs that suggest the presence of renal disease include edema and hypertension. Uremic signs and symptoms may be present if the patient presents with very advanced disease. The clinical manifestations of the different types of lupus nephritis are listed in the table below.

Clinical Manifestations of the Different Types of Lupus Nephritis

Type of Lupus Nephritis	Clinical Manifestations
Mesangial	Seen in 10% to 20% of lupus nephritis patients Microscopic hematuria and/or proteinuria may be present (mild) Hypertension uncommon Renal function is normal Nephrotic syndrome very unusual
Focal proliferative	Seen in 10% to 20% of lupus nephritis patients Hematuria and proteinuria in almost all patients Some may have the nephrotic syndrome Hypertension not uncommon Some have an elevated serum creatinine level

Clinical Manifestations of the Different Types of Lupus Nephritis *(continued)*

Type of Lupus Nephritis	Clinical Manifestations
Diffuse proliferative	Most common type of lupus nephritis Most severe form of lupus nephritis Hematuria and proteinuria in all patients Nephrotic syndrome commonly present Hypertension commonly present Renal insufficiency common Hypocomplementemia usually present Anti-ds-DNA antibodies usually present
Membranous	Seen in 10% to 20% of lupus nephritis patients Proteinuria in all patients Nephrotic syndrome common Microscopic hematuria may be present Hypertension may be present Serum creatinine usually normal but may be mildly increased

In addition to the glomerulopathies described above, renal insufficiency in SLE can also be due to tubulointerstitial disease. This type of renal disease should be suspected when a SLE patient presents with an unremarkable urinalysis or one that is minimally remarkable (few RBCs or WBCs). Another clue is the presence of metabolic acidosis due to renal tubular acidosis. Other causes of renal insufficiency in SLE patients include NSAID use, vasculitis, and thrombotic microangiopathy.

Although the clinical manifestations and laboratory testing may provide clues to the type of lupus nephritis present, the definitive diagnosis of lupus nephritis can only be established by renal biopsy. However, not all SLE experts are proponents of renal biopsy in patients suspected of having lupus nephritis. Those who are in favor of performing renal biopsy maintain that it is needed for the following reasons:

1. To exclude other causes of renal dysfunction
2. To precisely determine the patient's lupus nephritis class (see box above), which has bearing on the therapy selected
3. To assess the degree of chronicity, which has bearing on the aggressiveness of therapy

Those who are not advocates of renal biopsy believe that the diagnosis can be established with confidence from the patient's clinical presentation and laboratory testing. Empiric treatment can be started in these patients, who are thus spared the risks of renal biopsy.

The type of lupus nephritis identified on renal biopsy also provides information regarding prognosis. Mesangial and focal proliferative lupus nephritis have a better prognosis. Renal insufficiency does not develop in these patients unless their disease transforms into the diffuse or membranous forms. Without treatment, renal failure develops in patients with diffuse proliferative lupus nephritis.

Disease Activity

Levels of anti-ds-DNA, along with complement, often reflect disease activity. Disease exacerbation is usually associated with an increase in the anti-ds-DNA titer, along with a decrease in the serum complement level. A considerable decline in or even absence of anti-ds-DNA levels accompanied by normalization of serum complement level has been noted to occur with clinical improvement in patients with SLE. Once it has been shown that a patient has an increase in titer with disease flares followed by a decrease with remission, anti-ds-DNA antibodies can be used to follow disease activity. In approximately 15% of patients, however, disease exacerbations are not accompanied by an increase in the anti-ds-DNA titer and hypocomplementemia. In these patients, anti-ds-DNA levels usually cannot be used to gauge response to therapy.

Other Laboratory Test Abnormalities

Other laboratory test abnormalities that may be noted in patients with SLE include:

- Elevated ESR/CRP
- Increased gamma globulin levels
- False-positive VDRL test

  A false-positive VDRL test is typically due to the presence of anticardiolipin antibodies.
- Antiphospholipid antibodies

  Antiphospholipid antibodies include lupus anticoagulant and anticardiolipin antibodies. These antibodies may manifest with a prolonged PTT.

References

Gill JM, Quisel AM, Rocca PV, et al, "Diagnosis of Systemic Lupus Erythematosus," *Am Fam Physician*, 2003, 68(11):2179-86.

Lane SK and Gravel JW Jr, "Clinical Utility of Common Serum Rheumatologic Tests," *Am Fam Physician*, 2002, 65(6):1073-80.

RHEUMATOID ARTHRITIS

Rheumatoid arthritis is a symmetric polyarthritis of unclear etiology. If the disease is not treated, erosion of the cartilage and bone can lead to joint destruction and deformity.

Criteria for Diagnosis

The criteria for the diagnosis of rheumatoid arthritis are listed in the following box.

AMERICAN COLLEGE OF RHEUMATOLOGY 1987 REVISED CRITERIA FOR RHEUMATOID ARTHRITIS*
Morning stiffness
>1 hour for ≥6 weeks
Arthritis of ≥3 or more joint areas
Soft tissue swelling in elbows, wrists, knee, ankle, PIPs, MCPs, or MTPs for 6 weeks
Arthritis of hand joints
Swelling in one area (MCPs, PIPs, or wrist) for ≥6 weeks
Symmetric arthritis
Involving the joints outlined above for ≥6 weeks
Rheumatoid nodules
Serum rheumatoid factor
Radiographic changes typical of rheumatoid arthritis
Erosions and bony decalcification in areas adjacent to involved joints

*In order to establish the diagnosis of rheumatoid arthritis, the patient must have 4 of the 7 criteria.

The criteria listed above may not be as helpful in patients who present early in their disease course. There is no laboratory test that can establish the diagnosis of rheumatoid arthritis. Laboratory test findings can, however, support the diagnosis in a patient who has clinical manifestations consistent with rheumatoid arthritis. These lab test findings will be discussed in the remainder of this chapter.

Rheumatoid Factor

Rheumatoid factor is an autoantibody that reacts with the Fc portion of IgG. It is found in approximately 80% of patients with rheumatoid arthritis. While a positive rheumatoid factor test alone cannot be used to make the diagnosis of rheumatoid arthritis, in the presence of symptoms and signs consistent with rheumatoid arthritis, a positive test result can provide support for the diagnosis.

Rheumatoid factor is not specific for the diagnosis of rheumatoid arthritis, as it can be appreciated in many other diseases, as well as in "normal persons." Indeed, the percentage of normal persons with a positive rheumatoid factor increases with age. It is estimated that between 10% and 20% of people over the age of 65 have a positive test result.

Approximately 20% to 25% of rheumatoid arthritis patients have a negative rheumatoid factor test result. Therefore, a negative test result does not exclude the diagnosis. It is also important to note that the test may be negative early in the course of the disease.

The rheumatoid factor titer is also important. In most patients with nonrheumatic conditions, the titer is much lower than that appreciated in rheumatoid arthritis. Therefore, specificity increases with increasing serum titer. Higher titers are thought to be associated with aggressive joint disease, poor prognosis, and an increased risk for the development of extra-articular manifestations.

Once a patient is found to be rheumatoid factor positive, there is no need to repeat testing since the test is not useful in following disease activity.

Two other autoantibodies that may be present in rheumatoid arthritis patients include antikeratin and antiperinuclear antibodies. These autoantibodies are specific for the diagnosis.

Hematologic Disease in RA

Anemia is commonly found in RA patients, especially in those with active disease. It is usually due to the anemia of chronic disease. The anemia tends to correlate with disease activity. Hemoglobin levels typically do not fall below 9-10 g/dL. Levels lower than this should prompt consideration of other causes of anemia (alone or superimposed on the anemia of chronic disease) such as iron deficiency anemia, folate deficiency, vitamin B_{12} deficiency, and drug-induced anemia (methotrexate, azathioprine). An autoimmune hemolytic anemia has rarely been described, mainly in patients with Felty's syndrome.

The presence of neutropenia should prompt consideration of Felty's syndrome, which is characterized by the triad of rheumatoid arthritis, neutropenia, and splenomegaly. Anemia and thrombocytopenia may also be noted. Felty's syndrome needs to be differentiated from other causes of neutropenia in rheumatoid arthritis patients such as medications (methotrexate, gold salts, penicillamine, sulfasalazine, azathioprine). Also in the differential diagnosis is the large granular lymphocyte syndrome, which is also known as pseudo-Felty's syndrome. In contrast to Felty's syndrome, patients with the large granular lymphocyte syndrome are at increased risk for the development of leukemia. In fact, 3% to 14% of patients with this syndrome ultimately develop leukemia.

The clinical manifestations of these two conditions are similar and cannot be used to reliably differentiate between them. To differentiate between these two conditions, it is necessary to examine the peripheral blood and bone marrow for expansion of the lymphocyte population with large granular lymphocytes. Immunophenotyping of the lymphocytes may also be helpful in establishing the diagnosis since the presence of certain surface makers is more common in the large granular lymphocyte syndrome.

Leukocytosis is not uncommon in rheumatoid arthritis patients. Although it is often due a disease flare, it is wise to exclude infection. It may also be due to corticosteroid therapy. Thrombocytosis is also common and there is some evidence to suggest that the platelet count correlates with disease activity. A low platelet count is uncommon but can occur due to medication use (gold salts, methotrexate, azathioprine, penicillamine) or Felty's syndrome.

Renal Disease in Rheumatoid Arthritis

The kidney is not a commonly affected organ in rheumatoid arthritis. Renal disease is usually due to drug nephrotoxicity. NSAIDs are probably the most common cause. Membranous nephropathy may occur, usually due to either the use of gold salts or penicillamine. However, there are some reports that suggest rheumatoid arthritis itself is associated with a higher incidence of membranous nephropathy. Other types of renal disease in this population include amyloidosis, analgesic nephropathy, rheumatoid vasculitis, and focal mesangial proliferative glomerulonephritis.

Other Laboratory Test Findings

Other laboratory test abnormalities include hypoalbuminemia (correlates with disease activity), elevated ESR, elevated C-reactive protein, and positive antinuclear antibodies (30% to 40%). The ESR and C-reactive protein can be monitored periodically to gauge disease activity. ANCA testing may also yield positive results. In fact, ANCA is positive in 75% of patients with Felty's syndrome.

Laboratory Testing During Treatment

A number of medications are available for the treatment of rheumatoid arthritis. The use of many of these medications may be complicated by the development of adverse effects, some of which can be detected with laboratory test monitoring.

Laboratory Test Monitoring During the Treatment of Rheumatoid Arthritis

Medication	Recommended Laboratory Test Monitoring
Sulfasalazine	CBC every 2-4 weeks for the first 3 months Thereafter, every 3 months
Methotrexate	CBC/platelet count/AST/albumin/creatinine every 4-8 weeks
Gold (intramuscular)	CBC/platelet count/urine dipstick every 1-2 weeks for first 20 weeks Thereafter, with each (or every other) injection
Gold (oral)	CBC/platelet count/urine dipstick for protein every 4-12 weeks
D-penicillamine	CBC/urine dipstick for protein every 2 weeks until dosage stable Thereafter, every 1-3 months
Azathioprine	CBC/platelet count every 1-2 weeks with changes in dosage Thereafter, every 1-3 months
Cyclophosphamide	CBC/platelet count every 1-2 weeks with changes in dosage Thereafter, every 1-3 months Urinalysis and urine cytology every 6-12 months after cessation
Cyclosporine	Creatinine every 2 weeks until dose is stable Thereafter, monthly Periodic CBC, LFTs, potassium
Chlorambucil	CBC/platelet count every 1-2 weeks with changes in dosage Thereafter, every 1-3 months

From "Guidelines for Monitoring Drug Therapy in Rheumatoid Arthritis, American College of Rheumatology Ad Hoc Committee on Clinical Guidelines," *Arthritis Rheum*, 1996, 39:723.

References

Lee DM and Weinblatt ME, "Rheumatoid Arthritis," *Lancet*, 2001, 358(9285):903-11.

SCLERODERMA

Scleroderma is a disorder of connective tissue that is characterized by skin thickening. This disease may also affect internal organs. The three major forms of scleroderma include:

1. Diffuse disease

   Patients typically present with skin involvement extending above the elbows or knees. The diffuse form is the most serious type of scleroderma and usually has a rapid onset. These patients are more likely to have pulmonary renal, or cardiac complications. Evidence of organ failure often manifests within 5 years of symptom onset.

2. Limited disease

   Skin fibrosis of limited disease is usually confined to the distal extremities but may affect the face. Limited disease is also known as the CREST syndrome, which stands for:

   C = calcinosis
   R = Raynaud's phenomenon
   E = esophageal dysmotility
   S = sclerodactyly
   T = telangiectasia

   While the limited form may be complicated by visceral involvement, it occurs very late in the course of the disease.

3. Localized disease (morphea or linear scleroderma)

The following table compares limited and diffuse scleroderma.

Comparison Between Limited and Diffuse Forms of Scleroderma

Manifestation	Limited	Diffuse
Site of skin involvement	Distal, face only	Distal and proximal
Pace of skin involvement	Slow	Rapid
Telangiectasias	+++	+ (late)
Calcinosis	+++	+ (late)
Tendon friction rubs	0	+++ (early)
Pulmonary hypertension	++	(+/-)
"Renal crisis"	0	++
Anticentromere antibody	+++	0
Anti-Scl 70	0	+
Survival (10 years)	>70%	<50%

From Brasington RD Jr, Kahl LE, Ranganathan P, et al, "Immunologic Rheumatic Disorders," *J Allergy Clin Immunol*, 2003, 111(2 Suppl):S593-601 (review).

Laboratory Test Findings

Antinuclear antibodies are present in >95% of scleroderma patients. Antibodies that are characteristic for scleroderma include anticentromere and antitopoisomerase-1 (Scl-70) antibodies. Anticentromere antibodies are present in many patients with the CREST syndrome (44% to 98%). Although antitopoisomerase-1 antibodies occur in just 30% of scleroderma patients (diffuse form), they are highly specific for the diagnosis. Other antibodies that may be present in scleroderma patients include anti-RNA polymerase and U3-RNP antibodies.

Autoantibodies in Scleroderma

Antibodies	Diffuse Disease	Limited (CREST) Disease
Antinuclear	95% often speckled or nucleolar	95% often speckled or nucleolar
Anticentromere	Negative	44% to 98% good prognosis
Antitopoisomerase-1 (Scl-70)	30% poor prognosis for pulmonary and peripheral vascular disease; correlates with ethnicity	Negative
Anti-RNA polymerase 1	4% quite specific	Negative
Anti-RNA polymerase 2	Rare	Rare
Anti-RNA polymerase 3	45% severe skin disease; poor prognosis for renal crisis and cardiac involvement; better prognosis for pulmonary disease	6%

From *Textbook of Autoimmune Diseases*, Lahita RG, N Chiorazzi, and WH Reeves, eds, Philadelphia, PA: Lippincott Williams and Wilkins, 2000, 563.

Because of the low sensitivity of these antibodies, negative serologic test results do not exclude the diagnosis of scleroderma.

Anemia is not uncommon in scleroderma patients. It is most often due to the anemia of chronic disease. Iron deficiency anemia due to gastrointestinal bleeding (NSAID use) and vitamin B_{12} deficiency secondary to bacterial overgrowth are other causes of anemia in this population. Microangiopathic hemolytic anemia can occur in patients with scleroderma renal crisis. Scleroderma renal crisis is discussed below. Other laboratory test abnormalities include elevated ESR, hypergammaglobulinemia, and positive rheumatoid factor (25%).

Renal Disease in Scleroderma

Severe renal disease, termed the "scleroderma renal crisis," occurs in about 10% to 15% of patients. This complication of scleroderma typically occurs early in the disease course. In fact, most patients (75%) develop renal disease within the first four years. Late cases have been reported, however, even 20 years after disease onset. Risk factors for renal disease include diffuse skin involvement, rapid progression of the disease, disease duration less than 4 years, presence of anti-RNA polymerase III antibody, and high dose corticosteroid therapy. African Americans are at higher risk as well.

Renal crisis presents with acute renal failure, moderate to severe hypertension that develops abruptly, and a relatively bland urinalysis (mild proteinuria but few cells or casts). Urine protein excretion usually does not exceed 2.5 g/day. Microscopic hematuria and granular casts may be noted if patients have malignant hypertension. The peripheral blood smear may reveal findings consistent with microangiopathic hemolytic anemia (occurs in 43% of cases). Platelet counts rarely fall below 50,000/mm^3. Without treatment, patients with scleroderma renal crisis usually progress to end-stage renal disease in 1-2 months.

Many experts advocate screening for renal disease with the following:

- Measurement of blood pressure every month
- Determination of serum creatinine level every 3-6 months
- Dipstick testing for protein or urine protein to creatinine ratio every 3-6 months

Screening is especially important during the first five years of the illness since most cases of renal disease will manifest at some point during this time. Hypertension, raised serum creatinine level, decrease in creatinine clearance, or the development of persistent proteinuria (>500 mg/day) should prompt an evaluation for scleroderma renal disease along with appropriate therapy.

References

Steen VD, "Scleroderma Renal Crisis," *Rheum Dis Clin North Am*, 2003, 29(2):315-33.

Valentini G, "The Assessment of the Patient With Systemic Sclerosis," *Autoimmun Rev*, 2003, 2(6):370-6.

POLYMYOSITIS / DERMATOMYOSITIS

Polymyositis and dermatomyositis are inflammatory diseases characterized by proximal muscle weakness. Histologically, there is inflammation and damage to the skeletal muscle, which are detected biochemically be elevations in creatine kinase (CK) and other muscle enzymes. Dermatomyositis differs from polymyositis in that the former is characterized by the presence of skin lesions.

Criteria for Diagnosis

The criteria of Bohan and Peter have been widely used in the diagnosis of polymyositis and dermatomyositis.

CRITERIA FOR THE DIAGNOSIS OF POLYMYOSITIS / DERMATOMYOSITIS
Muscle weakness (symmetrical muscle weakness developing over weeks to months)
Elevated serum muscle enzymes
EMG findings consistent with polymyositis/dermatomyositis
Muscle biopsy findings consistent with polymyositis/dermatomyositis
For dermatomyositis, dermatologic features consistent with the diagnosis (eg, Gottron's papules, heliotrope rash, erythematous and/or poikilodermatous rash)

Modified from Bohan A and Peter JB, "Polymyositis and Dermatomyositis (Parts I and II)," *New Engl J Med*, 1975, 292:344-7, 403-7.

Laboratory Testing

Serum muscle enzymes should be obtained in patients suspected of having polymyositis or dermatomyositis. These include creatine kinase (CK), lactate dehydrogenase (LDH), aspartate aminotransferase (AST), alanine aminotransferase (ALT), aldolase, and myoglobin. One or more of these enzymes are increased at some point in the patient's illness.

Serum CK levels are elevated in 80% to 90% of patients at the time of presentation with >95% of patients having an elevation noted at some point in their disease course. In adult patients, the mean increase of CK is about ten times the upper limit of normal. Cases have been described, however, in which CK levels were 100 times the upper limit of normal.

CK levels may be normal in some patients despite active myositis. This may occur early in the disease course or in advanced or chronic disease, particularly when severe atrophy is present. It is preferable to measure serum muscle enzymes before an EMG is performed because the procedure itself can result in an elevation of the enzyme levels.

To some extent, the CK level correlates with disease activity. It should not be used alone, however, to assess disease activity. An increase in the CK level may be appreciated several weeks before the disease flares. Normalization of the CK level suggests successful treatment of the disease and can precede recovery of strength by 3-4 weeks. When CK levels increase in a patient who is being treated, recurrent myositis should be considered. Other causes of CK elevation should be excluded.

Measurement of the CK isozymes will usually reveal an increase in the CK-MM fraction. However, CK-MB levels can be elevated in patients with myositis. In these cases, the increased CK-MB fraction may be due to the enhanced expression of the CK B chain by the inflamed muscles. Another consideration is that the elevated CK-MB fraction reflects disease of the myocardium, which can occur in patients with polymyositis or dermatomyositis. When the CK-MB fraction is increased, it can lead to considerable diagnostic confusion, with myocardial infarction being the major concern. If such a situation arises, the clinician can choose to measure cardiac troponin I. Troponin I levels will be normal if the source of the CK-MB elevation is inflamed skeletal muscle. An elevated cardiac troponin I should prompt an evaluation for cardiac disease.

The other serum muscle enzymes (AST, ALT, aldolase, LDH) are often elevated in patients with polymyositis or dermatomyositis. They may be particularly useful in following disease activity in patients who have normal CK levels. It is important to realize that disease of non-muscle can also lead to elevations in these enzymes. Serum myoglobin also seems to vary with disease activity. In some patients, an increase in the serum myoglobin may herald an exacerbation.

Antinuclear antibodies are positive in 50 to 80% of patients with polymyositis or dermatomyositis. The presence of antinuclear antibodies, however, is not specific for these conditions. This limits their diagnostic usefulness. However, the presence of high titer antinuclear antibodies in a patient with a clinical presentation consistent with polymyositis or dermatomyositis is useful in differentiating these inflammatory myopathies from other considerations in the differential diagnosis such as muscular dystrophies and nonautoimmune myopathies. One autoantibody that is specific for myositis is the anti-histidyl-tRNA synthetase (anti-Jo-1 antibody), which is present in about 20% to 30% of cases. Patients with myositis who have this antibody have a greater tendency to develop interstitial lung disease, polyarticular arthritis, and Raynaud's phenomenon.

Other laboratory test abnormalities in dermatomyositis and polymyositis include elevated ESR, positive rheumatoid factor (50%), and decreased hemoglobin.

There are a number of conditions that should be considered in the differential diagnosis of polymyositis and dermatomyositis. Lab testing can help exclude some of these conditions. Lab tests that are often obtained include TSH (hypothyroidism), differential white blood cell count looking for eosinophilia (hypereosinophilic syndrome), electrolytes (hypokalemia, hypophosphatemia, hyponatremia, hypocalcemia, hypernatremia), 24-hour urine cortisol (Cushing's syndrome), and anti-acetylcholine receptor antibodies (myasthenia gravis).

Establishing the Diagnosis

An EMG is usually obtained in the evaluation of these patients. While it is abnormal in most cases, about 10% of affected patients have normal findings. EMG findings can only be consistent with the diagnosis – they are not diagnostic. In fact, similar findings have been noted in other myopathies.

The gold standard for the diagnosis of polymyositis or dermatomyositis is muscle biopsy. Not only can this test establish the diagnosis but it can also exclude other considerations in the differential diagnosis. A muscle biopsy should not be performed at the site of the EMG needle insertion because inflammatory cells may be found in the muscle due to the procedure.

References

Amato AA and Barohn RJ, "Idiopathic Inflammatory Myopathies," *Neurol Clin*, 1997, 15(3):615-48.

Dalakas MC and Hohlfeld R, "Polymyositis and Dermatomyositis," *Lancet*, 2003, 362(9388):971-82.

SJÖGREN'S SYNDROME

Sjögren's syndrome is a slowly progressive autoimmune inflammatory disorder characterized by keratoconjunctivitis sicca and xerostomia, due to dysfunction of lacrimal and salivary gland secretion. Sjögren's syndrome may be divided into primary and secondary forms. Secondary Sjögren's syndrome occurs in patients with underlying disease.

CONDITIONS ASSOCIATED WITH SECONDARY SJÖGREN'S SYNDROME	
Rheumatoid arthritis	Vasculitis
Scleroderma	Mixed essential cryoglobulinemia
Systemic lupus erythematosus	Thyroiditis
Mixed connective tissue disease	Primary biliary cirrhosis
Polymyositis/dermatomyositis	HIV
	Hepatitis C

Clinical Manifestations

The initial manifestations of primary Sjögren's syndrome are listed in the following box.

INITIAL MANIFESTATIONS OF PRIMARY SJÖGREN'S SYNDROME	
Subjective xerophthalmia (47%)	Raynaud's phenomenon (21%)
Subjective xerostomia (42%)	Fever / fatigue (10%)
Arthralgia/arthritis (28%)	Dyspareunia (5%)
Parotid gland enlargement (24%)	

From Pavlidirs NA, Karsh J, and Moutsotoulos HM, "The Clinical Picture of Primary Sjögren's Syndrome: A Retrospective Study," *J Rheumatol*, 1982, 9:685-90.

As shown above, xerophthalmia and xerostomia are the two most commonly encountered symptoms. Xerophthalmia often manifests with a foreign body sensation, itchiness, redness, and photosensitivity. Xerostomia should be suspected when a patient presents with difficulty swallowing dry food, changes in the taste of food, a burning sensation in the mouth, or an increase in dental caries.

Laboratory Testing

In patients suspected of having Sjögren's syndrome, it is reasonable to measure autoantibodies such as anti-Ro (SSA), anti-La (SSB), rheumatoid factor, and antinuclear antibodies. A positive ANA is seen in approximately 60% to 80% of patients. Antibodies to Ro and La are seen in about 50% of patients. Sixty percent of Sjögren's syndrome patients have a positive rheumatoid factor. Other laboratory test abnormalities that may be appreciated include elevated ESR, hypergammaglobulinemia (50%), and mildly decreased hemoglobin level (normocytic, normochromic anemia).

Sjögren's syndrome patients may develop an interstitial nephritis characterized by a mildly increased serum creatinine level and tubular dysfunction. The tubular dysfunction may manifest as the Fanconi syndrome, nephrogenic diabetes insipidus, or type 1 renal tubular acidosis (distal). Patients with type 1 renal tubular acidosis present with a normal anion gap metabolic acidosis that is usually mild. Cases have been reported, however, in which the serum bicarbonate was less than 10 mEq/L. Because type 1 renal tubular acidosis can be the initial presentation of Sjögren's syndrome, it is important to recognize this relationship. If a patient is diagnosed with type 1 renal tubular acidosis and no etiology can be found, an evaluation for Sjögren's syndrome is reasonable. An evaluation for Sjögren's syndrome should also be performed in patients with unexplained nephrogenic diabetes insipidus.

Although interstitial involvement is more common, glomerular disease has been described. Of the glomerulopathies found in these patients, membranous nephropathy and membranoproliferative glomerulonephritis are the most common.

Establishing the Diagnosis

Patients who complain of dry eyes and/or dry mouth should be evaluated for Sjögren's syndrome. A thorough evaluation should be performed to exclude other illness that can present with these symptoms. Tear production can be tested with the Schirmer test. In this test, absorbent paper strips are inserted into the lower palpebral fold to measure the amount of moisture. After 5 minutes, moisture or wetting <5 mm argues strongly for decreased tear production. A positive test result is suggestive, but not diagnostic, of the illness. Lip gland biopsy can be performed to demonstrate the characteristic lymphocytic infiltration that is found in patients with Sjögren's syndrome.

References

Mahoney EG and Spiegel JH, "Sjögren's Disease," *Otolaryngol Clin North Am*, 2003, 36(4):733-45.

MIXED CONNECTIVE TISSUE DISEASE (MCTD)

Mixed connective tissue disease, also known as the overlap syndrome, is a connective tissue disease characterized by the presence of antibodies to U1 ribonucleoprotein (RNP) in high titers along with clinical features of SLE, scleroderma, and polymyositis.

Clinical Manifestations

Clinical manifestations of MCTD at the onset of the disease are listed in the following box.

CLINICAL MANIFESTATIONS AT THE ONSET OF MCTD	
JOINT SYMPTOMS (93%)	HEPATOMEGALY (21%)
SWELLING OF THE HANDS (71%)	SPLENOMEGALY (21%)
RAYNAUD'S PHENOMENON (93%)	SEROSITIS (29%)
LYMPHADENOPATHY (71%)	MUSCLE INVOLVEMENT (50%)

Criteria for Diagnosis

Several groups have proposed diagnostic criteria for MCTD. The criteria of Alarcon-Segovia have been found to have a sensitivity and specificity of 63% and 86%, respectively.

CRITERIA FOR MCTD*

CLINICAL
- Swollen hands
- Synovitis
- Raynaud's phenomenon
- Myositis
- Acrosclerosis + proximal systemic sclerosis

SEROLOGIC
- Anti-RNP antibodies > 1:1600 (hemagglutination titer)

*The diagnosis of MCTD is established if the serologic criteria and at least 3 of the 5 clinical criteria are met.

From Alarcon-Segovia, D and Cardiel MH, "Comparison Between 3 Diagnostic Criteria for Mixed Connective Tissue Disease. Study of 593 Patients," *J Rheumatol*, 1989, 16:328.

Laboratory Testing

An alternative diagnosis should be considered in patients with clinical features of MCTD who do not have high titers of antibodies to RNP. It is also important to realize that the mere presence of these antibodies is not synonymous with the diagnosis.

Hematologic abnormalities are common. Anemia, usually mild in severity, is found in about 75% of patients. Leukopenia and lymphopenia are other common findings. Less frequently encountered are thrombocytopenia, Coombs' positive hemolytic anemia, red cell aplasia, and thrombotic thrombocytopenic purpura. Other laboratory test abnormalities include positive rheumatoid factor (50% to 70%), hypergammaglobulinemia, and elevated ESR. Renal disease is not common but, if present, is not severe. In these patients, histology often reveals membranous nephropathy.

GOUT

The clinical manifestations of gout are the result of the deposition of monosodium urate crystals. The prevalence of gout increases with advancing age and it is considered to be the most common cause of inflammatory arthritis in men over the age of 40.

Clinical Manifestations

Patients with acute gouty arthritis (acute attack of gout) typically present with an acute monoarticular arthritis. The involved joint is very painful, red, warm, and swollen. Over 50% of first attacks affect the first metatarsophalangeal joint (MTP) of the great toe (podagra). This joint is involved at some point in the disease course in over 90% of patients. Patients who have had an acute gout attack are at risk for future attacks and the time between acute gout attacks is termed the intercritical period (intercritical gout). If the disease is untreated, tophaceous gout may develop, characterized by the presence of tophi (deposits of monosodium urate crystals commonly located in the synovium, olecranon bursa, Achilles tendon, extensor surfaces of forearm, digits of hands/feet).

Laboratory Test Findings

Although hyperuricemia is not always present in gout patients, at some point in the disease course, it can be demonstrated. The clinician should realize, however, that there are many hyperuricemic patients who never develop manifestations of gout.

In patients who develop acute gouty arthritis, laboratory testing may reveal leukocytosis and elevated ESR. These findings, however, are nonspecific. For example, patients with septic arthritis, which is a major consideration in the differential diagnosis of acute gouty arthritis, can also present with these lab test abnormalities. To establish the diagnosis of acute gouty arthritis, it is necessary obtain synovial fluid for analysis. Measurement of the synovial fluid white blood cell count typically reveals counts between 20,000 and 100,000/mm^3. If intracellular monosodium urate crystals (needle-shaped and negatively birefringent) can be demonstrated using polarized light microscopy, a diagnosis of acute gouty arthritis can be made with confidence. In fact, the sensitivity of this test is at least 85%. The clinician should realize, however, that, on occasion, acute gout may co-exist with another cause of acute monoarticular arthritis such as pseudogout or septic arthritis. Patients with acute gouty arthritis may have normal serum uric acid levels during the attack.

Not uncommonly, clinicians will encounter asymptomatic patients who carry a diagnosis of gout but lack confirmation of the diagnosis. Patients who have had an episode of acute gout are clearly at risk for another episode in the future. In fact, only 7% are free of subsequent gout attacks when followed for >10 years. If the diagnosis has not been definitively established, the clinician may choose to wait until another attack occurs before establishing the diagnosis with certainty. The diagnosis can still be made, however, in asymptomatic patients who are in the intercritical period. In these cases, it is appropriate to pursue the diagnosis so that other causes of joint disease can be excluded and the patient can be spared from using medications that are not necessary and potentially toxic. During the intercritical period, joint aspiration and examination of the synovial fluid can help establish the diagnosis. This is because extracellular urate crystals can still be found in the synovial fluid (from a previously affected joint) of asymptomatic gout patients. This is especially true if the patient has not received chronic gout therapy but even in patients on uric acid lowering agents, urate crystals are appreciated in approximately 70% of patients.

In the patient with tophaceous gout, the clinician can choose to aspirate material directly from the tophaceous deposit. Examination of the specimen under polarized light microscopy will reveal the presence of urate crystals.

Renal disease in gout patients is discussed below.

Renal Disease in Gout

Patients with gout may develop two types of renal disease – uric acid nephrolithiasis and chronic urate nephropathy. Renal insufficiency is not uncommon in gout patients but is usually due a concomitant condition such as diabetes mellitus or hypertension. At times, however, the renal insufficiency may be due to the deposition of urate in the renal interstitium. This has been termed chronic urate nephropathy and is characterized by mild proteinuria, bland urine sediment, and isothenuria. A clue to the diagnosis is the presence of hyperuricemia that is out of proportion to the degree of renal insufficiency.

References

Rott T and Agudelo CA, "Gout," *JAMA*, 2003, 289(21):2857-60.

Terkeltaub RA, "Clinical Practice. Gout," *N Engl J Med*, 2003, 349(17):1647-55.

PSEUDOGOUT

Pseudogout is a form of calcium pyrophosphate dihydrate disease (CPDD), which presents similar to acute gouty arthritis. In contrast to gout, the disease is characterized by synovitis from the deposition of calcium pyrophosphate dihydrate crystals in the joint space.

Clinical Manifestations

Attacks of pseudogout are typically acute and affect one joint. Occasionally, several extremity joints may be involved. These attacks resemble those seen in acute gout and it is not possible to reliably distinguish between these two diseases from the clinical presentation alone. Pseudogout should be in the differential diagnosis of all patients presenting with an acute arthritis, especially if a large joint is involved.

Criteria for Diagnosis

Criteria for the diagnosis of pseudogout are listed in the following box.

CRITERIA FOR THE DIAGNOSIS OF PSEUDOGOUT

CPPD crystal deposition disease is diagnosed if:

- CPPD crystals are demonstrated in tissue or synovial fluid
  OR
- Weakly positive birefringent crystals are demonstrated by polarized light microscopy and the characteristic joint capsule calcification is noted on the radiograph

The diagnosis is probable if:

- Weakly positive birefringent crystals are demonstrated by polarized light microscopy
  OR
- The characteristic joint capsule calcification is noted on the radiograph

Laboratory Testing

Like gout, pseudogout can present with a leukocytosis with left shift. An elevated ESR is common. In usual clinical practice, the diagnosis is established when examination of the synovial fluid using polarized light microscopy reveals the presence of weakly positive birefringent crystals. The clinician should realize, however, that it is not uncommon for both urate and CPPD crystals to be present together.

There are a number of diseases that are associated with CPPD disease. These include hemochromatosis, hypomagnesemia, hyperparathyroidism, hypothyroidism, hypophosphatasia, and familial hypocalciuric hypercalcemia. As a result, it is reasonable to obtain lab tests to diagnose or exclude these conditions. Lab tests that should be obtained include serum calcium, magnesium, phosphate, alkaline phosphatase, iron, TIBC, ferritin, and TSH.

References

Joseph J and McGrath H, "Gout or Pseudogout: How to Differentiate Crystal-Induced Arthropathy," *Geriatrics*, 1995, 50(4):33-9.

Pascual E, "The Diagnosis of Gout and CPPD Crystal Arthropathy," *Br J Rheumatol*, 1996, 35(4):306-8.

Schumacher HR, "Crystal-Induced Arthritis: An Overview," *Am J Med*, 1996, 100(2A):46S-52S.

Siva C, Velazquez C, Mody A, et al, "Diagnosing Acute Monoarthritis in Adults: A Practical Approach for the Family Physician," *Am Fam Physician*, 2003, 68(1):83-90.

GIANT CELL ARTERITIS

Giant cell arteritis, also known as temporal arteritis, is a vasculitis that affects medium and large vessels. Arteries of the head and neck are classically involved although vessels elsewhere may be affected.

Criteria for Diagnosis

Criteria for the diagnosis of giant cell arteritis are listed in the following box.

CRITERIA FOR TEMPORAL ARTERITIS*
Age at disease onset >50 years
New onset headache
New onset of or new type of localized pain in the head
Temporal artery abnormality
Temporal artery tender to palpation or decreased pulsation, unrelated to atherosclerosis of cervical arteries
Erythrocyte sedimentation rate
>50 mm/hour by Westergren method
Abnormal artery on biopsy
An artery showing predominance of mononuclear cells or granulomatous inflammation, usually with multinucleated giant cells

*Sensitivity and specificity are 94% and 91%, respectively, if at least 3 of the 5 criteria are fulfilled

From Hunder GG, Bloch DA, Michel BA, et al, "American College of Rheumatology 1990 Criteria for the Classification of Giant Cell Arteritis," *Arthritis Rheum*, 1990, 33(8):1122-8.

The most feared complication of giant cell arteritis is the development of vision loss, which is due to optic nerve ischemia from arteritis affecting the ocular vessels.

Giant cell arteritis and polymyalgia rheumatica are related disorders. Although either may be present alone, at times, they develop together. In other cases, manifestations of one may precede that of the other. Polymyalgia rheumatica patients often complain of pain and stiffness all over. These symptoms tend to be more pronounced at the limb girdles, low back, and neck. Constitutional symptoms are commonly present (fatigue, malaise, weight loss, fever). Criteria for the diagnosis of polymyalgia rheumatica are listed in the following box.

CRITERIA FOR THE DIAGNOSIS OF POLYMYALGIA RHEUMATICA*
1. Age >50 years
2. Three of the following: Pain in the neck, shoulder, or pelvic girdle Marked morning stiffness for >1 hour Elevated ESR Rapid response to prednisone (20 mg/day)
3. Negative tests for rheumatoid factor and antinuclear antibodies

*All 3 criteria must be met to confirm a diagnosis of polymyalgia rheumatica.

From Puttick MP, "Rheumatology: 11. Evaluation of the Patient With Pain All Over," *CMAJ*, 2001, 164(2):223-7.

Laboratory Testing

Most patients with temporal arteritis have an elevated ESR. At times, the degree of elevation is impressive with levels exceeding 100 mm/h not uncommon. The clinician should realize, however, that a normal ESR does not exclude the diagnosis. An increase in other acute phase reactants such as C-reactive protein and fibrinogen is frequently seen.

CBC abnormalities include a normocytic, normochromic anemia and thrombocytosis. Microscopic hematuria has been noted in up to 33% of patients. Despite this, the presence of renal insufficiency or heavy degrees of proteinuria should prompt consideration of other conditions. Antinuclear antibodies are not usually found but, on occasion, titers may be increased. Up to 35% of patients have liver function test abnormalities (abnormal AST, alkaline phosphatase). The degree of elevation is mild to moderate.

Establishing the Diagnosis

Temporal arteritis deserves consideration in patients who present with headache, unexplained fever, abrupt loss of vision, polymyalgia rheumatica, unexplained anemia, and elevated ESR or CRP. If even one of these features is present, the diagnosis should be considered. To establish the diagnosis, a temporal artery biopsy is needed. Since the inflammation of temporal arteritis is often focal, it is important to biopsy a segment of the artery that has signs of inflammation such as tenderness or swelling. If the physical exam does not reveal any signs of inflammation, a longer portion of the artery may need to be biopsied. It is preferable to perform biopsy before starting therapy because treatment can alter the histologic findings. However, an improvement in the inflammation does take time, which is why the biopsy may be revealing even up to several weeks after institution of therapy. In patients suspected of having temporal arteritis, treatment should not be delayed while arrangements are being made for a temporal artery biopsy.

Response to Therapy

Corticosteroid therapy is indicated in patients with temporal arteritis. The initial starting dose of corticosteroid therapy is usually continued until all symptoms and signs of the illness disappear (if reversible) and laboratory test abnormalities normalize. Once the patient is free of disease manifestations, tapering of the therapy is started. How a patient is tapered will depend upon periodic monitoring of the patient's symptoms and changes in the ESR. An ESR rise during treatment, especially if it is sudden, should prompt a thorough evaluation of the patient, inquiring about signs and symptoms of the disease. Alternative causes of the ESR increase should be considered as well.

References

Calvo-Romero JM, "Giant Cell Arteritis," *Postgrad Med J*, 2003, 79(935):511-5.

Salvarani C, Cantini F, Boiardi L, et al, "Polymyalgia Rheumatica and Giant-Cell Arteritis," *N Engl J Med*, 2002, 347(4):261-71.

Weyand CM and Goronzy JJ, "Giant-Cell Arteritis and Polymyalgia Rheumatica," *Ann Intern Med*, 2003, 139(6):505-15.

POLYARTERITIS NODOSA (PAN)

Polyarteritis nodosa is a multisystem disorder characterized by inflammation and necrosis of medium sized arteries leading to various organ manifestations.

Criteria for Diagnosis

In 1990, the American College of Rheumatology developed criteria for the diagnosis of PAN. These criteria are listed in the following box.

CRITERIA FOR POLYARTERITIS NODOSA*
Weight loss ≥4 kg
Livedo reticularis
Testicular pain/tenderness
Myalgia/weakness/leg tenderness
Mononeuropathy/mononeuropathy multiplex/polyneuropathy
Diastolic blood pressure >90 mm Hg
BUN >40 mg/dL or Cr >1.5 mg/dL
Hepatitis B viral infection
Arteriographic abnormalities
Aneurysms or occlusions of the visceral arteries, not due to atherosclerosis, fibromuscular dysplasia, or other noninflammatory causes
Biopsy of small-medium sized artery consistent with PAN
Histologic changes showing the presence of granulocytes with or without mononuclear cells in the artery wall

*Sensitivity and specificity are 82% and 87%, respectively, if at least 3 of the 10 criteria are present.

Lightfoot RW, Michel BA, Bloch DA, et al, "American College of Rheumatology Criteria for the Classification of Polyarteritis Nodosa," *Arthritis Rheum*, 1990, 33:1088-93.

Laboratory Testing

No laboratory test finding is pathognomonic for the diagnosis of PAN. Laboratory test findings that may be appreciated in PAN patients are listed in the following box.

LABORATORY TEST FINDINGS IN PAN
ELEVATED ESR
ANEMIA OF CHRONIC DISEASE
THROMBOCYTOPENIA
HEPATITIS B SURFACE ANTIGENEMIA*
URINALYSIS ABNORMALITIES (hematuria, red blood cell casts)†
ELEVATED SERUM CREATININE
POSITIVE RHEUMATOID FACTOR

*In patients with polyarteritis nodosa, hepatitis B serology is indicated because hepatitis B accounts for a small percentage of cases (7% to 22% of cases) and the treatment of hepatitis B-associated cases differs. When PAN is due to hepatitis B, the illness usually occurs within five months of the onset of hepatitis B viral infection. PAN can also occur in the setting of hepatitis C or HIV.

†Although red blood cells and red blood cell casts may be noted, the urinalysis in PAN patients is usually normal or near normal. This is because PAN tends to present as a primary vascular nephropathy.

ANCA testing usually reveals negative results in PAN patients. Positive ANCA test results should prompt consideration of other possibilities such as microscopic polyarteritis or Wegener's granulomatosis.

Establishing the Diagnosis

The diagnosis of PAN can be confirmed by biopsy of an affected organ. Because peripheral nerve and skin involvement are common in PAN, one of these two sites is usually biopsied. Mesenteric or renal arteriography can also be performed to establish the diagnosis. Angiographic findings suggestive of the diagnosis include microaneurysms, stenoses, and alternating areas of arterial narrowing and dilation.

References

Hughes LB and Bridges SL Jr, "Polyarteritis Nodosa and Microscopic Polyangiitis: Etiologic and Diagnostic Considerations," *Curr Rheumatol Rep*, 2002, 4(1):75-82.

MICROSCOPIC POLYANGIITIS

Microscopic polyangiitis (MPA) is a systemic, necrotizing vasculitis that affects small vessels. Because it was only recently differentiated from polyarteritis nodosa, there is less information available about this disease.

Clinical Manifestations

Patients may present with an acute or subacute onset of symptoms. Even in those with acute disease, history will often reveal the presence of constitutional symptoms (fatigue, malaise, weight loss, fever) for weeks to months prior to the development of acute disease. The clinical manifestations of MPA are listed in the following box, in descending order of frequency.

CLINICAL MANIFESTATIONS OF MICROSCOPIC POLYANGIITIS

RPGN
CONSTITUTIONAL SYMPTOMS
ARTHRALGIAS / MYALGIAS
CUTANEOUS INVOLVEMENT
MONONEURITIS MULTIPLEX
GI INVOLVEMENT
PULMONARY HEMORRHAGE / HEMOPTYSIS
OCULAR INVOLVEMENT
CARDIAC INVOLVEMENT
UPPER AIRWAY INVOLVEMENT

The major differences between MPA and polyarteritis nodosa are listed in the following table.

Comparison of Microscopic Polyangiitis and Polyarteritis Nodosa

	Microscopic Polyangiitis	Polyarteritis Nodosa
Renal vasculature with infarcts and microaneurysms	No	Yes
RPGN	Yes	No
Lung hemorrhage	Yes	No
Hepatitis B infection	No	Yes (7% to 22%)
p-ANCA	50% to 80%	<20%
Abnormal angiogram	No	Yes
Histology	Necrotizing vasculitis	Necrotizing vasculitis

From Clotte F and Guillevin L, "Polyarteritis Nodosa, Microscopic Arteritis, and Churg-Strauss Syndrome: Clinical Aspects and Treatment," *Rheum Dis Clin North Am*, 1995, 21:911-48.

Laboratory Testing

Laboratory test findings in microscopic polyangiitis are listed in the following box.

LABORATORY TEST FINDINGS IN MICROSCOPIC POLYANGIITIS	
Elevated ESR	Urinalysis abnormalities
Anemia of chronic disease	p-ANCA (50% to 75%)
Elevated platelets	c-ANCA (10% to 15%)
Renal insufficiency (70% to 100%)*	Positive rheumatoid factor (25% to 50%)

*Renal function can rapidly decline in these patients. Microscopic polyangiitis deserves consideration in any patient who presents with rapidly progressive glomerulonephritis.

Establishing the Diagnosis

In patients who have a clinical presentation compatible with microscopic polyangiitis, biopsy can be performed to support the diagnosis. Biopsy will reveal a necrotizing vasculitis of small vessels. The disease is not characterized by the presence of granulomas. If granulomas are present, another diagnosis should be considered.

References

Hughes LB and Bridges SL Jr, "Polyarteritis Nodosa and Microscopic Polyangiitis: Etiologic and Diagnostic Considerations," *Curr Rheumatol Rep*, 2002, 4(1):75-82.

WEGENER'S GRANULOMATOSIS

Wegener's granulomatosis is a systemic inflammatory disorder characterized by granulomatous inflammation of the upper and lower respiratory tracts, as well as necrotizing glomerulonephritis. The classic triad of Wegener's granulomatosis is disease affecting the lungs, kidneys, and upper respiratory tract.

Criteria for Diagnosis

In 1990, the American College of Rheumatology developed criteria for the diagnosis of Wegener's granulomatosis. These criteria are listed in the following box.

CRITERIA FOR WEGENER'S GRANULOMATOSIS
NASAL OR ORAL INFLAMMATION
Development of painful or painless oral ulcers or purulent/bloody nasal discharge
ABNORMAL CHEST X-RAY
Nodules
Fixed infiltrates
Cavities
URINARY SEDIMENT ABNORMALITIES
Hematuria/RBCs/RBC casts
GRANULOMATOUS INFLAMMATION ON BIOPSY
Histology showing granulomatous changes within the wall of an artery or in the perivascular or extravascular area

*Sensitivity and specificity for the criteria listed above are 88% and 92%, respectively, if at least 2 of the 4 criteria are present.

Leavitt RY, Fauci AS, Bloch DA, et al, "American College of Rheumatology 1990 Criteria for the Classification of Wegener's Granulomatosis," *Arthritis Rheum*, 1990, 33:1101-7.

It is important to note that ANCA testing is not part of the criteria because the criteria were developed before the ANCA testing became available. This is one of the limitations of the above criteria.

Laboratory Test Findings

Laboratory test findings that may be noted in Wegener's granulomatosis patients are listed in the following box.

LABORATORY TEST FINDINGS IN WEGENER'S GRANULOMATOSIS	
Positive ANCA*	Anemia of chronic disease
Elevated white blood cell count	Urinalysis abnormalities (red blood cells, red blood cell casts, white blood cells, proteinuria)
Elevated platelet count	Elevated serum creatinine
Elevated ESR	
Elevated C-reactive protein	
Positive rheumatoid factor (50% to 60%)	

*Most patients (75% to 80%) have c-ANCA, which refers to antineutrophil cytoplasmic antibodies directed against proteinase-3. Not all patients with Wegener's granulomatosis will have circulating c-ANCA, however. 10% to 15% will have p-ANCA and 5% to 10% will have negative ANCA test results. Therefore, the absence of ANCA should not exclude the diagnosis. The sensitivity of this test depends, to a certain extent, on the activity of the disease. Those with active disease usually have positive test results (90%) while those with inactive or limited disease may have negative test results (sensitivity of c-ANCA in the latter is 65% to 70%). The specificity of c-ANCA is high (90%) but, on occasion, c-ANCA test results may be positive in other diseases such as microscopic polyangiitis and Churg-Strauss syndrome.

Establishing the Diagnosis

A diagnosis of Wegener's granulomatosis can be confirmed by performing a renal biopsy. Biopsy must be done on an area that is affected. Some argue that biopsy is not necessary in all Wegener's granulomatosis patients, particularly in those who have a classic clinical presentation and are c-ANCA positive.

References

Bartunkova J, Tesar V, and Sediva A, "Diagnostic and Pathogenetic Role of Antineutrophil Cytoplasmic Autoantibodies," *Clin Immunol*, 2003, 106(2):73-82.

Kamesh L, Harper L, and Savage CO, "ANCA-Positive Vasculitis," *J Am Soc Nephrol*, 2002, 13(7):1953-60.

Langford CA, "Vasculitis," *J Allergy Clin Immunol*, 2003, 111(2 Suppl):S602-12.

Wilk A, "Rational Use of ANCA in the Diagnosis of Vasculitis," *Rheumatology (Oxford)*, 2002, 41(5):481-3.

SARCOIDOSIS

Sarcoidosis is a systemic noncaseating granulomatous disease of unclear etiology.

Clinical Manifestations

The disease typically presents between the ages of 10-40 years. Fifty percent of cases are diagnosed when a routine chest radiograph, obtained for one reason or another, reveals radiographic manifestations consistent with the disease. In those who are symptomatic, pulmonary symptoms are common (cough, shortness of breath, chest pain). Nonspecific symptoms that may be present include weakness, malaise, weight loss, and fatigue. Signs of pulmonary or extrapulmonary involvement may be noted on physical examination.

Laboratory Testing

Laboratory test findings in sarcoidosis patients are listed in the following box.

LABORATORY TEST FINDINGS IN SARCOIDOSIS	
Anemia*	Hypercalciuria (up to 50%)‡
Leukopenia (5% to 10%)*	Hypercalcemia (10% to 20%)‡
Thrombocytopenia*	Elevated alkaline phosphatase§
Eosinophilia	Hypergammaglobulinemia (30% to 80%)
Elevated ESR	Positive rheumatoid factor
Elevated ACE level†	Arterial blood gas abnormalities#

*Although it is not common, anemia can occur in sarcoidosis patients. Most often, it is due to the anemia of chronic disease. Other causes of anemia in sarcoidosis patients include autoimmune hemolytic anemia and hypersplenism. Hypersplenism can also lead to the development of leukopenia or thrombocytopenia.

†Approximately 75% of sarcoidosis patients have an elevated serum ACE level. It is more likely to be elevated when the disease is active. However, there are many other conditions that are associated with increased levels as well. Serum ACE levels may be normal in sarcoidosis patients, especially when the disease is chronic. Some patients treated with corticosteroids will have a fall in the serum ACE level. Therefore, the test is neither sensitive nor specific for the diagnosis of sarcoidosis.

‡The macrophages present in the sarcoid granulomas are able to produce calcitriol. This can lead to hypercalciuria and hypercalcemia with the former being more common than the latter. Renal disease in sarcoidosis patients can be due to interstitial nephritis, membranous nephropathy, focal glomerulosclerosis, or crescentic glomerulonephritis. Sarcoidosis is also a cause of diabetes insipidus (central and nephrogenic).

§An elevated serum alkaline phosphatase level should prompt consideration of infiltrative liver disease due to sarcoidosis.

#While arterial blood gas analysis may reveal normal findings, some patients may have hypoxemia and/or hypocarbia.

None of the above laboratory test findings can be considered to be pathognomonic for the diagnosis of sarcoidosis.

Establishing the Diagnosis

The definitive diagnosis of sarcoidosis requires biopsy of involved tissue. Some argue that a tissue diagnosis is not necessary if the patient presents with classic features of sarcoidosis. The most easily accessible lesion should be chosen for biopsy. If an easily accessible lesion (ie, skin lesion, lymph node) is not present, then the clinician should consider performing bronchoscopy. During the procedure, a transbronchial lung biopsy can be done and the tissue obtained can be histologically examined. Acid-fast and fungal stains and cultures can be performed to exclude infectious etiologies that may present similarly.

Bronchoalveolar lavage can also yield results consistent with sarcoidosis. Lavage fluid lymphocytosis is common but does not have sufficient sensitivity or specificity to be useful for the diagnosis of sarcoidosis. Other lavage findings found in sarcoidosis include an increased number of CD4 cells, decreased number of CD8 cells, and an increased CD4 to CD8 ratio. If the bronchoalveolar lavage fluid has neutrophils or eosinophils exceeding 2% and 1%, respectively, then diagnoses other than sarcoidosis should be considered.

References

Baughman RP, Lower EE, and du Bois RM, "Sarcoidosis," *Lancet*, 2003, 361(9363):1111-8.

Newman LS, Rose CS, and Maier LA, "Sarcoidosis," *N Engl J Med*, 1997, 336(17):1224-34.

Thomas KW and Hunninghake GW, "Sarcoidosis," *JAMA*, 2003, 289(2):3300-3.

CRYOGLOBULINEMIA

STEP 1 – *What Are Cryoglobulins?*

Cryoglobulins are immunoglobulins that spontaneously precipitate at lower temperatures. In may instances, cryoglobulins become soluble as the temperature climbs.

Proceed to Step 2.

STEP 2 – *Who Should Be Tested for Cryoglobulinemia?*

The signs and symptoms of cryoglobulinemia are listed in descending order of frequency in the following box.

CRYOGLOBULINEMIA CLINICAL FEATURES
SKIN LESIONS*
LIVER DISEASE
RENAL DISEASE
ARTHRALGIA / ARTHRITIS
RAYNAUD'S PHENOMENON
NEUROLOGIC MANIFESTATIONS
ACROCYANOSIS
HEMORRHAGE

*Skin manifestations include palpable purpura, changes in pigmentation, petechiae, telangiectasias, urticaria, livedo, and leg ulcers.

Laboratory Features of Cryoglobulinemia

The laboratory features of cryoglobulinemia are listed in the following box.

CRYOGLOBULINEMIA LABORATORY FEATURES
RHEUMATOID FACTOR POSITIVITY (>90%)
INCREASED ERYTHROCYTE SEDIMENTATION RATE (70%)
HYPOCOMPLEMENTEMIA (80%)
ABNORMAL URINALYSIS (>60%)
Hematuria
Pyuria
Proteinuria
ANEMIA (70%)
RENAL INSUFFICIENCY (>40%)
INCREASED TRANSAMINASES (50%)
MONOCLONAL GAMMOPATHY (5%)

If the patient has suggestive signs and symptoms or laboratory findings of cryoglobulinemia, testing should be performed to establish the diagnosis. The presence of a disease associated with cryoglobulinemia strengthens the argument.

Proceed to Step 3.

STEP 3 – *How is Testing for Cryoglobulinemia Performed?*

Testing begins with the collection of serum. Ten to 20 mL of blood should be collected in a prewarmed (37°C) tube. The sample should be kept at this temperature for up to 1 hour to allow for clotting. The serum is then separated from the clot by centrifuging warm for 10 minutes at 2500 rpm. After separation, the serum is incubated at 4°C for 7 days. There should be daily inspection of the specimen in an effort to detect a cryoprecipitate. After a precipitate is detected, the concentration of the cryoglobulin can be measured using one of the following methods:

- Measurement of the packed volume of precipitate (cryocrit)
- Spectrophotometric determination of the protein concentration

The collection process includes a number of steps in which errors can be made, seriously impacting on the ability to detect the presence of cryoglobulins. As a result, misleading information may be obtained in the patient suspected of having cryoglobulinemia if proper care is not exercised.

If cryoglobulins are detected, ***proceed to Step 4.***

If cryoglobulins are not detected, ***consider alternative diagnoses.***

STEP 4 – *What Are the Results of the Serum Protein Electrophoresis?*

Every patient who is found to have cryoglobulinemia requires a serum protein electrophoresis. A serum protein electrophoresis is essential in establishing the presence of a monoclonal protein. The presence of a tall narrow peak on the densitometer tracing and a dense localized band on the gel, indicates that a monoclonal protein is present.

If the serum protein electrophoresis is positive, ***proceed to Step 6.***

If the serum protein electrophoresis is negative, ***proceed to Step 5.***

STEP 5 – *What Are the Results of the Serum Immunofixation Study?*

Every patient with cryoglobulinemia and a negative serum protein electrophoresis should have a serum immunofixation study. This test is more sensitive than the serum protein electrophoresis in the detection of a monoclonal protein. This study will establish the presence of the monoclonal protein, and will also characterize its heavy chain class and light chain type.

If the serum immunofixation test is negative, ***proceed to Step 10.***

If the serum immunofixation test is positive, ***proceed to Step 7.***

STEP 6 – *What Are the Results of the Serum Immunofixation Study?*

When a monoclonal protein is identified on serum protein electrophoresis, it is essential to perform a serum immunofixation study. This study will confirm the presence of the monoclonal protein, and will also characterize its heavy chain class and light chain type.

Proceed to Step 7.

STEP 7 – *What Other Studies Should Be Performed in the Patient With Cryoglobulinemia Found to Have a Monoclonal Protein?*

When a monoclonal protein is identified on serum protein electrophoresis and/or serum immunofixation, the patient has either type I or type II cryoglobulinemia. Further evaluation involves characterization and typing of the cryoglobulins. While immunofixation is useful in typing, other helpful tests include immunoblot and capillary zone electrophoresis. In type I cryoglobulinemia, these tests will demonstrate the presence of a single monoclonal immunoglobulin. Type II cryoglobulinemia is characterized by a mixed picture, consisting of a monoclonal immunoglobulin directed against polyclonal IgG.

If the patient has type I cryoglobulinemia, ***proceed to Step 8***.

If the patient has type II cryoglobulinemia, ***proceed to Step 9***.

STEP 8 – *What Is the Differential Diagnosis of Type I Cryoglobulinemia?*

The differential diagnosis of type I cryoglobulinemia is listed in the following box.

TYPE I CRYOGLOBULINEMIA DIFFERENTIAL DIAGNOSIS
MULTIPLE MYELOMA
WALDENSTRÖM'S MACROGLOBULINEMIA
OTHER LYMPHOPROLIFERATIVE DISORDERS WITH M COMPONENTS

For further information regarding specific disorders associated with type I cryoglobulinemia, the reader is referred to the appropriate chapter.

End of Section.

STEP 9 – *What Is the Differential Diagnosis of Type II Cryoglobulinemia?*

The differential diagnosis of type II cryoglobulinemia is listed in the following box.

TYPE II CRYOGLOBULINEMIA DIFFERENTIAL DIAGNOSIS
WALDENSTRÖM'S MACROGLOBULINEMIA
CHRONIC LYMPHOCYTIC LEUKEMIA
NON-HODGKIN'S LYMPHOMA
COLD AGGLUTININ DISEASE
SJÖGREN'S SYNDROME
OTHER AUTOIMMUNE DISEASES
CHRONIC HEPATITIS C

Hepatitis C viral infection accounts for a considerable number of cryoglobulinemia type II cases. As such, testing for hepatitis C virus should be performed. Testing should be done irrespective of liver function test results. Many patients with hepatitis C viral infection have minimally or intermittently elevated liver function tests. Normal liver function tests, therefore, should not dissuade the clinician from pursuing the diagnosis.

End of Section.

STEP 10 – *What Is the Differential Diagnosis of Type III Cryoglobulinemia?*

In the patient with cryoglobulinemia, a normal serum protein electrophoresis and immunofixation study establishes a diagnosis of type III cryoglobulinemia. The differential diagnosis of type III cryoglobulinemia is listed in the following box.

CAUSES OF TYPE III CRYOGLOBULINEMIA DIFFERENTIAL DIAGNOSIS

- CHRONIC INFECTIONS
  - VIRAL
    - Hepatitis viruses
    - Cytomegalovirus
    - HIV
    - Epstein-Barr virus
  - BACTERIAL
    - Subacute bacterial endocarditis
    - Leprosy
  - SPIROCHETAL
  - FUNGAL
  - PARASITIC
- AUTOIMMUNE DISEASES
  - SYSTEMIC LUPUS ERYTHEMATOSUS
  - RHEUMATOID ARTHRITIS
- INFLAMMATORY BOWEL DISEASE
- BILIARY CIRRHOSIS

Testing for hepatitis C should be performed in every patient found to have type III cryoglobulinemia, since hepatitis C viral infection is a major cause.

End of Section.

References

Dammacco F, Sansonno D, Piccoli C, et al, "The Cryoglobulins: An Overview," *Eur J Clin Invest*, 2001, 31(7):628-38.

Della Rossa A, Trevisani G, and Bombardieri S, "Cryoglobulins and Cryoglobulinemia. Diagnostic and Therapeutic Considerations," *Clin Rev Allergy Immunol*, 1998, 16(3):249-64.

Dispenzieri A and Gorevic PD, "Cryoglobulinemia," *Hematol Oncol Clin North Am*, 1999, 13(6):1315-49.

Ferri C, Zignego AL, and Pileri SA, "Cryoglobulins," *J Clin Pathol*, 2002, 55(1):4-13.

Lunel F and Musset L, "Hepatitis C Virus Infection and Cryoglobulinemia," *J Hepatol*, 1998, 29(5):848-55.

AMYLOIDOSIS

There are four major forms of amyloidosis. These include primary (AL) amyloidosis, secondary (AA) amyloidosis, the heredofamilial form of amyloidosis, and dialysis-related (β_2-microglobulin) amyloidosis.

Clinical Manifestations

The clinical manifestations of AL amyloidosis are listed in the following box.

AMYLOIDOSIS (TYPE AL) CLINICAL FEATURES
NEPHROTIC SYNDROME PERIPHERAL NEUROPATHY AUTONOMIC NEUROPATHY MUSCLE WEAKNESS RESTRICTIVE CARDIOMYOPATHY CARPAL TUNNEL SYNDROME GIANT HEPATOMEGALY MALABSORPTION CUTANEOUS PURPURA (particularly periorbital) MACROGLOSSIA

AA amyloidosis should be suspected in the patient who develops significant proteinuria (nephrotic syndrome) in the setting of a long-standing chronic inflammatory disorder. Some of these inflammatory disorders include osteomyelitis, tuberculosis, rheumatoid arthritis, and inflammatory bowel disease.

Renal Disease in Amyloidosis

In primary (AL) amyloidosis, >50% of patients have significant proteinuria (>1 g/day). At the time of diagnosis, approximately 33% of patients have nephrotic range proteinuria, often accompanied by hyperlipidemia and hypoalbuminemia. Between 10% and 20% of patients have renal insufficiency defined as a serum creatinine >2.0 mg/dL at the time of presentation.

Secondary (AA) amyloidosis is also characterized by renal disease. In fact, renal disease is the most common manifestation of this type of amyloidosis. Proteinuria or renal insufficiency, or both, may occur in these patients. When a patient with a chronic inflammatory disorder develops proteinuria, AA amyloidosis should be a consideration.

Hematologic Disease in Amyloidosis

In primary amyloidosis, the serum monoclonal protein is usually small. In many cases, the concentration is <1 g/dL. It is possible to identify a monoclonal protein in about 95% of patients with primary amyloidosis, using serum and urine electrophoresis / immunofixation.

Anemia is often present but seldom does the patient require transfusion. With the development of renal failure, however, a transfusion-dependent anemia may occur. Thrombocytosis and the presence of Howell-Jolly bodies may herald the presence of functional hyposplenism.

Abnormalities of the coagulation system include a prolonged thrombin time (up to 50% of cases) and factor X deficiency (10% of cases).

Establishing the Diagnosis

The diagnosis of amyloidosis is established through biopsy of any one of the following sites.

1. Abdominal fat pad

   Tissue biopsy forms the cornerstone of diagnosis. The subcutaneous tissue of the abdominal fat pad is quite accessible and amyloid deposits are commonly found here. For these reasons, an abdominal fat pad aspirate is the initial test of choice. In various studies, it has been found to be positive in 80% to 95% of patients with amyloidosis. An abdominal fat aspirate is useful in establishing the diagnosis of AL, AA, and familial ATTR forms of the disease. However, it is not useful in those patients suspected of having β_2-microglobulin amyloidosis.

2. Bone marrow biopsy

   In many patients with amyloidosis, a bone marrow biopsy is done to determine not only the number of plasma cells, but also the clonality of the cells. Bone marrow staining for amyloid is positive in 50% to 60% of patients with amyloidosis.

3. Rectal biopsy

   If neither the abdominal fat aspirate or bone marrow biopsy provides the diagnosis in a patient suspected of having amyloidosis, the clinician should proceed to rectal biopsy. Rectal biopsy is positive in 75% of cases of patients with AL amyloidosis.

If all of the above sites are negative, the clinician should direct attention to an organ that is clinically affected by the systemic process. Affected organs that have high yield in the diagnosis include liver, kidney, and heart.

Before performing a biopsy, it is important to ensure that the patient does not have an abnormality of the clotting system. Even when patients with amyloidosis do not have laboratory evidence of a clotting abnormality, they remain at increased risk of bleeding because of the deposition of amyloid fibrils in the walls of small blood vessels.

Once a biopsy is obtained, the specimen should be stained with Congo red. Amyloid fibrils display apple-green birefringence when observed under polarized light.

References

Falk RH and Skinner M, "The Systemic Amyloidoses: An Overview," *Adv Intern Med*, 2000, 45:107-37.

Gertz MA, Lacy MQ, and Dispenzieri A, "Amyloidosis," *Hematol Oncol Clin North Am*, 1999, 13(6):1211-33, ix.

Sezer O, Eucker J, Jakob C, et al, "Diagnosis and Treatment of AL Amyloidosis," *Clin Nephrol*, 2000, 53(6):417-23.

PART IX:

INFECTIOUS DISEASE

CELLULITIS

Cellulitis is a commonly encountered infection, affecting the skin and subcutaneous fat. Patients often report redness, swelling, and pain of the involved skin. Fever may or may not be present. Physical examination usually reveals erythema, tenderness, edema, and warmth of the affected area. Although most cases are diagnosed clinically, laboratory testing does have a role in certain situations (see table below).

Laboratory Test Findings in Patients With Cellulitis

Lab Test	Clinical Significance
Blood cultures	Do not need to be obtained in most cases of cellulitis since the yield is typically low. In patients who present with severe disease, high grade fever, marked leukocytosis, toxic presentation, or immunocompromised state, cultures should be obtained.
Serologic testing for group A streptococcus	Group A streptococcus is a common cause of cellulitis Positive serologic tests (antistreptolysin O, antideoxyribonuclease B, antihyaluronidase, Streptozyme antibody assay) support the diagnosis. Results are not often available at a time when treatment needs to be instituted.
Needle aspiration cultures of the leading edge	Not performed in most cases, since the yield of a positive test result is <20%. Should be considered in immunocompromised patients, those who have a lack of response to therapy, or when infection due to an atypical organism is suspected. Skin biopsy cultures have been found to have higher yield then needle aspiration.
Radiologic imaging	Not necessary in most cases. Plain radiographs may identify foreign body, presence of gas, or involvement of bones. CT or MRI can be obtained if deeper infection is suspected.

References

Morris A, "Cellulitis and Erysipelas," *Clin Evid*, 2002, (7):1483-7.

Stulberg DL, Penrod MA, and Blatny RA, "Common Bacterial Skin Infections," *Am Fam Physician*, 2002, 66(1):119-24.

URINARY TRACT INFECTION

Usually, it is the history and physical examination that prompts the clinician to consider the possibility that a patient has a urinary tract infection. In almost all cases, laboratory testing is obtained to support or confirm the diagnosis. Urinalysis abnormalities found in patients with urinary tract infection are described in the following table.

Urinalysis Abnormalities in the Patient With Urinary Tract Infection

Lab Test	Clinical Significance
Urine WBCs	Pyuria is one of the key urinalysis findings in patients with UTI. In fact, the absence of pyuria should prompt consideration of other causes of the patient's symptoms (urethritis or vaginitis). Significant pyuria is said to be present when examination of spun urine sediment reveals the presence of >10 WBC/hpf. A more accurate technique is the counting chamber method, in which unspun urine is examined. With this method, significant pyuria is defined as $>10/mm^3$. Pyuria is not synonymous with urinary tract infection although there is a high association between the two. Presence of white blood cell casts signifies upper urinary tract infection. Pyuria can occur in the absence of bacterial infection. Causes of "sterile pyuria" include the acute urethral syndrome, urinary tuberculosis, foreign body of the urinary tract, urinary tract malignancy, interstitial cystitis, contamination of the urine with vaginal leukocytes, nephrolithiasis, and chronic interstitial nephritis. In patients with renal abscess, pyuria may be lacking if the abscess is not in communication with the collecting system. This is not uncommon with abscesses that are the result of hematogenous spread (eg, those due to *Staphylococcus*).
Urine leukocyte esterase	Can be used as an alternative to the microscopic examination of the urine sediment for WBCs (pyuria). Sensitivity for the detection of pyuria is 75% to 95% Specificity for the detection of significant pyuria is 94% to 98% Microscopic examination of the urine for WBCs is recommended when the leukocyte esterase test is negative but the patient has symptoms/signs consistent with urinary tract infection.
Urine bacteria	Microscopic examination of the urinary sediment may demonstrate bacteriuria in patients with UTI. In order to see bacteria (in unspun urine), higher colony counts are necessary (usually $>10^5$/mL). Avoid any delays in the processing of the urine specimen for culture because colony counts can increase if the specimen is allowed to sit at room temperature for a long period of time (>1-2 hours). When bacteria are present in the urine in the absence of pyuria, it usually is the result of contamination. However, some patients may have asymptomatic bacteriuria, which is important to identify in certain settings (pregnancy, before and after urologic instrumentation or manipulation, after removal of chronic indwelling Foley catheter).

Urinalysis Abnormalities in the Patient With Urinary Tract Infection *(continued)*

Lab Test	Clinical Significance
Urine Gram stain	Particularly useful in the evaluation and management of patients with urosepsis, severe pyelonephritis, and those at risk for enterococcal UTI. If the Gram stain reveals gram-positive cocci, enterococcal UTI should be a major consideration. This should be taken into account when selecting appropriate antibiotic therapy. If the Gram stain reveals gram-negative organisms, it is not necessary to treat the patient for enterococcal UTI.
Urine red blood cells (hematuria)	Hematuria is noted in 50% of women with acute cystitis. Hematuria is uncommonly present in patients with vaginitis or urethritis, two major considerations in the differential diagnosis of acute cystitis.
Urine nitrite	Will be positive if infection is due to Enterobacteriaceae and the organism is present in colony counts $>10^5$/mL. These organisms have the ability to convert nitrate to nitrite. May be negative with lower colony counts of *Enterobacteriaceae.* Negative if enterococcal or staphylococcal organism is causing UTI.
Urine culture	Urine culture is not always necessary. For example, women with uncomplicated urinary tract infections can be treated without culture. This approach has been shown in studies to be cost-effective. Culture should be obtained, however, in patients with complicated UTI and pyelonephritis. It is important to exercise proper care in the collection of the urine specimen for culture (should be clean-catch, midstream urine). This will help avoid urethral, vaginal, or perineum contamination of the specimen. Avoid delays in the processing of the urine specimen for culture because bacteria present in urine that is left to stand for a long period of time at room temperature will proliferate (leading to an increase in colony counts). If necessary, the specimen can be stored in the refrigerator for up to 48 hours without significant change or proliferation. Traditionally, urine colony counts $>10^5$/mL were considered significant while counts $<10^4$/mL were considered to be contaminants. It is now known that 1/3 of women with lower UTI have lower colony counts (10^2 to 10^4/mL). With this being the case, the growth of a single or predominant uropathogen in colony counts $>10^2$/mL should be considered significant. In men with dysuria, colony counts $>10^3$/mL of a single or predominant uropathogen is considered to be significant. Colony counts $>10^2$/mL are considered significant when the specimen for urine culture is obtained by straight catheterization or suprapubic aspiration. The growth of lactobacilli, diphtheroids, *Staphylococcus epidermidis*, and *Gardnerella vaginalis* generally reflects contamination. When culture results reveal the growth of two or more species, it usually signifies contamination, especially if the patient has a normal urinary tract. In these cases, another culture should be obtained.

Blood cultures are not necessary in every patient with urinary tract infection. Blood cultures are not required in patients with lower urinary tract infection. In patients with upper urinary tract infection (pyelonephritis), blood cultures should be obtained if the patient is febrile, has rigors, or if the illness requires hospitalization. In patients with pyelonephritis, leukocytosis (often with a left shift) is commonly present.

SEPSIS

Sepsis is defined as the systemic inflammatory response to infection. It is said to be present when both of the following are present:

- Systemic inflammatory response syndrome (2 or more of the following):
  - Temperature >38°C or <36°C
  - Heart rate >90 beats/minute
  - Tachypnea (respiratory rate >20 /minute) or hyperventilation ($PaCO_2$ <32 mm Hg)
  - WBC >12,000 /microliter or <4,000/ microliter or >10% immature neutrophils (bands)
- Infection (definitive evidence for infection present)

It needs to be differentiated from the systemic inflammatory response syndrome (defined above), bacteremia, severe sepsis, and septic shock. In 1992, the American College of Physicians defined these various terms, as shown in the following table.

Sepsis-Related Definitions

Term	Definition
Bacteremia	Presence of viable bacteria in the blood
Systemic inflammatory response syndrome	See text above
Severe sepsis	Sepsis + organ dysfunction or hypotension or hypoperfusion
Septic shock	Severe sepsis + sepsis-induced hypotension (not responsive to adequate volume resuscitation) + perfusion abnormalities

Laboratory Testing

The evaluation of the patient with or suspected of having sepsis begins with a thorough history and physical exam. Laboratory testing is also an essential part of the evaluation. Diagnostic studies should be obtained expeditiously without delaying the institution of antibiotic therapy in seriously ill patients.

The following box describes key information about blood culture testing in these patients.

SOME IMPORTANT POINTS ABOUT BLOOD CULTURES IN THE PATIENT WITH SEPSIS
• Blood cultures are an essential part of the evaluation of the patient with or suspected of having sepsis.
• The clinician should realize that negative blood cultures will be found in a considerable number of sepsis patients. Some possible reasons include the administration of prior antimicrobial therapy, inadequate volume of blood cultured (at least 10 mL should be cultured but 20 mL is preferable), and infection due to fastidious or slow-growing pathogens (notify laboratory if suspected to maximize recovery of organism).
• False-positive blood culture results are common. The challenge lies in differentiating true pathogens from contaminants.
• Avoid the still common practice of obtaining a single blood culture. Instead, collect 2-3 sets of blood cultures (taken from separate venipuncture sites).

(continued)

(continued)

SOME IMPORTANT POINTS ABOUT BLOOD CULTURES IN THE PATIENT WITH SEPSIS
• If possible, avoid obtaining blood from the femoral vessels because of the higher contamination rate (when compared to upper extremity vessels).
• If possible, avoid obtaining cultures through intravenous or intra-arterial catheters. If cultures are obtained through an intravenous line, be sure to obtain another culture via peripheral venipuncture.
• Blood cultures are usually discarded after 5-7 days of incubation (if negative). The clinician should notify the laboratory if a fastidious pathogen is suspected. Some of these pathogens require a longer incubation period. Fungal and mycobacterial blood cultures are routinely incubated for 4-6 weeks.
• The recovery of certain organisms is highly suggestive of the presence of true bloodstream infection (*N. meningitides*, *N. gonorrhoeae*, *E. coli*, *Enterobacteriaceae P. aeruginosa*, *Histoplasma capsulatum*, *Cryptococcus neoformans*, *Streptococcus pneumoniae*, and *Staphylococcus aureus*).
• Some organisms rarely cause bloodstream infection and their recovery usually suggests contamination. These organisms include *Corynebacterium* species, *Bacillus* species, and *Propionibacterium acnes*. Please note that even an organism typically recognized as a contaminant can cause true bloodstream infection. An example would be the isolation of *Corynebacterium jekeium* in the neutropenic patient with an indwelling catheter.
• Coagulase-negative staphylococci (ie, *S. epidermidis*) is a common contaminant but can also be a true pathogen (catheter infection, joint prosthesis infection, prosthetic heart valve endocarditis). This underscores the importance of always evaluating the culture result in the context of the patient's clinical presentation.

In addition to blood cultures, many other laboratory tests may be abnormal in the sepsis patient. These abnormalities and their clinical significance are noted in the following table.

Laboratory Test Abnormalities in the Sepsis Patient

Lab Test	Clinical Significance
Blood culture	See table above
WBC count	Leukocytosis with left shift (presence of immature WBCs) suggestive of infection. Normal WBC count does not rule out infection (left shift may be revealing in these cases). Low WBC count does not rule out infection and may occur in severe sepsis (left shift may be revealing in these cases). Neutropenia is a risk factor for bacterial and fungal infection. Review of the peripheral blood smear may reveal the presence of vacuolization, toxic granulations, or Döhle bodies in PMNs.
Hemoglobin / hematocrit	Should be obtained to ensure that the patient has adequate oxygen delivery. Maintain hemoglobin >10 g/dL
Platelet count	Infection can be associated with reactive thrombocytosis. Sepsis can cause thrombocytopenia, which may be severe. Sepsis is also a cause of disseminated intravascular coagulation. A DIC panel should be obtained in the septic patient with thrombocytopenia.
Prothrombin time	Elevated when sepsis is complicated by DIC

(continued)

Laboratory Test Abnormalities in the Sepsis Patient *(continued)*

Lab Test	Clinical Significance
Partial thromboplastin time	Elevated when sepsis is complicated by DIC
BUN Serum creatinine	When elevated, consider volume depletion as well as acute tubular necrosis due to sepsis
Electrolytes	Electrolyte abnormalities can certainly occur in sepsis patients. Low serum bicarbonate suggests the presence of metabolic acidosis. Elevated anion gap in the setting of metabolic acidosis is not uncommon in sepsis and is usually due to lactic acidosis. Other causes of metabolic acidosis should also be considered (ie, diabetic ketoacidosis precipitated by infection).
Liver function test abnormalities	Common in patients with severe sepsis and may be due to the sepsis itself. Abnormalities may also be due to liver (ie, liver abscess) or biliary infection (ie, cholecystitis/cholangitis).
Amylase Lipase	Elevated levels (in the absence of shock) should prompt consideration of acute pancreatitis, which can present with some of the same features found in sepsis. It is important to realize that both are causes of the systemic inflammatory response syndrome. In patients with septic shock, however, elevated amylase and lipase levels may be a reflection of end-organ damage.
C-reactive protein	Often elevated in infection/sepsis but is not specific. Levels do not correlate with severity of the illness. Can be used to assess response to therapy (levels should normalize with successful therapy).
Arterial blood gas analysis	Essential part of the evaluation of the septic patient. Helpful in assessing the need for intubation/ventilatory support. Metabolic acidosis is common, often due to lactic acidosis. Respiratory alkalosis (from hyperventilation) is an early sign. Lung / CNS evaluation indicated in patients with respiratory acidosis.
Urinalysis	Urinary tract infection is a major cause of sepsis. If urinalysis is consistent with infection, urine culture is warranted. If acute tubular necrosis due to sepsis has developed, urinalysis abnormalities of acute tubular necrosis may be noted.

Laboratory Test Abnormalities in the Sepsis Patient *(continued)*

Lab Test	Clinical Significance
Gram stain/acid-fast stain/other stains of appropriate specimens	If possible, obtain Gram stain before starting antimicrobial therapy. Acid-fast stains should be obtained if tuberculous or nontuberculous mycobacterial infection is suspected. In some labs, mycobacterial species can now be identified more rapidly with the use of gene probe testing Direct fluorescent antibody stains are available for the detection of certain pathogens (ie, *Legionella*) Fungal stains should be obtained when fungal infection is suspected. The above stains can often provide important information well before culture results become available.
Cultures	In addition to blood cultures, other appropriate cultures should be obtained, depending on the patient's clinical presentation (ie, urine, sputum, CSF, catheter, wound). Positive culture results allow the clinician to identify the etiologic organism and determine antibiotic susceptibility. If fastidious organisms are suspected, it is important to communicate this to the laboratory.
Stool studies	Fecal leukocytes and stool cultures should be performed in the sepsis patient with diarrhea. *C. difficile* toxin testing may also be obtained, depending on the patient's clinical presentation (recent antibiotic usage).
Serology	Serologic testing that may be useful in the sepsis patient includes the following: – Testing for the presence of the *Legionella pneumophilia* serogroup 1 antigen in the urine (if Legionella infection suspected) – Testing for the cryptococcal antigen (if *C. neoformans* infection suspected) – Acute and convalescent antibody titers
Lumbar puncture/CSF analysis	Perform lumbar puncture if the patient has altered mental status or other manifestations of CNS infection (be sure that the patient does not have any contraindications to the procedure)

References

Aird WC, "The Hematologic System as a Marker of Organ Dysfunction in Sepsis," *Mayo Clin Proc*, 2003, 78(7):869-81.

HELICOBACTER PYLORI

Helicobacter pylori is a curved, microaerophilic Gram-negative bacillus. It is a motile organism with flagella at one end. The prevalence of infection increases with advancing age. In developing countries, most individuals have acquired the infection by late adolescence or young adulthood. In developed countries, however, the prevalence of infection is much lower.

H. pylori infection and NSAID use have been found to be the two major risk factors for the development of peptic ulcer disease (both gastric and duodenal ulcers). In fact, over 90% of patients with duodenal ulcer disease have been found to have infection (excluding those taking NSAIDs). It is quite clear that the eradication of *H. pylori* in patients with peptic ulcer disease significantly decreases the recurrence rate of the ulcer disease.

Who Should Be Tested?

Although *H. pylori* infection is a major risk factor for the development of peptic ulcer disease, most patients with infection do not develop disease. In fact, only about 20% of infected patents develop ulcer disease at some point during their life. At the current time, it is not clear why some patients develop ulcer disease while others do not. In the following table, indications for testing are listed.

Patient with.....	Is Testing Indicated?	Clinical Significance
Duodenal ulcer (active)	Yes	*H. pylori* infection and NSAIDs use are the two major causative factors. Eradication of the organism decreases the rate of ulcer recurrence
Gastric ulcer (active)	Yes	*H. pylori* infection and NSAIDs use are the two major causative factors. Eradication of the organism decreases the rate of ulcer recurrence
Past history of peptic ulcer disease (documented by radiography or endoscopy)	Yes (especially if the patient has not been treated for *H. pylori*)	Eradication of the organism decreases the rate of ulcer recurrence
No symptoms	No	Possible exceptions to this rule may be in patients with family history of gastric cancer or those who live in geographic areas with an increased incidence of gastric cancer
Nonulcer dyspepsia	Controversial	Many clinicians are testing patients with nonulcer dyspepsia for *H. pylori* infection but the data to support this is not convincing. The position of the American College of Gastroenterology is as follows: "There is no conclusive evidence that eradication of *H. pylori* infection will reverse the symptoms of nonulcer dyspepsia. Patients may be tested for *H. pylori* on a case-by-case basis, and treatment offered to those with a positive result."

Establishing the Diagnosis

The diagnosis of *Helicobacter pylori* infection can be made invasively or noninvasively.

DIAGNOSTIC TESTING FOR *H. pylori* INFECTION
Invasive (requiring endoscopy)
Culture
Campylobacter-like organism (Clo) test
Histology
Noninvasive
Urea breath test
Serology
Stool antigen test
13C-bicarbonate assay

These tests will be discussed in more detail in the remainder of this chapter.

Invasive Testing

Invasive tests are those that require endoscopy for their performance and are listed in the following table.

Invasive Test	Clinical Significance
Culture	Not usually performed because the procedure/technique is difficult Used in research studies to obtain susceptibility of *H. pylori* to antibiotics Should be considered in patients with refractory disease (not responding to standard antimicrobial regimens) to assess for resistance
Histology	Multiple biopsies of the body and fundus of the stomach are recommended because the organism may have a patchy distribution More expensive than the Clo test (see below) False-negative test results may occur because of sampling error or because of interobserver variability Sensitivity of the test may also be decreased if the patient is taking antisecretory therapy
Clo test	Clo (*Campylobacter*-like organism) test is one type of biopsy urease testing In this test, tissue obtained by endoscopy is added to a solution of urea and phenol red. If *H. pylori* is present, its urease enzyme will metabolize the urea to ammonia, resulting in an increased pH (>6.0). The increase in the pH will lead to a color change (pink), which is easily detected. Results are often available within one hour of inoculation although a final reading should take place at 24 hours Sensitivity and specificity are 90% to 95% and 95% to 100%, respectively False-negative test results can occur with gastrointestinal bleeding or with the use of proton pump inhibitors, H_2-blockers, bismuth-containing compounds, or antibiotics. If a negative test result is thought to be a false-negative, another type of *H. pylori* test should be obtained (histology, serology).

Noninvasive Testing

Noninvasive tests available for the diagnosis of *H. pylori* infection are listed in the following table.

Noninvasive Test	Clinical Significance
Urea breath test	American College of Gastroenterology has identified this test as the noninvasive test of choice for the diagnosis of *H. pylori* infection Sensitivity and specificity are 88% to 95% and 95% to 100%, respectively Useful not only for the diagnosis but also in assessing the effectiveness of therapy In this test, carbon 13- or 14-labeled urea solution is ingested. If *H. pylori* is present, its urease enzyme will metabolize the urea, leading to the formation of ammonia and radiolabeled CO_2. This CO_2 is absorbed into the bloodstream and expired in the breath, where it can be detected. If the test is being performed for the initial diagnosis of *H. pylori* infection, to avoid false-negative test results, antibiotics and proton pump inhibitors should be discontinued for at least 4 and 2 weeks, respectively (before testing) Because false-negative test results can occur with the use of antimicrobial agents and proton pump inhibitors, the urea breath test should not be performed until at least 4 weeks have passed after completion of *H. pylori* therapy (when performing testing to assess the effectiveness of therapy).
Serology	Relatively inexpensive Sensitivity and specificity range from 90% to 100% and 76% to 96%, respectively Accuracy of the test is diminished in elderly and cirrhotic patients. In these two groups, alternative testing should be considered. Can be used for assessing effectiveness of *H. pylori* therapy but not in the short-term or in the early follow-up of treated patients. Titers must be followed for a long period of time because the rate of decline is not rapid. Some patients have detectable antibodies for months to years after eradication therapy (therefore serology can be considered to be less useful than some of the other tests for assessing the response to therapy).
Stool antigen assay	Patients with *H. pylori* infection excrete the organism in their stools Sensitivity and specificity of fecal/stool assays are 94% and 86% to 92%, respectively False-positive test results have been reported in patients with acute upper gastrointestinal bleeding Can be used for initial diagnosis as well as assessing the effectiveness of therapy but false-negative test results have been reported in patients who are taking or who have recently been on bismuth-containing compounds or proton pump inhibitors. When assessing response to therapy, testing should not be performed until at least 4-6 weeks have passed after completion of therapy
13C bicarbonate assay	In this test, a serum specimen is obtained before and then 60 minutes after the ingestion of 13C-urea rich meal Sensitivity and specificity of 92% and 96%, respectively (when compared to the urea breath test)

References

Anderson J and Gonzalez J, "*H. pylori* Infection. Review of the Guideline for Diagnosis and Treatment," *Geriatrics*, 2000, 55(6):44-9.

Braden B and Caspary WF, "Detection of *Helicobacter pylori* Infection: When to Perform Which Test?" *Ann Med*, 2001, 33(2):91-7.

Ho B and Marshall BJ, "Accurate Diagnosis of *Helicobacter pylori*. Serologic Testing," *Gastroenterol Clin North Am*, 2000, 29(4):853-62.

McColl K, "Should Noninvasive *Helicobacter pylori* Testing Replace Endoscopy in Investigation of Dyspepsia?" *Helicobacter*, 2000, 5(Suppl 1):S11-5; discussion S27-31.

Monteiro L, de Mascarel A, Sarrasqueta AM, et al, "Diagnosis of *Helicobacter pylori* Infection: Noninvasive Methods Compared to Invasive Methods and Evaluation of Two New Tests," *Am J Gastroenterol*, 2001, 96(2):353-8.

Nakamura RM, "Laboratory Tests for the Evaluation of *Helicobacter pylori* Infections," *Ann Med*, 2001, 15(6):301-7.

Roberts AP, Childs SM, Rubin G, et al, "Tests for *Helicobacter pylori* Infection: A Critical Appraisal From Primary Care," *Fam Pract*, 2000, Suppl 2:S12-20.

SYPHILIS

SEROLOGIC TESTS

Which Serologic Tests Are Available for Diagnosing Syphilis?

The serologic tests available for the diagnosis of syphilis include the nontreponemal and treponemal tests. Of the nontreponemal tests, the most useful are the Venereal Disease Research Laboratory (VDRL) and the Rapid Plasmin Reagin (RPR) tests. These tests depend on the appearance of antibodies (reagin) found in the serum. These antibodies, usually IgG and IgM, are directed against cardiolipin-lecithin-cholesterol antigens. The results of these tests are reported as reactive, weakly reactive, or nonreactive. When nontreponemal tests are reactive, specimens are diluted and the test is repeated to give a quantitative result.

A positive test result may not occur until 3-5 weeks after initial infection. In fact, these tests are only positive in 75% of patients with primary syphilis. VDRL and RPR are quantitative tests. As a result, these tests are useful in following the activity of the disease, as well as response to therapy. These tests become negative or decrease in titer with appropriate treatment.

Which Conditions Are Associated With a False-Positive VDRL or RPR Test?

A false-positive VDRL or RPR may result from laboratory error, after infection with other treponemal organisms (such as those responsible for conditions such as yaws, bejel, and pinta), or it may represent an acute or chronic biological false-positive.

What Conditions Are Associated With a Biological False-Positive VDRL or RPR Test?

Biological false-positive test results may be divided into acute and chronic types. Typically, the antibody titer in patients with a false-positive serologic is low (often <1:8). An acute biological false-positive test result is said to be present when it persists for <6 months. Causes of an acute biological false-positive test result are listed in the following box.

FALSE-POSITIVE VDRL RESULTS ACUTE BIOLOGICAL CAUSES	
VIRAL INFECTION	IMMUNIZATION
Measles	Typhoid
Chickenpox	Yellow fever
Mumps	PREGNANCY
Herpes simplex viral infection	MALARIA
Viral pneumonia	

A chronic false-positive serologic test is defined as one that persists for 6 months. It may last for years, or even the lifetime of the individual. Causes of a chronic false-positive nontreponemal serologic test are listed in the following box.

FALSE-POSITIVE VDRL RESULT CHRONIC BIOLOGICAL CAUSES
SYSTEMIC LUPUS ERYTHEMATOSUS
HEMOLYTIC ANEMIA
MEDICATIONS (antihypertensive agents)
THYROIDITIS
RHEUMATOID ARTHRITIS
DRUG ADDICTION
LEPROSY
MALIGNANCY
ADVANCING AGE

At times, the VDRL or RPR may be positive even before signs of the above conditions are present.

What Treponemal Testing Is Available for the Diagnosis of Syphilis?

Treponemal tests are highly sensitive and specific for the diagnosis of syphilis. These tests are usually ordered to confirm diagnosis. They can also establish the presence of a false-positive nontreponemal test. The most widely used treponemal tests include the fluorescent treponemal antibody – absorption test (FTA-ABS) and the microhemagglutination assay for *T. pallidum* (MHA-TP). The degree of fluorescence dictates the reporting of the FTA-ABS. Results may be reported as negative, minimally reactive (equivocal), or positive.

Since this is a qualitative test, the degree of positivity does not indicate the stage of the illness. Any treponemal test that is equivocal should be repeated. If the repeat test is equivocal or negative, then syphilis is unlikely. A positive test result connotes either past or present infection.

How Do the Sensitivities of the Treponemal and Nontreponemal Tests Compare in Detecting the Various Stages of Syphilis?

Treponemal tests are more sensitive than nontreponemal tests for all stages of syphilis.

	Nontreponemal (VDRL or RPR)	Treponemal (FTA-ABS)
Primary syphilis	75%	85%
Secondary syphilis	99% to 100%	99% to 100%
Latent syphilis	75%	95%
Late syphilis	75%	95%

Because treponemal tests are very sensitive and specific, they are of particular use in patients suspected of having early primary syphilis or tertiary syphilis. At these times, in the course of the syphilitic infection, nontreponemal tests may be negative.

FTA-ABS is the first serologic test to become positive in patients with primary syphilis. As a result, it may be the only serologic test that is positive in patients with early primary disease. The clinician, however, must not forget that all serologic tests may be unrevealing in primary syphilis. It is also important to realize that these treponemal tests can only differentiate treponemal from nontreponemal disease. They are unable to differentiate between illnesses due to different spirochetal organisms. Treponemal tests remain positive for an individual's lifetime, despite appropriate treatment of syphilis.

How Should the Clinician Proceed With the Workup of a Positive Nontreponemal Test in an Asymptomatic Patient?

A commonly encountered problem is the workup of an asymptomatic patient who has a positive nontreponemal test. The first step is to repeat the test to exclude the possibility of laboratory error. If the repeat test remains positive, a treponemal test should be obtained to exclude the possibility of a false-positive nontreponemal test. If the treponemal test is also positive, consider the following possibilities:

- The patient has treated or untreated syphilis.
- The patient has an alternative treponemal infection (ie, yaws, bejel, pinta).

Nontreponemal Test	Treponemal Test	Significance
Positive	Positive	Untreated syphilis Other spirochetal infection (not syphilis)
Negative	Positive	Adequately treated syphilis Untreated early syphilis Untreated late syphilis False-positive teponemal test (rare) Lyme disease (antibody to *Borrelia burgdorferi* may cross react with *T. pallidum* antigens)
Positive	Negative	False-positive test result
Negative	Negative	Very early syphilis Syphilis not present Patient with HIV

PRIMARY SYPHILIS

What Are the Clinical Features of Primary Syphilis?

Primary syphilis is the disease phase in which infection first manifests. Usually, a lesion on the skin or mucous membranes, known as a chancre, appears. More often than not, the chancre is located in the genital region. The clinician should diligently examine the rectum, cervix, anus, and intraurethral areas for the chancre. Extragenital areas may also be affected, including the mouth. The time between exposure and appearance of the lesion is typically 3-5 weeks, but may range from 10-90 days.

How Is the Diagnosis of Primary Syphilis Established?

The diagnosis of primary syphilis may be established using darkfield microscopy from material taken from the lesion. Three separate specimens should be obtained from the lesion for microscopy. Darkfield microscopy should be repeated on 3 consecutive days if the initial examination is unremarkable. Darkfield microscopy is an important test in the diagnosis of primary syphilis, as serologic tests are not always positive at this point in the disease course. Darkfield microscopy requires considerable experience. The clinician should realize that darkfield microscopy is not useful when the chancre is in the mouth, because of the presence of nonpathologic treponemes in the oral cavity. In these cases, direct fluorescence antibody staining for *T. pallidum* may be used instead.

Serology is also important in the diagnosis of primary syphilis. Between 60% and 75% of patients have a positive serologic test. In those with a negative test result, the infection has been present for too short a time period for the development of a sufficient antibody titer. If the initial serologic test (RPR or VDRL) is negative, treatment may be instituted if suspicion for syphilis is high. This should be followed by repeat serologic testing at weekly intervals for 1 month. Alternatively, the clinician may elect to order a treponemal test (FTA-ABS) because of its greater sensitivity in patients with primary syphilis.

SECONDARY SYPHILIS

What Are the Clinical Characteristics of Secondary Syphilis?

Secondary syphilis usually develops 1-2 months after the chancre appears. In approximately 33% of cases, the primary lesion is still present. The lesions of secondary syphilis are usually generalized and affect the skin and mucous membranes. The rash, which is symmetrical in nature, may be macular, papular, maculopapular, papulosquamous, or rarely pustular. The papular lesions may coalesce to form large masses known as condylomata lata. Nonspecific constitutional symptoms including fever, malaise, and anorexia often accompany the other findings. Generalized lymphadenopathy is not uncommon. Since secondary syphilis is characterized by spirochetemia, other findings may be present, reflecting disease at other sites.

How Is the Diagnosis of Secondary Syphilis Established?

As in primary syphilis, darkfield microscopy may be diagnostic in material taken from mucous membrane lesions, condylomata lata, and lymph node puncture. Rarely, material taken from the skin lesion may reveal the spirochetes. In almost every case, the serologic testing for both nontreponemal and treponemal antibodies will be strongly reactive. A negative test result excludes the diagnosis. The clinician should be aware, however, of a phenomenon known as the "prozone reaction" that can occur in secondary syphilis. This reaction refers to a false-negative nontreponemal antibody test that may result from insufficient dilution of the serum.

LATENT SYPHILIS

Latent syphilis follows secondary syphilis. It may be classified as either early or late disease. Early disease refers to latent syphilis of less than 2 years in duration, whereas late latent syphilis exceeds this period of time. Early or late latent syphilis can only be diagnosed if all of the following are present:

- No overt signs and symptoms in an untreated patient
- Positive serologic tests
- No CSF findings consistent with neurosyphilis

SYPHILIS IN HIV

What Are the Limitations of Nontreponemal and Treponemal Testing in HIV Patients?

False-positive and false-negative serologic test results are not uncommon in HIV patients with syphilis. This, coupled with atypical clinical presentations of syphilis, can make the diagnosis of syphilis extremely difficult in HIV patients. However, in most patients with syphilis, the nontreponemal and treponemal antibody tests remain reliable in establishing diagnosis.

The sensitivity of nontreponemal antibody tests is high in HIV patients infected with syphilis. In general, RPR and VDRL titers are higher in HIV patients when compared to immunocompetent patients with syphilis. However, negative RPR or VDRL test results may occur in HIV patients. This suggests that some patients with HIV may not be able develop an immune response to infection.

Of note, the specificity of nontreponemal tests may be diminished in HIV patients with syphilis. High titers (>1:64) have been reported in HIV patients without syphilis. In general, it is wise to consider a positive nontreponemal antibody test as a marker of active syphilis in an HIV patient until proven otherwise.

Sensitivity of treponemal tests in HIV patients with syphilis remains very high, particularly in patients beyond the primary syphilis stage. A negative treponemal test result obtained in the evaluation of asymptomatic HIV patient having a positive nontreponemal test is strong evidence against the diagnosis of syphilis.

RESPONSE TO THERAPY

With adequate treatment, the titer of the nontreponemal test decreases. A fourfold decline in antibody titer reflects adequate treatment. After treatment, the nontreponemal antibody titer should be followed at 3 and 6 months until titers stabilize or disappear. Relapse or reinfection is heralded by a rise in the nontreponemal antibody titer. It is essential to use the same nontreponemal antibody test (either RPR or VDRL) for assessing the response to therapy.

References

Birnbaum NR, Goldschmidt RH, and Buffett WO, "Resolving the Common Clinical Dilemmas of Syphilis," *Am Fam Physician*, 1999, 59(8):2233-40, 2245-6.

Clyne B and Jerrard DA, "Syphilis Testing," *J Emerg Med*, 2000, 18(3):361-7.

Goldmeier D and Guallar C, "Syphilis: An Update," *Clin Med*, 2003, 3(3):209-11.

Singh AE and Romanowski B, "Syphilis: Review With Emphasis on Clinical, Epidemiologic, and Some Biologic Features," *Clin Microbiol Rev*, 1999, 12(2):187-209.

Wicher K, Horowitz HW, and Wicher V, "Laboratory Methods of Diagnosis of Syphilis for the Beginning of the Third Millennium," *Microbes Infect*, 1999, 1(12):1035-49.

Young H, "Syphilis. Serology," *Dermatol Clin*, 1998, 16(4):691-8.

TUBERCULIN SKIN TESTING

What Is the Basis Behind Tuberculin Skin Testing?

Tuberculin skin testing is an essential test that should be performed on every patient suspected of having tuberculosis. A positive tuberculin skin test signifies infection with tubercle organisms.

The tuberculin used for testing is obtained from cultures of the organism. The injection of this material subcutaneously is followed by examination of the skin 48-72 hours later. Induration of the skin exceeding a certain cutoff level is considered a positive result.

This test is based on delayed hypersensitivity. Following infection with tuberculous organisms, sensitization of T lymphocytes takes approximately 2 months. When an infected patient receives a subcutaneous injection of tuberculin, the previously sensitized lymphocytes are restimulated. Infiltration of the skin site occurs with these activated T lymphocytes, resulting in induration. The reaction is maximal at 48-72 hours after injection.

What Does PPD Stand For?

PPD (purified protein derivative) is a type of tuberculin preparation. There are three different dosage strengths of purified protein derivative. Of the three strengths, the standard test dose involves the use of 5 TUs (tuberculin units).

Who Should Be Skin Tested for Tuberculosis?

Skin testing should be performed on the population groups listed in the following box.

CANDIDATES FOR PPD SCREENING
SIGNS AND SYMPTOMS CONSISTENT WITH TUBERCULOSIS
RADIOGRAPHIC FINDINGS SUGGESTIVE OF TUBERCULOSIS
HIV INFECTION
RECENT CONTACT WITH ACTIVE TUBERCULOSIS
CONDITIONS ASSOCIATED WITH INCREASED RISK OF TB
Diabetes mellitus
Silicosis
End-stage renal disease
Immunosuppressive treatment (including steroids)
Intravenous drug use
Lymphoreticular malignancies
IMMIGRANTS FROM AFRICA, ASIA, LATIN AMERICA, AND OCEANIA
HOSPITAL EMPLOYEES
NURSING HOME RESIDENTS / WORKERS
PRISON EMPLOYEES / INMATES
RESIDENTS / WORKERS IN MENTAL HEALTH INSTITUTIONS

What Degree of Reaction Is Considered a Positive PPD Result?

A reaction ≥5 mm of induration is considered positive in population groups listed in the following box.

PATIENTS IN WHOM A ≥5 mm INDURATION INDICATES PPD POSITIVITY
HIV POSITIVE
HIGH RISK FOR HIV (unknown HIV status)
CHEST X-RAY CONSISTENT WITH OLD INACTIVE TUBERCULOSIS
RECENT, CLOSE CONTACT WITH ACTIVE TUBERCULOSIS
S/P ORGAN TRANSPLANTATION
CORTICOSTEROID THERAPY (greater than the equivalent of 15 mg/day of prednisone for >1 month)

A reaction >10 mm is considered positive in the population groups listed in the following box.

PATIENTS IN WHOM A ≥10 mm INDURATION INDICATES PPD POSITIVITY
INTRAVENOUS DRUG USERS
FOREIGN BORN INDIVIDUALS FROM AREAS ENDEMIC FOR TB
Africa
Asia
Latin America
HIGH-RISK RACIAL GROUPS / ETHNIC MINORITIES
Hispanics
Native Americans
African Americans
INDIVIDUALS IN PRISON
RESIDENTS OF NURSING HOMES
RESIDENTS OF MENTAL INSTITUTIONS
HEALTHCARE WORKERS
SILICOSIS
DIABETES MELLITUS
GASTRECTOMY
HEMATOLOGIC MALIGNANCIES
IMMUNOSUPPRESSIVE TREATMENT
RESIDENTS OF SHELTERS
CHRONIC RENAL FAILURE
JEJUNOILEAL BYPASS
WEIGHT LOSS >10% OF IDEAL BODY WEIGHT
CHILDREN <4 YEARS OF AGE

A reaction >15 mm is considered positive in all other patients.

Does a Negative Skin Test Reaction Exclude the Diagnosis of Tuberculosis?

A negative skin test reaction to tuberculin does not exclude the diagnosis. While a negative reaction may signify the absence of tuberculous infection, there are many reasons why a skin test may be negative in a patient with active tuberculosis. These factors are listed in the following box.

FACTORS CAUSING FALSE-NEGATIVE PPD SKIN TESTS
IMPROPER STORAGE OF TUBERCULIN
POOR TECHNIQUE
Not enough antigen administered
Injection given too deep
MISTAKES IN READING THE TEST
HIV INFECTION (33% of patients)
VIRAL INFECTION
Measles
Varicella
BACTERIAL INFECTION
IMMUNOSUPPRESSIVE MEDICATIONS / CORTICOSTEROIDS
SARCOIDOSIS
CHRONIC RENAL FAILURE
LIVE VIRUS VACCINATION
MALNUTRITION
LYMPHORETICULAR MALIGNANCIES
Hodgkin's disease
OVERWHELMING *M. TUBERCULOSIS* INFECTION
OVERWHELMING ILLNESS OF ANY TYPE

What Is the Booster Effect?

Waning of skin test reactivity often occurs with advancing age. This can result in false-negative skin testing in the patient with tuberculosis. This false-negative skin testing can be overcome by repeat testing 1-3 weeks after the initial test. This will help to unmask a positive result by enhancing the reaction. This is known as the booster effect. The second skin test result is considered to be the patient's baseline response. If a patient with an initially negative skin test is tested 1 year rather than several weeks later, the booster effect may be misconstrued as a recent conversion. Performing a second skin test shortly after the initial negative test will avoid this misinterpretation. This is particularly useful in the patient who will receive serial skin testing.

References

Ciesielski SD, "BCG Vaccination and the PPD Test: What the Clinician Needs to Know," *J Fam Pract*, 1995, 40(1):76-80.

Curley C, "New Guidelines: What to Do About an Unexpected Positive Tuberculin Skin Test," *Cleve Clin J Med*, 2003, 70(1):49-55.

Huebner RE, Schein MF, and Bass JB Jr, "The Tuberculin Skin Test," *Clin Infect Dis*, 1993, 17(6):968-75.

Jasmer RM, Nahid P, and Hopewell PC, "Clinical Practice. Latent Tuberculosis Infection," *N Engl J Med*, 2002, 347(23):1860-6.

Mackin LA, "Screening for Tuberculosis in the Primary Care Setting," *Lippincotts Prim Care Pract*, 1998, 2(6):599-610.

Ortona L and Fantoni M, "Tuberculin Skin Test and Chemoprophylaxis of Tuberculosis," *Rays*, 1998, 23(1):218-24.

Pickwell SM, "Positive PPD and Chemoprophylaxis for Tuberculosis Infection," *Am Fam Physician*, 1995, 51(8):1929-34, 1937-8.

PART X:

CARDIOLOGY

CARDIAC MARKERS

Although many patients with an acute myocardial infarction (AMI) will present with the classic history of severe chest pain and have EKG findings of ST elevation and pathologic Q waves, approximately 25% of patients will not. Approximately 50% of patients who come through the emergency room with a myocardial infarction have nondiagnostic EKGs. It is for this reason that when a patient is suspected of having myocardial damage, in addition to close hemodynamic monitoring, a good physical exam, and serial EKGs, a set of cardiac markers should be obtained.

The cardiac markers include myoglobin, creatine kinase (CK), the MB fraction of creatine kinase (CK-MB), aspartate aminotransferase (AST), lactate dehydrogenase (LDH), and troponin. These are intracellular cardiac markers normally detectable in the blood at very low levels. As the myocytes become necrotic, the cardiac markers will leak out of these cells and ultimately into the vasculature where they can be detected by routine laboratory testing.

Myoglobin

Myoglobin is an oxygen binding protein that is released from myocardial cells when they are injured. Since it has the lowest molecular weight of the marker proteins, it is released into the circulation first. It can be detected 1-4 hours after the insult and peaks at 4-12 hours. Therefore, it is a useful marker for early myocardial damage. Also, it is usually cleared from the circulation within 24 hours and therefore is not a very helpful marker thereafter. Additionally, it is not specific for myocardial damage as it is present not only in cardiac tissue but in skeletal and smooth muscle as well.

Creatine Kinase

Creatine kinase (CK) is another protein that is released from the myocardial cell when it is damaged. Its activity is greatest in striated muscle, brain, and heart tissue. It is a dimer composed of two subunits, B (brain) and M (muscle), with three resulting combinations of BB, MB, and MM. It is the CK-MB dimer that is primarily found in the heart and to a lesser degree in the brain and skeletal muscle, making it the preferred dimer to be measured during suspected cardiac damage. Total CK and CK-MB levels are detectable at 4-6 hours postinjury, peak at 24 hours and begin to fall after that time usually reaching basal levels by 48-72 hours after the acute insult. Therefore, it is important to follow the levels over time to establish this classic rise and fall characteristic of myocardial infarction. Additionally, as there may be variability among laboratories, it is important to calculate the ratio of the CK-MB mass to the total CK activity. This is known as the relative index and is calculated as follows:

RELATIVE INDEX FOR CREATININE KINASE
Relative index = CK-MB mass / total CK activity x 100

If the relative index is >4, then suspicion for myocardial infarction should be high.

Because CK-MB is present in striated cardiac muscle and skeletal muscle, any injury can potentially cause a leak of the CK enzyme. In addition to the aforementioned myocardial infarction, the disorders listed below have all been associated with an increased CK-MB.

DISORDERS ASSOCIATED WITH INCREASED CK-MB
CARDIAC ORIGIN
S/P angioplasty
S/P cardiac surgery
Blunt trauma
Left ventricular hypertrophy
Myocarditis
Pericarditis
SEVERE RHABDOMYOLYSIS*
CHRONIC MUSCLE DISEASE
Polymyositis
Duchenne's muscular dystrophy
MARATHON RUNNERS
CHRONIC RENAL FAILURE REQUIRING DIALYSIS

*Total CK levels can be very high, often in the thousands, with significant elevations of CK-MB. However, the percentage of the total CK is usually <1%.

Many of these disorders listed above will be apparent on history, but can cause confusion in the setting of chest pain. Again, it is for this reason that a single measurement of CK and CK-MB can be misleading. It is the trend over time (rise and fall) that proves most instructive.

Aspartate Aminotransferase

Aspartate aminotransferase is an enzyme that is also released with myocardial infarction. Like CK, in an acute MI, AST rises to a maximum at 24 hours and declines to normal levels at about 48 hours postinfarction. However, it is not specific to cardiac disease in that it may reflect disease of the lung, liver, or skeletal muscle. Therefore, it is not a reliable marker and is now rarely used in diagnosis.

Lactate Dehydrogenase

Like CK, lactate dehydrogenase is an enzyme that is released during myocardial infarction. There are five isoenzymes which include LDH_1, LDH_2, LDH_3, LDH_4 and LDH_5, with LDH_1 and LDH_2 being most abundant in the heart. Under normal conditions, serum LDH_2 levels are higher than LDH_1 levels. During acute myocardial infarction, there is a characteristic "LDH flip" that occurs in which LDH_1 levels increase to a greater degree than LDH_2 thus altering the usual LDH_1 to LDH_2 ratio. This change in the usual ratio should, therefore, raise suspicion for an infarction.

LDH levels do not begin to rise until 12-18 hours, do not peak until 48-72 hours postinfarction and are therefore of little help in early diagnosis. They are primarily used if a myocardial infarction is suspected to have occurred more than 24 hours prior to admission, when the CK enzyme levels are declining. The LDH isoenzyme levels remain elevated up to 10 days postinfarction.

Additionally, LDH isoenzymes are not specific for myocardial damage and can be elevated in hemolysis, megaloblastic anemia, liver, renal, and skeletal muscle disease.

With the advent of more specific cardiac markers, such as troponin described below, the use of LDH has fallen out of favor. Its only use, therefore, would be in facilities where troponin is not available.

Troponin

Troponin is the most sensitive and specific of the commercially available cardiac markers. It is a protein complex that regulates contraction of striated muscle. It exists in three forms: troponin C, troponin I, and troponin T, which are expressed in myocardial cells. The majority of the troponin is incorporated into the troponin complex, with the remaining 3% to 6% existing unbound in the cytosol.

The troponin C that is expressed in the heart is identical to that expressed in skeletal muscle, and, therefore, is not useful clinically. In contrast, the genes coding for troponin T and I differ in the heart and skeletal muscle. Specific monoclonal antibodies to the cardiac variety of each have been developed. Below, we answer commonly asked questions about cardiac troponin.

Question	Answer
Is cardiac troponin more sensitive than CK-MB?	Yes
Is cardiac troponin more specific than CK-MB?	Yes
When do cardiac troponin levels increase in acute myocardial infarction/injury patients?	Levels begin to rise 3-6 hours after myocardial infarction, roughly about the same time as CK-MB (Troponin I is slightly more sensitive than troponin T within the first 6 hours)
Are cardiac troponins always necessary for the diagnosis of acute myocardial infarction?	When the EKG reveals ST-segment elevation in the patient presenting with ischemic chest pain, cardiac markers, including troponin, can be obtained but the clinician should not wait until results come back before making treatment decisions. In this type of patient, thrombolytic therapy or primary angioplasty should be considered. In other patients with acute coronary syndrome (unstable angina, non-ST segment MI), serial cardiac marker testing, including troponin, is necessary for the diagnosis of acute myocardial infarction.
If the initial cardiac troponin levels are normal in the patient suspected of having an acute myocardial infarction, why is further testing necessary?	Not all myocardial infarction patients will have elevated levels at the time of initial testing. In patents suspected of having unstable angina/ NSTEMI who are presenting to the ER, the ACC/ AHA recently recommended that clinicians obtain a baseline test at the time of the patient's arrival followed by repeat testing 8-12 hours after symptom onset. Acute myocardial infarction is essentially excluded if cardiac markers are negative 12 hours after symptom onset.
How long do troponin levels remain elevated in acute myocardial infarction patients?	In contrast to CK-MB, troponin may be detectable for up to 14 days after the event, which makes it particularly useful in patients who present some time after their event.
Do cardiac troponin results provide information about prognosis in patients presenting with unstable angina/NSTEMI?	Elevated levels have been associated with increased mortality
Is acute myocardial injury or infarction the only cause of troponin elevation?	No. Elevations have been reported with other types of disease, including myocarditis, myocardial contusion, tachyarrhythmias, acute/ chronic congestive heart failure, s/p cardiac surgery, subarachnoid hemorrhage, pulmonary embolism, sepsis, and shock.

References

Collinson PO and Chamberlain L, "Cardiac Markers in the Diagnosis of Acute Coronary Syndromes," *Curr Cardiol Rep*, 2001, 3(4):280-8.

Donaldson A and Cove-Smith R, "Cardiac Troponin Levels in Patients With Impaired Renal Function," *Hosp Med*, 2001, 62(2):86-9.

Galvani M, Ferrini D, Ghezzi F, et al, "Cardiac Markers and Risk Stratification: An Integrated Approach," *Clin Chim Acta*, 2001, 311(1):9-17.

Karras DJ and Kane DL, "Serum Markers in the Emergency Department Diagnosis of Acute Myocardial Infarction," *Emerg Med Clin North Am*, 2001, 19(2):321-37.

Lewandrowski K, Chen A, and Januzzi J, "Cardiac Markers for Myocardial Infarction. A Brief Review," *Am J Clin Pathol*, 2002, 1(18 Suppl):S93-9.

Lindahl B, "Markers of Myocardial Damage in Acute Coronary Syndromes - Therapeutic Implications," *Clin Chim Acta*, 2001, 311(1):27-32.

Malasky BR and Alpert JS, "Diagnosis of Myocardial Injury by Biochemical Markers: Problems and Promises," *Cardiol Rev*, 2002, 10(5):306-17.

Newby LK, Goldmann BU, and Ohman EM, "Troponin: An Important Prognostic Marker and Risk-stratification Tool in Non-ST-segment Elevation Acute Coronary Syndrome," *J Am Coll Cardiol*, 2003, 41(4 Suppl S):31S-36S.

Penttila I, Penttila K, and Rantenen T, "Laboratory Diagnosis of Patients With Acute Chest Pain," *Clin Chem Lab Med*, 2000, 38(3):187-97.

Pollack CV Jr and Gibler WB, "2000 ACC/AHA Guidelines for the Management of Patients With Unstable Angina and non-ST-Segment Elevation Myocardial Infarction: A Practical Summary for Emergency Physicians".

COST-EFFECTIVE WORK-UP FOR ACUTE CHEST PAIN

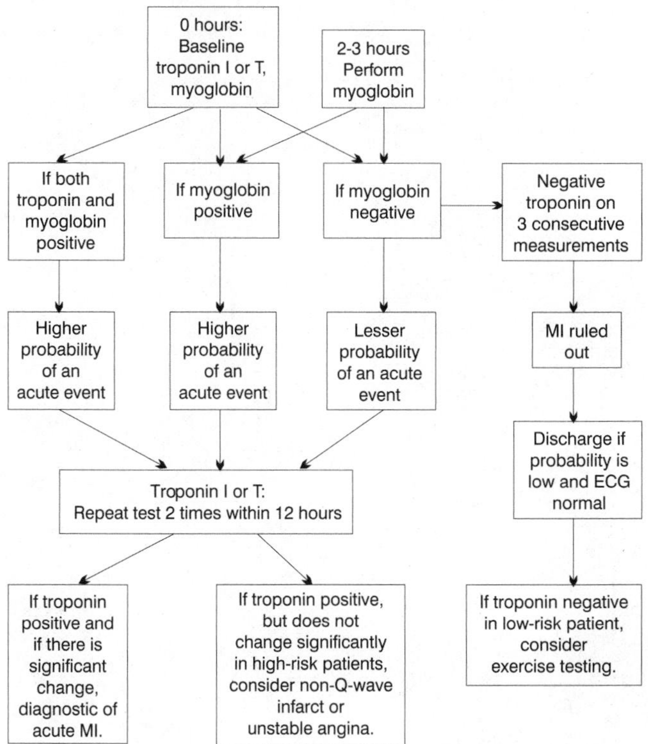

ECG = electrocardiogram
MI = myocardial infarction

Adapted from Khan F, Sachs HJ, Pechet L, et al, *Guide to Diagnostic Testing*, Philadelphia, PA: Lippincott Williams & Wilkins, 2002, 35.

BNP

Congestive heart failure (CHF) is the most common cause of hospitalization in Americans who are 65 years of age or older. It is also the most common reason that these patients present to the emergency department.

For many years, the diagnosis of CHF has largely rested on the history, physical examination, and diagnostic testing (nonlaboratory testing such as echocardiography, cardiac catheterization, etc). Because the signs and symptoms of CHF are not specific, differentiating CHF from other conditions that may present with the same manifestations has always been challenging. For example, dyspnea, one of the most common manifestations of CHF, can also be a symptom of acute pulmonary disease, such as pulmonary embolism, chronic obstructive pulmonary disease (COPD), and pneumonia.

In 2000, the Food and Drug Administration approved the use of a rapid assay for B-type natriuretic peptide (BNP). Its arrival in November 2000 marked the first time a blood test would be available for the diagnosis and management of CHF in the United States. The availability of this as well as other rapid BNP assays has had a profound effect on the diagnosis and management of CHF patients. Below we answer some of the common questions clinicians have about BNP levels in CHF patients.

Answering Common Questions About the Role of the Rapid BNP Assay in the Diagnosis and Management of CHF

Question	Answer
What is BNP?	BNP is one type of natriuretic hormone involved in the regulation of blood pressure and fluid volume. It is an antagonist of the renin-angiotensin-aldosterone system. It is secreted by the ventricles in response to volume expansion and pressure overload.
How should the BNP level be used in the diagnosis of CHF?	Without the use of BNP testing, some patients with CHF will be incorrectly diagnosed as having another condition and some without CHF will be incorrectly diagnosed as having CHF. Using the rapid BNP assay together with the clinical presentation, almost all of these patients will be correctly diagnosed. This was shown in a study of patients who presented to the emergency department with dyspnea (performed by Maisel and colleagues). The sensitivity and specificity of the assay for CHF diagnosis was 98% and 92%, respectively (using a level >80 pg/mL). The negative predictive value at this level was found to be 98%. In other words, CHF is unlikely to be the diagnosis in the patient presenting with dyspnea when the BNP level is <80 pg/mL. It is important to note that many of the studies have used a cutoff level of 100 pg/mL rather than 80 pg/mL.
How specific is BNP for the diagnosis of CHF?	Although quite useful for the diagnosis of CHF, the clinician must realize that the level may be elevated in other conditions (abdominal surgery, thoracic surgery, trauma, subarachnoid hemorrhage, primary hyperaldosteronism, Cushing syndrome, renal failure, cirrhosis, primary pulmonary hypertension, myocarditis, myocardial infarction, lung cancer)

Answering Common Questions About the Role of the Rapid BNP Assay in the Diagnosis and Management of CHF *(continued)*

Question	Answer
Do BNP levels correlate with disease severity?	Studies have shown that there is correlation between the degree of elevation and the severity of the CHF: • BNP <100 pg/mL = normal • BNP 100-300 pg/mL = mild CHF • BNP 300-700 pg/mL = moderate CHF • BNP >700 pg/mL = severe CHF BNP levels also correlate directly with the NYHA classification system for CHF.
Does the BNP level have prognostic significance?	Several studies have suggested that the BNP level has prognostic value in CHF patients. In a study performed by Harrison and colleagues, BNP levels were measured in over 300 patients presenting to the emergency department with dyspnea. These patients were then followed for six months. The probability of having a CHF event (another hospital admission for CHF, emergency department visit for CHF, CHF death) over the six month period was 51% in patients whose BNP level was >480 pg/mL but only 2.5% in those whose levels were <230 pg/mL. Higher levels are associated with poorer prognosis and warrant more aggressive therapy.
Is the BNP level useful for the diagnosis of diastolic CHF?	The degree of elevation cannot be used to differentiate systolic from diastolic CHF. However, an elevated level in the setting of normal left ventricular systolic function can be attributed to diastolic failure, especially if echocardiography is supportive of the diagnosis and no other cause of an increased level can be identified.
Does the BNP level predict outcomes for patients with acute coronary syndrome?	In a study of patients with unstable angina and non-ST-elevation myocardial infarction, elevated BNP levels were associated with an increased six-month mortality, independent of the troponin level. The risk of MI and development of CHF are higher in acute coronary syndrome patients with elevated BNP levels, again independent of the troponin level.
Can serial BNP levels be used to monitor the response to therapy?	Decreasing BNP levels suggest that the therapy is effective. Some studies suggest that BNP levels may be used to help titrate dosages of heart failure medications.

Although the rapid BNP assay is clearly useful for the diagnosis and management of CHF, clinicians should always interpret the level in the context of the patient's clinical presentation. As an example, consider the patient with CHF exacerbation due to pneumonia. In this type of patient, the BNP is likely to be elevated but if it is used alone (without consideration of the patient's clinical presentation), the diagnosis of CHF may be established but pneumonia may be missed. Another example is in the COPD patient who is having an exacerbation. Although COPD exacerbation often does not lead to a BNP elevation, if the illness results in worsening cor pulmonale/right ventricular volume overload, BNP levels may rise. Patients with small pulmonary emboli may not present with BNP elevation but with larger emboli, it is known that BNP levels may increase into the 200-300 pg/mL range.

References

Bhatila V, Nayyar P, and Dhindsa S, "Brain Natriuretic Peptide in Diagnosis and Treatment of Heart Failure," *J Postgrad Med*, 2003, 49(2):182-5.

Cardarelli R and Lumicao TG Jr, "B-type Natriuretic Peptide: A Review of Its Diagnostic, Prognostic, and Therapeutic Monitoring Value in Heart Failure for Primary Care Physicians," *J Am Board Fam Pract*, 2003, 16(4):327-33.

Cowie MR, Jourdain P, Maisel A, et al, "Clinical Applications of B-type Natriuretic Peptide (BNP) Testing," *Eur Heart J*, 2003, 24(19):1710-8.

Peacock WF 4th, "The B-type Natriuretic Peptide Assay: A Rapid Test for Heart Failure," *Cleve Clin J Med*, 2002, 69(3):243-51.

Ruskoaho H, "Cardiac Hormones as Diagnostic Tools in Heart Failure," *Endocr Rev*, 2003, 24(3):341-56.

Shapiro BP, Chen HH, Burnet JC Jr, et al, "Use of Plasma Brain Natriuretic Peptide Concentration to Aid in the Diagnosis of Heart Failure," *Cleve Clin J Med*, 2002, 69(3):243-51.

PART XI:

OBSTETRICS & GYNECOLOGY

OVARIAN CANCER

In females, ovarian cancer is the fifth most common cancer. Although most ovarian cancers are epithelial in origin, ovarian cancer can also be derived from other cell types (ie, germ cell, etc).

Clinical Presentation

Most patients who are diagnosed with ovarian cancer are found to have advanced disease. Advanced ovarian cancer often presents with abdominal distention, early satiety, anorexia, weight loss, and nausea. These symptoms are often manifestations of ascites and metastases to the omentum or bowel. Although early stage ovarian cancer is often symptomatic, the symptoms are often subtle or vague. In patients suspected of having ovarian cancer, the physical examination may reveal the presence of a pelvic mass. Not uncommonly, a patient is initially suspected of having ovarian cancer when an adnexal mass is palpated during a routine pelvic examination. In advanced disease, findings of metastases such as ascites may be present.

Laboratory Testing

In addition to a thorough history and physical examination, the patient suspected of having ovarian cancer should have routine laboratory testing, including complete blood count, chemistries, and urinalysis. Although these tests do not confirm the diagnosis of ovarian cancer, the results may help exclude other conditions in the differential diagnosis of the patient's symptoms. In addition, lab test abnormalities consistent with metastatic ovarian cancer may be noted. In a woman of reproductive age, a pregnancy test (serum B-HCG) should certainly be obtained.

CA-125 levels are often obtained in the evaluation of suspected ovarian cancer. CA-125 is a serum marker that is often elevated in patients with ovarian cancer (80% of women with epithelial ovarian cancer). The sensitivity of the test does vary depending upon the stage of the disease, with levels more commonly being normal in early stage disease (sensitivity 50% for stage I, 90% for stage II). The clinician should realize, however, that an elevated level does not confirm the diagnosis because benign conditions may also present with increased levels. In fact, elevated levels have been described in patients with pelvic inflammatory disease, ovarian cysts, endometriosis, hepatitis, cirrhosis, pancreatitis, renal failure, pneumonia, and congestive heart failure. CA-125 levels may also be increased in patients with other malignancies including endometrial and pancreatic cancer. The usefulness of the test also depends on the age of the patient. It is of little benefit in the premenopausal woman in whom an elevated CA-125 level is much more likely to be due to a benign condition since ovarian cancer is less common in this age group. In postmenopausal women, however, the positive predictive value is 97% for malignancy. It is also important to recognize that normal levels do not exclude the diagnosis of ovarian cancer. In patients who are found to have ovarian cancer, the degree of preoperative serum CA-125 elevation does provide additional information. Higher levels have been found to correlate with advanced stage and high grade disease. Of note, the pretreatment CA-125 level in patients with advanced disease is not predictive of survival in patients who respond to treatment.

Other tumor markers such as alpha-fetoprotein (AFP), human chorionic gonadotropin (hCG), and LDH can also be obtained. These are particularly useful when a germ cell tumor is suspected (see table).

Ovarian Germ Cell Tumors and Their Respective Markers

Tumor	HCG	AFP	LDH
Dysgerminoma	+	–	++
Immature teratoma	–	+	+
Embryonal carcinoma	++	++	+
Endodermal sinus tumor	+	++	+

– - not usually elevated

+ - occasionally elevated

++ - frequently elevated

From Chalas E and Valea FA, " Diagnosis and Surgery for Malignant Ovarian Disease," *Gynecologic Surgery*, Mann WJ and Stovall TG (eds), New York, NY: Churchill Livingstone, 1996, 691.

CA-125 testing certainly has a role in the follow-up of patients who are treated for ovarian cancer. In these patients, serial determination of the serum CA-125 level can provide information on the response to treatment and serve as a marker for the early detection of disease recurrence. Once the patient with ovarian cancer has been successfully treated, follow-up evaluations should take place at least every three months. At each visit, in addition to a history and physical examination, it is recommended that the clinician obtain a serum CA-125 level. The risk of recurrence is lower in patients who have a normal CA-125 level and unremarkable clinical evaluation. When serum CA-125 levels rise significantly, the patient is at higher risk for the development of clinical recurrence. Sometimes, patients are encountered who have a milder rise to a level that plateaus (<100 units). These patients are often observed, especially if the clinical evaluation reveals no findings consistent with disease recurrence. During serial follow-up, these patients should continue to be evaluated for any signs and symptoms of disease recurrence as well as further rise in the serum CA-125 level.

Imaging is often performed in patients suspected of having or who are diagnosed with ovarian cancer. The role of ultrasound, CT, MRI, and other radiologic imaging tests are beyond the scope of this chapter.

References

Markman M, "Limitations to the Use of the CA-125 Antigen Level in Ovarian Cancer," *Curr Oncol Rep*, 2003, 5(4):263-4.

Miralles C, Orea M, Espana P, et al, "Cancer Antigen 125 Associated With Multiple Benign and Malignant Pathologies," *Ann Surg Oncol*, 2003, 10(2):150-4.

Partridge EE and Barnes MN, "Epithelial Ovarian Cancer: Prevention, Diagnosis, and Treatment," *CA Cancer J Clin*, 1999, 49(5):297-320.

Sevinc A, Camci C, Turk HM, et al, "How to Interpret Serum CA 125 Levels in Patients With Serosal Involvement: A Clinical Dilemma," *Oncology*, 2003, 65(1):1-6.

Vaidya AP and Curtin JP, "The Follow-Up of Ovarian Cancer," *Semin Oncol*, 2003, 30(3):401-12.

PELVIC INFLAMMATORY DISEASE

Pelvic inflammatory disease is an infection of the female genital tract that primarily occurs in sexually, active women. *C. trachomatis* and/or *N. gonorrhoeae* are the most common etiologic agents but other organisms have been reported, either alone or in combination.

Clinical Presentation

The disease classically presents with the acute onset of fever and pelvic pain. Quite often, the symptoms begin during or after a menstrual period. Many patients, however, do not present with the classic symptoms. In fact, pelvic inflammatory disease that is the result of chlamydial infection often presents with a more gradual course. In these patients, the disease also tends to be less severe.

Fever and tachycardia are typically present. The degree of tachycardia can vary from mild to severe. Bilateral lower abdominal tenderness tends to be the rule in this disease. Upper abdominal tenderness may also be noted, especially in patients with the Fitz-Hugh-Curtis syndrome. With severe illness, the clinician may note rebound and/or guarding. The classic physical exam finding of pelvic inflammatory disease is cervical motion tenderness (chandelier sign). Tenderness is also elicited upon palpation of the uterus and adnexa. If a tubo-ovarian abscess is present, a unilateral adnexal mass may be appreciated. Speculum examination typically reveals the presence of a mucopurulent cervical discharge.

Criteria for Diagnosis

Criteria for the diagnosis of pelvic inflammatory disease are listed in the following box.

CRITERIA FOR THE DIAGNOSIS OF PELVIC INFLAMMATORY DISEASE

All three of the following minimal criteria must be met:

- History of lower abdominal pain and presence of abdominal tenderness, with or without rebound tenderness
- Tenderness with motion of the cervix and uterus
- Adnexal tenderness

These additional criteria may be used to enhance specificity of the diagnosis:

- Oral temperature >38°C
- Elevated ESR >15 mm/hour
- Abnormal vaginal or cervical discharge
- Elevated C-reactive protein
- Laboratory documentation of endocervical *N. gonorrhoeae* and/or *C. trachomatis*

Definitive criteria:

- Tubo-ovarian abscess on pelvic ultrasound
- Histopathologic evidence of endometritis by endometrial biopsy
- Laparoscopic abnormalities consistent with PID

From "1998 Guidelines for Treatment of Sexually Transmitted Diseases," *MMWR Morb Mortal Wkly Rep*, 1998, 47(RR-1):1.

Laboratory Testing

Laboratory testing performed in patients with pelvic inflammatory disease is described in the following table.

Laboratory Testing Often Performed in the Patient With Pelvic Inflammatory Disease

Test	Importance
Pregnancy test	Necessary to exclude ectopic pregnancy as well as complications of intrauterine pregnancy Patients with ectopic pregnancy are often misdiagnosed as having pelvic inflammatory disease. Rarely, pelvic inflammatory disease occurs in a pregnant woman (more likely before 12 week of pregnancy)
Urinalysis	Presence of abnormalities should prompt consideration of another etiology such as cystitis or pyelonephritis
Fecal occult blood test of stool	Abnormal test result should prompt consideration of another etiology
CBC	Of limited value - <50% of patients have leukocytosis
Gram stain / microscopic examination of vaginal discharge	Increased number of PMNs (in vaginal secretions) is known as leukorrhea. Leukorrhea is found in almost all patients with pelvic inflammatory disease. Not all patients with leukorrhea, however, have pelvic inflammatory disease. Therefore, the absence of leukorrhea is helpful in arguing against the diagnosis.
Cervical Gram stain	Probability of pelvic inflammatory disease increases if the Gram stain reveals the presence of gram-negative intracellular diplococci. A negative test result does not rule out the diagnosis.
Tests for chlamydia and gonococcus	Cultures or assays (DNA probes, ELISA, fluorescent antibody tests) should be obtained for these organisms since they are the major etiologic agents of pelvic inflammatory disease.

Imaging tests such as ultrasound may also be performed, especially in patients suspected of having tubo-ovarian abscess. Discussion regarding the role of radiologic testing in the patient with pelvic inflammatory disease is beyond the scope of this chapter.

References

Beigi RH and Wiesenfeld HC, "Pelvic Inflammatory Disease: New Diagnostic Criteria and Treatment," *Obstet Gynecol Clin North Am*, 2003, 30(4):777-93.

Peipert JF, "Clinical Practice. Genital Chlamydial Infections," *N Engl J Med*, 2003, 349(25):2424-30.

Watson EJ, Templeton A, Russell I, et al, "The Accuracy and Efficacy of Screening Tests for *Chlamydia trachomatis*: A Systematic Review," *J Med Microbiol*, 2002, 51(12):1021-31.

Zeger W and Holt K, "Gynecologic Infections," *Emerg Med Clin North Am*, 2003, 21(3):631-48.

PRENATAL CARE

Women who are pregnant may or may not have symptoms or signs of pregnancy. Most commonly, the pregnant woman will report missing one or two menstrual periods. Other early manifestations of pregnancy include nausea, fatigue, and breast fullness/tenderness. Quite often, women who suspect that they are pregnant will have performed a home pregnancy test. Even if the test is positive, laboratory testing is recommended to establish that the woman is truly pregnant. This testing as well as other testing performed as part of prenatal care is the focus of this chapter.

Diagnosis of Pregnancy

The gold standard for the diagnosis of pregnancy is testing for the beta subunit of human chorionic gonadotropin. The laboratory uses immunologic techniques to detect the presence of the beta subunit of human chorionic gonadotropin (hCG). This testing can be performed on either urine or serum samples. Sensitive ELISA tests can detect hCG as early as one week after fertilization. The sensitivity and specificity of hCG testing are 97% to 100% if testing is performed in the laboratory.

When testing is performed at home using easily available pregnancy kits, the sensitivity is lower. False-negative test results are not uncommon in this setting, most often due to testing being performed too soon after ovulation. If pregnancy is suspected but the test result is negative, it is reasonable to repeat testing one week later.

Routine Tests to Be Performed at Initial Visit (Prenatal Care)

Tests that should be routinely performed at the patient's initial visit are listed in the following box.

TESTS THAT SHOULD BE ROUTINELY PERFORMED AT THE INITIAL PRENATAL CARE
HEMOGLOBIN OR HEMATOCRIT BLOOD TYPE AND Rh STATUS ANTIBODY SCREEN SEROLOGIC TEST FOR SYPHILIS Hb_sAg (HEPATITIS B SURFACE ANTIGEN) HIV ANTIBODY (WITH CONSENT) RUBELLA HEMAGGLUTINATION-INHIBITION TITER PAP SMEAR URINALYSIS (INCLUDING DIPSTICK AND SCREEN FOR BACTERIURIA)

The importance of the above testing is described in the following table.

The Importance of Routine Laboratory Testing at the Initial Prenatal Care Visit

Test	Importance
Hemoglobin / hematocrit	Blood loss is to be expected during delivery and is usually between 500 and 1000 cc. Therefore, it is important to detect anemic patients so that they can be treated before delivery. Patients with high hematocrits (>40%) also need to be identified because these patients may be at risk for preeclampsia/other conditions.

Test	Importance
Serologic test for syphilis	All patients should have VDRL or RPR testing. FTA-ABS testing should follow in patients who have a positive test result.
Rubella titer	Although congenital rubella syndrome is rare (due to widespread vaccination), it is now known that 10% to 15% of adults are seronegative and therefore susceptible to the infection. Seronegative patients should be immunized postpartum.
Hepatitis B surface antigen	Chronic carriers of hepatitis B can transmit the infection to their offspring during or after birth.
Blood type and antibody screening test	It is necessary to identify women who are Rh-negative so that Rh immune globulin can be administered at 28-30 weeks and within 72 hours of delivery.
Pap smear	A PAP smear should be done if it has not been performed in the preceding 6-12 months.
Urinalysis	The urinalysis should be complete (microscopy, screen for infection). It is not necessary to perform urine culture but one should be done (to identify organism and determine antibiotic sensitivity) if the urinalysis reveals bacteriuria or other findings suggestive of bacteriuria (positive nitrite and/or leukocyte esterase). In pregnant women, identification and treatment of asymptomatic bacteriuria is important in preventing the development of pyelonephritis.
HIV	American College of Gynecology recommends that all pregnant women be tested for HIV (with consent). In patients who are deemed to be at high risk for the disease, retesting should occur at about 36 weeks of gestation (if the initial test was negative).

Routine Tests to Be Performed Later in Pregnancy

There are other tests that need to be routinely performed later in pregnancy. The importance of this testing is described in the following table.

Tests That Should Routinely Be Performed Later in Pregnancy

Test	When?	Importance
Triple marker test (AFP, estriol, hCG)	15-20 weeks of gestation	Assesses risk for certain fetal anomalies and chromosomal abnormalities. Those who have abnormal test results should undergo counseling (interpretation of the test is very dependent on accurate dating of the pregnancy). Testing for identification of the specific disorder should be offered.
Glucose screen	24-28 weeks of gestation	To screen for gestational diabetes mellitus Plasma glucose level should be measured one hour after a 50 g oral glucose load has been administered. Levels >140 mg/dL should be followed by a 100 g oral glucose tolerance test (after fasting). Using the oral glucose tolerance test, gestational diabetes mellitus is diagnosed if two or more of the following plasma venous glucose values are exceeded : – 95 mg/dL (fasting) – 180 mg/dL (1 hour) – 155 mg/dL (2 hour) – 140 mg/dL (3 hour)

Test	When?	Importance
Group B beta-hemolytic streptococcus culture	35 weeks of gestation	Swabs of both lower vagina and rectum should be obtained to detect colonization. Patients who have positive culture results should be treated during labor to prevent the development of neonatal sepsis (group B streptococcus is a major cause of neonatal sepsis)
Hematocrit	28 and 36 weeks of gestation	To identify anemia (Hct <32%) or elevated hematocrit (>40%)
Urine dipstick	Every visit	If patient has significant proteinuria, consider urinary tract infection, preeclampsia, or renal disease. If patient has glucosuria, consider gestational diabetes mellitus. If + nitrite and/or leukocyte esterase, evaluate and treat for urinary tract infection or asymptomatic bacteriuria.
Antibody screening test	28 weeks of gestation (in Rh-negative patients)	If Rh-negative, administer Rh immune globulin

Recommended Testing in At-risk Population

Some tests are not recommended in all pregnant women. These tests are indicated if the patient is at risk for certain diseases or illnesses.

RECOMMENDED TESTING IN AT-RISK POPULATION (PRENATAL CARE)
N. gonorrhoeae culture *Chlamydia trachomatis* PCR Wet preparation Tuberculin skin test Sickledex

The importance of this testing is discussed in the following table.

Testing That Should Be Performed in the At-risk Population (Prenatal Care)

Test	Importance
N. gonorrhoeae culture	Testing should be performed if risk factors for the infection are present (obtain cervical culture for *N. gonorrhoeae*). Of note, some experts recommend routine testing of all pregnant women. Retest in the third trimester if the patient is at high risk for acquiring the infection.
Chlamydia trachomatis PCR	Testing should be performed if risk factors for the infection are present (obtain PCR testing for *C. trachomatis*). Of note, some experts recommend routine testing of all pregnant women. Retest in the third trimester if the patient is at high risk for acquiring the infection.
Wet preparation of vaginal secretions	An association between some forms of lower genital tract infection (ie, bacterial vaginosis) and spontaneous preterm birth has been described (although controversial). Since symptoms are often lacking in infected patients, testing can identify the presence of infection in at-risk individuals.

(continued)

Testing That Should Be Performed in the At-risk Population (Prenatal Care) *(continued)*

Test	Importance
Tuberculin skin test	Tuberculin skin test (PPD) recommended in patients who are at risk for infection. If the test is positive (and the patient is asymptomatic with no HIV risk factors), perform chest radiograph after the 12th week of gestation to assess for presence of active disease. If the patient is symptomatic or has risk factors for HIV, do not delay performance of the chest radiograph.
Sickledex	The sickledex test will be positive in patients who have hemoglobin S. Hemoglobin S is responsible for the sickling disorder seen in sickle cell anemia, sickle cell-hemoglobin C disease, sickle cell-thalassemia, and other hemoglobinopathies. A positive test result should prompt performance of hemoglobin electrophoresis to identify the specific hemoglobinopathy that is present. If both the mother and father have sickle cell trait, there is a 25% chance that the newborn will have sickle cell anemia. Prenatal diagnosis of the fetus is now available.

GESTATIONAL DIABETES MELLITUS

Gestational diabetes mellitus (GDM) is diabetes mellitus that is diagnosed during pregnancy. It occurs in up to 5% of all pregnancies.

Risk Factors

Risk factors for gestational diabetes mellitus are listed in the following box.

RISK FACTORS FOR GESTATIONAL DIABETES MELLITUS
Age >30 years
Obesity
Ethnicity (African American, Native American, Hispanic American, Asian American, Pacific Islander)
Family history of type II diabetes mellitus (first-degree relatives)
Insulin resistance
Polycystic ovarian syndrome
History of large-for-age-gestational infant during previous pregnancy (>9 lbs)
History of GDM during previous pregnancy
History of abnormal glucose tolerance
Abnormal maternal birth weight (<6 lbs or >9 lbs)
History of unexplained perinatal loss or birth of malformed child

Screening

Although it is important to assess the pregnant woman's risk for developing GDM, a considerable number of cases would go undiagnosed if only women with risk factor(s) for the disease were screened. Despite this, many organizations recommend selective screening.

For example, the American Diabetes Association does not advocate routine screening of all pregnant women. The group maintains that screening is not necessary in women at low risk for GDM. Those at low risk are women who meet all of the following criteria:

- Age <25 years
- No family history of diabetes mellitus (first degree relatives)
- Normal maternal birth weight (>6 lbs and <9 lbs)
- Body mass index <25
- No history of abnormal glucose tolerance
- Ethnicity not associated with high prevalence of diabetes mellitus (ethnicities associated with high prevalence include African Americans, Native Americans, Hispanic Americans, Asian Americans, and Pacific Islanders)
- No history of adverse pregnancy outcomes often associated with GDM

Others recommend universal rather than selective screening, citing that selective screening is not sufficiently sensitive and less practical. This is an issue that continues to be debated.

Establishing the Diagnosis

Screening for gestational diabetes mellitus usually takes place between 24 and 28 weeks. Most perform an initial screen using a 50 g oral glucose challenge. This challenge can be performed at any time of the day (does not need to be fasting). Pregnant women who have a 1-hour glucose level >140 mg/dL require further evaluation. The sensitivity of this test can be increased if testing is performed in the fasting state or a lower cut-off value is used. For example, using a cut-off value of 130 mg/dL will detect 90% of GDM cases (rather than 80% that will be diagnosed using a cut-off of 140 mg/dL).

An abnormal initial screen should be followed by a 3-hour oral glucose tolerance test. Prior to performing this test, the patient should be fasting for at least 8 hours (patient should not fast for >14 hours). Dietary carbohydrate intake should not be restricted over the previous three days. A venous blood sample should be obtained (baseline value) followed by the administration of 100 g glucose orally. Thereafter, hourly glucose levels should be obtained for the next three hours while the patient continues to fast. The patient should remain seated during the test and instructed not to smoke.

Criteria for a positive oral glucose tolerance test are listed in the following table. For the 100 g oral glucose tolerance test, either the criteria of the National Diabetes Data Group or Carpenter and Coustan are used.

The clinician should realize that a 2-hour oral glucose tolerance test is also available (using 75 g oral glucose). Please note that the following table also contains criteria (WHO and ADA) for a positive 75 g oral glucose tolerance test.

Criteria for an Abnormal Oral Glucose Tolerance Test for the Diagnosis of GDM

Time	National Diabetes Data Group* (>2 abnormal results)	Carpenter and Coustan* (>2 abnormal results)	WHO† (>1 abnormal result)	ADA† (≥2 abnormal results)
0 hour (fasting)	≥105 mg/dL (5.8 mmol/L)	≥95 mg/dL (5.3 mmol/L)	≥125 mg/dL (7.0 mmol/L)	≥95 mg/dL (5.3 mmol/L)
1 hour	≥190 mg/dL (10.6 mmol/L)	≥180 mg/dL (10.0 mmol/L)		≥180 (10.0 mmol/L)
2 hour	≥165 mg/dL (9.2 mmol/L)	≥155 mg/dL (8.6 mmol/L)	≥140 mg/dL (7.8 mmol/L)	≥155 mg/dL (8.6 mmol/L)
3 hour	≥145 mg/dL (8.1 mmol/L)	≥140 mg/dL (7.8 mmol/L)		

*Using 100 g oral glucose

†Using 75 g oral glucose

References

American Diabetes Association, "Gestational Diabetes Mellitus," *Diabetes Care*, 2001, 24:S77.

Carpenter MW and Coustan DR, "Criteria Screening Tests for Gestational Diabetes," *Am J Obstet Gynecol*, 1982, 144:768.

National Diabetes Data Group, "Classification and Diagnosis of Diabetes Mellitus and Other Categories of Glucose Tolerance," *Diabetes*, 1979, 18:1039.

O'Brien and Carpenter M, "Testing for Gestational Diabetes," *Clin Lab Med*, 2003, 101(6):1197-203.

Sacs DA, Chen W, Wolde-Tsadik G, et al, "Fasting Plasma Glucose Test at the First Prenatal Visit as a Screen for Gestational Diabetes," *Obstet Gynecol*, 2003, 101(6):1197-203.

WHO Consultation, "Definition, Diagnosis and Classification of Diabetes Mellitus and Its Complications: Report of a WHO Consultation. Part I: Diagnosis and Classification of Diabetes Mellitus," WHO/NCD/NCS/99.2, World Health Organization, Geneva, 1999.

PREECLAMPSIA

Preeclampsia occurs in up to 8% of all pregnancies. It is associated with increased maternal and fetal mortality. In this chapter, the risk factors, clinical presentation, and laboratory testing of patients with preeclampsia will be described.

Risk Factors

Risk factors for preeclampsia are listed in the following box.

RISK FACTORS FOR PREECLAMPSIA
Positive family history Nulliparity
Chronic hypertension
History of preeclampsia during previous pregnancy
Obesity
Diabetes mellitus
Hyatidiform mole
Renal disease
Multiple gestation

Clinical Presentation

Preeclampsia is diagnosed when hypertension and proteinuria (systolic blood pressure >140 mm Hg or diastolic blood pressure >90 mm Hg AND urinary protein excretion >0.3 g/day) develop after 20 weeks of gestation in a woman who has been previously normotensive. Preeclampsia needs to be differentiated from chronic hypertension, which is defined as an elevated blood pressure (systolic >140 mm Hg and/or diastolic >90 mm Hg) that began before pregnancy, during pregnancy but before the 20 week of gestation, or that which persists for >12 weeks postpartum.

Because patients with chronic hypertension are at increased risk for the development of preeclampsia, the clinician must also be comfortable making the diagnosis of this illness in the chronic hypertensive patient (superimposed preeclampsia). The chronic hypertensive patient is said to have superimposed preeclampsia if new onset proteinuria develops after 20 weeks of gestation. In women with chronic hypertension who had preexisting proteinuria, superimposed preeclampsia can still be diagnosed if there is significant worsening of the blood pressure (systolic blood pressure >180 mm Hg and/or diastolic blood pressure >110 mm Hg) in the last half of pregnancy, especially if the elevation is associated with symptoms.

Laboratory Testing

As stated above, the diagnosis of preeclampsia is based not only on the blood pressure but also on the presence of significant proteinuria (proteinuria may be a late finding, however). Significant proteinuria is defined as the excretion of >0.3 g of protein/day (or urine protein to creatinine ratio >0.19). Although some clinicians consider urine dipstick testing that reveals >30 mg/dL or + 1 protein to be synonymous with the excretion of >0.3 g of protein/day, such dipstick findings are only suggestive of this degree of urinary protein excretion. An abnormal dipstick should be followed by a quantitative measure of urinary protein excretion (ie, 24-hour urine collection for protein or urine protein to creatinine ratio on a random urine specimen). The degree of proteinuria varies considerably in preeclampsia patients, ranging from slightly abnormal to frankly nephrotic.

Other laboratory tests that are often performed in the preeclampsia patient along with their clinical significance are listed in the following table.

Laboratory Testing in Preeclampsia

Laboratory Test	Clinical Significance
Hemoglobin / hematocrit	Presence of hemoconcentration (high hematocrit) is supportive of the diagnosis and suggests that the patient has more severe disease Low levels may be seen if hemolysis occurs (microangiopathic hemolytic anemia)
Platelet count	Low platelet count suggests the presence of severe preeclampsia
LDH	Elevated when preeclampsia is complicated by hemolysis and/or hepatic involvement Elevated LDH levels suggest severe preeclampsia
Peripheral blood smear	Findings consistent with microangiopathic hemolytic anemia supports the diagnosis
Serum creatinine	Mild elevation is not uncommon but rising levels suggestive of severe preeclampsia
Uric acid	Hyperuricemia is common in preeclampsia, with uric acid levels usually >5.5-6.0 mg/dL Patients with essential hypertension usually have uric acid levels less than this, unless they are receiving diuretic therapy.
AST / ALT	Elevated levels suggest hepatic involvement and more severe disease

HELLP Syndrome

HELLP is an acronym for a syndrome characterized by the presence of hemolysis (microangiopathic blood smear), elevated liver enzymes, and a low platelet count. It occurs in 10% to 20% of patients with preeclampsia. This is a severe illness that usually requires prompt delivery of the fetus. The features of this syndrome are listed in the following box.

FEATURES OF THE HELLP SYNDROME
Microangiopathic hemolytic anemia
Thrombocytopenia (platelet count <100,000/microliter)
Serum LDH >600 IU/L or bilirubin >1.2 mg/dL
AST >70 IU/L

Of note, clinical and laboratory findings of disseminated intravascular coagulation may be present in up to 20% of patients.

Differentiating among the causes of thrombocytopenia during pregnancy can be challenging. The following table provides information to aid the clinician in differentiating preeclampsia and HELLP syndrome from other causes of thrombocytopenia during pregnancy.

Differentiation of Pregnancy-Associated Microangiopathies

Condition	↓ PLT Count	Coagu-lopathy	HTN	Renal Disease	CNS Disease	MAHA	Peak Time of Onset
Preeclampsia	+	±	+++	+	+	+	3rd trimester
HELLP	+++	+	±	+	±	++	3rd trimester
HUS	++	±	±	+++	±	++	Postpartum
TTP	+++	±	±	+ / ±	+++	+++	2nd trimester, term

(continued)

Differentiation of Pregnancy-Associated Microangiopathies *(continued)*

Condition	↓ PLT Count	Coagu-lopathy	HTN	Renal Disease	CNS Disease	MAHA	Peak Time of Onset
SLE	+	±	±	+ / ++	+	+	Anytime
APS	+	±	±	±	+	±	Anytime
AFLP	+ / ±	+++	±	±	+	+	3rd trimester

± = variably present

+ = mild

++ = moderate

+++ = severe

MAHA = microangiopathic hemolytic anemia

From McCrae KR and Cines DB, "Thrombotic Microangiopathy During Pregnancy," *Semin Hematol*, 1997, 34(2):148-58 (review); also from McCrae KR, "Thrombocytopenia in Pregnancy: Differential Diagnosis, Pathogenesis, and Management," *Blood Rev*, 2003, 17(1):7-14 (review).

References

Garovic VD, "Hypertension in Pregnancy: Diagnosis and Treatment," *Mayo Clin Proc*, 2000, 75(10):1071-6.

Longo SA, Dola CP, and Pridjian G, "Pre-eclampsia and Eclampsia Revisited," *South Med J*, 2003, 96(9):891-9.

Sibal BM, "Diagnosis and Management of Gestational Hypertension and Pre-eclampsia," *Obstet Gynecol*, 2003, 102(1):181-92.

LABORATORY RANGES

Chemistry

Analyte	MGH Unit	SI Unit
Adrenocorticotropin	6.0-76.0 pg/mL	1.3-16.7 pmol/L
Alanine aminotransferase (ALT/SGPT)		
female	7-30 units/L	0.12-0.50 μkat/L
male	10-55 units/L	0.17-0.92 μkat/L
Albumin	3.1-4.3 g/dL	31-43 g/L
Aldosterone (adults)		
supine, normal-sodium diet	2-9 ng/dL	55-250 pmol/L
upright, normal-sodium diet	2-5 times supine value with normal-sodium diet	
Alkaline phosphatase (adults)		
female	30-100 units/L	0.5-1.67 μkat/L
male	45-115 units/L	0.75-1.92 μkat/L
Alpha-fetoprotein (nonmaternal)	<12.8 IU/mL	<9.92 μg/L
Ammonia	12-48 μmol/L	12-48 μmol/L
Amylase	53-123 units/L	0.88-2.05 nkat/L
Angiotensin-converting enzyme		
female	19-79 units/L	19-79 units/L
male	19-95 units/L	19-95 units/L
Aspartate aminotransferase (AST, SGOT)		
female	9-25 units/L	0.15-0.42 μkat/L
male	10-40 units/L	0.17-0.67 μkat/L
$Beta_2$-microglobulin	1.2-2.8 mg/L	1.2-2.8 mg/L
Bicarbonate (HCO_3^-)	22-26 mEq/L	22-26 mmol/L
Bilirubin, direct	0.0-0.4 mg/dL	0-7 μmol/L
Bilirubin, total	0.0-1.0 mg/dL	0-17 μmol/L
C-peptide (adults)	0.5-2.0 ng/mL	0.17-0.66 nmol/L
Calcium	8.5-10.5 mg/dL	2.1-2.6 mmol/L
Calcium, ionized	1.14-1.30 mmol/L	1.14-1.30 mmol/L
Carbon dioxide, partial pressure, arterial ($PaCO_2$)	35-45 mm Hg	4.7-6.0 kPa
Carboxyhemoglobin	<5% of total hemoglobin	<0.05 fraction of total hemoglobin saturation
Catecholamines (adults)		
epinephrine	2-24 μg/24 h	11-131 nmol/24 h
norepinephrine	15-100 μg/24 h	89-591 nmol/24 h
total (epinephrine + norepinephrine)	26-121 μg/24 h	142-660 nmol/24 h
Cerebrospinal fluid (adults)		
albumin	11-48 mg/dL	0.11-0.48 g/L
cell count	0-5 mononuclear cells/μL	0-5 x 10^6cells/L
glucose	50-75 mg/dL	2.8-4.2 mmol/L
IgG	8.0-8.6 mg/dL	0.08-0.086 g/L
pressure	70-180 mm of water	70-180 arbitrary units
protein, lumbar	15-45 mg/dL	0.15-0.45 g/L
Ceruloplasmin	27-50 mg/dL	270-500 mg/L
Chloride	100-108 mmol/L	100-108 mmol/L
Cholesterol		
desirable	<200 mg/dL	<5.17 mmol/L
borderline high	200-239 mg/dL	5.17-6.18 mmol/L
high	>239 mg/dL	>6.18 mmol/L
Cortisol		
fasting, 8 AM - noon	5-25 μg/dL	138-690 nmol/L
noon - 8 PM	5-15 μg/dL	138-414 nmol/L
8 PM - 8 AM	0-10 μg/dL	0-276 nmol/L
Cortisol, free in urine	20-70 μg/24 h	55-193 nmol/24 h

Chemistry *(continued)*

Analyte	MGH Unit	SI Unit
Creatine kinase (CK)		
female	40-150 units/L	0.67-2.50 μkat/L
male	60-400 units/L	1.00-6.67 μkat/L
Creatinine kinase isoenzyme index	0%-2.5% relative index	None
Creatinine kinase isoenzymes, MB fraction	0-5 ng/mL	0-5 μg/L
Creatinine		
plasma	0.6-1.5 mg/dL	53-133 μmol/L
urine	15-25 mg/kg/day	0.13-0.22 mmol/kg/day
Dehydroepiandrosterone (DHEA) (adults)		
female	130-980 ng/dL	4.5-34.0 nmol/L
male	180-1250 ng/dL	6.24-43.3 nmol/L
Dehydroepiandrosterone (DHEA) sulfate (adults)		
female		
premenopausal	12-535 μg/dL	120-5350 μg/L
postmenopausal	30-260 μg/dL	300-2600 μg/L
male	10-619 μg/dL	100-6190 μg/L
1,25-Dihydroxyvitamin D	18-62 pg/mL	43.2-148.8 pmol/L
Follicle-stimulating hormone (FSH)		
female		
menstruating		
follicular phase	3.0-20.0 units/L	3.0-20.0 units/L
ovulatory phase	9.0-26.0 units/L	9.0-26.0 units/L
luteal phase	1.0-12.0 units/L	1.0-12.0 units/L
postmenopausal	18.0-153.0 units/L	18.0-153.0 units/L
male	1.0-12.0 units/L	1.0-12.0 units/L
Globulin	2.6-4.1 g/dL	26-41 g/L
Glucose, fasting	70-110 mg/dL	3.9-6.1 mmol/L
γ-Glutamyltransferase (GGT)		
female	1-70 units/L	1-70 units/L
male	1-94 units/L	1-94 units/L
Growth hormone (resting)	2-5 ng/mL	2-5 μg/L
Hemoglobin A_{1C}	3.8%-6.4%	0.038-0.064
High-density lipoprotein cholesterol, as major risk factor	<35 mg/dL	<0.91 mmol/L
Human chorionic gonadotropin (hCG) (nonpregnant women)	<5 mIU/mL	<5 IU/L
25-Hydroxyvitamin D	8-42 ng/mL	20-105 nmol/L
Insulin	2-20 μunits/mL	14.35-143.5 pmol/L
Ketone (acetone)	Negative	Negative
Lactate dehydrogenase (LDH)	110-210 units/L	1.83-3.50 μkat/L
Lipase	3-19 units/dL	0.5-3.17 μkat/L
Lipoprotein (a)	0-30 mg/dL	0-300 mg/L
Low-density lipoprotein cholesterol		
desirable	<130 mg/dL	<3.36 mmol/L
borderline high risk	130-159 mg/dL	3.36-4.11 mmol/L
high risk	≥160 mg/dL	≥4.13 mmol/L
Luteinizing hormone (LH)		
female		
menstruating		
follicular phase	2.0-15.0 units/L	2.0-15.0 units/L
ovulatory phase	22.0-105.0 units/L	22.0-105.0 units/L
luteal phase	0.6-19.0 units/L	0.6-19.0 units/L
postmenopausal	16.0-64.0 units/L	16.0-64.0 units/L
male	2.0-12.0 units/L	2.0-12.0 units/L
Magnesium	1.4-2.0 mEq/L	0.7-1.0 mmol/L

Chemistry *(continued)*

Analyte	MGH Unit	SI Unit
Metanephrines		
metanephrine	45-290 μg/24 h	245-1583 nmol/24 h
normetanephrine	82-500 μg/24 h	448-2730 nmol/24 h
total	120-700 μg/24 h	655-3821 nmol/24 h
Microalbumin, random urine	<20 μg/mL	<20 mg/L
5′-Nucleotidase	0-11 units/L	0.02-0.18 μkat/L
Osmolality	280-296 mOsm/kg of water	280-296 mmol/kg of water
Oxygen, partial pressure, arterial (PaO_2) (room air, age dependent)	80-100 mm Hg	10.7-13.3 kPa
Parathyroid hormone	10-60 pg/mL	10-60 ng/L
pH, arterial	7.35-7.45 pH units	7.35-7.45 pH units
Phosphorus, inorganic (adults)	2.6-4.5 mg/dL	0.84-1.45 mmol/L
Potassium	3.4-4.8 mmol/L	3.4-4.8 mmol/L
Prolactin		
female		
premenopausal	0-20 ng/mL	0-20 μg/L
postmenopausal	0-15 ng/mL	0-15 μg/L
male	0-15 ng/mL	0-15 μg/L
Prostate-specific antigen (PSA)		
male		
<40 y	0.0-2.0 ng/mL	0.0-2.0 μg/L
≥40 y	0.0-4.0 ng/mL	0.0-4.0 μg/L
Prostate-specific antigen (PSA), free; in males 45-75 y, with PSA values between 4 and 20 ng/mL	>25% associated with benign prostatic hyperplasia	>0.25 associated with benign prostatic hyperplasia
Protein, total	6.0-8.0 g/dL	60-80 g/dL
Renin		
supine	0.3-3.0 ng/mL/h	0.08-0.83 ng/(L - sec)
upright	1.0-9.0 mg/mL/h	0.28-2.5 ng/(L - sec)
Sodium	135-145 mmol/L	135-145 mmol/L
Somatomedin C		
16-24 y	182-780 ng/mL	182-780 μg/L
25-39 y	114-492 ng/mL	114-492 μg/L
40-54 y	90-360 ng/mL	90-360μg/L
>54 y	71-290 ng/mL	71-290 μg/L
Testosterone, total		
female	6-86 ng/dL	0.21-2.98 nmol/L
male	270-1070 ng/dL	9.36-37.10 nmol/L
Testosterone, unbound		
female		
20-40 y	0.6-3.1 pg/mL	20.8-107.5 pmol/L
41-60 y	0.4-2.5 pg/mL	13.9-86.7 pmol/L
61-80 y	0.2-2.0 pg/mL	6.9-69.3 pmol/L
male		
20-40 y	15.0-40.0 pg/mL	520-1387 pmol/L
41-60 y	13.0-35.0 pg/mL	451-1213 pmol/L
61-80 y	12.0-28.0 pg/mL	416-971 pmol/L
Thyroglobulin	0-60 ng/mL	0-60 μg/L
Thyroid hormone-binding index	0.77-1.23	0.77-1.23
Thyroid-stimulating hormone	0.5-5.0 μU/mL	0.5-5.0 μU/mL
Thyroxine, total (T_4)	4.5-10.9 μU/dL	58-140 nmol/L
Transferrin	191-365 mg/dL	1.91-3.65 g/L
Triglycerides (fasting)	40-150 mg/dL	0.45-1.69 mmol/L
Triiodothyronine, total (T_3)	60-181 ng/dL	0.92-2.78 nmol/L
Troponin I	<0.6 ng/mL	<0.6 μg/L
Urea nitrogen (BUN) (adults)	8-25 mg/dL	2.9-8.9 mmol/L
Uric acid		
female	2.3-6.6 mg/dL	137-393 μmol/L

Chemistry *(continued)*

Analyte	MGH Unit	SI Unit
male	3.6-8.5 mg/dL	214-506 μmol/L
Urinalysis		
pH	5.0-9.0	5.0-9.0
specific gravity	1.001-1.035	1.001-1.035
Urine sediment		
white cells	0-2/hpf	0-2/hpf
red cells	0-2/hpf	0-2/hpf
Xylose	4-9 g/5 h	4-9 g/5 h

Toxicology and Therapeutic Drug Monitoring

Analyte	MGH Unit	SI Unit
Acetaminophen, toxicity	>120 μg/mL at 2-4 h	>794 μmol/L at 2-4 h
Amikacin		
trough	1.7 μg/mL	1.7-12 μmol/L
peak	15-25 μg/mL	26-43 μmol/L
Carbamazepine (adults)	4-12 μg/mL	17-51 μmol/L
Digoxin	0.9-2.0 ng/mL	1.2-2.6 nmol/L
Ethanol	>1000 mg/L	>1 g/L
Gentamicin		
trough	<2.1 μg/mL	<4.4 μmol/L
peak	4-8 μg/mL	8.4-16.7 μmol/L
Lithium	0.5-1.5 mmol/L	0.5-1.5 mmol/L
Phenobarbital	15-50 μg/mL	65-216 μmol/L
Phenytoin	5-20 μg/mL	20-79 μmol/L
Salicylate intoxication	>500 mg/L	>3.62 mmol/L
Theophylline	10-20 μg/mL	56-111 μmol/L
Tobramycin		
trough	<2.0 μg/mL	<4.3 μmol/L
peak	4.0-8.0 μg/mL	8.6-17.1 μmol/L
Valproic acid	50-100 μg/mL	347-693 μmol/L
Vancomycin		
trough	<10.1 μg/mL	<7.0 μmol/L
peak (2 hours postinfusion)	18-26 μg/mL	12-18 μmol/L

Immunology

Analyte	MGH Unit	SI Unit
Alpha$_1$-antitrypsin (adults)	76-189 mg/dL	0.76-1.89 g/L
Antiglomerular basement membrane antibodies		
qualitative	Negative	Negative
quantitative	<5 units/mL	<5 kU/L
Antineutrophil cytoplasmic autoantibodies, cytoplasmic (C-ANCA)		
qualitative	Negative	Negative
quantitative (antibodies to proteinase 3)	<2.8 units/mL	<2.8 kU/L
Antineutrophil cytoplasmic autoantibodies, perinuclear (P-ANCA)		
qualitative	Negative	Negative
quantitative (antibodies to myeloperoxidase)	<1.4 units/mL	<1.4 k units/L
Autoantibodies		
antiadrenal antibody	Negative at 1:10 dilution	NA
anti-double-stranded (native) DNA	Negative at 1:10 dilution	NA
antigranulocyte antibody	Negative	NA
anti-Jo-1 antibody	Negative	NA
anti-La antibody	Negative	NA
antimitochondrial antibody	Negative	NA
antinuclear antibody	Negative at 1:40 dilution	NA
antiparietal-cell antibody	Negative at 1:20 dilution	NA
anti-Ro antibody	Negative	NA
anti-RNP antibody	Negative	NA
anti-Scl-70 antibody	Negative	NA
anti-Smith antibody	Negative	NA
antismooth-muscle antibody	Negative at 1:20 dilution	NA
antithyroglobulin antibody	Negative	NA
antithyroid antibody	<0.3 IU/mL	<0.3 kIU/L
Bence Jones protein	None detected	NA
qualitative	None detected in a 50-fold concentration	NA
quantitative		
kappa	<2.5 mg/dL	<0.03 g/L
lambda	<5.0 mg/dL	<0.05 g/L
Complement		
C3 (adults)	86-184 mg/dL	0.86-1.84 g/L
C4 (adults)	20-58 mg/dL	0.20-0.58 g/L
total complement (adults)	63-145 units/mL	63-145 kU/L
CSF		
agarose electrophoresis	No banding seen in an 80-fold concentration	NA
quantitation of albumin (adults)	11.0-50.9 mg/dL	0.11-0.51 g/L
quantitation of IgG (adults)	0.0-8.0 mg/dL	0.0-0.08 g/L
Haptoglobin	16-199 mg/dL	0.16-1.99 g/L

Immunology *(continued)*

Analyte	MGH Unit	SI Unit
Immunoglobulin (adults)		
IgA	60-309 mg/dL	0.60-3.09 g/L
IgE	10-179 IU/mL	24-430 μg/L
IgG	614-1295 mg/dL	6.14-12.95 g/L
IgM	53-334 mg/dL	0.53-3.34 g/L
Rheumatoid factor	<30 IU/mL	<30 kIU/L
Viscosity	1.4-1.8 relative viscosity units, as compared with water	1.4-1.8 relative viscosity units, as compared with water

NA = not applicable.

Hematology and Coagulation

Analyte	MGH Unit	SI Unit
Activated protein C resistance (factor V Leiden)	Ratio >2.0	NA
Antiphospholipid-antibody panel		
partial thromboplastin time - lupus anticoagulant screen	Negative	Negative
platelet-neutralization procedure	Negative	Negative
anticardiolipin antibody		
IgG	0-15 GPL units	0-15 arbitrary units
IgM	0-15 MPL units	0-15 arbitrary units
Antithrombin III		
immunologic	22-39 mg/dL	220-390 mg/L
functional	80%-130%	0.8-1.30 units/L
Bleeding time (adults)	2-9.5 min	2-9.5 min
D-dimer	<0.5 μg/mL	<0.5 mg/L
Differential blood count		
neutrophils	45%-75%	0.45-0.75
bands	0%-5%	0.0-0.05
lymphocytes	16%-46%	0.16-0.46
monocytes	4%-11%	0.04-0.11
eosinophils	0%-8%	0.0-0.8
basophils	0%-3%	0.0-0.03
Erythrocyte count (adults)		
female	4.10-5.10 x 10^6/mm^3	4.50-5.30 x 10^{12}/L
male	4.50-5.30 x 10^6/mm^3	4.10-5.10 x 10^{12}/L
Erythrocyte sedimentation rate		
female	1-25 mm/h	1-25 mm/h
male	0-17 mm/h	0-17 mm/h
Factor II, prothrombin	60%-140%	0.60-1.40
Factor V	60%-140%	0.60-1.40
Factor VII	60%-140%	0.60-1.40
Factor VIII	50%-200%	0.50-2.00
Factor IX	60%-140%	0.60-1.40
Factor X	60%-140%	0.60-1.40
Factor XI	60%-140%	0.60-1.40
Factor XII	60%-140%	0.60-1.40
Factor XIII screen	No deficiency detected	NA
Factor-inhibitor assay	<0.5 Bethesda unit	<0.5 Bethesda unit
Ferritin		
female	10-200 ng/mL	10-200 μg/L
male	30-300 ng/mL	30-300 μg/L
Fibrin(ogen)-degradation products	<2.5 μg/mL	<2.5 mg/L
Fibrinogen	175-400 mg/dL	1.75-4.00 μmol/L
Folate (folic acid)		
normal	3.1-17.5 ng/mL	7.0-39.7 nmol/L
borderline deficient	2.2-3.0 ng/mL	5.0-6.8 nmol/L
deficient	<2.2 ng/mL	<5.0 nmol/L
excessive	>17.5 ng/mL	>39.7 nmol/L
Hematocrit (adults)		
female	36.0-46.0	0.36-0.46
male	37.0-49.0	0.37-0.49
Hemoglobin (adults)		
female	12.0-16.0 g/dL	7.4-9.9 mmol/L
male	13.0-18.0 g/dL	8.1-11.2 mmol/L
Hemoglobin A_2	<3.5%	<0.04
Hemoglobin F	<0.02%	<0.0002
Iron	30-160 μg/dL	5.4-28.7 μmol/L
Iron-binding capacity	228-428 μg/dL	40.8-76.7 μmol/L
Leukocyte count (WBC)	4.5-11.0 x 10^3/mm^3	4.5-11.0 x 10^9/L

Hematology and Coagulation *(continued)*

Analyte	MGH Unit	SI Unit
Mean corpuscular hemoglobin (MCH)	25.0-35.0 pg/cell	25.0-35.0 pg/cell
Mean corpuscular hemoglobin concentration (MCHC)	31.0-37.0 g/dL	310-370 g/L
Mean corpuscular volume (MCV) (adults)		
female	78-102 μm^3	78-100 fL
male	78-100 μm^3	78-102 fL
Partial thromboplastin time, activated	22.1-34.1 sec	22.1-34.1 sec
Plasminogen		
antigen	8.4-140 mg/dL	84-140 mg/L
functional	80%-130%	0.80-1.30
Platelet count	150-350 x $10^3/mm^3$	150-350 x $10^9/L$
Platelet, mean volume	6.4-11.0 μm^3	6.4-11.0 fL
Protein C		
total antigen	70%-140%	0.70-1.40
functional	70%-140%	0.70-1.40
Protein S		
total antigen	70%-140%	0.70-1.40
functional	70%-140%	0.70-1.40
free antigen	70%-140%	0.70-1.40
Prothrombin time	11.2-13.2 sec	11.2-13.2 sec
Red cell distribution width	11.5%-14.5%	0.115-0.145
Reptilase time	16-24 sec	16-24 sec
Reticulocyte count	0.5%-2.5% red cells	0.005-0.0025 red cells
Ristocetin cofactor (functional von Willebrand factor)		
blood group O	75% mean of normal	0.75 mean of normal
blood group A	105% mean of normal	1.05 mean of normal
blood group B	115% mean of normal	1.15 mean of normal
blood group AB	125% mean of normal	1.25 mean of normal
Sucrose hemolysis	<10%	<0.1
Thrombin time	16-24 sec	16-24 sec
Vitamin B_{12}		
normal	>250 pg/mL	>184 pmol/L
borderline	125-250 pg/mL	92-184 pmol/L
deficient	<125 pg/mL	<92 pmol/L
von Willebrand factor (vWF) antigen		
blood group O	75% mean of normal	0.75 mean of normal
blood group A	105% mean of normal	1.05 mean of normal
blood group B	115% mean of normal	1.15 mean of normal
blood group AB	125% mean of normal	1.25 mean of normal
von Willebrand factor multimers	Normal distribution	Normal distribution

TOPIC INDEX

A

B

C

D

P

NOTES

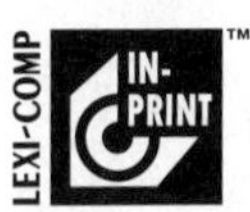

Other books offered by
LEXI-COMP

PHARMACOGENOMICS HANDBOOK

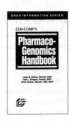

Perfect Bound / Book Size: 4.25" x 7"
by Humma, Ellingrod, Kolesar

This exciting new title by Lexi-Comp, introduces Pharmacogenomics to the forward-thinking healthcare professional and student! It presents information concerning key genetic variations that may influence drug disposition and/or sensitivity. Brief introductions to fundamental concepts in genetics and genomics are provided in order to bring the reader up-to-date on these rapidly emerging sciences. This book provides a foundation for all clinicians who will be called on to integrate rapidly expanding genomic knowledge into the management of drug therapy. A great introduction to pharmacogenetic principles as well as a concise reference on key polymorphisms known to influence drug response!

DRUG-INDUCED NUTRIENT DEPLETION HANDBOOK

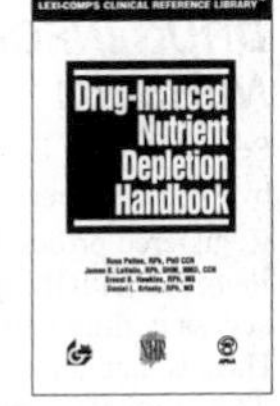

Perfect Bound / Book Size: 4.25" x 7"
by Pelton, LaValle, Hawkins, Krinsky

A complete and up-to-date listing of all drugs known to deplete the body of nutritional compounds.

This book is alphabetically organized and provides extensive cross-referencing to related information in the various sections of the book. Drug monographs identify the nutrients depleted and provide cross-references to the nutrient monographs for more detailed information on effects of depletion, biological function & effect, side effects & toxicity, RDA, dosage range, and dietary sources. this book also contains a studies & abstracts section, a valuable appendix, and alphabetical & pharmacological indexes.

NATURAL THERAPEUTICS POCKET GUIDE

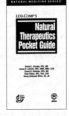

Perfect Bound / Book Size: 4.375" x 8"
by Krinsky, LaValle, Hawkins, Pelton, Ashbrook Willis

Provides condition-specific information on common uses of natural therapies. Each condition discussed includes the following: review of condition, decision tree, list of commonly recommended herbals, nutritional supplements, homeopathic remedies, lifestyle modifications, and special considerations.

Provides herbal/nutritional/nutraceutical monographs with over 10 fields including references, reported uses, dosage, pharmacology, toxicity, warnings & interactions, and cautions & contraindications. The Appendix includes: drug-nutrient depletion, herb-drug interactions, drug-nutrient interaction, herbal medicine use in pediatrics, unsafe herbs, and reference of top herbals.

To order call toll free anywhere in the U.S.: 1-800-837-LEXI (5394)
Outside of the U.S. call: 330-650-6506 or online at www.lexi.com

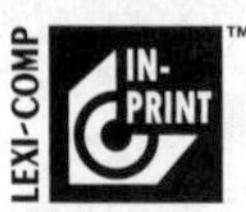

Other books offered by LEXI-COMP

DRUG INFORMATION HANDBOOK FOR ADVANCED PRACTICE NURSING

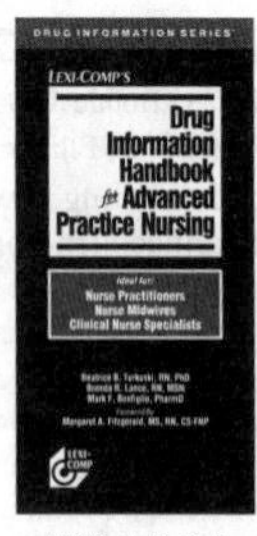

1999 "Book of the Year"
American Journal of Nursing

Perfect Bound / Book Size: 4.5" x 9"

by Turkoski, Lance, Bonfiglio

Designed specifically to meet the needs of nurse practitioners, clinical nurse specialists, nurse midwives, and graduate nursing students. The handbook is a unique resource for detailed, accurate information, which is vital to support the advanced practice nurse's role in patient drug therapy management. Over 4750 U.S., Canadian, and Mexican medications are covered in the 1000 monographs. Drug data is presented in an easy-to-use, alphabetically-organized format covering up to 46 key points of information (including dosing for pediatrics, adults, and geriatrics). Appendix contains over 230 pages of valuable comparison tables and additional information. Also included are two indexes, Pharmacologic Category and Controlled Substance, which facilitate comparison between agents.

DRUG INFORMATION HANDBOOK FOR NURSING

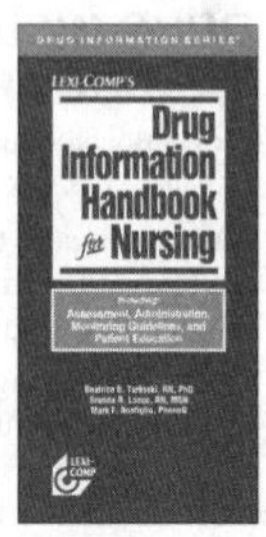

Perfect Bound / Book Size: 4.5" x 9"

by Turkoski, Lance, Bonfiglio

Registered professional nurses and upper-division nursing students involved with drug therapy will find this handbook provides quick access to drug data in a concise easy-to-use format. Over 4000 U.S., Canadian, and Mexican medications are covered with up to 43 key points of information in each monograph. The handbook contains basic pharmacology concepts and nursing issues such as patient factors that influence drug therapy (ie, pregnancy, age, weight, etc) and general nursing issues (ie, assessment, administration, monitoring, and patient education). The Appendix contains over 230 pages of valuable information.

DRUG INTERACTIONS HANDBOOK

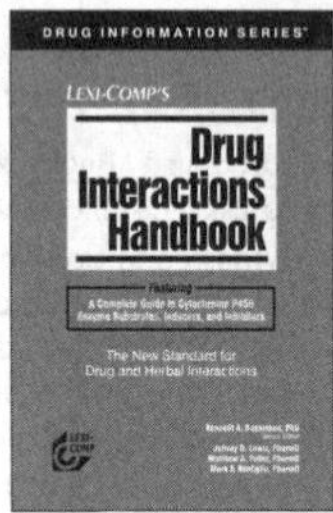

Perfect Bound / Book Size: 5.5" x 8.5"

by Bachmann, Lewis, Fuller, Bonfiglio

The New Standard for Evaluating Drug and Herbal Interactions

A comprehensive table of Cytochrome P450 enzyme substrates, inducers and inhibitors. Each interaction monograph contains the following ratings: **Reliability Rating** - indicating the quantity and nature of documentation for an interaction: **A** - No Known Interaction, **B** - No Action Needed, **C** - Monitor Therapy, **D** - Consider Therapy Modification, and **X** - Avoid Combination; **Severity Rating** - indicating the reported or possible magnitude of an interaction outcome. This book also contains the following: detailed patient management suggestions, full reference citations, discussion of published reports and potential mechanisms, identifies the greatest number of potential interactions compared to any other available references, user-friendly structure, over 3,000 brand names, includes interactions data on the most commonly used herbs, and "tall man" letters to identify between "look-a-like" medications

To order call toll free anywhere in the U.S.: 1-800-837-LEXI (5394)

Outside of the U.S. call: 330-650-6506 or online at www.lexi.com

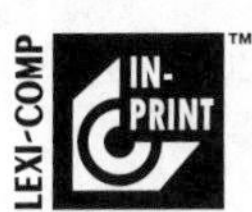

Other books offered by LEXI-COMP

DRUG INFORMATION HANDBOOK FOR ONCOLOGY

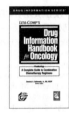

Perfect Bound / Book Size: 4.25" x 7"

by Solimando

Presented in a concise and uniform format, this book contains the most comprehensive collection of oncology-related drug information available. Organized like a dictionary for ease of use, drugs can be found by looking up the *brand or generic name!* This book contains individual monographs for both antineoplastic agents and ancillary medications. The fields of information per monograph include: Use, U.S. Investigational, Bone Marrow/Blood Cell Transplantation, Vesicant, Emetic Potential. A Special Topics Section, Appendix, and Therapeutic Category & Key Word Index are valuable features of this book, as well.

INFECTIOUS DISEASES HANDBOOK

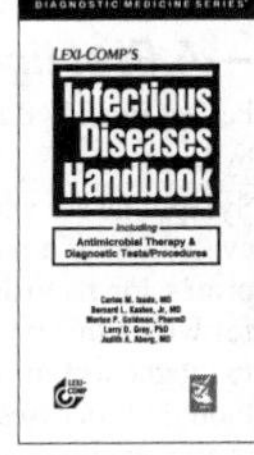

Perfect Bound / Book Size: 4.375" x 8"

by Isada, Kasten, Goldman, Gray, Aberg

A four-in-one quick reference concerned with the identification and treatment of infectious diseases. Each of the four sections of the book contains related information and cross-referencing to one or more of the other three sections. The Disease Syndrome section provides the clinical presentation, differential diagnosis, diagnostic tests, and drug therapy recommended for treatment of more common infectious diseases. The Organism section presents the microbiology, epidemiology, diagnosis, and treatment of each organism. The Laboratory Diagnosis section describes performance of specific tests and procedures. The Antimicrobial Therapy section presents important facts and considerations regarding each drug recommended for specific diseases of organisms. Also contains an International Brand Name Index with names from 58 different countries.

DIAGNOSTIC PROCEDURES HANDBOOK

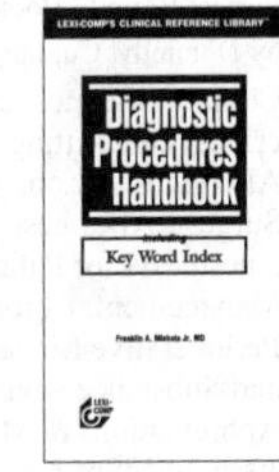

Perfect Bound / Book Size: 4.375" x 8"

by Michota

A comprehensive, yet concise, quick reference source for physicians, nurses, students, medical records personnel, or anyone needing quick access to diagnostic procedure information. This handbook is an excellent source of information in the following areas: allergy, rheumatology, and infectious disease; cardiology; computed tomography; diagnostic radiology; gastroenterology; invasive radiology; magnetic resonance imaging; nephrology, urology, and hematology; neurology; nuclear medicine; pulmonary function; pulmonary medicine and critical care; ultrasound; and women's health.

To order call toll free anywhere in the U.S.: 1-800-837-LEXI (5394)

Outside of the U.S. call: 330-650-6506 or online at www.lexi.com

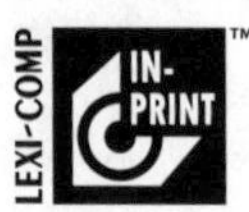

CLINICIAN'S GUIDE TO INTERNAL MEDICINE—A Practical Approach

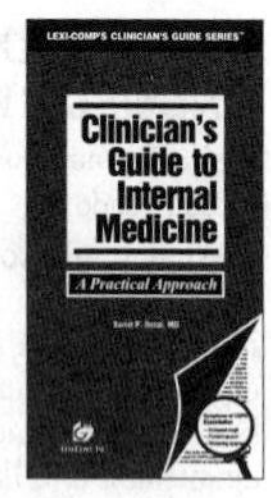

Perfect Bound / Book Size: 4.375" x 8"
by Desai

Provides quick access to essential information covering diagnosis, treatment, and management of commonly encountered patient problems in Internal Medicine. This up-to-date and clinically-relevant information is in an easy-to-read format and is easily accessible. Provides practical approaches that are not readily available in standard textbooks. Contains algorithms to help you establish the diagnosis and select the appropriate therapy. There are numerous tables and boxes that summarize diagnostic and therapeutic strategies. An ideal reference for use at the point-of-care. This is a reference companion that will provide you with the tools necessary to tackle even the most challenging problems in Internal Medicine.

CLINICIAN'S GUIDE TO DIAGNOSIS —A Practical Approach

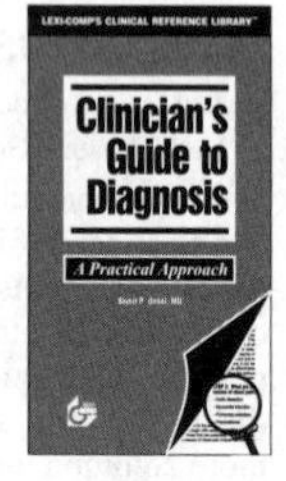

Perfect Bound / Book Size: 4.375" x 8"
by Desai

Symptoms are what prompt patients to seek medical care. In the evaluation of a patient's symptom, it is not unusual for healthcare professionals to ask "What do I do next?" This is precisely the question for which this book provides the answer. It will lead you from symptom to diagnosis through a series of steps designed to mimic the logical thought processes of seasoned clinicians. For the young clinician, this is an ideal book to help bridge the gap between the classroom and actual patient care. For the experienced clinician, this concise handbook offers rapid answers to the questions that are commonly encountered on a day-to-day basis. Let this guide become your companion, providing you with the tools necessary to tackle even the most challenging symptoms.

ANESTHESIOLOGY & CRITICAL CARE DRUG HANDBOOK

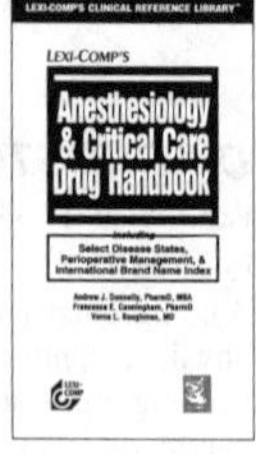

Perfect Bound / Book Size: 4.375" x 8"
by Donnelly, Cunningham, Baughman

Contains the most commonly used drugs in the perioperative and critical care setting and also Special Issues and Topics including: Allergic Reaction, Anesthesia for Cardiac Patients in Noncardiac Surgery, Anesthesia for Obstetric Patients in Nonobstetric Surgery, Anesthesia for Patients With Liver Disease, Chronic Pain Management, Chronic Renal Failure, Conscious Sedation, Perioperative Management of Patients on Antiseizure Medication, and Substance Abuse and Anesthesia. The Appendix includes Abbreviations & Measurements, Anesthesiology Information, Assessment of Liver & Renal Function, Comparative Drug Charts, Infectious Disease-Prophylaxis & Treatment, Laboratory Values, Therapy Re-commendations, Toxicology information, *and much more.* International Brand Name Index with names from over 58 different countries is also included.

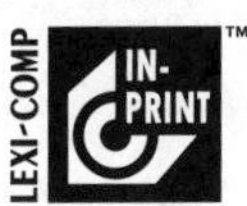

Other books offered by LEXI-COMP

DRUG INFORMATION HANDBOOK FOR DENTISTRY

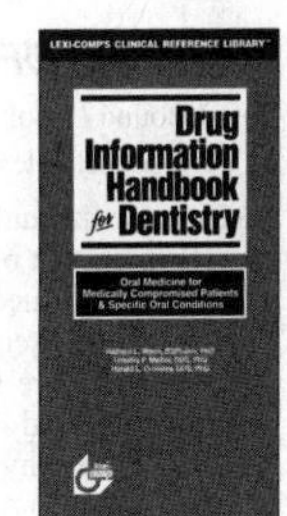

Perfect Bound / Book Size: 4.5" x 9"

by Wynn, Meiller, Crossley

For all dental professionals requiring quick access to concisely-stated drug information pertaining to medications commonly prescribed by dentists and physicians.

Designed and written by dentists for all dental professionals as a portable, chair-side resource. Includes drugs commonly prescribed by dentists or being taken by dental patients and written in an easy-to-understand format. There are 24 key points of information for each drug including Local Anesthetic/Vasoconstrictor, Precautions, Effects on Dental Treatment, and Drug Interactions. Includes information on dental treatment for medically-compromised patients and dental management of specific oral conditions. Also contains Canadian & Mexican brand names.

CLINICIAN'S ENDODONTIC HANDBOOK

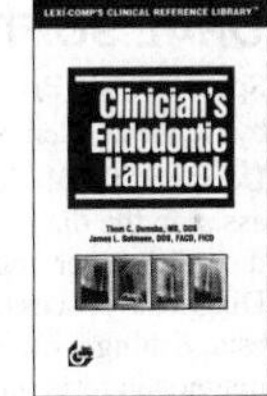

Perfect Bound / Book Size: 4.25" x 7"

by Dumsha and Gutmann

Designed for all general practice dentists.

- A quick reference addressing current endodontics
- Easy-to-use format and alphabetical index
- Latest techniques, procedures, and materials
- Root canal therapy: why's and why nots
- A guide to diagnosis and treatment of endodontic emergencies
- Facts and rationale behind treating endodontically-involved teeth
- Straight-forward dental trauma management information
- Pulpal histology, access openings, bleaching, resorption, radiology, restoration, and periodontal / endodontic complications
- Frequently asked questions (FAQ) section and "clinical notes" sections throughout

DENTAL OFFICE MEDICAL EMERGENCIES

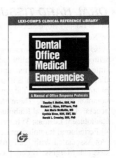

Spiral Bound / Book Size: 8.5" x 11"

by Meiller, Wynn, McMullin, Crossley

Designed specifically for general dentists during times of emergency. A tabbed paging system allows for quick access to specific crisis events. Created with urgency in mind, it is spiral bound and drilled with a hole for hanging purposes.

- Basic Action Plan for Stabilization
- Allergic / Drug Reactions
- Management of Acute Bleeding
- Altered Sensation / Changes in Affect
- Loss of Consciousness / Respiratory Distress / Chest Pain
- Office Preparedness / Procedures and Protocols
- Automated External Defibrillator (AED)
- Oxygen Delivery

To order call toll free anywhere in the U.S.: 1-800-837-LEXI (5394)

Outside of the U.S. call: 330-650-6506 or online at www.lexi.com

Patient Education Desk Charts

(Flip Charts)

A PATIENT GUIDE TO MENTAL HEALTH ISSUES

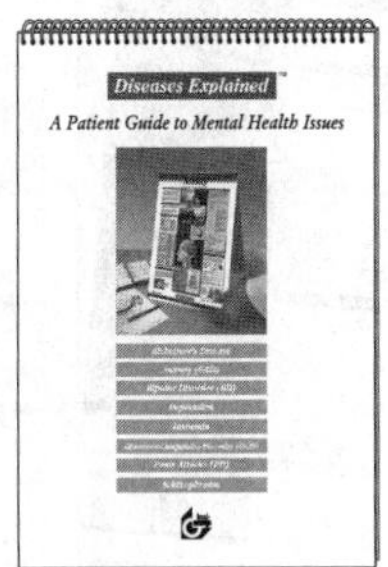

- Alzheimer's Disease
- Anxiety (GAD)
- Bipolar Disorder (BD)
- Depression
- Insomnia
- Obsessive-Compulsive Disorder (OCD)
- Panic Attacks (PD)
- Schizophrenia

A PATIENT GUIDE TO ROOT CANAL THERAPY

Contributor Thom C. Dumsha, M.S., D.D.S., M.S.

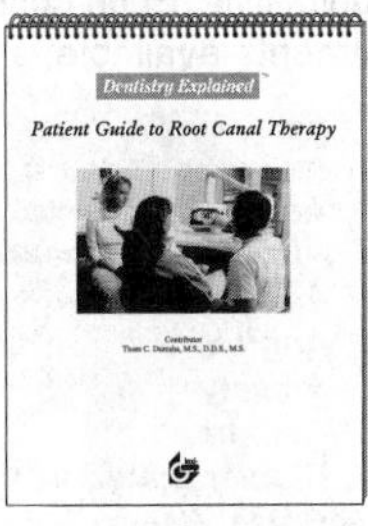

- An ideal tool used to educate and explain to your patients about root canals
- 8 1/2" x 11" colorful tabbed flip chart explaining each of the steps involved in a root canal
- Actual clinical photographs, radiographs, and diagrams

PATIENT GUIDE TO DENTAL IMPLANTS

Contributor Marvin L. Baer, D.D.S., M.Sc.

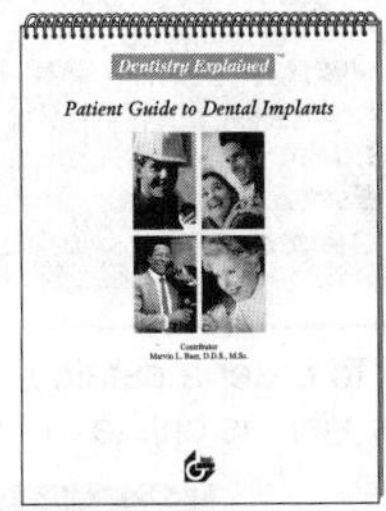

- An ideal tool used to educate and explain to your patients about dental implants
- 8 1/2" x 11" colorful tabbed flip chart explaining each of the steps involved in:

  1.) Single tooth restoration
  2.) Replacement of several teeth
  3.) Implants supported overdenture (4 implants/2 implants)
  4.) Screw-retained denture

To order call toll free anywhere in the U.S.: 1-800-837-LEXI (5394)

Outside of the U.S. call: 330-650-6506 or online at www.lexi.com